Arthropod Venom Components and Their Potential Usage

Arthropod Venom Components and Their Potential Usage

Special Issue Editors

Katsuhiro Konno
Gandhi Rádis-Baptista

MDPI • Basel • Beijing • Wuhan • Barcelona • Belgrade • Manchester • Tokyo • Cluj • Tianjin

Special Issue Editors
Katsuhiro Konno
Institute Natural Medicine,
University of Toyama
Japan

Gandhi Rádis-Baptista
Laboratory of Biochemistry and Biotechnology,
Institute for Marine Sciences,
Federal University of Ceara
Brazil

Editorial Office
MDPI
St. Alban-Anlage 66
4052 Basel, Switzerland

This is a reprint of articles from the Special Issue published online in the open access journal *Toxins* (ISSN 2072-6651) (available at: https://www.mdpi.com/journal/toxins/special_issues/arthropod_venom_usage).

For citation purposes, cite each article independently as indicated on the article page online and as indicated below:

LastName, A.A.; LastName, B.B.; LastName, C.C. Article Title. *Journal Name* **Year**, *Article Number*, Page Range.

ISBN 978-3-03928-540-2 (Pbk)
ISBN 978-3-03928-541-9 (PDF)

Contents

About the Special Issue Editors ix

Gandhi Rádis-Baptista and Katsuhiro Konno
Arthropod Venom Components and Their Potential Usage
Reprinted from: *Toxins* **2020**, *12*, 82, doi:10.3390/toxins12020082 1

Justin O. Schmidt
Pain and Lethality Induced by Insect Stings: An Exploratory and Correlational Study
Reprinted from: *Toxins* **2019**, *11*, 427, doi:10.3390/toxins11070427 5

Jimena I. Cid-Uribe, Erika P. Meneses, Cesar V. F. Batista, Ernesto Ortiz and Lourival D. Possani
Dissecting Toxicity: The Venom Gland Transcriptome and the Venom Proteome of the Highly Venomous Scorpion *Centruroides limpidus* (Karsch, 1879)
Reprinted from: *Toxins* **2019**, *11*, 247, doi:10.3390/toxins11050247 19

Douglas Oscar Ceolin Mariano, Úrsula Castro de Oliveira, André Junqueira Zaharenko, Daniel Carvalho Pimenta, Gandhi Rádis-Baptista and Álvaro Rossan de Brandão Prieto-da-Silva
Bottom-Up Proteomic Analysis of Polypeptide Venom Components of the Giant Ant *Dinoponera Quadriceps*
Reprinted from: *Toxins* **2019**, *11*, 448, doi:10.3390/toxins11080448 41

Naoki Tani, Kohei Kazuma, Yukio Ohtsuka, Yasushi Shigeri, Keiichi Masuko, Katsuhiro Konno and Hidetoshi Inagaki
Mass Spectrometry Analysis and Biological Characterization of the Predatory Ant *Odontomachus monticola* Venom and Venom Sac Components
Reprinted from: *Toxins* **2019**, *11*, 50, doi:10.3390/toxins11010050 69

Rogério Coutinho das Neves, Márcia Renata Mortari, Elisabeth Ferroni Schwartz, André Kipnis and Ana Paula Junqueira-Kipnis
Antimicrobial and Antibiofilm Effects of Peptides from Venom of Social Wasp and Scorpion on Multidrug-Resistant *Acinetobacter baumannii*
Reprinted from: *Toxins* **2019**, *11*, 216, doi:10.3390/toxins11040216 85

Marcia Perez dos Santos Cabrera, Marisa Rangel, João Ruggiero Neto and Katsuhiro Konno
Chemical and Biological Characteristics of Antimicrobial α-Helical Peptides Found in Solitary Wasp Venoms and Their Interactions with Model Membranes
Reprinted from: *Toxins* **2019**, *11*, 559, doi:10.3390/toxins11100559 103

Carolina Nunes da Silva, Flavia Rodrigues da Silva, Lays Fernanda Nunes Dourado, Pablo Victor Mendes dos Reis, Rummenigge Oliveira Silva, Bruna Lopes da Costa, Paula Santos Nunes, Flávio Almeida Amaral, Vera Lúcia dos Santos, Maria Elena de Lima and Armando da Silva Cunha Júnior
A New Topical Eye Drop Containing LyeTxI-b, A Synthetic Peptide Designed from A *Lycosa erithrognata* Venom Toxin, Was Effective to Treat Resistant Bacterial Keratitis
Reprinted from: *Toxins* **2019**, *11*, 203, doi:10.3390/toxins11040203 121

Elias Ferreira Sabiá Júnior, Luis Felipe Santos Menezes, Israel Flor Silva de Araújo and Elisabeth Ferroni Schwartz
Natural Occurrence in Venomous Arthropods of Antimicrobial Peptides Active against Protozoan Parasites
Reprinted from: *Toxins* **2019**, *11*, 563, doi:10.3390/toxins11100563 . . . . **137**

Danielle Bruno de Carvalho, Eduardo Gonçalves Paterson Fox, Diogo Gama dos Santos, Joab Sampaio de Sousa, Denise Maria Guimarães Freire, Fabio C. S. Nogueira, Gilberto B. Domont, Livia Vieira Araujo de Castilho and Ednildo de Alcântara Machado
Fire Ant Venom Alkaloids Inhibit Biofilm Formation
Reprinted from: *Toxins* **2019**, *11*, 420, doi:10.3390/toxins11070420 . . . . **165**

Douglas W. Whitman, Maria Fe Andrés, Rafael A. Martínez-Díaz, Alexandra Ibáñez-Escribano, A. Sonia Olmeda and Azucena González-Coloma
Antiparasitic Properties of Cantharidin and the Blister Beetle *Berberomeloe majalis* (Coleoptera: Meloidae)
Reprinted from: *Toxins* **2019**, *11*, 234, doi:10.3390/toxins11040234 . . . . **179**

Haejoong Kim, Soo-Yeon Park and Gihyun Lee
Potential Therapeutic Applications of Bee Venom on Skin Disease and Its Mechanisms: A Literature Review
Reprinted from: *Toxins* **2019**, *11*, 374, doi:10.3390/toxins11070374 . . . . **189**

Jan Lubawy, Arkadiusz Urbański, Lucyna Mrówczyńska, Eliza Matuszewska, Agata Światły-Błaszkiewicz, Jan Matysiak and Grzegorz Rosiński
The Influence of Bee Venom Melittin on the Functioning of the Immune System and the Contractile Activity of the Insect Heart—A Preliminary Study
Reprinted from: *Toxins* **2019**, *11*, 494, doi:10.3390/toxins11090494 . . . . **219**

Seunghwan Choi, Hyeon Kyeong Chae, Ho Heo, Dae-Hyun Hahm, Woojin Kim and Sun Kwang Kim
Analgesic Effect of Melittin on Oxaliplatin-Induced Peripheral Neuropathy in Rats
Reprinted from: *Toxins* **2019**, *11*, 396, doi:10.3390/toxins11070396 . . . . **231**

Craig A. Doupnik
Identification of *Aethina tumida* Kir Channels as Putative Targets of the Bee Venom Peptide Tertiapin Using Structure-Based Virtual Screening Methods
Reprinted from: *Toxins* **2019**, *11*, 546, doi:10.3390/toxins11090546 . . . . **241**

Yashad Dongol, Fernanda Caldas Cardoso and Richard J Lewis
Spider Knottin Pharmacology at Voltage-Gated Sodium Channels and Their Potential to Modulate Pain Pathways
Reprinted from: *Toxins* **2019**, *11*, 626, doi:10.3390/toxins11110626 . . . . **259**

Daniele Chaves-Moreira, Fernando Hitomi Matsubara, Zelinda Schemczssen-Graeff, Elidiana De Bona, Vanessa Ribeiro Heidemann, Clara Guerra-Duarte, Luiza Helena Gremski, Carlos Chávez-Olórtegui, Andrea Senff-Ribeiro, Olga Meiri Chaim, Raghuvir Krishnaswamy Arni and Silvio Sanches Veiga
Brown Spider (*Loxosceles*) Venom Toxins as Potential Biotools for the Development of Novel Therapeutics
Reprinted from: *Toxins* **2019**, *11*, 355, doi:10.3390/toxins11060355 . . . . **299**

Sébastien Nicolas, Claude Zoukimian, Frank Bosmans, Jérôme Montnach, Sylvie Diochot, Eva Cuypers, Stephan De Waard, Rémy Béroud, Dietrich Mebs, David Craik, Didier Boturyn, Michel Lazdunski, Jan Tytgat and Michel De Waard
Chemical Synthesis, Proper Folding, Na_v Channel Selectivity Profile and Analgesic Properties of the Spider Peptide Phlotoxin 1
Reprinted from: *Toxins* **2019**, *11*, 367, doi:10.3390/toxins11060367 . . . . **321**

Carmen Hernández, Katsuhiro Konno, Emilio Salceda, Rosario Vega, André Junqueira Zaharenko and Enrique Soto
Sa12b Peptide from Solitary Wasp Inhibits ASIC Currents in Rat Dorsal Root Ganglion Neurons
Reprinted from: *Toxins* **2019**, *11*, 585, doi:10.3390/toxins11100585 . . . . **343**

Paula A. L. Calabria, Lhiri Hanna A. L. Shimokava-Falcao, Monica Colombini, Ana M. Moura-da-Silva, Katia C. Barbaro, Eliana L. Faquim-Mauro and Geraldo S. Magalhaes
Design and Production of a Recombinant Hybrid Toxin to Raise Protective Antibodies against *Loxosceles* Spider Venom
Reprinted from: *Toxins* **2019**, *11*, 108, doi:10.3390/toxins11020108 . . . . **359**

Yusuke Yoshimoto, Masahiro Miyashita, Mohammed Abdel-Wahab, Moustafa Sarhan, Yoshiaki Nakagawa and Hisashi Miyagawa
Isolation and Characterization of Insecticidal Toxins from the Venom of the North African Scorpion, *Buthacus leptochelys*
Reprinted from: *Toxins* **2019**, *11*, 236, doi:10.3390/toxins11040236 . . . . **381**

About the Special Issue Editors

Katsuhiro Konno received his Ph.D. in Organic Chemistry from Hokkaido University (Sapporo, Japan) in 1986, and continued as a Postdoctoral Fellow in the Department of Chemistry, Columbia University (New York, NY, USA) in 1986–1989. He was appointed assistant professor at Teikyo University (Kanagawa, Japan) in 1989. He moved to Brazil and worked as a research fellow at Sao Paulo State University and Butantan Institute in 1998–2007. He has been a professor of Institute of Natural Medicine, University of Toyama (Toyama, Japan) since being appointed in 2008. His main interest is chemical and biological characterization of natural toxins from mushrooms and venomous animals (wasps, spiders, etc.).

Gandhi Rádis-Baptista received his master degree in Technology of Fermentation in 1996, and his Ph.D in Life Sciences (Biochemistry) in 2002, both from University of São Paulo. He was appointed associate researcher (postdoctoral fellow) in the Laboratory of Molecular Toxinology at Butantan Institute in 2002–2003. He has Participated in several scientific missions to the National Institute of Advanced Industrial Science and Technology (Tokyo, Japan). He was a former associate professor in Department of Biochemistry at Federal University of Pernambuco (2005–2008). Presently, he is an associate professor in Institute of Marine Sciences at Federal University of Ceara. His main scientific interests are polypeptides from terrestrial and marine organims, cell receptors, molecular interactions, recombinant DNA technology and molecular diagnostic, etc.

toxins

MDPI

Editorial

Arthropod Venom Components and Their Potential Usage

Gandhi Rádis-Baptista [1,*] and Katsuhiro Konno [2,*]

[1] Laboratory of Biochemistry and Biotechnology, Institute for Marine Sciences, Federal University of Ceara, Fortaleza CE 60165-081, Brazil
[2] Institute of Natural Medicine, University of Toyama, 2630 Sugitani, Toyama, Toyama 930-0194, Japan
* Correspondence: gandhi.radis@ufc.br (G.R.-B.); kkgon@inm.u-toyama.ac.jp (K.K.)

Received: 17 January 2020; Accepted: 21 January 2020; Published: 25 January 2020

check for updates

Arthropods comprise a predominant and well-succeeded phylum of the animal kingdom that evolved and diversified in millions of species grouped in four subphyla, namely, Chelicerata (arachnids), Crustacea, Myriapoda (centipedes), and Hexapoda (insects). It is agreed that the success of the arthropods' flourishment and evolutionary story are in great part due to the diversification of venom apparatus and venom usage [1,2]. Thousands of arthropod species, ranging from arachnids (spiders and scorpions) to hymenopterans (ants, bees, and wasps) and myriapods (centipedes), are venomous and utilize their venoms for chemical ecological warfare that includes individual and colonial defense, predation, and paralysis of coexistent species to nourish their brood. Despite arthropods' venoms are invariably harmful to humans, and some may cause serious injuries, e.g., those from scorpions, spiders, and wasps, they are potentially useful molecular scalpels to dissect and modulate cellular processes and, consequently, they can be converted into biopharmaceuticals and biotools. In this respect, arthropod venoms have attracted the attention of toxin researchers for years, seeking to characterize biologically active compounds of these rich venom sources. Especially in the last decades, venom component analysis has progressed more than ever because of the great advances of analytical techniques; in particular, mass spectrometry and next-generation deep (DNA and RNA) sequencing. As such, proteomic and peptidomic analyses utilizing LC–MS, as well as transcriptomics (alone or in combination with proteomics), have made it possible to fully analyze venom components, revealing a variety of novel peptide and protein toxin sequences and scaffolds. These are potentially useful as pharmacological research tools and for the development of highly selective peptide ligands and therapeutic leads. Moreover, because of their specificity for numerous ion-channel subtypes, including voltage- and ligand-gated ion channels, arthropod neurotoxins have been investigated to dissect and treat neurodegenerative diseases and control epileptic syndromes. This Special Issue collects information on such progress.

Considering the natural history of the evolutionary success of arthropods based on the molecular arsenal contained in their venom, a study reported here by Justin Schmidt explores and correlates the pain and lethality induced by hundreds of insect stings, pointing the direction to screen pharmacologically active venom components of pharmaceutical interest [3]. To dissect venom cocktails, particularly when limited amounts of crude venom are available from tiny animals, as in the case of most arthropod species, omics technologies have demonstrated to be an essential collection of robust strategies. Indeed, transcriptome and proteome, alone or in combination with functional analysis, has been applied to disclose and resolve the toxin peptide complexity of the venom, as described from the highly venomous Mexican scorpion *Centruroides limpidus* [4], the predatory giant ant *Dinoponera quadriceps* [5], and the predatory ant *Odontomachus monticola* [6]. In a later study published in this special issue, the authors also investigated the components of the *O. monticola* venom sac, besides the crude venom. Apart of numerous structural and functional classes of polypeptides found in a given venom proteome and peptidome, short membrane active peptides with or without definitive characterized antimicrobial activity have also been found in the venom of these species of ant and scorpion, like in other arthropods. The structural and molecular characterization of antimicrobial peptides are the focus of four articles: the antimicrobial and antibiofilm effects of peptides agelaia-MPI, polybia-MPII, polydim-I from the venom of social wasps, and the peptides Con10 and NDBP5.8 from scorpion venom against multidrug-resistant *Acinetobacter baumannii*, investigated and reported by das Neves and colleagues [7]; a detailed study on the chemical, biological, and biophysical properties of antimicrobial alpha-helical peptides from solitary wasp venoms, presented by dos Santos Cabrera and collaborators [8]; the formulation of a new topical eye drop containing a synthetic peptide designed from a spider *A. lycosa erithrognata* venom toxin, LyeTxI-b, that is effective in treating bacterial keratitis caused by drug-resistant Staphylococcus aureus, reported by Nunes da Silva et al. [9]; the arthropod venoms as a source of antimicrobial peptides that kill diverse life-threating parasites, reviewed by Sabia-Junio et al. [10]. In addition to antimicrobial and antiparasitic peptides from arthropod venom, low molecular weight compounds are also shown to be active against a broad spectrum of microbes. For instance, the anti-biofilm effect of alkaloids (solenopsins) isolated from the venom of the fire ants *Solenopsis invicta* was evaluated by de Carvalho and colleagues [11]. Cantharidin, a toxic monoterpene from the hemolymph of the blister beetles *Berberomeloe majalis* (Coleoptera: Meloidae), was demonstrated by Whitman and coworkers to display an important effect against distinct class of parasites [12].

One of the most studied animal venoms, bee venom, still has many interesting aspects to be discovered and explored. Crude venom and isolated components were reexamined in a review dealing with the potential therapeutic applications of bee venom to treat skin diseases [13], and in three different research articles dealing with bee venom peptides, melittin and tertiapin, from the view of immunology, molecular neurobiology and physiology. Indeed, Lubawy and collaborators studied the immunotropic and cardiotropic effects of melittin on the physiology of beetle *Tenebrio molitor* [14], while Choi and coworkers investigated the use of melittin as an analgesic to treat peripheral neuropathy caused by oxaliplatin (an anticancer drug), demonstrating the molecular basis of this particular melittin effect, which was mediated by the activation of the spinal $\alpha1$- and $\alpha2$-adrenergic receptors [15]. In another work, the Kir channel subtypes of the small hive beetle *Aethina tumida* were identified by Doupnik [16] as molecular targets of the bee venom peptide tertiapin, based on structure-guided virtual screening methods.

Neural receptors on excitable tissues, particularly ion channels, are a sort of preferential targets for arthropod venom components, notably from spider and wasps. Dongol and coworkers reviewed the structural determinants of diverse spider knottins (inhibitor cystine knot toxins) that influence voltage-gated sodium (Nav) channel activity on neuronal signaling, their role in the modulation of pain, and as a platform to develop analgesics [17]. In the same line, Chaves-Moreira and collaborators explored the potential of distinct structural and functional classes of toxins from brown spider (*Loxoceles*) to be developed into therapeutics [18]. The purification and preparation of fully bioactive peptide toxins, particularly folded and constrained by disulfide bonds, are critical for functional analysis and development as biopharmaceuticals. Nicolas and colleagues synthesized and characterized in a structural and functional basis a spider peptide toxin, phlotoxin-1, that was specifically selective to Nav channel and, consequently, useful to investigate the involvement of sodium channel in pain and analgesia [19]. Acid-sensing ion channels (ASICs) comprise another family of proton-gated ion channel expressed in the nervous system and with multiples roles in organism physiology and neurological diseases. Hernández and colleagues reported the effect of two peptides purified from the solitary wasp *Sphex argentatus*, Sa12b and Sh5b, on ASIC currents in rat dorsal root ganglion neuron, contributing with the first discovery of a wasp peptide toxin that acts on such a kind of ion channel [20]. The preparation of toxin with sizes exceeding those of peptides can be achieved by recombinant procedures instead of solid phase peptide synthesis chemistry. An example of this alternative in the present special issue is the production of recombinant hybrid toxin/immunogen. Taking phospholipase D from the spider *Loxoceles* as toxin moiety, a chimeric hybrid was produced by Calabria and colleagues to raise protective antibodies in *Loxoceles* antivenom therapy [21]. Last but not least, the use of arthropod toxins as bioinsecticide is continuously showed to be a promising application of this classes of animal venom. Yoshimoto and collaborators described the isolation and molecular characterization of insecticidal toxins from the venom of the North African scorpion, *Buthacus leptochelys* [22]. These new toxins were shown to be similar to scorpion α- and β-toxins and probably acted via sodium ion channels.

Overall, the compilation of such special articles highlights the huge potential of the discovery of arthropod venom. The diversity of peptide scaffolds and structures found in the numerous species of arthropods are amenable to be developed into specific and selective ligands and biotools. These, apart from being useful in basic research, are usable for precise intervention and modulation of the physio-pathological processes of diseases such as neurological disorders, or even for pest control, such as in the preparation and use of environmentally friendly biopesticides. So far, the future is bright for the usage of selective arthropod peptides.

Funding: This research received no external funding.

Conflicts of Interest: The authors declare no conflict of interest.

References

1. Laxme, R.R.S.; Suranse, V.; Sunagar, K. Arthropod venoms: Biochemistry, ecology and evolution. *Toxicon* **2019**, *158*, 84–103. [CrossRef] [PubMed]
2. Herzig, V. Arthropod assassins: Crawling biochemists with diverse toxin pharmacopeias. *Toxicon* **2019**, *158*, 33–37. [CrossRef] [PubMed]
3. Schmidt, J.O. Pain and Lethality Induced by Insect Stings: An Exploratory and Correlational Study. *Toxins* **2019**, *11*, 427. [CrossRef] [PubMed]
4. Cid-Uribe, J.I.; Meneses, E.P.; Batista, C.V.F.; Ortiz, E.; Possani, L.D. Dissecting Toxicity: The Venom Gland Transcriptome and the Venom Proteome of the Highly Venomous Scorpion Centruroides limpidus (Karsch, 1879). *Toxins* **2019**, *11*, 247. [CrossRef] [PubMed]
5. Mariano, C.; Oscar, D.; de Oliveira, Ú.C.; Zaharenko, A.J.; Pimenta, D.C.; Rádis-Baptista, G.; Prieto-da-Silva, Á.R.D. Bottom-Up Proteomic Analysis of Polypeptide Venom Components of the Giant Ant Dinoponera Quadriceps. *Toxins* **2019**, *11*, 448. [CrossRef]
6. Tani, N.; Kazuma, K.; Ohtsuka, Y.; Shigeri, Y.; Masuko, K.; Konno, K.; Inagaki, H. Mass Spectrometry Analysis and Biological Characterization of the Predatory Ant Odontomachus monticola Venom and Venom Sac Components. *Toxins* **2019**, *11*, 50. [CrossRef]
7. Neves, R.C.d.; Mortari, M.R.; Schwartz, E.F.; Kipnis, A.; Junqueira-Kipnis, A.P. Antimicrobial and Antibiofilm Effects of Peptides from Venom of Social Wasp and Scorpion on Multidrug-Resistant Acinetobacter baumannii. *Toxins* **2019**, *11*, 216. [CrossRef]
8. dos Santos Cabrera, M.P.; Rangel, M.; Ruggiero Neto, J.; Konno, K. Chemical and Biological Characteristics of Antimicrobial α-Helical Peptides Found in Solitary Wasp Venoms and Their Interactions with Model Membranes. *Toxins* **2019**, *11*, 559. [CrossRef]
9. Silva, C.N.D.; Silva, F.R.D.; Dourado, L.F.N.; Reis, P.V.M.D.; Silva, R.O.; Costa, B.L.D.; Nunes, P.S.; Amaral, F.A.; Santos, V.L.D.; de Lima, M.E.; et al. A New Topical Eye Drop Containing LyeTxI-b, A Synthetic Peptide Designed from A Lycosa erithrognata Venom Toxin, Was Effective to Treat Resistant Bacterial Keratitis. *Toxins* **2019**, *11*, 203. [CrossRef]
10. Júnior, E.F.S.; Menezes, L.F.S.; de Araújo, I.F.S.; Schwartz, E.F. Natural Occurrence in Venomous Arthropods of Antimicrobial Peptides Active against Protozoan Parasites. *Toxins* **2019**, *11*, 563. [CrossRef]
11. Carvalho, D.B.D.; Fox, E.G.P.; Santos, D.G.D.; Sousa, J.S.D.; Freire, D.M.G.; Nogueira, F.; Domont, G.B.; Castilho, L.V.A.D.; Machado, E.D.A. Fire Ant Venom Alkaloids Inhibit Biofilm Formation. *Toxins* **2019**, *11*, 420. [CrossRef] [PubMed]
12. Whitman, D.W.; Andrés, M.F.; Martínez-Díaz, R.A.; Ibáñez-Escribano, A.; Olmeda, A.S.; González-Coloma, A. Antiparasitic Properties of Cantharidin and the Blister Beetle Berberomeloe majalis (Coleoptera: Meloidae). *Toxins* **2019**, *11*, 234. [CrossRef] [PubMed]

13. Kim, H.; Park, S.-Y.; Lee, G. Potential Therapeutic Applications of Bee Venom on Skin Disease and Its Mechanisms: A Literature Review. *Toxins* **2019**, *11*, 374. [CrossRef] [PubMed]
14. Lubawy, J.; Urbański, A.; Mrówczyńska, L.; Matuszewska, E.; Światły-Błaszkiewicz, A.; Matysiak, J.; Rosiński, G. The Influence of Bee Venom Melittin on the Functioning of the Immune System and the Contractile Activity of the Insect Heart—A Preliminary Study. *Toxins* **2019**, *11*, 494. [CrossRef] [PubMed]
15. Choi, S.; Chae, H.K.; Heo, H.; Hahm, D.-H.; Kim, W.; Kim, S.K. Analgesic Effect of Melittin on Oxaliplatin-Induced Peripheral Neuropathy in Rats. *Toxins* **2019**, *11*, 396. [CrossRef]
16. Doupnik, C.A. Identification of Aethina tumida Kir Channels as Putative Targets of the Bee Venom Peptide Tertiapin Using Structure-Based Virtual Screening Methods. *Toxins* **2019**, *11*, 546. [CrossRef]
17. Dongol, Y.; Cardoso, F.C.; Lewis, R.J. Spider Knottin Pharmacology at Voltage-Gated Sodium Channels and Their Potential to Modulate Pain Pathways. *Toxins* **2019**, *11*, 626. [CrossRef]
18. Chaves-Moreira, D.; Matsubara, F.H.; Schemczssen-Graeff, Z.; de Bona, E.; Heidemann, V.R.; Guerra-Duarte, C.; Gremski, L.H.; Chávez-Olórtegui, C.; Senff-Ribeiro, A.; Chaim, O.M.; et al. Brown Spider (Loxosceles) Venom *Toxins* as Potential Biotools for the Development of Novel Therapeutics. *Toxins* **2019**, *11*, 355. [CrossRef]
19. Nicolas, S.; Zoukimian, C.; Bosmans, F.; Montnach, J.; Diochot, S.; Cuypers, E.; de Waard, S.; Béroud, R.; Mebs, D.; Craik, D.; et al. Chemical Synthesis, Proper Folding, Nav Channel Selectivity Profile and Analgesic Properties of the Spider Peptide Phlotoxin 1. *Toxins* **2019**, *11*, 367. [CrossRef]
20. Hernández, C.; Konno, K.; Salceda, E.; Vega, R.; Zaharenko, A.J.; Soto, E. Sa12b Peptide from Solitary Wasp Inhibits ASIC Currents in Rat Dorsal Root Ganglion Neurons. *Toxins* **2019**, *11*, 585. [CrossRef]
21. Calabria, P.A.L.; Shimokawa-Falcão, L.H.A.L.; Colombini, M.; Moura-da-Silva, A.M.; Barbaro, K.C.; Faquim-Mauro, E.L.; Magalhaes, G.S. Design and Production of a Recombinant Hybrid Toxin to Raise Protective Antibodies against Loxosceles Spider Venom. *Toxins* **2019**, *11*, 108. [CrossRef] [PubMed]
22. Yoshimoto, Y.; Miyashita, M.; Abdel-Wahab, M.; Sarhan, M.; Nakagawa, Y.; Miyagawa, H. Isolation and Characterization of Insecticidal Toxins from the Venom of the North African Scorpion, Buthacus leptochelys. *Toxins* **2019**, *11*, 236. [CrossRef] [PubMed]

toxins

MDPI

Article

Pain and Lethality Induced by Insect Stings: An Exploratory and Correlational Study

Justin O. Schmidt

Southwestern Biological Institute, 1961 W. Brichta Dr., Tucson, AZ 85745, USA; ponerine@dakotacom.net; Tel.: +1-520-884-9345

Received: 3 July 2019; Accepted: 16 July 2019; Published: 21 July 2019

check for updates

Abstract: Pain is a natural bioassay for detecting and quantifying biological activities of venoms. The painfulness of stings delivered by ants, wasps, and bees can be easily measured in the field or lab using the stinging insect pain scale that rates the pain intensity from 1 to 4, with 1 being minor pain, and 4 being extreme, debilitating, excruciating pain. The painfulness of stings of 96 species of stinging insects and the lethalities of the venoms of 90 species was determined and utilized for pinpointing future directions for investigating venoms having pharmaceutically active principles that could benefit humanity. The findings suggest several under- or unexplored insect venoms worthy of future investigations, including: those that have exceedingly painful venoms, yet with extremely low lethality—tarantula hawk wasps (*Pepsis*) and velvet ants (Mutillidae); those that have extremely lethal venoms, yet induce very little pain—the ants, *Daceton* and *Tetraponera*; and those that have venomous stings and are both painful and lethal—the ants *Pogonomyrmex*, *Paraponera*, *Myrmecia*, *Neoponera*, and the social wasps *Synoeca*, *Agelaia*, and *Brachygastra*. Taken together, and separately, sting pain and venom lethality point to promising directions for mining of pharmaceutically active components derived from insect venoms.

Keywords: venom; pain; ants; wasps; bees; Hymenoptera; envenomation; toxins; peptides; pharmacology

Key Contribution: Insect venom-induced pain and lethal activity provide a roadmap of what species and venoms are promising to investigate for development of new pharmacological and research tools.

1. Introduction

Stinging insects in the immense order Hymenoptera display a dazzling array of lifestyles and natural histories. These complex life histories offer a wealth of opportunities for the discovery of new natural products and pharmaceuticals to benefit the human endeavor. Each of the multitude of independent biological paths followed by stinging ants, social wasps, social bees, and solitary wasps and bees has resulted in evolutionary complex—and often unique—blends of venom constituents. Compared with the venoms of snakes, scorpions, medically important spiders, and a variety of other marine and terrestrial venomous animals, the venoms of most stinging insects are understudied. The reason for fewer investigations of insect venoms is explained, in part, by their general low potential for causing severe acute or long-term medical damage and partly by their small size. Additional complicating factors contributing to less emphasis on investigations of stinging insect venoms are the difficulties of identifying the insects and obtaining enough venom for study. Much of the recent research on insect venoms has focused on the relatively small number of species that are responsible for inducing human allergic reactions to insect stings [1]. The topic of sting allergy will not be addressed here.

Venoms of stinging insects have a variety of biologically important activities including the abilities to induce pain, cause cellular or organ toxicity, be lethal, produce paralysis, plus others [2–5]. These activities are the result of a wide variety of venom components, especially peptides and proteins, but also other categories of constituents [6–8]. The ability to cause pain is fundamental to most insect venoms that are used for defense against predators [9]. Pain is the body's warning system that damage has occurred, is occurring, or is about to occur. In essence, pain informs the inflicted organism that it should immediately act to limit injury, or potential injury. The envenomated animal often releases the offending stinging insect and flees the area [9]. The net effect is that the stinging insect frequently survives the ordeal with minimal, or no, injury and for a social species enhances the survival of her nest mates (personal observation).

An understanding of the biology and use of the venom by a stinging insect species helps to guide strategies for discovery of new pain-inducing materials. Venoms used offensively for prey capture are predicted to produce little or no pain in the envenomated prey. The induction of pain in a prey animal would likely be detrimental to the predator by causing heightened flight, resistance, and potential for prey escape. Pain can also cause stress and increased physiological activity in the prey that, in turn, might reduce its survival time as a paralyzed food source for the young of the stinging insect. In a few species that use venom for paralyzing prey, the venom might also be used for defense. These venoms could contain pain-inducing constituents that would be predicted to be non-paralytic, but might be toxic or lethal to potential predators [9,10].

Pain sensation in humans is a subjective feeling ultimately registered by the brain. Consequently, quantitative and reliable assays for measuring conscious pain induced by individual venom components are scarce, though a variety of assays for measuring pain response in animals, including the rat paw lifting and/or licking assays have been developed [11,12]. Additionally, a variety of in vivo assays for nociception of pain by receptors, especially TRPV1 and other members of the transient receptor potential family of receptors, and the Nav channels, are known [13–16]. The shortage of simple metrics for measuring pain in humans has hampered our scientific ability to analyze the pain-causing properties of insect venom components. The result is that the evaluation of venom-induced human pain is often indirect and by inference. Investigators sometimes rely on personally testing the material on themselves, a procedure with inherent disadvantages and possible risks [17]. The limited number of human-based assays is partly responsible for the small number of characterized insect venom algogens reported in the literature. To help quantify painfulness of an insect sting, our group and colleagues developed the semi-quantitative stinging insect pain scale that rates the pain produced by an insect sting on a scale of 1 to 4 [18]. In the scale, 1 represents minor, almost trivial, pain and 4 represents the most extreme pain experienced. This insect sting pain rating can assist in choosing promising insect venoms for discovery of new algogens and medical products.

Two major components, phospholipases (A_1 and/or A_2) and hyaluronidases are nearly universally present in insect venoms. Additionally, several insect venoms contain esterases and lipases and sometimes acid phosphatases [19]. In addition to these major components, insect venoms contain a vast diversity of proteins and peptides in trace levels [6,8,20,21]. Known algogens in insect venoms include, among others, the peptide melittin from honeybee venom [16], wasp kinins in social wasp venoms [22], poneratoxin from the ant *Paraponera clavata* [23], peptide MIITX$_1$-Mg1a from a bulldog ant [24], piperidine alkaloids in fire ants [25], barbatolysin in harvester ant venom [26], and possibly bombolitin in bumblebee venom [27]. Stings of virtually all social wasps, social bees, and ants cause at least some pain in humans. A few solitary wasp and bee species can also sting painfully. In most of the species of stinging insects, the properties of the pain-causing venom components are unknown. The intensity of the pain caused by an insect sting depends upon several factors, including the size of the stinging insect, the amount of venom it injects and, most importantly, on the chemical properties of the pain-inducing constituent(s). The purpose of this investigation was to explore as wide a diversity of stinging insects as possible to determine their ability to cause pain, and to pinpoint species that hold promise for discovering new pain-producing products that might be of benefit for science or medical investigations. The secondary purpose was to explore the lethality of venoms, again having in mind pinpointing potential species that hold promise for new scientific or medical discoveries. Several new species of stinging insects whose venoms hold promise are highlighted.

2. Results and Discussion

2.1. Pain Ratings of Insect Stings

Table 1 is a complete listing of all 115 stinging insects in 67 genera that were evaluated for the painfulness of their stings and/or the lethality of their venoms. Of these, sting pain determinations were made for 96 species in 62 genera including 38 ants in 27 genera, 25 social wasps in 12 genera, 6 social bees in 2 genera, 12 solitary bees in 10 genera, and 15 solitary wasps in 11 genera. The average pain level among the groups was: ants—1.62, social wasps—2.18, social bees—1.92, solitary bees—1.25, and solitary wasps—1.63. The members of each group do not necessarily represent the overall group in the natural world, instead represent those taxa that were often targeted for investigation, were historically known for painful stings, or were available. In many examples, the species were also among the largest in their respective genus, or the usual size of the individuals in the genus was large compared to their grouping in general. This was particularly true for the solitary bees and solitary wasps, most of which represent some of the largest known individuals in those categories. Given the targeted search for the most painful and lethal species of stinging insects, a general prediction is that most species not evaluated will deliver less painful stings than those represented in Table 1, or if they are in a genus that is listed in the table, their pain rating will be similar. The prediction of similarity of stings within a genus is based upon the sting pain values among the several species within the genera in Table 1. An extreme example of this similarity within a genus is found within the ant genus *Pogonomyrmex* in which all 21 species have the same rating of 3 on the sting pain scale. Similar results are found among the ant genera *Myrmecia* and *Solenopsis*, the social wasp genus *Vespula*, and the honeybee genus *Apis*.

Table 1. Sting pain rating on a scale of 1 to 4 and venom lethality of ant, social wasp, social bee, and solitary species of stinging Hymenoptera. The data are arranged by increasing pain level from the lowest rated species in each genus, followed by those genera unrated for pain and, within a pain level, arranged by highest to lowest lethality. Blanks in the table columns indicate no data are available for the assay.

Species (Common Name)	Sting Pain	LD_{50} (mg/kg)
Ants		
Solenopsis invicta (red fire ant)	1	
S. xyloni (southern fire ant)	1	
S. geminata (tropical fire ant)	1	
Tetraponera sp. (Old World twig ant)	1	0.35
Daceton armigerum (trap-jawed ant)	1	1.1
Myrmica rubra (European fire ant)	1	6.1
Bothroponera strigulosa	1	9.2
Leptogenys kitteli	1	10
Pseudomyrmex gracilis (twig ant)	1	12
P. nigrocinctus (bullhorn acacia ant)	1.5	1.9
Ectatomma ruidum,	1	15
E. tuberculatum	1.5	0.3
E. quadridens	1.5	17
Ectatomma sp.		17
Opthalmopone berthoudi (big-eye ant)	1	32
Harpegnathos venator	1	52
Brachyponera chinensis (needle ant)	1	
B. sennaarensis (Samsum ant)	1.5	5.6
Myrmecia gulosa (red bulldog ant)	1.5	0.18
M. browning (bulldog ant)		0.18

Table 1. *Cont.*

Species (Common Name)	Sting Pain	LD_{50} (mg/kg)
M. tarsata (bulldog ant)		0.18
M. simillima (bulldog ant)	1.5	0.21
M. rufinodis (bulldog ant)	1.5	0.35
M. pilosula (Jack jumper ant)	2	5.7
Eciton burchelli (army ant)	1.5	10
Anochetus inermis (a trap-jaw ant)	1.5	12
Dinoponera gigantea (giant ant)	1.5	14
Paltothyreus tarsatus (giant stink ant)	1.5	38
Megaponera analis (Matabele ant)	1.5	128
Pachycondyla crassinoda	2	2.8
Neoponera villosa	2	7.5
N. commutate (termite-hunting ant)	2	11
Streblognathus aethiopicus (African giant ant)	2	8
Diacamma rugosum	2	8
Platythyrea lamellose	2	11
P. cribrinodis		42
Odontoponera transversa	2	29
Rhytidoponera metallica	2	
Odontomachus bauri (trap-jaw ant)	2.5	23
O. infandus (trap-jaw ant)		33
O. chelifer (trap-jaw ant)		37
Pogonomyrmex cunicularius (Argentine harvester ant)	3	0.088
Pogonomyrmex (North American harvester ants) (20 spp.)	3	0.12–0.7
Paraponera clavata (bullet ant)	4	1.4
Manica bradleyi		6
Social Wasps		
Polybia occidentalis (polybia wasp)	1	5
P. rejecta (polybia wasp)	1.5	16
P. simillima (polybia wasp)	2.5	4.1
P. sericea (polybia wasp)		6.1
Ropalidia flavobrunnea	1	5.9
Ropalidia sp.	1	10
Ropalidia (Icarielia) sp.		14
Belonogaster sp. (thin paper wasp)	1.5	
B. juncea colonialis (fire-tail wasp)	2	3
Brachygastra mellifica (honey wasp)	2	1.5
Vespula germanica (yellowjacket wasp)	2	2.8
V. vulgaris (yellowjacket wasp)	2	5.4
V. pensylvanica (yellowjacket wasp)	2	6.4
V. vidua (yellowjacket wasp)		2.6
V. consobrina (yellowjacket wasp)		2.8
Polistes instabilis (paper wasp)	2	1.6
P. arizonicus (paper wasp)	2	2
P. infuscatus (paper wasp)	3	1.3
P. erythrocephalus (paper wasp)	3	1.5
P. canadensis. (paper wasp)	3	2.4
P. tepidus (paper wasp)	3	7.7
P. annularis (paper wasp)	3	11
Parachartergus fraternus (artistic wasp)	2	5.3
Dolichovespula maculata (baldfaced hornet)	2	6.1
D. arenaria (aerial yellowjacket)	2	8.7
Mischocyttarus sp. (a paper wasp)	2	
Agelaia myrmecophila (fire wasp)	2.5	5.6
Provespa sp. (nocturnal hornet)	2.5	
Synoeca septentrionalis (warrior wasp)	4	3
Vespa luctuosa (hornet)		1.6
V. tropica (hornet)		2.8

Table 1. *Cont.*

Species (Common Name)	Sting Pain	LD_{50} (mg/kg)
V. simillima (hornet)		3.1
V. mandarinia (giant hornet)		4.1
Apoica pallens (night wasp)		13.5
Social Bees		
Apis florea (dwarf honey bee)	1.5	2.8
A. mellifera (honey bee)	2	2.8
A. dorsata (giant honey bee)	2	2.8
A. cerana (Eastern honey bee)	2	3.1
Bombus impatiens (bumble bee)	2	11
B. sonorus (bumble bee)	2	12
Solitary Bees		
Dieunomia heteropoda (giant sweat bee)	0.5	25
Triepeolus sp. (cuckoo bee)	0.5	
Xenoglossa angustior (squash bee)	1	12
Habropoda pallida (white-faced bee)	1	70
Diadasia rinconis (cactus bee)	1	76
Emphoropsis pallida	1	
Lasioglossum spp. (sweat bee)	1	
Ericrocis lata (cuckoo bee)	1	
Euglossa dilemma (orchid bee)	1.5	
Xylocopa rufa (nocturnal carpenter bee)	2	11
X. californica (carpenter bee)	2	14
X. veripuncta (carpenter bee)		33
Xylocopa sp. (giant Bornean bee)	2.5	
Centris pallida (palo verde bee)		56
Solitary Wasps		
Sapyga pumila (club-horned wasp)	0.5	
Eumeninae spp. (potter wasps)	1	
Sphecius convallis (cicada killer wasp)	1	
S. grandis (cicada killer wasp)	1.5	46
Sphex pensylvanicus (great black wasp)	1	
Chlorion cyaneum (cockroach-hunter wasp)	1	
Triscolia ardens (scarab-hunter wasp)	1	
Sceliphron caementarium (mud dauber wasp)	1	
Euodynerus crypticus (water walking wasp)	1	
Dasymutilla thetis (little velvet ant)	1	
D. gloriosa (velvet ant)	2	
D. klugii (cow killer velvet ant)	3	70
Pepsis grossa (tarantula hawk wasp)	4	90
P. thisbe (tarantula hawk wasp)	4	120
Mutillidae sp. (small nocturnal velvet ant)	1.5	
Crioscolia flammicoma (scoliid wasp)		62

2.2. Lethality of Stinging Insect Venoms

The venom lethalities for 90 stinging insects in 50 genera are listed in Table 1. Lethalities were determined for 40 ants in 26 genera, 31 social wasps in 12 genera, 6 social bees in 2 genera, 8 solitary bees in 6 genera, and 5 solitary wasps in 4 genera. Overall, the venom lethalities of social bees and social wasps were higher than those of their solitary counterparts, with average values for the groupings: social wasps—5.38 mg/kg; social bees—5.75 mg/kg; solitary bees—37.1 mg/kg; and solitary wasps—77.6 mg/kg. The small number of solitary bees and solitary wasps is mainly because the venom of many individuals needed to be pooled for the lethality determinations. In addition, the general low overall lethality of solitary bees and wasps precluded extensive research on venom toxicity of these two groups. The ants presented a much higher variability in their venom lethalities: 13 taxa having lethalities of < 5 mg/kg, 10 in the range of 5–10 mg/kg, 8 in the range of 10–20 mg/kg, 7 in the range of 20–50 mg/kg, and 2 in the range of 50–128 mg/kg. This large range of values did not depend upon the body size of the ants: some ants of similar body weights had high lethalities (*Tetraponera* sp., 15 mg; *Pogonomyrmex* spp., 16 mg), medium lethalities (*Anochetus inermis*, 15 mg), or low lethalities (*Ectatomma ruidum*, 20 mg; *Harpegnathos venator*, 20 mg). The same contrast in lethalities was also observed among the largest ants, with the venoms of some species being highly lethal (*Myrmecia gulosa*, 80 mg; *Paraponera clavata*, 200 mg), some being moderately lethal (*Dinoponera gigantea*, 400 mg), and some being of low lethality (*Megaponera analis*, 90 mg) (weights, unpublished data).

2.3. Relationship between Sting Pain Level and Lethality of Stinging Insect Venoms

The question addressed here is the possible connection between the painfulness of a sting and the lethality of the venom delivered by the stinging insect. Of the 115 taxa investigated, data for both the sting pain rating and for the lethality are available for 71 stinging insects (Figure 1). The data are scattered throughout both the range of pain levels and lethalities with no apparent pattern or relationship, and no significant regression was found ($r^2 = 0.013$; $P = 0.356$; line drawn only for visual reference). To obtain visual representations and possible relationships among the different stinging insect groups, the data were plotted separately for the ants, the social wasps, the social bees, and the solitary bees and wasps (Figure 2). The ant data scatter throughout Figure 2A and parallel the entire range found for all stinging species. Again, no relationship between sting painfulness and lethality was observed ($r^2 = 0.028$; $P = 0.354$). The social wasp data clump in the middle range of lethalities and rang from lowest to highest in painfulness (Figure 2B) with no relationship observed ($r^2 = 0.095$; $P = 0.162$). The sting and venom activities of the six social bees exhibit midranges for both activities (Figure 2C). The data for social bees are limited in part because all stinging social bees reside in only two genera and the species within each genus have similar values. The solitary bees and wasps represent a wide variety of families and genera that have little in common biologically except for their solitary lifestyles. The 10 species share in common a comparatively low lethality, but have a maximal range from trivial to extreme in ability to deliver pain (Figure 2D). The relationship between pain and lethality among the solitary species, though not statistically significant, appears inverse, with those species delivering the most painful stings generally also trending towards having the least lethal venoms ($r^2 = 0.398$; $P = 0.0504$).

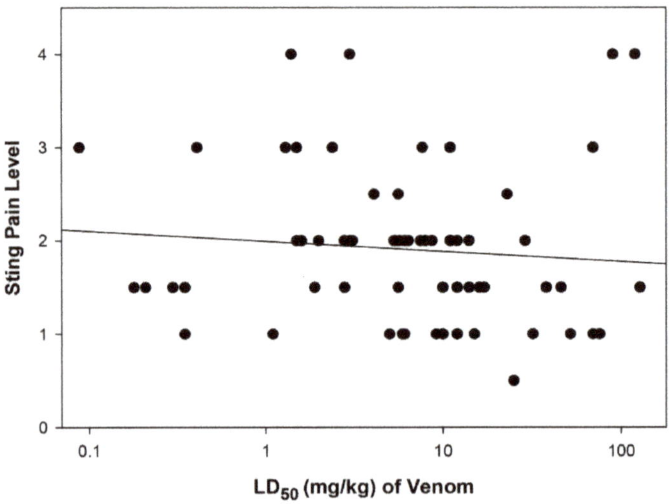

Figure 1. Scatter diagram of sting pain level and lethality of all 71 species of Hymenoptera for which both values are available. The trendline is provided only for reference, as no significant trend was observed ($r^2 = 0.013$; $P = 0.356$).

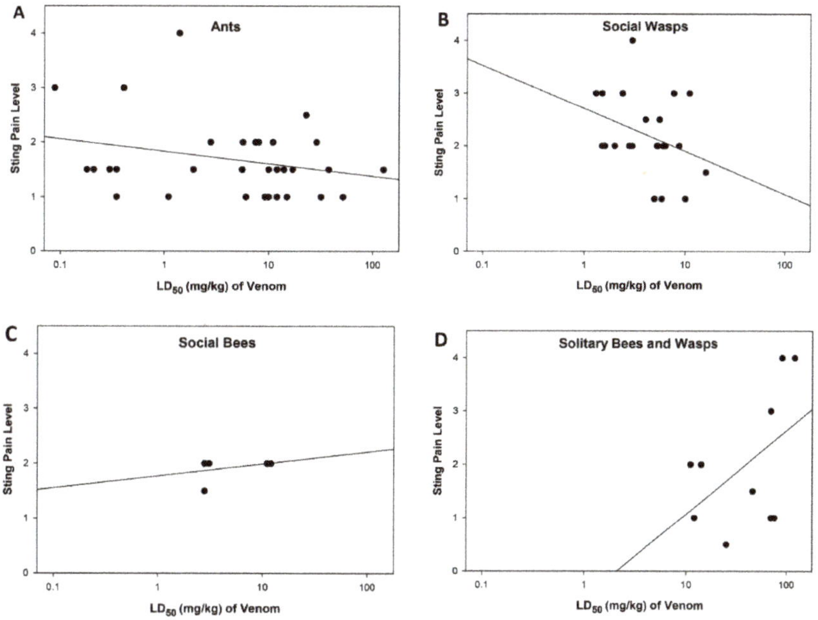

Figure 2. Scatter diagrams of sting pain level and lethality showing potential trends among the taxa within the individual groupings of stinging Hymenoptera. (**A**) The 33 species of ants, (**B**) the 22 species of social wasps, (**C**) the 6 species of social bees, and (**D**) the 10 species of solitary bees and wasps. The ants exhibit the broadest range of values, while the values of the other groupings are more tightly clustered. The trendlines are provided only for reference, as no significant relationship between sting pain level and lethality was observed for any of the groups ((**A**) $r^2 = 0.028$. $P = 0.354$; (**B**) $r^2 = 0.095$, $P = 0.162$; (**C**) $r^2 = 0.105$, $P = 0.532$; (**D**) $r^2 = 0.398$, $P = 0.0504$).

2.4. Relationship between Sting Pain Level, Lethality, and Sociality of Stinging Insects

Field observations and the data presented here tend to indicate that stings of social insect are more painful than those of solitary species. On average, the sting pain level the social species in Table 1 is 1.85 ± 0.71 (S.D.; n = 69) compared to 1.46 ± 0.94 (S.D.; n = 27) for solitary species (P = 0.032, t-test). Some exceptions to this trend exist and will be the discussed in detail later.

The overall lethality of venoms of social species of stinging insects is higher than for solitary species. On average the lethality of social insects is 10.6 ± 17.3 mg/kg (S.D.; n = 77) compared to 52.7 ± 33.2 mg/kg (S.D.; n = 13) for solitary species, a highly significant difference (P = 0.0001, t-test).

Although both the painfulness of stings and the lethality of the venoms of social insects are greater than for solitary insects, the two factors combined do not result in a significant correlation between them and sociality. This might seem counterintuitive but the presence of sociality appears not simply based on venom lethality alone, but rather a combination of venom lethality and the amount venom delivered in a sting, in combination with the number of individuals available to deliver stings. When the amount of venom delivered per sting is considered, the result is a significant correlation between sting pain and venom potency (P < 0.001) [28]. Venom lethality also strongly correlates with the population in a colony, and with the overall weight of the individuals within a colony (P < 0.001), thus indicating that higher sociality evolved in concert with increased effectiveness of their venoms with more populated colonies [28]. These factors of venom quantity per insect and colony weight and number of individuals will not be discussed further here as they do not relate directly to questions of identification of venom peptides and proteins or their activities.

2.5. Natural History of Stinging Insects and How It Can Help Guide Discovery of Interesting Venom Peptides, Proteins, and Other Natural Pharmaceuticals

The functions and activities of the venoms of stinging insects evolved in concert with their natural history. If the natural history of a species is mainly based upon procuring prey for feeding their young, as occurs in most solitary wasps, then the primary activity of the venom would be expected to be paralysis, or sometimes death, of the prey. Most solitary species of wasps do not have serious predation pressure exerted by large predators, especially vertebrate predators, and hence their stings and venoms are only rarely used for defense. Their stings and tend not to be highly painful or toxic to vertebrates. In contrast, social wasps never use their stings and venom for subduing prey. Powerful mandibles are used for prey capture and dismemberment and the sting is used only for defense (and in some situations for release of pheromones or other activities) [29]. Thus, in general, solitary and social wasps would be expected to have different venom chemistries and activities.

All ants are social. Ants also have an extreme breath of behaviors and natural histories. Some ants use their stings to paralyze or subdue prey, whereas others rarely use their venom for prey capture. All stinging ants use their stings and venom for defense against potential predators, whether the predators are small arthropods or large vertebrates. These diverse natural histories of ants provide a wealth of potential opportunities for discovery of new and exciting peptides, proteins, and other active constituents.

All bees are vegetarians, with the exception of a few species that scavenge dead animals. Bees, therefore, have no need to use their venom for prey capture and their stings and venoms are only used for defense against predators. In the case of solitary bees, their main predators are also small animals, mainly spiders, other arachnids, and insects, especially ants. Solitary bees rarely experience strong predation pressure vertebrates and their stings and venoms have not evolved to be especially painful or toxic to vertebrates. Social bees, mainly honeybees and bumblebees, live in colonies rich in resources including honey, pollen, and larvae and pupae that provide an enticing nutritional reward for mammals and birds. In response to this heightened predation pressure experience by social bees, their venoms have evolved to be lethal to vertebrates and to induce pain.

2.6. Targeting Promising Species of Stinging Insects for Discovery of New Pharmaceuticals Based upon Sting Pain and Lethality

Species of stinging insects that exhibit extreme values of either sting painfulness or lethality may be promising for further investigation. Especially interesting might be those species whose stings are extraordinarily painful but have little lethal activity, or species that are the opposite with extremely lethal venoms that are not particularly painful. A third category of species that might be of interest are those that have both painful stings and are highly lethal. Species in a fourth category that have stings of low painfulness and their venoms are of low lethality likely have minimal potential for discovery of new interesting peptides or pharmaceuticals that relate to human biology or welfare. However, those species that are low in both categories might have high potential for discovery of peptides or other active principles that target insects and other invertebrates and could be of benefit for agriculture. Species in this category include many of the solitary wasps, with noteworthy species being the cicada killer wasps in the genus *Sphecius*, the potter wasps in the subfamily Eumeninae, and any of the species that routinely paralyze or kill insect or spider prey. The sting painfulness and/or venom lethality of many of these wasps is *Terra incognita* and is well worth investigating. Solitary wasp species such as velvet ants in the family Mutillidae that use their stings only for defense are likely to show no potential for discovering new agricultural materials. The main disadvantage of investigating solitary hunting wasps is the problem of obtaining enough individuals for study.

Solitary bees use their stings and venom strictly for defense, and even for defense most of them have ineffective venoms that produce little pain and low toxicity. The activity of their venoms towards insects is basically unknown. Thus, solitary bees likely represent a group that have little or no potential for discovery of new peptides or materials useful for either agriculture or other human endeavors. The one exception to this generalization might be the large carpenter bees in the genus *Xylocopa* that have venoms that produce moderate pain and moderate lethality. An additional benefit of these bees is that they are large and easy to obtain.

Species whose stings produce extreme pain, yet have low venom lethality provide a promising starting point for the development of bioassays for screening of potential analgesic pharmaceuticals. They have active components that can readily induce pain, while not causing tissue toxicity. Tarantula hawks in the genus *Pepsis* and the velvet ants the family Mutillidae, both of which produce extraordinary painful stings, yet have almost no vertebrate lethality, are candidates for further study. One species that produces the most painful stings of any hymenopteran is the bullet ant *Paraponera clavata*. The venom of this species is also highly lethal and both activities appear to be caused mainly by the single peptide poneratoxin that has been well studied [23]. A promising pain-inducing venom that has potential for new meaningful discoveries is that of the warrior wasps in the genus *Synoeca*. The stings of these wasps are intensely painful for at least an hour and have a sting pain rating of 4. The venom is also highly lethal. This small genus of six species is widespread and common throughout much of tropical Latin America and their venoms have been studied to a limited extent [30]. These large wasps live in populist colonies and produce 270 μg venom/wasp (Schmidt, unpublished). A final promising group of wasps with painful stings and lethal venoms worthy of investigation of the fire wasps in the genus *Agelaia*. The genus of about two dozen species of small wasps live in populist colonies of many thousands of individuals and range throughout much of the New World tropics.

Stings that are highly lethal, yet induce low pain levels are relatively uncommon. Most impressive example of this is an unidentified species in the ant genus *Tetraponera* from Malaysia. The stings of this species produce only the mild pain level of 1, yet have the exquisite lethality of 0.35 mg/kg. This venom could be useful for assays designed to determine the mechanism of lethality while producing little pain. Another species of similar potential is that of the trap-jaw ant *Daceton armigerum* that is a common arboreal species in the tree canopy of the rain forests of northern South America. Other promising species include the common Latin American ant *Ectatomma tuberculatum* and many of the Australian bulldog ants in the genus *Myrmecia* that have been subject to a variety of studies [24,31]. The venoms of the social wasps in the enormous Old-World genus *Ropalidia* have been neglected and appear to have potential for new discoveries.

The final category of stinging insects that have promising venoms are those that are both painful and lethal. In addition to the already mentioned bullet ants, the new world harvester ants in the genus *Pogonomyrmex* present ideal opportunities. Their venoms are the most toxic known from any of the Hymenoptera and produce intense waves of deep, agonizing pain that lasts 4–8 h, plus induce piloerection and localized sweating at sting site [29,32]. These ants are abundant over large areas of North and South America and are easy to maintain in the laboratory. The Neotropical ants in the genus *Neoponera*, including *N. villosa* and the termite-hunting ant, *N. commutata* are large species whose stings are painful and venom is lethal to mammals and paralytic to insects [33,34]. The venoms of honey wasps in the Neotropical genus *Brachygastra*, have not been studied and represent a good opportunity for discovery of interesting venom activities and constituents. Likewise, many of the paper wasps in the large worldwide genus *Polistes* possess both painful stings and lethal venoms and their venoms are worthy of further investigation.

3. Materials and Methods

3.1. Insects

Stinging ants, wasp, and bees were live collected from their natural environments, typically from their nests in the soil, in trees, sometimes in urban areas, or from their normal foraging locations on flowers, vegetation, or soil surface. Species were determined with keys to the various taxa, with difficult identifications made by experts in the specific taxa. Once collected, the insects were cooled on ice, and in most situations the iced insects were brought to the laboratory where they were frozen and stored at −20 °C until their use. In some field situations where access to a freezer was unavailable, the insects were maintained on ice until dissected for venom. In situations where the insects were maintained on ice, the insect tissues were fresh, appeared the same as live dissected individuals, and the venom reservoirs were intact and contained venom that was clear and transparent.

3.2. Pain Measurement

Since human perception of sting pain cannot be easily measured instrumentally or with great precision, a pain scale for the immediate, acute pain caused by a sting was developed [18,35]. The scale ranges in values from 1–4 and is anchored by the value of a single honeybee sting (*Apis mellifera*), which is defined as a 2 on the scale. The honeybee is a convenient reference point because honeybees exist worldwide, are abundant, and most people have been stung by a honeybee. They are also about midway within the range of pain intensities produced by hymenopterous stings. Sting pain induced by a single sting can vary depending upon how much venom was delivered with the sting, where on the body the sting occurred (for example stings to the nose, lips, or palms of hands are considerably more painful than stings to lower legs or arms; see also [19]), the age of the insect, the time of day the sting was received, and other factors [36]. For these reasons, the scale was limited to 4 values, plus a trivial value of 0 for insects that are incapable of penetrating human skin. The criteria distinguishing between pain levels is that the pain of the lower level is substantially less than the pain in the upper level and that the evaluating person would clearly know that one of the stings hurt considerably more than the other. When comparing species, the evaluator compares the current sting pain with memory of the pain of previous stings by a honeybee or other species for which the pain was rated previously. In most cases the reference point for the value of 2 that is used to stabilize the scale is quite robust because the evaluator has been stung many times by honeybees and can sense the amount of pain in an average honeybee sting. The number of stings for other species evaluated can vary from a low of a single sting to a high of many stings depending upon the species; consequently, some values have greater potential subjectivity than others. In some cases, values halfway between whole numbers are assigned where the pain appears greater than the lower level, yet less than the higher level. This evaluation system works remarkably well as witnessed by nearly identical ratings for stings by various colleagues (personal observations) [35]. Stings of many different species have the same numerical value; this does not imply that they are identical in feeling, but that they fall into the same general range of acute painfulness, and presumed effectiveness as predation deterrents. Pain that arises at or near the sting site hours or days after the initial sting pain has receded is not considered for this pain scale because it is caused by immunological or physiological reactions to the venom or its damage [37].

Most measurements of pain were scored in the field from live stings as they naturally occurred. In exceptional situations where normal stings were not received during the course of working with or collecting the species, or when the species does not normally sting as a primary defense, intentional stings were received by forcing the insect to sting the medial side of the forearm. This area was chosen because the low hair density allows better observation and that area is a convenient and relatively non-specialized part of the skin.

3.3. Venom

Pure venom was obtained by the method of Schmidt [36]. In brief, frozen ants or bees were thawed, their sting apparatuses removed to a spot of distilled water, the venom reservoir (minus filamentous glands) was pinched off at the duct and removed from the rest of the sting apparatus, twice rinsed with distilled water, and placed in clean distilled water (Figure 3). Depending upon the number of insects available and their size, up to 100 reservoirs were collected into an approximately 50 µL droplet of distilled water, after which the venom was squeezed from the reservoirs and the empty chitinous reservoirs were discarded. The pure venom was either lyophilized and stored at −20 °C until used, or dried over molecular sieves 5A (Supelco, Bellefonte, PA, USA) and then stored in a freezer −20 °C until used.

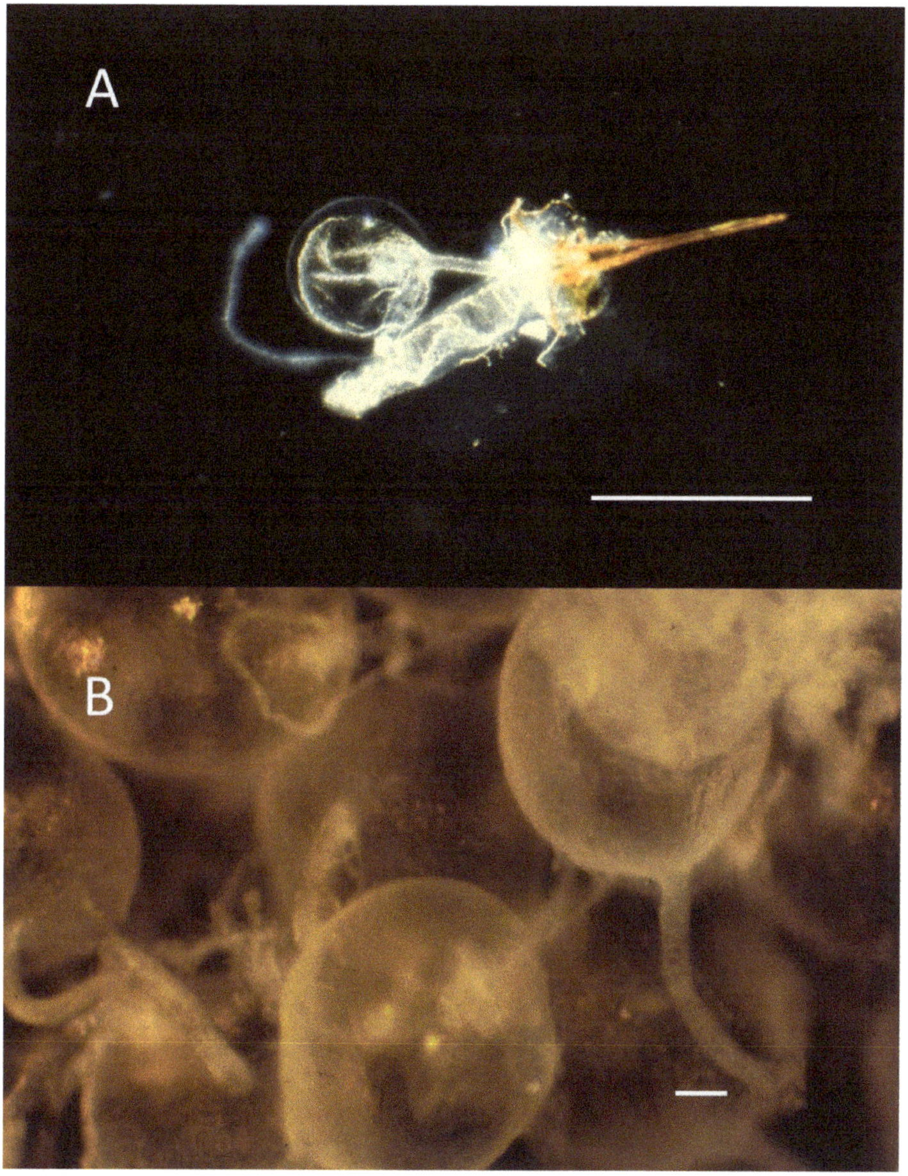

Figure 3. (**A**) Sting apparatus of *Pogonomyrmex badius* showing sting shaft, tubular Dufour's gland, and spherical venom reservoir with a long venom duct leading to the base of the sting shaft (scale bar = 1 mm). (**B**) Isolated venom reservoirs of *Pogonomyrmex maricopa* in a droplet of distilled water ready for the venom to be drained and the empty membranous reservoirs discarded (scale bar = 0.1 mm). Photos taken with an Olympus PM-10-A camera attached to an Olympus JM Zoom Stereo Microscope.

For wasps, venom was collected by expression through the sting shaft into the space (by capillary action) between the tines of fine forceps. Often, in order to accomplish this, one or two terminal sternites of the abdomen needed to be removed to allow the sting apparatus including the muscular venom reservoir to be removed. To facilitate venom expression gentle squeezing pressure was applied via broad forceps to the venom reservoir. After the venom was collected, it was released into the bottom of a small polyethylene microtube by opening the forceps and allowing the venom to be deposited in the microtube. The venom from several individuals could be combined a single microtube before the venom was frozen, lyophilized and stored at −20 °C.

3.4. *Physiological Measurements*

Animal experiments were approved by the Southwestern Biological Institute Ethics Committee (SWBIEC/0017_29, 29 June 2016). Dried venom was used in all tests. Venoms were weighed to the nearest 1.0 µg on a 7-place microbalance (Model 1-912, Mettler, Zurich, Switzerland). Damage potential of an insect sting was measured as lethality of the venom to ICR white mice of mixed sex and ranging in weight from 18 to 22 g, as described previously [38]. Generally, four groups of six mice were used for each experiment, though in some situations where venom availability was limited only three groups of four mice were used.

For each analysis the calculated and measured weight of venom was dissolved in 0.15 M NaCl saline and injected in the volume of 0.6% of the animal body weight. Venoms were intravenously (i.v.) injected into the tail veins of the mice. Median lethal amount of venom to kill 50% of the individuals (LD_{50}) in 24 h were calculated according to the rapid 50% endpoint method that interpolates between the 25% and 75% values to obtain a reliable 50% lethality value [39].

Funding: This research received no external funding.

Conflicts of Interest: The author declares no conflict of interest.

References

1. Freeman, T.; Tracy, J. (Eds.) *Stinging Insect Allergy: A Clinician's Guide*; Springer: Heidelberg, Germany, 2017; p. 321, ISBN 978-3-319-46190-8.
2. Bettini, S. (Ed.) Arthropod Venoms. In *Handbook of Experimental Pharmacology*; Springer: Berlin, Germany, 1978; Volume 48, p. 978, ISBN 3-540-082228-X.
3. Maschwitz, U.; Hahn, M.; Schönegge, P. Paralysis of prey in ponerine ants. *Naturwissenschaften* **1979**, *66*, 213–214. [CrossRef]
4. Piek, T. (Ed.) *Venoms of the Hymenoptera: Biochemical, Pharmacological and Behavioral Aspects*; Academic Press: London, UK, 1986; p. 570, ISBN 0-12-554770-6.
5. Palma, M.S. Insect venom peptides. In *Handbook of Biologically Active Peptides*; Kastin, A.J., Ed.; Academic Press: Amsterdam, The Netherlands, 2006; pp. 409–416. ISBN 13: 978-0-12-369442-3.
6. Schmidt, J.O. Biochemistry of insect venoms. *Annu. Rev. Entomol.* **1982**, *27*, 339–368. [CrossRef] [PubMed]
7. Torres, A.F.C.; Quinet, Y.P.; Havt, A.; Rádis-Baptista, G.; Martins, A.M.C. Molecular pharmacology and toxinology of venom from ants. In *Analytical Procedures to Biomedical Applications*; Rádis Baptista, G., Ed.; IntechOpen: London, UK, 2013; pp. 207–222. [CrossRef]
8. Touchard, A.; Samira, R.; Aili, S.R.; Gonçalves, E.; Fox, P.; Escoubas, P.; Orivel, J.; Nicholson, G.M.; Dejean, A. The Biochemical Toxin Arsenal from Ant Venoms. *Toxins* **2016**, *8*, 30. [CrossRef] [PubMed]
9. Schmidt, J.O. Hymenopteran venoms: Striving toward the ultimate defense against vertebrates. In *Insect Defense: Adaptations and Strategies of Prey and Predators*; Evans, D.L., Schmidt, J.O., Eds.; SUNY Press: Albany, NY, USA, 1990; pp. 387–419, ISBN 0-88706-896-0.
10. Schmidt, J.O. Venom and the good life in tarantula hawks (Hymenoptera: Pompilidae): How to eat, not be eaten, and live long. *J. Kansas Entomol. Soc.* **2004**, *77*, 402–413. [CrossRef]
11. Pessini, A.C.; Kanashiro, A.; Malvar, D.C.; Machado, R.R.; Soares, D.M.; Figueiredo, M.J.; Kalapothakis, E.; Souza, G.E.P. Inflammatory mediators involved in the nociceptive and oedematogenic responses induced by Tityus serrulatus scorpion venom injected into rat paws. *Toxicon* **2008**, *52*, 729–736. [CrossRef]
12. Pucca, M.B.; Cerni, F.A.; Cordeiro, F.A.; Peigneur, S.; Cunha, T.M.; Tytgat, J.; Arantes, E.C. Ts8 scorpion toxin inhibits the Kv4.2 channel and produces nociception in vivo. *Toxicon* **2016**, *119*, 244–252. [CrossRef] [PubMed]

13. Julius, D. TRP channels and pain. *Annu. Rev. Cell Dev. Biol.* **2013**, *29*, 355–384. [CrossRef]
14. Min, J.W.; Liu, W.H.; He, X.H.; Peng, B.W. Different types of toxins targeting TRPV1 in pain. *Toxicon* **2013**, *71*, 66–75. [CrossRef]
15. Klint, J.K.; Smith, J.J.; Vetter, I.; Rupasinghe, D.B.; Er, S.Y.; Senff, S.; Herzig, V.; Mobli, M.; Lewis, R.J.; Bosmans, F.; et al. Seven novel modulators of the analgesic target NaV1.7 uncovered using a high-throughput venom-based discovery approach. *Br. J. Pharmacol.* **2015**, *172*, 2445–2458. [CrossRef]
16. Chen, J.; Guan, S.M.; Sun, W.; Fu, H. Melittin, the major pain-producing substance of bee venom. *Neurosci. Bull.* **2016**, *32*, 265–272. [CrossRef]
17. Smith, M.L. Honey bee sting pain index by body location. *PeerJ* **2014**, *2*, e338. [CrossRef] [PubMed]
18. Schmidt, J.O.; Blum, M.S.; Overal, W.L. Hemolytic activities of stinging insect venoms. *Arch. Insect Biochem. Physiol.* **1984**, *1*, 155–160. [CrossRef]
19. Schmidt, J.O.; Blum, M.S.; Overal, W.L. Comparative enzymology of venoms from stinging Hymenoptera. *Toxicon* **1986**, *24*, 907–921. [CrossRef]
20. Aili, S.R.; Touchard, A.; Koh, J.M.S.; Dejean, A.; Orivel, J.; Padula, M.P.; Escoubas, P.; Nicholson, G.M. Comparisons of protein and peptide complexity in poneroid and formicoid ant venoms. *J. Proteome Res.* **2016**, *15*, 3039–3054. [CrossRef] [PubMed]
21. Aili, S.R.; Touchard, A.; Petitclerc, F.; Dejean, A.; Orivel, J.; Padula, M.P.; Escoubas, P.; Nicholson, G.M. Combined peptidomic and proteomic analysis of electrically stimulated and manually dissected venom from the South American bullet ant Paraponera clavata. *J. Proteome Res.* **2017**, *16*, 1339–1351. [CrossRef] [PubMed]
22. Lee, S.H.; Baek, J.H.; Yoon, K.A. Differential properties of venom peptides and proteins in solitary vs. social hunting wasps. *Toxins* **2016**, *8*, 32. [CrossRef] [PubMed]
23. Johnson, S.R.; Rikli, H.G.; Schmidt, J.O.; Evans, M.S. A reexamination of poneratoxin from the bullet ant Paraponera clavata. *Peptides* **2017**, *98*, 51–62. [CrossRef]
24. Robinson, S.D.; Mueller, A.; Clayton, D.; Starobova, H.; Hamilton, B.R.; Payne, R.J.; Vetter, I.; King, G.F.; Undheim, E.B. A comprehensive portrait of the venom of the giant red bull ant, Myrmecia gulosa, reveals a hyperdiverse hymenopteran toxin gene family. *Sci. Adv.* **2018**, *4*, eaau4640. [CrossRef]
25. MacConnell, J.G.; Blum, M.S.; Fales, H.M. Alkaloid from fire ant venom: Identification and synthesis. *Science* **1970**, *168*, 840–841. [CrossRef]
26. Bernheimer, A.W.; Avigad, L.S.; Schmidt, J.O. A hemolytic polypeptide from the venom of the red harvester ant, Pogonomyrmex barbatus. *Toxicon* **1980**, *18*, 271–278. [CrossRef]
27. Argiolas, A.; Pisano, J.J. Bombolitins, a new class of mast cell degranulating peptides from the venom of the bumblebee Megabombus pennsylvanicus. *J. Biol. Chem.* **1985**, *260*, 1437–1444. [PubMed]
28. Schmidt, J.O. Evolutionary responses of solitary and social Hymenoptera to predation by primates and overwhelmingly powerful vertebrate predators. *J. Hum. Evol.* **2014**, *71*, 12–19.
29. Schmidt, J.O. *The Sting of the Wild*; Johns Hopkins Univ. Press: Baltimore, MD, USA, 2016; p. 280, ISBN 978-1-4214-1928-2.
30. Mortari, J.M.R.; do Couto, L.L.; dos Anjos, L.C.; Mourão, C.B.F.; Camargos, T.S.; Vargas, J.A.G.; Oliveira, F.N.; Gati, C.C.; Schwartz, C.A.; Schwartz, E.F. Pharmacological characterization of Synoeca cyanea venom: An aggressive social wasp widely distributed in the Neotropical region. *Toxicon* **2012**, *59*, 163–170. [CrossRef] [PubMed]
31. da Silva, J.R.; de Souza, A.Z.; Pirovani, C.P.; Costa, H.; Silva, A.; Dias, J.C.T.; Delabie, J.H.C.; Fontana, R. Assessing the proteomic activity of the venom of the ant Ectatomma tuberculatum (Hymenoptera: Formicidae: Ectatomminae). *Psyche* **2018**, *2018*, 7915464. [CrossRef]
32. Schmidt, J.O.; Blum, M.S. A harvester ant venom: Chemistry and pharmacology. *Science* **1978**, *200*, 1064–1066. [CrossRef] [PubMed]
33. Schmidt, J.O.; Snelling, G.C. Pogonomyrmex anzensis Cole: Does an unusual harvester ant species have an unusual venom? *J. Hymenopt. Res.* **2009**, *18*, 322–325.
34. Pessoa, W.F.B.; Silva, L.L.C.; Dias, L.O.; Delabie, J.H.C.; Costa, H.; Romano, C.C. Analysis of protein composition and bioactivity of Neoponera villosa venom (Hymenoptera: Formicidae). *Int. J. Mol. Sci.* **2016**, *17*, 513. [CrossRef]
35. Starr, C.K. A simple pain scale for field comparison of hymenopteran stings. *J. Entomol. Sci.* **1985**, *20*, 225–232. [CrossRef]

36. Schmidt, J.O. Chemistry, pharmacology and chemical ecology of ant venoms. In *Venoms of the Hymenoptera*; Piek, T., Ed.; Academic Press: London, UK, 1986; pp. 425–508, ISBN 0-12-554770-6.
37. Schmidt, J.O. Allergy to venomous insects. In *The Hive and the Honey Bee*; Graham, J.M., Ed.; Dadant and Sons: Hamilton, IL, USA, 2015; pp. 907–952, ISBN 978-0-915698-16-5.
38. Schmidt, J.O. Toxinology of venoms from the honeybee genus *Apis*. *Toxicon* **1995**, *33*, 917–927. [CrossRef]
39. Reed, L.J.; Muench, H. A simple method of estimating fifty per cent endpoints. *Am. J. Epidemiol.* **1938**, *27*, 493–497. [CrossRef]

toxins

MDPI

Article

Dissecting Toxicity: The Venom Gland Transcriptome and the Venom Proteome of the Highly Venomous Scorpion *Centruroides limpidus* (Karsch, 1879)

Jimena I. Cid-Uribe [1], Erika P. Meneses [2], Cesar V. F. Batista [2], Ernesto Ortiz [1,*] and Lourival D. Possani [1,*]

1 Departamento de Medicina Molecular y Bioprocesos, Instituto de Biotecnología, Universidad Nacional Autónoma de México, Avenida Universidad 2001, Cuernavaca, Morelos 62210, Mexico; jcidu@ibt.unam.mx

2 Laboratorio Universitario de Proteómica, Instituto de Biotecnología, Universidad Nacional Autónoma de México, Avenida Universidad 2001, Cuernavaca, Morelos 62210, Mexico; pkas@ibt.unam.mx (E.P.M.); fbatista@ibt.unam.mx (C.V.F.B.)

* Correspondence: erne@ibt.unam.mx (E.O.); possani@ibt.unam.mx (L.D.P.)

Received: 12 April 2019; Accepted: 26 April 2019; Published: 30 April 2019

check for updates

Abstract: Venom glands and soluble venom from the Mexican scorpion *Centruroides limpidus* (Karsch, 1879) were used for transcriptomic and proteomic analyses, respectively. An RNA-seq was performed by high-throughput sequencing with the Illumina platform. Approximately 80 million reads were obtained and assembled into 198,662 putative transcripts, of which 11,058 were annotated by similarity to sequences from available databases. A total of 192 venom-related sequences were identified, including Na^+ and K^+ channel-acting toxins, enzymes, host defense peptides, and other venom components. The most diverse transcripts were those potentially coding for ion channel-acting toxins, mainly those active on Na^+ channels (NaScTx). Sequences corresponding to β- scorpion toxins active of K^+ channels (KScTx) and λ-KScTx are here reported for the first time for a scorpion of the genus *Centruroides*. Mass fingerprint corroborated that NaScTx are the most abundant components in this venom. Liquid chromatography coupled to mass spectometry (LC-MS/MS) allowed the identification of 46 peptides matching sequences encoded in the transcriptome, confirming their expression in the venom. This study corroborates that, in the venom of toxic buthid scorpions, the more abundant and diverse components are ion channel-acting toxins, mainly NaScTx, while they lack the HDP diversity previously demonstrated for the non-buthid scorpions. The highly abundant and diverse antareases explain the pancreatitis observed after envenomation by this species.

Keywords: *Centruroides limpidus* Karch; proteome; scorpion; transcriptome; venom toxicity

Key Contribution: A detailed molecular dissection of the venom of the highly toxic buthid scorpion *Centruroides limpidus* through transcriptomic and proteomic analyses is reported. Ion channel-acting toxins are shown to be the most abundant and diverse components of the venom, especially the NaScTx. Two new families of KScTx are reported for the first time in a scorpion of the genus *Centruroides*: β-KScTx and λ-KScTx. Zn-metalloproteases of the antarease family are present in the venom, providing the molecular basis for the observed pancreatitis after envenomation by this species.

1. Introduction

Scorpion venoms are known to contain hundreds of pharmacologically active components, affecting many other animals, which constitute their preys, competitors and/or predators [1]. They have a cosmopolitan distribution with 2415 distinct species reported up to December 2018 [2], which are classified into twenty different families. The scorpions belonging to the family Butidae produce the most active toxins that affect mammals, including humans [3,4]. Mexico harbors approximately 12% of the world's diversity of scorpions, with 281 different species thus far described, of which 21 are dangerous to humans [5]. Their medical importance drove the initial research towards the isolation and biochemical characterization of the toxic compounds present in their venoms, and the identification of their physiological effects. The more recent development of high-throughput methods for massive sequencing and mass spectrometry has impacted the number of identified venom components [6–13].

In Mexico, the scorpions dangerous to humans belong to the genus *Centruroides*, comprising 42 different species [4,5]. The best studied species are: *Centruroides noxius*, *Centruroides suffusus*, *Centruroides tecomanus*, and *Centruroides limpidus*. *Centruroides limpidus* (Karsch, 1879) (Figure 1A) is widely distributed in densely populated areas of Central Mexico, including the States of Guerrero, Morelos, Mexico State, Michoacán, Queretaro, Hidalgo, and Puebla (Figure 1B) [14], and has a tendency to live side by side with humans [15]. It produces a potent venom which is highly toxic for mammals (the LD_{50} in mice is approximately 15 μg/20 g [16]) and poses a serious threat to human life. Even though it is practically impossible to single out the species involved in each envenomation case, *C. limpidus* and other closely related species of the *Centruroides* genus with which it shares its habitat, are responsible for over 120,000 reported accidents with humans in those states alone every year—a third of all scorpionism cases in the country [17]. Those high morbidity numbers alone justify the efforts made toward the characterization of the venom components responsible for human intoxication. The identification of the toxins present in this venom should impact, for example, the research aimed at the production of antivenoms [18]. Thus far, for *C. limpidus* alone, nine peptides have been biochemically characterized, and nine precursors for other putative toxins have been described [19–23]. It is clear, however, that the characterization of this venom is far from complete, as information on novel, potentially lethal toxins from this species continues to emerge [23]. A more comprehensive study was therefore required.

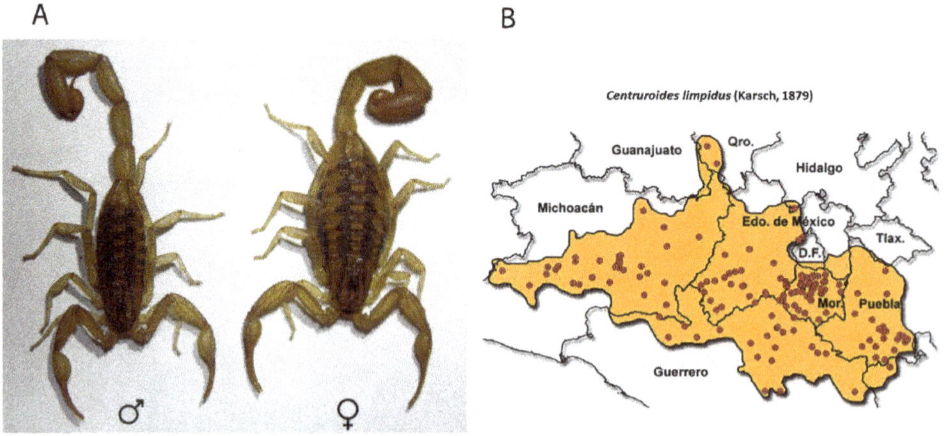

Figure 1. Habitus and distribution of *Centruroides limpidus*. (**A**) The morphology of *C. limpidus*, male (left) and female (right). (**B**) Geographical distribution of *C. limpidus* in 10 Mexican States (red dots indicate the places of sampling). (**B**) Reproduced with permission from [14] Copyright 2009, Universidad Nacional Autónoma de México.

This communication reports the transcriptomic and proteomic analyses of the venom glands and the soluble venom of the scorpion *C. limpidus*, respectively. The transcriptomic results showed 192 transcripts encoding proteins/peptides with sequences identified as authentic venom components. Among these sequences, five main categories of precursors were identified: toxins, host defense peptides (HDPs), protease inhibitors, enzymes, and other components. The peptides encoded by the 46 transcripts identified in the transcriptome analysis were confirmed to be expressed in the venom by LC-MS/MS sequencing. They showed sequence similarity with previously reported scorpion venom components.

The relative abundance and diversity of ion channel-acting toxins, in particular those active on Na^+ channels, is reported, confirming their responsibility in venom toxicity for mammals. The presence of several transcripts coding for antareases provide molecular support for the observed pancreatitis resulting from this species' envenomation. Toxins from families never before identified in *Centruroides* venoms are also reported.

2. Results and Discussion

2.1. RNA Isolation, Sequencing, and Assembly

Two groups of scorpions separated by gender (5 males and 5 females) were used for total RNA isolation. A total of 9 µg (males) and 8 µg (females) of RNA was obtained and its quality was assessed with a Bioanalyzer 2100 (Agilent), as reported in other transcriptomic analyses [7,10,12,24,25]. The results indicated that the RNA samples were not degraded, even though a single RNA band corresponding to the mitochondrial 18S was observed, an effect previously reported for other organisms [7,10,12,24,25]. Paired-end cDNA libraries were prepared for males and females separately and sequenced using the Illumina platform (2 × 72 bp reads). The two genders were sequenced independently to fulfill the requirements of a related project that focuses on the differential expression of venom components in both genders [26], and which the results of will be published elsewhere. Two datasets with 38,364,311 and 41,366,601 reads were obtained for males and females, respectively, which were submitted to the European Nucleotide Archive (ENA), under project PRJEB31683. In order to have a global, species–specific transcriptomic analysis, comparable with other published scorpion transcriptomes, both datasets were merged and jointly analyzed henceforth. After de novo RNA-seq assembly with the Trinity software, 198,662 putative transcripts were obtained, with an N50 of 1611. The annotation was performed with the Trinotate software, resulting in 11,058 annotated transcripts that were identified by sequence similarity with sequences deposited in the Uniprot database. The divergence between the large number of assembled transcripts and the smaller subset of sequences with annotation, reflects the lack of information on many scorpion venom components, and reinforces the need for further biochemical and functional characterization of the scorpion venoms. Among the annotated transcripts, 366 sequences had similarity with arachnid sequences, 227 were specific for scorpions, and 192 sequences were from components related to venom, in particular. The 192 venom-related sequences were analyzed by BLAST to identify the closest related matches by sequence. The transcripts described in this study were labeled following the previously suggested standard for transcript nomenclature [10]. The species code for *C. limpidus* was set to "Cli", the existing family and subtype codes were observed, and new ones were added for components not previously found in scorpion venoms. A complete listing of the 192 sequence IDs, organized by type/subtype, the ID of the closest matches (with E values), and their translated Open Reading Frame (ORF) is provided in Supplementary Materials Table S1. For the reference sequences, the original names found in the databases were honored.

2.2. *The Diversity of Transcripts Related to Venom Components in the Venom Gland of* C. limpidus

The identification of transcripts putatively coding for venom peptides/proteins in *C. limpidus* was initially based on Pfam domains [27]. The search for matching domains was not limited to scorpions, but broadened to include all venomous animals [28]. Four major categories were identified by this method: toxins, host defense peptides, enzymes, and protease inhibitors. A fifth heterogeneous category denominated as "other components" was designated to include annotated sequences without defined domain and function, as well as sequences with well-conserved domains, but without a defined function in venoms. Figure 2 shows the distribution of the annotated venom-related sequences grouped into these five categories, as percentages of the total 192. For this figure, the number of individual sequences was considered, rather than their relative abundance in the transcriptome (and therefore the term "Diversity" was used in the graph). Each major category was further divided into subcategories, determined by the more specific, putative structural or functional classification of the peptides/proteins. The transcripts were also globally classified in accordance to Gene Ontology (GO) terms [29] (Supplementary Materials Figure S1).

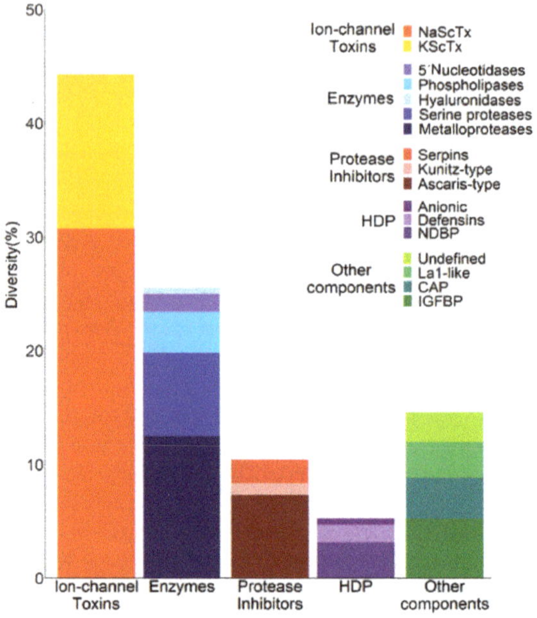

Figure 2. Relative diversity of transcripts related to venom components. For the graphic, only the number of different transcripts identified for each category.

2.2.1. Ion Channel-Acting Toxins

Hundreds of toxic components have been described to be present in scorpion venoms [1]. Many of these are peptides known to affect ion channels from mammals, birds or arthropods (e.g., arachnids, insects or crustaceans), including sodium, potassium, calcium and chloride ion channels [30].

As shown in Figure 2, this category was the most diverse in terms of sequence in the transcriptome of *C. limpidus*, which did not come as a surprise, given the known high toxicity of this species to animals from different taxa. Eighty-five distinct sequences with conserved motifs or domains for ion channel-acting toxins were found, including 59 transcripts potentially coding for sodium channel-acting toxins (NaScTx) and 26 for putative potassium channel-acting toxins (KScTx). This is by far the largest number of toxin sequences reported for a scorpion of any species to date. Supplementary Materials Table S2 contains all the transcripts putatively coding for ion channel-acting toxins, together with the reference protein/transcript (the best match by sequence similarity), the source of the reference, plus its function if known.

Toxins Active on Voltage-Gated Sodium Channels (NaScTx)

Due to their central role in the intoxication process following envenomation, the scorpion toxins that affect voltage-gated sodium channels are the best characterized venom components, both biochemically and functionally. They are broadly subdivided into α-NaScTx and β-NaScTx, the former being known for slowing down the Na^+ channel inactivation and binding to receptor site-3, while the latter shifts the channels' opening kinetics to more negative potentials and bind to receptor site-4 [31]. Scorpion β-NaScTx are further classified as classical (active on mammalian Na^+ channels), excitatory anti-insect, depressant anti-insect, and β-like (compete for binding sites on both insect and mammalian Na^+ channels) toxins [32].

The genome sequences from a scorpion of the same genus, *Centruroides sculpturatus*, have been recently released as BioProject PRJNA422877 on NCBI. As expected, many of the transcripts recovered in this study had sequence similarity with sequences from *C. sculpturatus*. Sequences matching those of other scorpions were also found, not only of the *Centruroides* genus, but also from old-world scorpions of the genera *Isometrus*, *Lychas* and *Parabuthus*. In the particular case of the putative NaScTx, 45 transcripts were found to be similar to sequences from *C. sculpturatus*, seven to previously reported sequences from *C. limpidus*, three to those from *C. noxius*, and one to a similar sequence from each of the following species, *C. exilicauda*, *Centruroides vittatus*, *Parabuthus transvaalicus*, and *Lychas mucronatus* (Supplementary Materials Table S2).

The NaScTx are usually more abundant in scorpions of the family Buthidae, which produce highly neurotoxic venoms. Three previous high-throughput sequencing-derived transcriptomic analyses with scorpions belonging to this family (*Tityus bahiensis*, *Centruroides hentzi*, and *C. noxius* [6,8,33]), reported 27 to 38 transcripts potentially coding for NaScTx. This study found 59 transcripts of this kind, which represents the largest diversity so far described for scorpions of this, or any other taxonomic family. Of them, 16 transcripts putatively code for α-NaScTx and 43 for β-NaScTx (Supplementary Materials Table S2).

Figure 3A shows, as an example, a multiple-sequence alignment of CliNaTAlp03 and CliNaTAlp08, both annotated as possible α-NaScTx, with their best matches in terms of sequence similarity. Only the sequence region corresponding to the predicted mature toxin was used for the alignment, since the signal and propeptide regions were missing in the sequences of the peptides obtained directly from the venom. The peptides encoded by CliNaTAlp03 and CliNaTAlp08 were confirmed to be present in the venom by the proteomic analysis, and were the α-NaScTx with the highest identification scores by that analysis. CliNaTAlp03 matched with "precursor alpha-like toxin CsEv5" (XP_023210703) and the peptide itself (P58779) [34]. CliNaTAlp08 matched with "precursor alpha-toxin CsE5" (XP_023242920) and the peptide itself (P46066) [35]. Here, and in all further alignments, the newly reported *C. limpidus* sequences are shown on top of the alignment for clarity.

```
A                                      10        20        30        40        50        60
                               ....|....|....|....|....|....|....|....|....|....|....|....|....|..   %Identity
CliNaTAlp08                    KKDGYIVDSGNCKYECL-RDDYCKDMCLKRKADDGYCFLGKFSCYCYGLPDNSPI--KTSGKCK---      100
CliNaTAlp03                    -....P..NKG..IS.VISGKF.DTE.KM...SS...Y--SL....E...E.AKVSG.ATST.G---       47
P46066 C. sculpturatus          .....P...........-K....N.L..E....K...YW..V............T--......NPA-       82
XP_023242920 C. sculpturatus   .....P...........-K....N.L..E....K...YW..V............T--......NPAR       82
XP_023210703 C. sculpturatus   -....P...KG..LS.V-ANN..DNQ.KMK..SG.H.Y--AM....E...E.AKVSDSATNI.G---       46
P58779 C. sculpturatus         -....P...KG..LS.V-ANN..DNQ.KMK..SG.H.Y--AM....E...E.AKVSDSATNI.----       45

B                                      10        20        30        40        50        60
                               ....|....|....|....|....|....|....|....|....|....|....|....|....|.   %Identity
CliNaTBet31                    KEGYLVNHSTGCKYECYKLGDNDYCLRECKQQYGKGAGGYCYAFGCWCTHLYEQAVVWPLPKKTCN     100
CliNaTBet32                    ....I..L.......F...................................................N.R.K      91
CliNaTBet33                    .......K.....G.FW..K.EN.DK...AKNQG.SY....S.A...EG.PDSTPTY...N.S.S      55
P59899 C. limpidus             ..................................................................     100
P59898 C. limpidus             ...............F..................................N...............      97
Q7Z1K7 C. limpidus             .......K.....G.FW..K.EN.DK...AKNQG.SY....S.A...EG.PDSTPTY...N.S.S      55
Q7YT61 C. limpidus             .......K.....G.FW..K.EN.DM...AKNQG.SY....S.A...EG.PDSTPTY...N.S.S      55
```

Figure 3. Examples of Na^+ channel-specific toxins. (**A**) Putative α-NaScTx and (**B**) Putative β-NaScTx. The transcript-derived peptides are aligned to their reference sequences. The percentage of identity was calculated considering only the mature sequences. Accession numbers and species' names of the references were taken from UniProt or GenBank. Conserved cysteine residues are highlighted in blue. Dots indicate identical residues, and dashes indicate gaps.

Three transcripts, CliNaTxBet31, CliNaTxBet32, and CliNaTxBet33 are shown in Figure 3B, aligned to the best matching reference sequences (mature peptides only). CliNaTxBet31 codes for Cll2b (P59899), a peptide found in the *C. limpidus* venom [21], which was confirmed by the proteomic analysis in this study (see below). Cll2b is toxic to mice and active on sodium and calcium channels in cultured chick dorsal root ganglion cells [21]. CliNaTxBet32 potentially codes for a peptide similar to Cll2b, but with six amino acid changes. Cll2b is very close in sequence to Cll2 (P59898), one of the major toxins of the *C. limpidus* venom [18,23], having only two differences at the amino acid level. Cll2 is a highly neurotoxic peptide for mammals [19]. CliNaTxBet33 matches the precursor of Cll5b (Q7Z1K7) and was here confirmed to be present in the venom by the proteomic analysis. A very similar sequence, Cll5c (Q7YT61), which differs from Cll5b by just one residue, is also included in the alignment. The remaining 40 transcripts found in this study are described in Supplementary Materials Table S2. These include four sequences with similarity to other previously reported sequences from *C. limpidus*.

Toxins Active on Potassium Channels (KScTx)

Potassium channels are the most widely distributed type of ion channels, found in basically all living organisms, where they play fundamental roles in the physiology of the cells [36–38]. Scorpion venoms contain toxins that affect these channels (KScTx), as demonstrated with insect and mammalian channels [37]. The KScTx have been classified into seven families (α, β, γ, δ, ε, κ, and λ) depending on their amino acid sequences, length, and 3D-structure [39–41]. They have been shown to be active on voltage-gated potassium channels (such as Kv1, Kv3, Kv4, Kv7, Kv11) and calcium-activated potassium channels (KCa1.1 or BK) [37].

This study reports 26 transcripts with sequence similarity to members of five families of KScTx: 15 sequences potentially coding for α-KScTx, 2 for β-KScTx, 3 for γ-KScTx, 3 for δ-KScTx, and 2 for λ-KScTx (Supplementary Materials Table S1).

Figure 4A shows two examples of the peptide sequences derived from the transcriptomic analysis in this study, which potentially correspond to α-KScTx. CliKTxAlp15 codes for a peptide confirmed to be expressed in the venom of *C. limpidus* by the proteomic analysis here reported. It is similar to alpha-KTx4.5 from *Tityus costatus* (Q5G8B6), a toxin found to inhibit with low potency the Kv1.1, Kv1.2, Kv1.3, and Kv11.1 (ERG1) channels [42]. CliKTxAlp07 potentially codes for a peptide similar to Noxiustoxin-2 (Q9TXD1), having only one difference at the amino acid level. Noxiustoxin-2 has a paralyzing effect on crickets but is not toxic to mice or crustaceans [43]. Two other similar sequences were included in the alignment, A0A218QXG2, a nucleotide sequence reported from *Tityus serrulatus* (only the predicted, translated mature region was included), and Noxiustoxin (P08815), a toxin from *C. noxius* that blocks several Kv and KCa channels [44]. The remaining 14 transcripts found in this study are summarized in Supplementary Materials Table S2, including CliKTxAlp10, which is similar to a previously reported toxin from this scorpion, CllTx1 (P45629).

One very relevant finding of this work is the description, for the first time, of potential β-KScTx in a scorpion from the *Centruroides* genus. Toxins of this family have been found in the venoms of buthid and non-buthid scorpions from the genera *Androctonus*, *Euscorpiops*, *Heterometrus*, *Hoffmannihadrurus*, *Liocheles*, *Mesobuthus*, *Pandinus*, and *Tityus*, but never before in *Centruroides*. Toxins of the β-KScTx family are active on Kv1.1, Kv1.3 or Kv4.2 mammalian channels [45]. Two transcripts were found in the venom gland of *C. limpidus* coding for peptides that were confirmed to be expressed in the venom by the proteomic analysis. CliKTxBet01 displayed sequence similarity with a DNA sequence from *C. sculpturatus* (XP_023220228) and with toxin TdiKIK (Q0GY43) from *Tityus discrepans*. CliKTxBet02 was similar to another DNA sequence from *C. sculpturatus* (XP_023220230) and to the "Scorpine-like peptide Tco 41.46-2" from *T. costatus*. The putative β-KScTx here described are shown aligned to the reference sequences (only the predicted mature sequences) in Figure 4B.

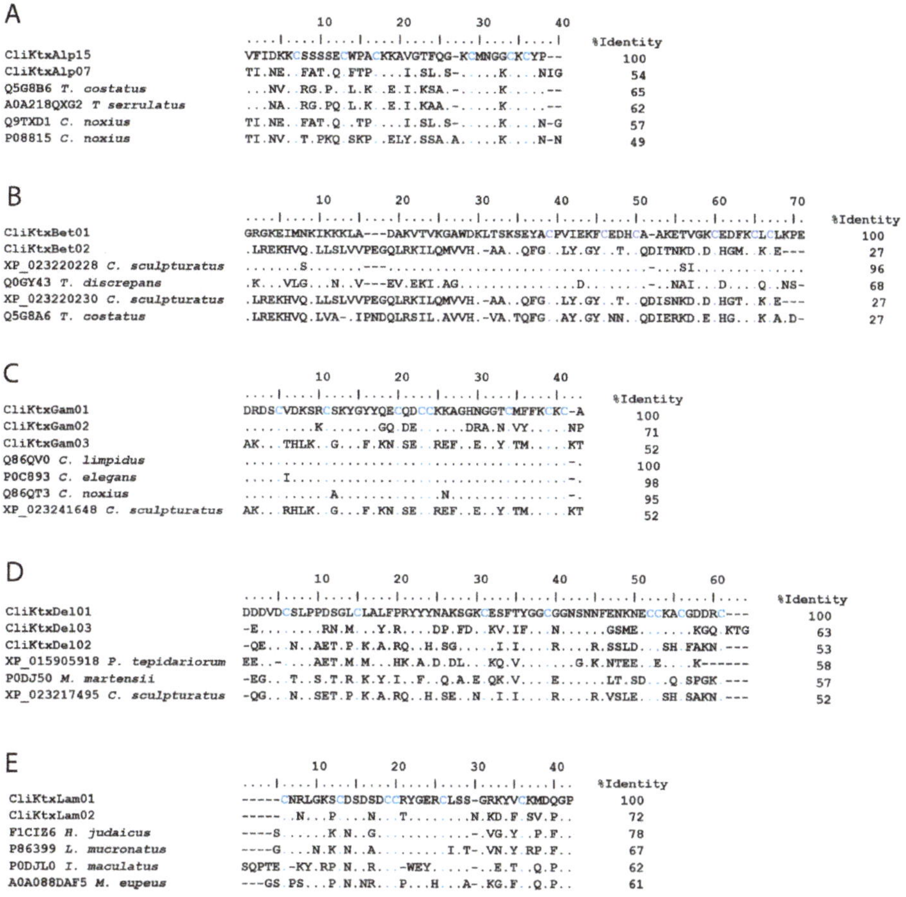

Figure 4. Examples of K^+ channel-specific toxins. (**A–E**) show the alignments of the transcript-derived sequences of members of the α, β, γ, δ, and λ-KScTx families, respectively, with the reference sequences. The percentage of identity was calculated considering only the mature sequences. Accession numbers and species' names of the references were taken from UniProt or GenBank. Conserved cysteine residues are highlighted in blue. Dots indicate identical residues, and dashes indicate gaps.

The γ-KScTx are short-chain peptides of 36–47 amino acid residues. Structurally, they have a cysteine-stabilized αβ (CSα/β) motif, with three or four disulfide bridges. The γ-KScTx are capable of blocking the ERG K^+ channels. Three new sequences, potentially coding for γ-KScTx are reported here (Figure 4). CliKTxGam01 codes for a peptide identical to CllErg1 (Q86QV0) isolated from the venom of *C. limpidus*, though never tested on ion channels. It is also closely related to CeErgTx5, from *Centruroides elegans*, differing in just one amino acid. CeErgTx5 is active on mammalian ERG K^+ channels [46]. CliKTxGam02 is similar to CnErg1 (Q86QT3) identified in the venom of *C. noxius*, a peptide with activity on mammalian ERG K^+ channels [47]. CliKTxGam03 is closest in sequence to "potassium channel toxin gamma-KTx 1.1-like" (XP_023241648), derived from the genome sequences of *C. sculpturatus* (only the predicted mature sequence was considered in the alignment in Figure 4C). The three putative sequences, here reported, contained the functionally relevant K13, involved in the interaction with the outer vestibule of the channel [48]. Two other residues, demonstrated to be relevant for the interaction of γ-KScTx with the channels, are Q18 and M35 [49]. Only CliKTxGam01 has those residues conserved (Figure 4C), which might have implications in the functionality of the peptides derived from CliKTxGam02 and CliKTxGam03 if they happen to be indeed expressed in the venom.

The δ-KScTx are peptides with 59–70 amino acid residues. They are structurally characterized by the presence of a CSα/β motif of the Kunitz type, stabilized by three disulfide bonds [50]. They display a dual activity: as serine protease inhibitors and as blockers of the Kv channels, mainly the Kv1.3, though other channels can also be weekly inhibited. Three different transcripts are here described, which are shown aligned to reference sequences in Figure 4D. CliKTxDel01 is similar to "Kunitz-type serine protease inhibitor BmKTT-2" (P0DJ50), a peptide from *M. martensii* which completely inhibits trypsin and blocks the murine Kv1.3. CliKTxDel02 shares sequence similarity with a genome sequence from *C. sculpturatus* labeled as "isoinhibitor K-like" (XP_023217495). CliKTxDel03 was found to be similar to a genome sequence from the spider *Paraestatoda tepidariorum* annotated as "hemolymph trypsin inhibitor B-like isoform X2" (XP_015905918). The genome-derived sequences used in the alignment in Figure 4 are limited to the predicted mature sequences.

It is very relevant that no transcripts coding for calcium channel-specific toxins of the calcin family (active on the ryanodine receptors of mammalian cardiac or skeletal muscle cells) were found in the analysis, while two transcripts are here reported for the phylogenetically related, insect-specific λ-KScTx family. The λ-KScTx are short (approximately 40 amino acids) peptides which adopt an inhibitor cystine knot (ICK) fold. Both CliKTxLam01 and CliKTxLam02 code for the first λ-KScTx ever described for the genus *Centruroides*. Their finding in a buthid scorpion confirms the proposition that calcins and λ-KScTx are specific for non-buthid families and the buthid family, respectively, being mutually exclusive in those venoms [51]. In order to confirm that CliKTxLam01 and CliKTxLam02 are indeed λ-KScTx and not the structurally related calcins, these two sequences were incorporated into a phylogenetic analysis with those in Reference [51] by Carlos Santibáñez-López (see Acknowledgements) and shown to group with other buthid λ-KScTx and not the non-buthid calcins (Supplementary Materials Figure S2). CliKTxLam01 has sequence similarity with "phi-buthitoxin-Hj1a" (F1CIZ6), derived from a transcript from *Hottentotta judaicus*. CliKTxLam02 matched by sequence similarity the "potassium channel blocker pMeKTx30-1" (A0A088DAF5), derived from a transcript from *Mesobuthus eupeus*. These sequences are shown aligned in Figure 4E. Only two tested K^+ channel blockers belonging to the λ-KScTx family have been reported thus far: ImKTx1 from *Isometrus maculatus* (P0DJL0) [52] and Neurotoxin lambda-MeuTx from *M. eupeus* (P86399) [53]. They are also included in the alignment for reference.

2.2.2. Host Defense Peptides (HDPs)

Arachnid venoms are rich sources of host defense peptides (HDPs) [54]. They are characterized by having a broad spectrum of biological activities, including antimicrobial [55–57], insecticidal [58], bradykinin-potentiating [59], antitumoral [60,61], and hemolytic [62], among others. Host defense peptides have been demonstrated to be abundant and highly diverse in the venoms of scorpions belonging to non-Buthidae families [7,24,25], though a previous study with high-throughput sequencing techniques also identified HDPs in the buthid *C. hentzi* [8]. Host defense peptides are divided into two categories: non-disulfide-bridged-peptides (NDBPs) and cysteine-stabilized β-sheet-rich peptides, which include the defensins and scorpines [54]. Though just one HDP (a defensin whose expression is induced in the hemolymph in response to septic injury) had been reported from *C. limpidus* [63], a mass fingerprint of the venom revealed components with lower molecular weights than KScTx, indicating the potential presence of HDPs [26]. This analysis confirms that conclusion. Ten transcripts coding for HDPs were found: six defensins, one NDBP-2, two NDBP-4, and one anionic peptide. Nevertheless, compared to the above referenced studies by massive RNA sequencing of non-buthid scorpions, the diversity here described for the HDPs was significantly lower, confirming the previous empiric observation that, contrary to the ion channel-acting toxins, HDP are more diverse in non-buthid scorpions than in buthids.

CliHDPDef01 is actually the transcript coding for Cll-dlp (Q6GU94), the previously reported hemolymph defensin. It is notable that the same defense peptide is expressed in both tissues. The remaining five defensin transcripts, CliHDPDef02–CliHDPDef06, have similarity to Defensin-1 (A0A0K0LBV1), a transcript from *Androctonus bicolor* [64]. Both CliHDPDef01 and CliHDPDef02 are shown in Figure 5A, aligned to the reference sequences. Since the complete precursors for all the sequences are available, they were used in the alignment and included in the calculated percentage of identity.

A

```
                                10        20        30        40        50        60
                       ....|....|....|....|....|....|....|....|....|....|....|....|..   %Identity
CliHDPDef01            MKAIVVLLILALILCLYAMTTVEG--ACQF--WSCNSSCISRGYRQGYCWGIQYKYCQCQ--    100
CliHDPDef02            ..IVA..FL..FVF.TLEIA...AGFG.P.NQGA.HKH.Q.IRK.G...D.FLKHR.R.Y--     39
Q6GU94 C.limpidus      ........................--....--............................--    100
A0A0K0LBV1 A. bicolor  ..T..L.FV...VF.TLE.GV..AGFG.P.NQGR.HRH.R.I.R.G...R..FKQT.A.YRK     46
```

B

```
                             10        20        30        40        50        60        70
                       ....|....|....|....|....|....|....|....|....|....|....|....|....|....|..   %Identity
CliHDPND201            MKGKTLLVVLLVALLIAEEVNGFKFGGFLKKMWKSKLAKKLRAKGREMIKDYANRVLEGPQEE-APPAERRR      100
A0A146CJE0 M. eupeus   .NK....IFI.TM..VD...S....S....V.............K.LL........N..E..A.A..K...       73
Q9Y0X4 M. martensii    .NK....IFF.TM..VD...S.R..S....V..........S..KQLL.....K..N..E..A.A......       69
```

C

```
                              10        20        30        40        50        60        70
                        ....|....|....|....|....|....|....|....|....|....|....|....|....|....|....|....   %Identity
CliHDPND401             MQFKKQLLVIFFAYFLVINESEAFLGSLFSLGSKLLPSVFKLFQRKKSRSINKRDLEDLYDPYQRNLEMERFLKQLPMY    100
CliHDPND402             ..I-.H.I.V..VVLI.ADHCH..F.LI----PS.VGGLISA.KGRRK.DLTA-Q.NQYRHLQK.EA.FRE..DN..I.     30
A0A1D3IXJ5 T. obscurus  ................V......F.T..K.....I.G.M...SK..E..LM..E.KN.......SV....L..E..L.     75
S6D3A7 T. serrulatus    ..I-.H.IT...LVLI.ADHCH...MI----PG.IGGLISA.KGRRK.E.TS-QI.QYRNLQK.EA.L.NL.AN..V.     33
```

D

```
                                  10        20        30        40        50        60        70
                            ....|....|....|....|....|....|....|....|....|....|....|....|....|....|....|   %Identity
CliHDPAni01                 MVRKSLIVLLLVSVLVSTFLTTDAYPASFDDDFDALDDMNDLDLDSLLDLEPADLVLLDMWANMLENSDFEDDFE    100
XP_023227050 C. sculpturatus ............................................D..............................     99
JK483720 T. stigmurus       ..S..............F..E..............LD.....D..................MDSQ...-...     87
```

Figure 5. Examples of host defense peptides (HDPs). The translated sequences from representative transcripts coding for HDPs found in the *C. limpidus* transcriptome are shown aligned to matching sequences from databases. The complete precursor sequences are shown and the complete precursor was considered in the calculation of the percentage of identity. (**A**) Defensins. (**B**) The unique NDBP-2 precursor found. (**C**) Two putative NDBP-4 precursors. (**D**) The unique precursor for the putative anionic peptide. Accession numbers and species' names of the references were taken from UniProt or GenBank. Conserved cysteine residues are highlighted in blue. The predicted mature sequences are indicated in bold typeface, the predicted signal peptides are underlined and the propeptides are indicated in italics. Dots indicate identical residues and dashes indicate gaps.

Transcripts with sequence similarity to members of families NDBP-2 and NDBP-4 were also found. CliHDPND201 had similarity to "venom toxin meuTx20" (A0A146CJE0) deduced from a transcript from *M. eupeus*, and with BmKbpp (Q9Y0X4), a peptide from *M. martensii* with antimicrobial and bradykinin-potentiating activities against bacteria and fungi [65]. The precursor sequence of these three molecules are shown aligned in Figure 5B. CliHDPND401 has similarity to ToAP2 (A0A1D3IXJ5), a transcript isolated from the venom of *Tityus obscurus*. Synthetic ToAP2 displayed antimicrobial activity, both in vitro and in vivo [66]. CliHDPND402 is similar to peptide TsAP2 (S6D3A7), an antibacterial, antifungal, anticancer, and hemolytic peptide isolated from *T. serrulatus* [61]. The precursor sequences of these NDBP-4 are shown aligned in Figure 5C.

A transcript for a putative anionic HDP without disulfide bridges is also reported. CliHDPAni01 shows similarities to the genome-derived sequence XP_023227050 from *C. sculpturatus*, and with TanP (GeneBank ID of the transcript: JK483720), a peptide isolated from the venom of *Tityus stigmurus* [67]. The predicted precursors translated from these sequences, are shown aligned in Figure 5D.

2.2.3. Enzymes

Enzymes are essential components of many animal venoms. Thought more abundant in snakes [68,69], enzymes have been discovered in venoms from many taxa, including ants [70], jellyfish [71], wasps [72], spiders [73], and scorpions [74]. Scorpions, in particular, were shown to contain proteases [75], phospholipases [76], and hyaluronidases [77] in their venoms by classical studies. More recently, high-throughput transcriptomic analyses with venom glands have reported the existence of transcripts putatively coding for other enzymes never before reported in scorpion venoms, e.g., 5′nucleotidases in non-buthid scorpions [10,12,24].

The venom gland of *C. limpidus* was found in this study to be rich in terms of transcripts putatively coding for enzymes. Forty-nine different sequences potentially coding for enzymes are here reported. Thirty-eight corresponded to proteases, seven to phospholipases, three to 5′nucleotidases, and one to a putative hyaluronidase. All of them were annotated by sequence similarity to genome-derived sequences from *C. sculpturatus*. They are all reported in detail in Supplementary Materials Tables S1 and S2, together with the reference genomic sequences.

The large number of protease-encoding sequences in this scorpion is remarkable. It is particularly rich in transcripts for metalloproteases, with 24 out of the 38 transcripts potentially coding for proteases, being for metalloproteases (the remaining 14 are for serine proteases). It is also noticeable that the most diverse metalloprotease transcripts are those coding for antarease-type Zn-metalloproteases, 14 out of 24. Antarease was first described in the venom of *T. serrulatus* [78]. The envenomation by *Tityus* species can lead to the development of acute pancreatitis [79–83]. Venoms from *Tityus* scorpions are potent secretagogues that can elicit the release of secretory proteins from the pancreas [80,84–86]. Antarease was shown to specifically cleave the soluble N-ethylmaleimide-sensitive factor attachment protein receptors (SNAREs) involved in pancreatic secretion, disrupting the normal vesicular traffic [78]. Antarease could, therefore, be responsible for the acute pancreatitis induced by the *T. serrulatus* venom. Antarease-like enzymes were shown thereafter to be ubiquitous in the venoms of different scorpion genera [74]. The venom from *C. limpidus* was also shown to elicit manifestations associated with pancreatitis and to act as a secretagogue for amylase in the mouse pancreas [87]. The abundance of transcripts coding for antareases in *C. limpidus* could be an indicative of the prominent role of these enzymes in the manifestation of pancreatitis after scorpion envenomation by this species. The presence of antareases in the venom was here confirmed by the proteomic analysis. The proteins encoded by CliEnzMtp15, CliEnzMtp19, CliEnzMtp20, and CliEnzMtp21 were found by LC-MS/MS.

The other found transcripts, potentially coding for disintegrins, reprolysins, an astacin, and an angiotensin-converting enzyme complete the picture of the metalloproteases putatively expressed in this venom (Supplementary Materials Table S2). The astacin (CliEnzMtp23) and the angiotensin-converting enzyme (CliEnzMtp24) were also confirmed to be present in the venom by LC-MS/MS.

It is intriguing that, even though transcripts potentially coding for phospholipases A2 and D2 were found in the transcriptomic analysis (Supplementary Materials Table S2), none were confirmed by the proteomic analysis. The inability to detect them in the proteome seems to correlate with the absence of phospholipase activity in the *C. limpidus* crude venom [26] as assayed by the egg-yolk method of Haberman and Hard, which detects phospholipases A, B, and C [88]. Nevertheless, it should be kept in mind that this transcriptomic analysis is descriptive and not quantitative. Therefore, no inferences can be derived from the transcript detection about the transcript and protein levels in the gland and the venom, respectively.

An interesting family of enzymes, just recently identified in scorpion venoms are the 5′nucleotidases. They were initially found in snake venoms where they seem to be ubiquitous [89]. They are known to endogenously liberate purines, which potentiate venom-induced hypotension and paralysis via purine receptors [89]. In addition, they can synergistically interact with other venom proteins, contributing to the overall effects of venoms [89]. The presence of 5′nucleotidases in non-buthid scorpion venoms was demonstrated for *Paravaejovis schwenkmeyeri*, *Thorellius atrox*, and *Megacormus gertschi* [10,12,24]. This study confirms that this enzyme could also be present in a buthid scorpion venom—at least its mRNA is transcribed in the gland—suggesting that these enzymes could also be ubiquitous in scorpion venoms. Three transcripts for *C. limpidus* 5′nucleotidases are reported in Supplementary Materials Table S2.

It was previously shown that the *C. limpidus* crude venom contains active hyaluronidases [26]. A single transcript encoding for a hyaluronidase, CliEnzHya01 (Supplementary Materials Table S2), was found in the present study. Noticeably, its presence in the venom was confirmed by the proteomic analysis. By degrading hyaluronic acid from the extracellular matrix [90], this enzyme could facilitate venom spreading [91].

2.2.4. Other Venom Components

Besides the ones described above, other components frequently found in scorpion venoms were also detected in this analysis (Supplementary Materials Table S1).

Protease inhibitors, which, in principle, protect the venom components from autogenous degradation by venom proteases [69], though might also inhibit enzymes in the targets' tissues with neurological consequences [92], were very diverse in terms of transcripts in *C. limpidus*. Nineteen precursors encoding potential protease inhibitors were found, 13 of the Ascaris-type [93], two of the Kunitz-type [94], and four serpins [95].

Ascaris-type protease inhibitors are serine protease inhibitors, which have a Trypsin-Inhibitor-Like (TIL) domain. They are long-chain peptides with approximately 60 amino acid residues, stabilized by five disulfide bonds [96]. Recombinant SjAPI was the first functionally characterized Ascaris-type protease inhibitor from animal venoms [93]. It inhibits chymotrypsin and elastase while being inactive on trypsin. Three transcripts described here (CliPInTIL01–CliPInTIL03) have sequence similarity with classical Ascaris-type protease inhibitors from scorpion venoms or transcriptomes. Ten others, (CliPInTIL04–CliPInTIL13), with conserved TIL domain, but which are larger (ca 14 kDa instead of the classical ca 6 kDa) and have more disulfide bridges than the classical inhibitors (up to five extra disulfides), are also reported. A fourteenth sequence with a TIL domain (annotated here as CliPInTIL14) was detected in the proteomic analysis but had no matching transcript. It was annotated within this group due to the presence of the TIL domain, but it is a much larger protein (ca 210 kDa).

Kunitz-type protease inhibitors have been described in scorpion venoms [94]. The transcripts here reported (CliPInKun01 and CliPInKun02) were similar to genome sequences from *C. sculpturatus*. Members of the superfamily of serine proteinase inhibitors (serpins) from venomous animals have been poorly studied [95,97]. Four transcripts encoding serpins, CliPInSrp01–CliPInSrp04 are here reported, which also have sequence similarities with genome sequences from *C. sculpturatus*.

The CAP superfamily proteins are well distributed in all organisms, where they display a variety of functions [98]. This superfamily includes three major groups of proteins: cysteine-rich secretory proteins (CRISP), antigen or allergen proteins from arthropod venoms, and pathogenesis-related proteins from plants (PR) [99]. The CRISP proteins and antigen/allergen proteins have been described in venoms [100]. There are reports showing that CRISP proteins can interact with ion channels [101,102]. Six precursors coding for CAP-like proteins are here reported, CliOthCAP01–CliOthCAP06 (Supplementary Materials Table S1). They all code for putative proteins with a Pfam domain corresponding to the CAP superfamily and the transcripts are similar to genome sequences from *C. sculpturatus*. Both CliOthCAP02 and CliOthCAP05 were confirmed to be expressed in the venom by the proteomic analysis.

Transcripts for Insuline Growth Factor Binding Proteins (IGFBPs) have been found in scorpion venom glands [7,8,12,33,64,103,104], though the function of IGFBPs in venoms has not been established. Ten putative IGFBP transcripts are reported for *C. limpidus* (Supplementary Materials Table S1). All of them matched genomic sequences from *C. sculpturatus*, except for CliOthIGF10, which was similar to a peptide annotated as "Venom toxin" (A0A1L4BJ69) from *Hemiscorpius lepturus*.

The first described La1 peptide was found in the venom of *Liocheles australiase* [105]. Peptides with similar amino acid sequences were thereafter annotated as "La1-like" peptides. They are usually long-chain peptides containing 73–100 amino acids, stabilized by four disulfide linkages, with a conserved single domain von Willebrand factor-type C (SVWC) structural motive. Transcripts for La1-like peptides have been identified in buthid [8] and non-buthid scorpions [7,10,12,24,104]. Six transcripts are here reported with those features, assumed to code for La1-like peptides

(Supplementary Materials Table S1). Of them, only CliOthLa106 was confirmed to be expressed as protein in the venom. Noticeably, CliOthLa106 is the only transcript among the six, which codes for a long-chain-type La1-like [24] (Supplementary Materials Table S1).

Other orphan transcripts with ORF coding for putative peptides with no conserved structural domains, nor a known function, were also found. Since similar sequences had been described in other scorpion transcriptomic analyses or were directly identified in the *C. limpidus* venom, they were grouped as "undefined peptides" and annotated as CliOthUnd01–CliOthUnd05. Not much information can be provided on them, except for the reference sequences they are similar with (Supplementary Materials Table S1).

2.3. *Proteomic Exploration of the Venom Components of* C. limpidus

2.3.1. Mass Fingerprint of the Soluble Venom

The soluble fraction of the whole venom from sixty scorpions of mixed gender was used for the proteomic analysis. An aliquot of the soluble venom was applied to an HPLC coupled to a mass spectrometer, as previously reported [26]. The mass fingerprint detected 395 individual masses, ranging from 800 to 19,000 Da (Supplementary Materials Table S3 and Figure 6). The mass range with the largest number of individual masses detected was the one which spans 7001 to 8000 Da, which is within the expected range for the Na^+ channel-acting scorpion toxins. This mass group was followed, in the number of independent masses, by the 4001 to 5000 Da range, which are the characteristic masses of K^+ channel-acting scorpion toxins. This mass distribution corroborates the findings by the transcriptomic analysis pointing to the ion channel-acting toxins as the most diverse components in the venom of the highly toxic *C. limpidus*. It is relevant to note that, although transcripts potentially coding for enzymes were highly diverse in accordance to the transcriptomic analysis, the used setup for the mass fingerprint cannot precisely detect the mass of high molecular weight components (approximately above 10,000 Da) [24], so all those components are shown grouped in Figure 6.

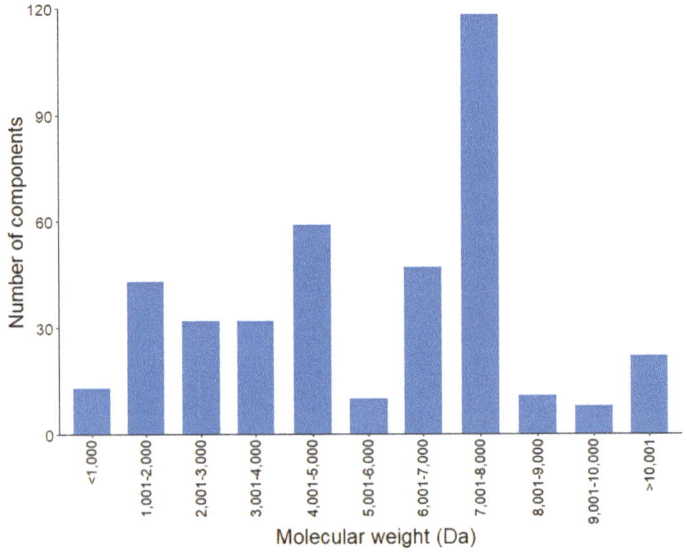

Figure 6. Distribution of the *C. limpidus* venom components detected by mass fingerprint with respect to their molecular masses.

2.3.2. Identification of Peptides by LC-MS/MS

The peptides identified by LC-MS/MS, which also matched the sequences discovered by the transcriptomic analysis, were mentioned above in the description of the corresponding transcripts. This section summarizes those findings (Supplementary Materials Table S4).

From a total of 52 identified sequences, 46 corresponded to molecular entities annotated as venom-related peptides/proteins. The remaining sequences corresponded to enzymes or proteins related to cellular processes, or without an identifiable conserved domain or structural motif. In correlation with the results of the transcriptomic and mass fingerprint analyses, the largest class of MS/MS-recovered sequences corresponded to toxins that affect ion channels, of which 26 were Na^+ channel-acting toxins (7 α-type and 19 β-type, by sequence similarity) and three K^+ channel-acting toxins. Tryptic peptides from eight enzymes were also recovered. Other venom components were also detected, but to a lesser extent. This includes two HDPs, one Ascaris-type protease inhibitor (though this is a protein much larger than the typical sequences of this kind, as discussed in the transcriptomic section), two proteins of the CAP superfamily, and one La1-like peptide of the long-chain type.

2.4. The Venom of the Highly Toxic C. limpidus *versus the Venoms of Non-buthid Scorpions*

Two other transcriptomic/proteomic analyses from scorpions of the genus *Centruroides* have already been published [6,8]. It would be interesting to compare these venoms in terms of their composition to try to define a possible pattern that would differentiate toxic from non-toxic species within this genus (*C. limpidus* and *C. noxius* are highly toxic to mammals while *C. hentzi* is not). However, even minor differences in sample preparation, cDNA library construction, cDNA sequencing protocol, MS/MS protocol or the bioinformatics analysis could lead to inaccurate conclusions. Nevertheless, the results here reported are comparable with those generated for other non-buthid scorpions under the exact same experimental protocol. That is the case for the analyses performed with *Serradigitus gertschi*, *Superstitionia donensis*, *T. atrox*, *P. schwenkmeyeri*, and *M. gertschi* [7,10,12,24,25]. As Figure 7A illustrates, the venom of *C. limpidus* is characterized by the highest diversity of toxins, in general. This is remarkable, considering also that no Ca^{2+} channel-acting toxins were recovered for the buthid species, so only two super-families, the NaScTx and the KScTx, are present in the venom. The fraction of recovered transcripts related to Na^+ channel-acting toxins equals or surpasses the fraction of all toxins in the non-buthids, taken together. It is also relevant that the fraction of NaScTx in *C. limpidus* is larger than the fraction of KScTx, while for the non-buthids it is the other way around. It is well established that the toxicity of the scorpion venoms is primordially related to the neurotoxic action of the NaScTx [16,18]. It is well known that the neutralization of the main NaScTx in scorpion venoms results in the neutralization of the whole venom toxicity [106,107]. It is remarkable that, in the highly toxic *C. noxius*, the NaScTx are also more abundant and diverse than the KScTx [6,108], while in the non-lethal *C. hentzi*, the transcripts for NaScTx and KScTx are more or less equally diverse [8] (although, in absolute numbers, not comparable with the abundances here reported, as indicated above).

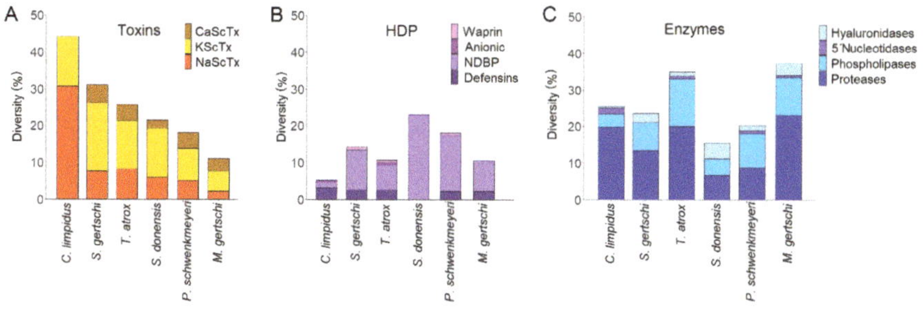

Figure 7. Comparative diversity of the transcripts coding for toxins (**A**), HDPs (**B**), and enzymes (**C**) found in *C. limpidus* versus those from non-buthid species reported in other transcriptomic analyses.

Figure 7B confirms that, on the contrary, the venoms from the non-toxic, non-buthid scorpions seem to be more diverse in terms of HDPs, with respect to the buthids, as proposed above in Section 2.2.2. Additionally, no direct link seems to exist between enzyme diversity and venom toxicity, according to the results charted in Figure 7C.

3. Conclusions

A total of 192 transcripts were identified in the present transcriptomic analysis. These sequences are assumed to code for Na^+ and K^+ channel-acting toxins, enzymes, HDPs, protease inhibitors, CAP-super-sfamily proteins, IGFBP, La-1-like peptides, and other orphan venom components. Mass fingerprint of the venom resulted in the detection of 395 individual components, the most abundant of which were peptides with molecular weights in the range of 7000 to 8000 Da, which are known to correspond to Na^+ channel-acting toxins. The LC-MS/MS of the tryptically-digested venom confirmed that at least 46 of the venom-related, transcript-encoded proteins are indeed expressed in the venom.

The molecular dissection of the venom components from the highly toxic buthid scorpion *C. limpidus* revealed that the most abundant (from the mass fingerprint) and most diverse (from the transcriptomic and MS/MS analyses) venom components are the neurotoxic NaScTx. The fraction of toxins (most notably, the NaScTx) is significantly higher in *C. limpidus* than in other non-toxic, non-buthid scorpions from different genera. These findings correlate with classical biochemical and physiological observations on the relevance of the neurotoxic NaScTx in the toxicity of the scorpion venoms for mammals. It also reveals that the efforts directed at generating neutralizing antivenoms from toxin-specific human antibodies or their fragments might require a larger number of antibodies in the cocktail, depending on their effective cross-reactivity.

Molecular support for the observed pancreatitis after envenomation by this species is also provided. The relative abundance and diversity of the antarease-like Zn-metalloproteases seem to confirm their relevant role in this pathology.

Two families of toxins are described here for the first time in a scorpion of the genus *Centruroides*. Transcripts coding for β-KScTx were found, and the presence of the expressed toxins in the venom was confirmed by the proteomic analysis. Transcripts putatively coding for members of the λ-KScTx family are here also reported, though their presence in the venom remains to be demonstrated.

4. Materials and Methods

4.1. Biological Material

Adult scorpions of the species *C. limpidus* were collected in Morelos and Guerrero States, with official permit from the Secretaría de Medio Ambiente, Recursos Naturales y Pesca (SEMARNAT, numbers SGPA/DGVS/07805/16 and 004474/18). The collected specimens were maintained in plastic boxes with water ad libitum. Sixty adult scorpions were milked by electrical stimulation for the proteomic analyses. The venom was immediately suspended in deionized water and centrifuged at 15,000 *g* for 15 min. The protein content of the soluble venom was estimated with a Nanodrop 1000 (Thermo Fisher Scientific, Waltham, MA, USA) based on absorbance at $\lambda = 280$ nm, assuming that one absorbance unit equaled 1 mg/mL of protein. The soluble fraction of the whole venom was lyophilized and kept at −20 °C until used.

Seven days after milking, 5 male and 5 female scorpions were processed for telson dissection to extract the total RNA. These specimens were thereafter euthanized and preserved in ethanol as vouchers. The remaining scorpions were kept alive and released thereafter in the same locations where they were collected.

4.2. RNA Isolation, Sequencing, and Assembly

Total RNA was isolated as previously described [7,10,12]. The SV Total RNA Isolation System Kit (Promega, Madison, WI, USA) was used for this purpose. The telsons from 5 males and 5 females were dissected separately, under RNAse-free conditions, in microcentrifuge tubes containing the RNA lysis buffer. The optional 70 °C heating step of the protocol was followed before column purification. Total RNA was quantitated with a NanoDrop 1000 (Thermo Fisher Scientific, Waltham, MA, USA) and its quality was assessed with a 2100 Bioanalyzer (Agilent Technologies, Santa Clara, CA, USA).

Two cDNA libraries were prepared from 1 µg of total RNA for each gender, using the TruSeq Stranded mRNA Sample Preparation Kit (Illumina, San Diego, CA, USA), according to the manufacturer's directions. DNA sequencing was performed at the Massive DNA Sequencing Facility of the Instituto de Biotecnología (Cuernavaca, Mexico) with a Genome Analyzer IIx (Illumina, San Diego, CA, USA) using a 72-bp paired-end sequencing scheme over cDNA fragments ranging 200–400 bp in size. The quality of the reads was verified with the FastQC program [109] after clipping off the adaptors.

The reads resulting from the sequencing of both male and female cDNA libraries were joined together for a de novo assembly into contigs using the Trinity software version 2.0.3 [110], employing the standard protocol. Basic statistics, such as the number of transcripts and contigs, were determined with the TrinityStats.pl script.

4.3. Bioinformatics

The assembled contigs were annotated as previously described [24], using the Uniprot/Uniref90 protein database for BLASTx and BLASTp. The prediction of ORFs were done with TransDecoderLongORfs. Putative signal peptides and propeptides were predicted with the ProP 1.0 server [111] and SpiderP from Arachnoserver [112]. Multiple sequence alignments were performed using MAFFT 7.0 online [113]. Alignments were edited in Bioedit [114] and in Adobe Illustrator CS6. All figures were generated with Rstudio [115]. The GO terms were quantified in WEGO [116].

4.4. Molecular Mass Fingerprint by LC-MS of the Venom

Eight micrograms of soluble venom was applied in an LC-MS system composed of an HPLC UltiMate 3000; Dionex, RSLCnano System (Thermo Fisher Scientific, San Jose, CA, USA) coupled to an LTQ-Orbitrap Velos mass spectrometer (Thermo Fisher Scientific, San Jose, CA, USA). Venom was fractionated through a 10-cm reversed-phase C18 in-house-made column (filled with Jupiter® 4 µm Proteo 90 Å resin, Phenomenex, Torrance, CA, USA), using a linear gradient of 5% to 90% of solvent B (0.1% formic acid in acetonitrile) in 240 min, with a flow rate of 300 nL/min. The resolved peptides were ionized by a nano-electrospray ion source. A full scan MS was used (400–2000 m/z) with a resolution of 60,000. The monoisotopic molecular mass is reported for components below 3000 Da, and the average molecular masses for those above 3000 Da.

4.5. Identification of Venom Components by LC-MS/MS

Three hundred micrograms of the venom soluble fraction were reduced with dithiothreitol (DTT) 10 mM (Sigma–Aldrich, Saint Louis, MO USA) and alkylated with iodoacetamide (IAA) 55 mM (Sigma–Aldrich, Saint Louis, MO USA). After that, the samples were digested with trypsin (Promega Sequencing Grade Modified Trypsin; Madison, WI, USA) using a 1:50 enzyme:protein ratio by weight, in 50 mM ammonium bicarbonate buffer (ABC). The samples were acidified with 10 µL of 10% formic acid (FA). The tryptic peptides were desalted with Sep-Pak tC18 cartridges (Waters, Milford, MA, USA) following the manufacturer's protocol, and dried in a SpeedVac (Savant SPD1010, Thermo Scientific, San Jose, CA, USA).

Samples containing 4 µg of tryptically digested venom in 10 µL of solution A (0.1% formic acid) were analyzed. The proteins were separated through a 15-cm in-house-made column (filled with the same C18, Jupiter 4 µm Proteo 90 Å resin) using a linear gradient of 5% to 75% of solvent B (0.1% formic acid in acetronitrile) in 270 min. Mass spectra were registered in a full scan of 350 m/z to 1400 m/z with a resolution of 60,000. The MS/MS spectra were analyzed with the Proteome Discoverer 1.4.1.14 suite (Thermo Fisher Scientific, San Jose, CA, USA), employing the Sequest HT search engine with the following parameters: two missed cleavages, dynamic modifications (methionine oxidation, glutamine and asparagine deamidation), static modifications (cysteine carbamidomethylation), precursor mass tolerance of 20 ppm, fragment mass tolerance 0.6 Da, and 1% false discovery rate. The database of the translated transcripts from Transdecoder was used for protein identification. An identification was considered positive when a minimum of two matching peptides were identified, and Sequest HT gave a global score (sum of all peptides' XCorr) of at least 20.

Supplementary Materials: The following are available online at http://www.mdpi.com/2072-6651/11/5/247/s1, Supplementary Figure S1: Distribution of the annotated transcripts in accordance to Gene Ontology (GO) terms, Supplementary Figure S2: Phylogenetic tree of scorpion toxins with the ICK fold. Supplementary Table S1: Translated sequences of the 192 venom-related transcripts obtained from the transcriptomic analysis of the *C. limpidus* venom gland, Supplementary Table S2: The 192 venom-related transcripts obtained from the *C. limpidus* venom gland and their reference proteins, Supplementary Table S3: Mass fingerprint results. The 395 masses identified in the *C. limpidus* venom by LC-MS, sorted by C18-RT-HPLC Retention Times (RT). Supplementary Table S4: LC-MS/MS results. The 52 transcripts that were identified in venom by LC-MS/MS. The parameters generated by the Proteome Discoverer software are shown for each identified fragment.

Author Contributions: Conceptualization, J.I.C.-U., E.O. and L.D.P.; methodology, J.I.C.-U., E.P.M. and E.O.; software, J.I.C.-U.; validation, J.I.C.-U., E.P.M., C.V.F.B., E.O. and L.D.P.; formal analysis, J.I.C.-U. and E.P.M.; investigation, J.I.C.-U.; resources, J.I.C.-U. and L.D.P.; data curation, J.I.C.-U. and E.P.M.; writing—original draft preparation, J.I.C.-U. and E.P.M.; writing—review and editing, C.V.F.B., E.O. and L.D.P.; visualization, J.I.C.-U.; supervision, E.O. and L.D.P.; project administration, L.D.P.; funding acquisition, L.D.P.

Funding: This research was funded by grants IN203416 and IN202619, from Dirección General de Personal Académico, UNAM and grant SEP-CONACyT 237864 from Consejo Nacional de Ciencia y Tecnología (CONACyT) awarded to Lourival D. Possani and Jimena I. Cid-Uribe was supported by scholarship No. 404460 from CONACyT.

Acknowledgments: Specimens were classified by Edmundo González-Santillán based on the available literature [14]. We are indebted to Carlos Santibáñez-López from the University of Wisconsin-Madison, for performing the phylogenetic analysis that allowed the classification of the λ-KScTx. We are grateful to Gloria T. Vázquez-Castro and Ricardo A. Grande-Cano from the Massive Sequencing Unit of the Instituto de Biotecnología-UNAM for their technical support. The computer analysis was performed using the cluster of the Instituto de Biotecnología-UNAM maintained by Jérôme Verleyen. The technical assistance of David S. Castañeda-Carreón, Roberto P. Rodríguez-Bahena, Jesús O. Arriaga-Pérez, Juan M. Hurtado-Ramírez, and Servando Aguirre-Cruz is also greatly acknowledged.

Conflicts of Interest: The authors declare no conflict of interest.

References

1. Possani, L.D.; Becerril, B.; Delepierre, M.; Tytgat, J. Scorpion toxins specific for Na^+-channels. *Eur. J. Biochem.* **1999**, *264*, 287–300. [CrossRef]
2. The Scorpion Files. Available online: https://www.ntnu.no/ub/scorpion-files/ (accessed on 29 April 2019).
3. Chippaux, J.-P.; Goyffon, M. Epidemiology of scorpionism: A global appraisal. *Acta Trop.* **2008**, *107*, 71–79. [CrossRef] [PubMed]
4. Santibáñez-López, C.E.; Francke, O.F.; Ureta, C.; Possani, L.D.; Lai, R. Scorpions from Mexico: From species diversity to venom complexity. *Toxins* **2016**, *8*, 2. [CrossRef]
5. González-Santillán, E.; Possani, L.D. North American scorpion species of public health importance with a reappraisal of historical epidemiology. *Acta Trop.* **2018**, *187*, 264–274. [CrossRef]
6. Rendón-Anaya, M.; Delaye, L.; Possani, L.D.; Herrera-Estrella, A. Global transcriptome analysis of the scorpion *Centruroides noxius*: New toxin families and evolutionary insights from an ancestral scorpion species. *PLoS ONE* **2012**, *7*, e43331. [CrossRef]
7. Santibáñez-López, C.E.; Cid-Uribe, J.I.; Batista, C.V.F.; Ortiz, E.; Possani, L.D. Venom gland transcriptomic and proteomic analyses of the enigmatic scorpion *Superstitionia donensis* (Scorpiones: *Superstitioniidae*), with insights on the evolution of its venom components. *Toxins* **2016**, *8*, 367. [CrossRef]
8. Ward, M.J.; Ellsworth, S.A.; Rokyta, D.R. Venom-gland transcriptomics and venom proteomics of the Hentz striped scorpion (*Centruroides hentzi; Buthidae*) reveal high toxin diversity in a harmless member of a lethal family. *Toxicon* **2018**, *142*, 14–29. [CrossRef] [PubMed]
9. Quintero-Hernández, V.; Ramírez-Carreto, S.; Romero-Gutiérrez, M.T.; Valdez-Velázquez, L.L.; Becerril, B.; Possani, L.D.; Ortiz, E. Transcriptome analysis of scorpion species belonging to the *Vaejovis Genus*. *PLoS ONE* **2015**, *10*, e0117188. [CrossRef] [PubMed]

10. Romero-Gutierrez, T.; Peguero-Sanchez, E.; Cevallos, M.A.; Batista, C.V.F.; Ortiz, E.; Possani, L.D. A deeper examination of *Thorellius atrox* Scorpion venom components with omic techonologies. *Toxins* **2017**, *9*, 399. [CrossRef]
11. Zhong, J.; Zeng, X.-C.; Zeng, X.; Nie, Y.; Zhang, L.; Wu, S.; Bao, A. Transcriptomic analysis of the venom glands from the scorpion *Hadogenes troglodytes* revealed unique and extremely high diversity of the venom peptides. *J. Proteom.* **2017**, *150*, 40–62. [CrossRef]
12. Santibáñez-López, C.E.; Cid-Uribe, J.I.; Zamudio, F.Z.; Batista, C.V.F.; Ortiz, E.; Possani, L.D. Venom gland transcriptomic and venom proteomic analyses of the scorpion *Megacormus gertschi Díaz-Najera*, 1966 (Scorpiones: *Euscorpiidae: Megacorminae*). *Toxicon* **2017**, *133*, 95–109. [CrossRef] [PubMed]
13. Luna-Ramírez, K.; Quintero-Hernández, V.; Juárez-González, V.R.; Possani, L.D. Whole transcriptome of the venom gland from *Urodacus yaschenkoi* Scorpion. *PLoS ONE* **2015**, *10*, e0127883. [CrossRef]
14. Ponce-Saavedra, J.; Francke, O.F.; Cano-Camacho, H.; Hernández-Calderón, E. Morphological and molecular evidence supporting specific status for *Centruroides tecomanus* (Scorpiones, *Buthidae*). *Rev. Mex. Biodivers.* **2009**, *80*, 71–84.
15. Chavez-Haro, A.L.; Ortiz, E. Scorpionism and Dangerous Species of Mexico. In *Scorpion Venoms*; Springer: Dordrecht, The Netherlands, 2014; pp. 201–213.
16. Riaño-Umbarila, L.; Rodríguez-Rodríguez, E.R.; Santibañez-López, C.E.; Güereca, L.; Uribe-Romero, S.J.; Gómez-Ramírez, I.V.; Cárcamo-Noriega, E.N.; Possani, L.D.; Becerril, B. Updating knowledge on new medically important scorpion species in Mexico. *Toxicon* **2017**, *138*, 130–137. [CrossRef]
17. Available online: https://www.gob.mx/cms/uploads/attachment/file/425972/sem52.pdf (accessed on 29 April 2019).
18. Riaño-Umbarila, L.; Olamendi-Portugal, T.; Morelos-Juárez, C.; Gurrola, G.B.; Possani, L.D.; Becerril, B. A novel human recombinant antibody fragment capable of neutralizing Mexican scorpion toxins. *Toxicon* **2013**, *76*, 370–376. [CrossRef]
19. Dehesa-Dávila, M.; Ramfrez, A.N.; Zamudio, F.Z.; Gurrola-Briones, G.; Liévano, A.; Darszon, A.; Possani, L.D. Structural and functional comparison of toxins from the venom of the scorpions *Centruroides infamatus infamatus*, *Centruroides limpidus limpidus* and *Centruroides noxius*. *Comp. Biochem. Physiol. Part B: Biochem. Mol. Boil.* **1996**, *113*, 331–339. [CrossRef]
20. Ramírz, A.N.; Martin, B.M.; Gurrola, G.B.; Possani, L.D. Isolation and characterization of a novel toxin from the venom of the scorpion *Centruroides limpidus limpidus* Karsch. *Toxicon* **1994**, *32*, 479–490. [CrossRef]
21. Alagon, A.; Guzmán, H.; Martin, B.; Ramírez, A.; Carbone, E.; Possani, L. Isolation and characterization of two toxins from the mexican scorpion *Centruroides limpidus limpidus* Karsch. *Comp. Biochem. Physiol. Part B: Comp. Biochem.* **1988**, *89*, 153–161. [CrossRef]
22. Lebreton, F.; Delepierre, M.; Ramírez, A.N.; Balderas, C.; Possani, L.D. Primary and NMR three-dimensional structure determination of a novel crustacean toxin from the venom of the scorpion *Centruroides limpidus limpidus* Karsch. *Biochemistry* **1994**, *33*, 11135–11149. [CrossRef]
23. Olamendi-Portugal, T.; Restano-Cassulini, R.; Riaño-Umbarila, L.; Becerril, B.; Possani, L.D. Functional and immuno-reactive characterization of a previously undescribed peptide from the venom of the scorpion *Centruroides limpidus*. *Peptides* **2017**, *87*, 34–40. [CrossRef]
24. Cid-Uribe, J.I.; Santibáñez-López, C.E.; Meneses, E.P.; Batista, C.V.; Jiménez-Vargas, J.M.; Ortiz, E.; Possani, L.D. The diversity of venom components of the scorpion species *Paravaejovis schwenkmeyeri* (Scorpiones: *Vaejovidae*) revealed by transcriptome and proteome analyses. *Toxicon* **2018**, *151*, 47–62. [CrossRef] [PubMed]
25. Romero-Gutiérrez, M.T.; Santibáñez-López, C.E.; Jiménez-Vargas, J.M.; Batista, C.V.F.; Ortiz, E.; Possani, L.D. Transcriptomic and proteomic analyses reveal the diversity of venom components from the vaejovid scorpion *Serradigitus gertschi*. *Toxins* **2018**, *10*, 359. [CrossRef] [PubMed]
26. Cid-Uribe, J.I.; Jiménez-Vargas, J.M.; Batista, C.V.F.; Zuñiga, F.Z.; Possani, L.D. Comparative proteomic analysis of female and male venoms from the Mexican scorpion *Centruroides limpidus*: Novel components found. *Toxicon* **2017**, *125*, 91–98. [CrossRef]
27. Pfam. Available online: https://pfam.xfam.org/ (accessed on 29 April 2019).
28. Venom Zone. Available online: https://venomzone.expasy.org/ (accessed on 29 April 2019).
29. Gene Ontology. Available online: http://geneontology.org/ (accessed on 29 April 2019).
30. Quintero-Hernandez, V.; Jimenez-Vargas, J.; Gurrola, G.; Valdivia, H.; Possani, L. Scorpion venom components that affect ion-channels function. *Toxicon* **2013**, *76*, 328–342. [CrossRef] [PubMed]

31. Gurevitz, M.; Froy, O.; Zilberberg, N.; Turkov, M.; Strugatsky, D.; Gershburg, E.; Lee, D.; Adams, M.E.; Tugarinov, V.; Anglister, J.; et al. Sodium channel modifiers from scorpion venom: Structure–activity relationship, mode of action and application. *Toxicon* **1998**, *36*, 1671–1682. [CrossRef]
32. Escalona, M.P.; Possani, L.D. Scorpion beta-toxins and voltage-gated sodium channels: Interactions and effects. *Front Biosci.* **2013**, *18*, 572–587. [CrossRef]
33. De Oliveira, U.C.; Candido, D.M.; Dorce, V.A.C.; Junqueira-De-Azevedo, I.D.L.M. The transcriptome recipe for the venom cocktail of *Tityus bahiensis* scorpion. *Toxicon* **2015**, *95*, 52–61. [CrossRef] [PubMed]
34. Jablonsky, M.J.; Jackson, P.L.; Krishna, N.R. Solution structure of an insect-specific neurotoxin from the new world scorpion *Centruroides sculpturatus Ewing*[†,‡]. *Biochemistry* **2001**, *40*, 8273–8282. [CrossRef] [PubMed]
35. Jablonsky, M.J.; Watt, D.D.; Krishna, N.R. Solution structure of an old world-like neurotoxin from the venom of the new world scorpion *Centruroides sculpturatus Ewing*. *J. Mol. Boil.* **1995**, *248*, 449–458. [CrossRef]
36. Kuang, Q.; Purhonen, P.; Hebert, H. Structure of potassium channels. *Cell. Mol. Life Sci.* **2015**, *72*, 3677–3693. [CrossRef] [PubMed]
37. Jiménez-Vargas, J.M.; Possani, L.D.; Luna-Ramírez, K. Arthropod toxins acting on neuronal potassium channels. *Neuropharmacology* **2017**, *127*, 139–160. [CrossRef] [PubMed]
38. Kim, D.M.; Nimigean, C.M. Voltage-gated potassium channels: A structural examination of selectivity and gating. *Cold Spring Harbor Perspect. Boil.* **2016**, *8*, a029231. [CrossRef]
39. Tytgat, J.; Chandy, K.; Garcia, M.L.; A Gutman, G.; Martin-Eauclaire, M.-F.; Van Der Walt, J.J.; Possani, L.D. A unified nomenclature for short-chain peptides isolated from scorpion venoms: α-KTx molecular subfamilies. *Trends Pharmacol. Sci.* **1999**, *20*, 444–447. [CrossRef]
40. Rodríguez De La Vega, R.C.; Possani, L.D. Current views on scorpion toxins specific for K^+-channels. *Toxicon* **2004**, *43*, 865–875. [CrossRef]
41. Cremonez, C.M.; Maiti, M.; Peigneur, S.; Cassoli, J.S.; Dutra, A.A.A.; Waelkens, E.; Lescrinier, E.; Herdewijn, P.; de Lima, M.E.; Pimenta, A.M.C.; et al. Structural and functional elucidation of peptide TS11 shows evidence of a novel subfamily of scorpion venom toxins. *Toxins* **2016**, *8*, 288. [CrossRef] [PubMed]
42. Correnti, C.E.; Gewe, M.M.; Mehlin, C.; Bandaranayake, A.D.; Johnsen, W.A.; Rupert, P.B.; Brusniak, M.-Y.; Clarke, M.; Burke, S.E.; De Van Der Schueren, W.; et al. Screening, large-scale production, and structure-based classification for cystine-dense peptides. *Nat. Struct. Mol. Boil.* **2018**, *25*, 270–278. [CrossRef] [PubMed]
43. Nieto, A.R.; Gurrola, G.B.; Vaca, L.; Possani, L.D. Noxiustoxin 2, a novel K^+ channel blocking peptide from the venom of the scorpion *Centruroides noxius Hoffmann*. *Toxicon* **1996**, *34*, 913–922. [CrossRef]
44. Valdivia, H.H.; Smith, J.S.; Martin, B.M.; Coronado, R.; Possani, L.D. Charybdotoxin and noxiustoxin, two homologous peptide inhibitors of the $K^+(Ca^{2+})$ channel. *FEBS Lett.* **1988**, *226*, 280–284. [CrossRef]
45. Kuzmenkov, A.I.; Krylov, N.A.; Chugunov, A.O.; Grishin, E.V.; Vassilevski, A.A. Kalium: A database of potassium channel toxins from scorpion venom. *Database* **2016**, *2016*. [CrossRef]
46. Restano-Cassulini, R.; Olamendi-Portugal, T.; Zamudio, F.; Becerril, B.; Possani, L.D. Two novel ergtoxins, blockers of K^+-channels, purified from the Mexican scorpion *Centruroides elegans elegans*. *Neurochem Res.* **2008**, *33*, 1525–1533. [CrossRef]
47. Hill, A.P.; Sunde, M.; Campbell, T.J.; Vandenberg, J.I. Mechanism of block of the hERG K^+ channel by the scorpion toxin CnErg1. *Biophys. J.* **2007**, *92*, 3915–3929. [CrossRef] [PubMed]
48. Torres, A.M.; Bansal, P.; Alewood, P.F.; A Bursill, J.; Kuchel, P.W.; I Vandenberg, J.; Vandenberg, J. Solution structure of CnErg1 (Ergtoxin), a HERG specific scorpion toxin. *FEBS Lett.* **2003**, *539*, 138–142. [CrossRef]
49. Jimenez-Vargas, J.; Restano-Cassulini, R.; Quintero-Hernandez, V.; Gurrola, G.; Possani, L. Recombinant expression of the toxic peptide ErgTx1 and role of Met35 on its stability and function. *Peptides* **2011**, *32*, 560–567. [CrossRef] [PubMed]
50. Chen, Z.-Y.; Hu, Y.-T.; Yang, W.-S.; He, Y.-W.; Feng, J.; Wang, B.; Zhao, R.-M.; Ding, J.-P.; Cao, Z.-J.; Li, W.-X.; et al. Hg1, Novel peptide inhibitor specific for Kv1.3 channels from first scorpion kunitz-type potassium channel toxin family*. *J. Boil. Chem.* **2012**, *287*, 13813–13821. [CrossRef]
51. Santibáñez-López, C.E.; Kriebel, R.; Ballesteros, J.A.; Rush, N.; Witter, Z.; Williams, J.; Janies, D.A.; Sharma, P.P.; Crandall, K. Integration of phylogenomics and molecular modeling reveals lineage-specific diversification of toxins in scorpions. *PeerJ* **2018**, *6*, e5902. [CrossRef]
52. Chen, Z.; Hu, Y.; Han, S.; Yin, S.; He, Y.; Wu, Y.; Cao, Z.; Li, W. ImKTx1, a new Kv1.3 channel blocker with a unique primary structure. *J. Biochem. Mol. Toxicol.* **2011**, *25*, 244–251. [CrossRef]

53. Gao, B.; Harvey, P.J.; Craik, D.J.; Ronjat, M.; De Waard, M.; Zhu, S. Functional evolution of scorpion venom peptides with an inhibitor cystine knot fold. *Biosci. Rep.* **2013**, *33*, 513–527. [CrossRef] [PubMed]
54. Wang, X.; Wang, G. Insights into Antimicrobial Peptides from Spiders and Scorpions. *Protein Pept. Lett.* **2016**, *23*, 707–721. [CrossRef]
55. Yan, L.; Adams, M.E. Lycotoxins, antimicrobial peptides from venom of the wolf spider *Lycosa carolinensis*. *J. Boil. Chem.* **1998**, *273*, 2059–2066. [CrossRef]
56. Torres-Larios, A.; Gurrola, G.B.; Zamudio, F.Z.; Possani, L.D.; Torres-Larios, A. Hadrurin, a new antimicrobial peptide from the venom of the scorpion *Hadrurus aztecus*. *JBIC J. Boil. Inorg. Chem.* **2000**, *267*, 5023–5031. [CrossRef]
57. Lorenzini, D.M.; Da Silva, P.I.; Fogaça, A.C.; Bulet, P.; Daffre, S. Acanthoscurrin: A novel glycine-rich antimicrobial peptide constitutively expressed in the hemocytes of the spider *Acanthoscurria gomesiana*. *Dev. Comp. Immunol.* **2003**, *27*, 781–791. [CrossRef]
58. Luna-Ramirez, K.; Skaljac, M.; Grotmann, J.; Kirfel, P.; Vilcinskas, A.; Possani, L.D. Orally delivered scorpion antimicrobial peptides exhibit activity against pea aphid (*Acyrthosiphon pisum*) and Its Bacterial Symbionts. *Toxins* **2017**, *9*, 261. [CrossRef]
59. Ferreira, L.; Alves, W.; Lucas, M.; Habermehl, G. Isolation and characterization of a bradykinin potentiating peptide (BPP-S) isolated from *Scaptocosa raptoria* venom. *Toxicon* **1996**, *34*, 599–603. [CrossRef]
60. Liu, Z.; Deng, M.; Xiang, J.; Ma, H.; Hu, W.; Zhao, Y.; Li, D.-C.; Liang, S. A novel spider peptide toxin suppresses tumor growth through dual signaling pathways. *Mol. Med.* **2012**, *12*, 1350–1360. [CrossRef]
61. Guo, X.; Ma, C.; Du, Q.; Wei, R.; Wang, L.; Zhou, M.; Chen, T.; Shaw, C. Two peptides, TsAP-1 and TsAP-2, from the venom of the Brazilian yellow scorpion, *Tityus serrulatus*: Evaluation of their antimicrobial and anticancer activities. *Biochimie* **2013**, *95*, 1784–1794. [CrossRef]
62. Zeng, X.-C.; Zhou, L.; Shi, W.; Luo, X.; Zhang, L.; Nie, Y.; Wang, J.; Wu, S.; Cao, B.; Cao, H. Three new antimicrobial peptides from the scorpion *Pandinus imperator*. *Peptides* **2013**, *45*, 28–34. [CrossRef]
63. De La Vega, R.R.; García, B.I.; D'Ambrosio, C.; Diego-García, E.; Scaloni, A.; Possani, L.D. Antimicrobial peptide induction in the haemolymph of the Mexican scorpion *Centruroides limpidus limpidus* in response to septic injury. *Cell. Mol. Life Sci.* **2004**, *61*, 1507–1519. [CrossRef] [PubMed]
64. Zhang, L.; Shi, W.; Zeng, X.-C.; Ge, F.; Yang, M.; Nie, Y.; Bao, A.; Wu, S.; E, G. Unique diversity of the venom peptides from the scorpion *Androctonus bicolor* revealed by transcriptomic and proteomic analysis. *J. Proteom.* **2015**, *128*, 231–250. [CrossRef] [PubMed]
65. Zeng, X.-C.; Wang, S.; Nie, Y.; Zhang, L.; Luo, X. Characterization of BmKbpp, a multifunctional peptide from the Chinese scorpion *Mesobuthus martensii Karsch*: Gaining insight into a new mechanism for the functional diversification of scorpion venom peptides. *Peptides* **2012**, *33*, 44–51. [CrossRef]
66. Marques-Neto, L.M.; Trentini, M.M.; Das Neves, R.C.; Resende, D.P.; Procopio, V.O.; Da Costa, A.C.; Kipnis, A.; Mortari, M.R.; Schwartz, E.F.; Junqueira-Kipnis, A.P. Antimicrobial and chemotactic activity of scorpion-derived peptide, ToAP2, against *Mycobacterium massiliensis*. *Toxins* **2018**, *10*, 219. [CrossRef]
67. Melo, M.M.; Daniele-Silva, A.; Teixeira, D.G.; Estrela, A.B.; Melo, K.R.; Oliveira, V.S.; Rocha, H.A.; Ferreira, L.D.S.; Pontes, D.L.; Lima, J.P.; et al. Structure and in vitro activities of a copper II-chelating anionic peptide from the venom of the scorpion *Tityus stigmurus*. *Peptides* **2017**, *94*, 91–98. [CrossRef]
68. Ramos, O.; Selistre-De-Araújo, H. Snake venom metalloproteases—structure and function of catalytic and disintegrin domains. *Comp. Biochem. Physiol. Part C: Toxicol. Pharmacol.* **2006**, *142*, 328–346. [CrossRef]
69. Lu, J.; Yang, H.; Yu, H.; Gao, W.; Lai, R.; Liu, J.; Liang, X. A novel serine protease inhibitor from *Bungarus fasciatus* venom. *Peptides* **2008**, *29*, 369–374. [CrossRef]
70. Touchard, A.; Aili, S.R.; Fox, E.G.P.; Escoubas, P.; Orivel, J.; Nicholson, G.M.; Dejean, A.; King, G.F. The biochemical toxin arsenal from ant venoms. *Toxins* **2016**, *8*, 30. [CrossRef] [PubMed]
71. Toom, P.M.; Chan, D.S. Enzymatic activities of venom from the jellyfish *Stomolophus meleagris*. *Comp. Biochem. Physiol. Part B: Comp. Biochem.* **1972**, *43*, 435–441. [CrossRef]
72. De Graaf, D.C.; Aerts, M.; Brunain, M.; Desjardins, C.A.; Jacobs, F.J.; Werren, J.H.; Devreese, B. Insights into the venom composition of the ectoparasitoid wasp *Nasonia vitripennis* from bioinformatic and proteomic studies. *Insect Mol. Boil.* **2010**, *19*, 11–26.
73. Trevisan-Silva, D.; Bednaski, A.V.; Gremski, L.H.; Chaim, O.M.; Veiga, S.S.; Senff-Ribeiro, A. Differential metalloprotease content and activity of three *Loxosceles* spider venoms revealed using two-dimensional electrophoresis approaches. *Toxicon* **2013**, *76*, 11–22. [CrossRef]

74. Ortiz, E.; Rendón-Anaya, M.; Rego, S.C.; Schwartz, E.F.; Possani, L.D. Antarease-like Zn-metalloproteases are ubiquitous in the venom of different scorpion genera. *Biochim. Biophys. Acta (BBA)—General Subj.* **2014**, *1840*, 1738–1746. [CrossRef]
75. Almeida, F.; Pimenta, A.; De Figueiredo, S.; Santoro, M.; Martin-Eauclaire, M.; Diniz, C.; De Lima, M.; Pimenta, A.M.D.C. Enzymes with gelatinolytic activity can be found in *Tityus bahiensis* and *Tityus serrulatus* venoms. *Toxicon* **2002**, *40*, 1041–1045. [CrossRef]
76. Conde, R.; Zamudio, F.Z.; Becerril, B.; Possani, L.D. Phospholipin, a novel heterodimeric phospholipase A2 from *Pandinus imperator* scorpion venom. *FEBS Lett.* **1999**, *460*, 447–450. [CrossRef]
77. Morey, S.S.; Kiran, K.; Gadag, J. Purification and properties of hyaluronidase from *Palamneus gravimanus* (Indian black scorpion) venom. *Toxicon* **2006**, *47*, 188–195. [CrossRef] [PubMed]
78. Fletcher, P.L.; Fletcher, M.D.; Weninger, K.; Anderson, T.E.; Martin, B.M. Vesicle-associated membrane protein (VAMP) cleavage by a new metalloprotease from the Brazilian scorpion *Tityus serrulatus*. *J. Biol. Chem.* **2010**, *285*, 7405–7416. [CrossRef] [PubMed]
79. Otero, R.; Navío, E.; Céspedes, F.; Núñez, M.; Lozano, L.; Moscoso, E.; Matallana, C.; Arsuza, N.; García, J.; Fernandez, D.; et al. Scorpion envenoming in two regions of Colombia: Clinical, epidemiological and therapeutic aspects. *Trans. Soc. Trop. Med. Hyg.* **2004**, *98*, 742–750. [CrossRef] [PubMed]
80. Fletcher, P.L., Jr.; Fletcher, M.D.; Possani, L.D. Characteristics of pancreatic exocrine secretion produced by venom from the brazilian scorpion, *Tityus serrulatus*. *Eur. J. Cell Biol.* **1992**, *58*, 259–270. [PubMed]
81. D'Suze, G.; Sevcik, C.; Ramos, M. Presence of curarizing polypeptides and a pancreatitis-inducing fraction without muscarinic effects in the venom of the Venezuelan scorpion *Tityus discrepans* (Karsch). *Toxicon* **1995**, *33*, 295. [CrossRef]
82. Borges, A.; Trejo, E.; Vargas, A.M.; Céspedes, G.; Hernández, A.; Alfonzo, M.J. Pancreatic toxicity in mice elicited by *Tityus zulianus* and *Tityus discrepans* scorpion venoms. *Investig. Clin.* **2004**, *45*, 269–276.
83. Bartholomew, C. Acute Scorpion Pancreatitis in Trinidad. *BMJ* **1970**, *1*, 666–668. [CrossRef]
84. Possani, L.D.; Martin, B.M.; Fletcher, M.D.; Fletcher, P.L. Discharge effect on pancreatic exocrine secretion produced by toxins purified from *Tityus serrulatus* scorpion venom. *J. Boil. Chem.* **1991**, *266*, 3178–3185.
85. Fletcher, M.D.; Possani, L.D.; Fletcher, P.L., Jr. Morphological studies by light and electron microscopy of pancreatic acinar cells under the effect of *Tityus serrulatus* venom. *Cell Tissue Res.* **1994**, *278*, 255–264. [CrossRef]
86. Fletcher, P.L.; Fletcher, M.D.; Fainter, L.K.; Terrian, D.M. Action of new world scorpion venom and its neurotoxins in secretion. *Toxicon* **1996**, *34*, 1399–1411. [CrossRef]
87. Jiménez-Ferrer, E.; Reynosa-Zapata, I.; Pérez-Torres, Y.; Tortoriello, J. The secretagogue effect of the poison from *Centruroides limpidus limpidus* on the pancreas of mice and the antagonistic action of the *Bouvardia ternifolia* extract. *Phytomedicine* **2005**, *12*, 65–71. [CrossRef]
88. Habermann, E.; Hardt, K. A sensitive and specific plate test for the quantitation of phospholipases. *Anal. Biochem.* **1972**, *50*, 163–173. [CrossRef]
89. Dhananjaya, B.L.; D'Souza, C.J.M. The pharmacological role of nucleotidases in snake venoms. *Cell Biochem.* **2010**, *28*, 171–177. [CrossRef]
90. Khan, N.; Niazi, Z.R.; Rehman, F.U.; Akhtar, A.; Khan, M.M.; Khan, S.; Baloch, N.; Khan, S. Hyaluronidases: A Therapeutic Enzyme. *Protein Pept. Lett.* **2018**, *25*, 663–676. [CrossRef] [PubMed]
91. Bordon, K.C.F.; Wiezel, G.A.; Amorim, F.G.; Arantes, E.C. Arthropod venom *Hyaluronidases*: Biochemical properties and potential applications in medicine and biotechnology. *J. Venom. Anim. Toxins Incl. Trop. Dis.* **2015**, *21*, 165. [CrossRef]
92. Almonte, A.G.; Sweatt, J.D. Serine proteases, serine protease inhibitors, and protease-activated receptors: Roles in synaptic function and behavior. *Brain Res.* **2011**, *1407*, 107–122. [CrossRef] [PubMed]
93. Chen, Z.; Wang, B.; Hu, J.; Yang, W.; Cao, Z.; Zhuo, R.; Li, W.; Wu, Y. SjAPI, the first functionally characterized ascaris-type protease inhibitor from animal venoms. *PLoS ONE* **2013**, *8*, e57529. [CrossRef] [PubMed]
94. Zhao, R.; Dai, H.; Qiu, S.; Li, T.; He, Y.; Ma, Y.; Chen, Z.; Wu, Y.; Li, W.; Cao, Z. SdPI, the first functionally characterized kunitz-type trypsin inhibitor from scorpion venom. *PLoS ONE* **2011**, *6*, e27548. [CrossRef] [PubMed]
95. Law, R.H.P.; Zhang, Q.; McGowan, S.; Buckle, A.M.; A Silverman, G.; Wong, W.; Rosado, C.J.; Langendorf, C.G.; Pike, R.N.; I Bird, P.; et al. An overview of the serpin superfamily. *Genome Boil.* **2006**, *7*, 216.

96. Gronenborn, A.M.; Nilges, M.; Peanasky, R.J.; Clore, G.M. Sequential resonance assignment and secondary structure determination of the ascaris trypsin inhibitor, a member of a novel class of proteinase inhibitors. *Biochemistry* **1990**, *29*, 183–189. [CrossRef]
97. Meekins, D.A.; Kanost, M.R.; Michel, K. Serpins in arthropod biology. *Semin. Cell Dev. Boil.* **2017**, *62*, 105–119. [CrossRef] [PubMed]
98. Gibbs, G.M.; Roelants, K.; O'Bryan, M.K. The CAP Superfamily: Cysteine-rich secretory proteins, antigen 5, and pathogenesis-related 1 proteins—Roles in reproduction, cancer, and immune defense. *Endocr. Rev.* **2008**, *29*, 865–897. [CrossRef]
99. Abraham, A.; Chandler, D.E. Tracing the evolutionary history of the CAP superfamily of proteins using amino acid sequence homology and conservation of splice sites. *J. Mol. Evol.* **2017**, *85*, 137–157. [CrossRef]
100. Fry, B.G.; Roelants, K.; Champagne, D.E.; Scheib, H.; Tyndall, J.D.; King, G.F.; Nevalainen, T.J.; Norman, J.A.; Lewis, R.J.; Norton, R.S.; et al. The toxicogenomic multiverse: Convergent recruitment of proteins into animal venoms. *Annu. Genom. Hum. Genet.* **2009**, *10*, 483–511. [CrossRef]
101. Wang, J.; Duan, Y.; Guo, M.; Huang, Q.; Liu, Q.; Niu, L.; Teng, M.; Hao, Q.; Shen, B.; Cheng, X.P.; et al. Blocking effect and crystal structure of natrin toxin, a cysteine-rich secretory protein from *Naja atra* Venom that Targets the BK Ca Channel†,‡. *Biochemistry* **2005**, *44*, 10145–10152. [CrossRef] [PubMed]
102. Gibbs, G.M.; Orta, G.; Reddy, T.; Koppers, A.J.; Martínez-López, P.; De La Vega-Beltràn, J.L.; Lo, J.C.Y.; Veldhuis, N.; Jamsai, D.; McIntyre, P.; et al. Cysteine-rich secretory protein 4 is an inhibitor of transient receptor potential M8 with a role in establishing sperm function. *Proc. Natl. Acad. Sci. USA* **2011**, *108*, 7034–7039. [CrossRef] [PubMed]
103. Ruiming, Z.; Yibao, M.; Yawen, H.; Zhiyong, D.; Yingliang, W.; Zhijian, C.; Wenxin, L. Comparative venom gland transcriptome analysis of the scorpion *Lychas mucronatus* reveals intraspecific toxic gene diversity and new venomous components. *BMC Genom.* **2010**, *11*, 452. [CrossRef]
104. Rokyta, D.R.; Ward, M.J. Venom-gland transcriptomics and venom proteomics of the black-back scorpion (*Hadrurus spadix*) reveal detectability challenges and an unexplored realm of animal toxin diversity. *Toxicon* **2017**, *128*, 23–37. [CrossRef] [PubMed]
105. Miyashita, M.; Otsuki, J.; Hanai, Y.; Nakagawa, Y.; Miyagawa, H. Characterization of peptide components in the venom of the scorpion *Liocheles australasiae* (*Hemiscorpiidae*). *Toxicon* **2007**, *50*, 428–437. [CrossRef]
106. Possani, L.D.; Becerril, B.; Riaño-Umbarila, L.; Juárez-González, V.R.; Olamendi-Portugal, T.; Ortíz-León, M.; Riaño-Umbarila, L.; Juárez-González, V.R.; Olamendi-Portugal, T.; Ortiz-León, M. A strategy for the generation of specific human antibodies by directed evolution and phage display. *FEBS J.* **2005**, *272*, 2591–2601.
107. Riaño-Umbarila, L.; Rudiño-Piñera, E.; Becerril, B.; Torres-Larios, A.; Canul-Tec, J.C.; Possani, L.D. Structural basis of neutralization of the major toxic component from the scorpion *Centruroides noxius Hoffmann* by a human-derived single-chain antibody fragment. *J. Boil. Chem.* **2011**, *286*, 20892–20900.
108. Zamudio, F.; Saavedra, R.; Martin, B.M.; Gurrola-Briones, G.; Herion, P.; Possani, L.D. Amino acid sequence and immunological characterization with monoclonal antibodies of two toxins from the venom of the scorpion *Centruroides noxius Hoffmann*. *JBIC J. Boil. Inorg. Chem.* **1992**, *204*, 281–292. [CrossRef]
109. Fastqc. Available online: https://www.bioinformatics.babraham.ac.uk/projects/fastqc/ (accessed on 29 April 2019).
110. Grabherr, M.G.; Haas, B.J.; Yassour, M.; Levin, J.Z.; Thompson, D.A.; Amit, I.; Adiconis, X.; Fan, L.; Raychowdhury, R.; Zeng, Q.; et al. Full-length transcriptome assembly from RNA-Seq data without a reference genome. *Nat. Biotechnol.* **2011**, *29*, 644–652. [CrossRef] [PubMed]
111. ProP. Available online: http://www.cbs.dtu.dk/services/ProP/ (accessed on 29 April 2019).
112. SpiderP. Available online: http://www.arachnoserver.org/spiderP.html (accessed on 29 April 2019).
113. Mafft. Available online: https://www.ebi.ac.uk/Tools/msa/mafft/ (accessed on 29 April 2019).
114. Hall, T.A. BioEdit: A user-friendly biological sequence alignment editor and analysis program for Windows 95/98/NT. *Nucleic Acids Symp. Ser.* **1999**, *41*, 95–98.
115. Rstudio. Available online: https://www.rstudio.com/ (accessed on 29 April 2019).
116. Wego. Available online: http://wego.genomics.org.cn/ (accessed on 29 April 2019).

toxins

MDPI

Article

Bottom-Up Proteomic Analysis of Polypeptide Venom Components of the Giant Ant *Dinoponera Quadriceps*

Douglas Oscar Ceolin Mariano [1], Úrsula Castro de Oliveira [2], André Junqueira Zaharenko [3], Daniel Carvalho Pimenta [1], Gandhi Rádis-Baptista [4,*] and Álvaro Rossan de Brandão Prieto-da-Silva [3,*]

1 Laboratory of Biochemistry and Biophysics, Instituto Butantan, São Paulo SP 05503-900, Brazil
2 Laboratory of Applied Toxinology, CeTICS, Instituto Butantan, São Paulo SP 05503-900, Brazil
3 Laboratory of Genetics, Instituto Butantan, São Paulo SP 05503-900, Brazil
4 Laboratorio of Biochemistry and Biotechnology, Institute for Marine Sciences, Federal University of Ceara, Fortaleza CE 60165-081, Brazil
* Correspondence: gandhi.radis@ufc.br (G.R.-B.); alvaro.prieto@butantan.gov.br (Á.R.d.B.P.-d.-S.); Tel.: +55-85-3229-8718 (ext. 25) (G.R.-B.); +55-11-2627-9300 (Á.R.d.B.P.-d.-S.)

Received: 2 June 2019; Accepted: 26 July 2019; Published: 29 July 2019

check for updates

Abstract: Ant species have specialized venom systems developed to sting and inoculate a biological cocktail of organic compounds, including peptide and polypeptide toxins, for the purpose of predation and defense. The genus *Dinoponera* comprises predatory giant ants that inoculate venom capable of causing long-lasting local pain, involuntary shaking, lymphadenopathy, and cardiac arrhythmias, among other symptoms. To deepen our knowledge about venom composition with regard to protein toxins and their roles in the chemical–ecological relationship and human health, we performed a bottom-up proteomics analysis of the crude venom of the giant ant *D. quadriceps*, popularly known as the "false" tocandiras. For this purpose, we used two different analytical approaches: (i) gel-based proteomics approach, wherein the crude venom was resolved by denaturing sodium dodecyl sulfate-polyacrylamide gel electrophoresis (SDS-PAGE) and all protein bands were excised for analysis; (ii) solution-based proteomics approach, wherein the crude venom protein components were directly fragmented into tryptic peptides in solution for analysis. The proteomic data that resulted from these two methodologies were compared against a previously annotated transcriptomic database of *D. quadriceps*, and subsequently, a homology search was performed for all identified transcript products. The gel-based proteomics approach unequivocally identified nine toxins of high molecular mass in the venom, as for example, enzymes [hyaluronidase, phospholipase A1, dipeptidyl peptidase and glucose dehydrogenase/flavin adenine dinucleotide (FAD) quinone] and diverse venom allergens (homologous of the red fire ant *Selenopsis invicta*) and venom-related proteins (major royal jelly-like). Moreover, the solution-based proteomics revealed and confirmed the presence of several hydrolases, oxidoreductases, proteases, Kunitz-like polypeptides, and the less abundant inhibitor cysteine knot (ICK)-like (knottin) neurotoxins and insect defensin. Our results showed that the major components of the *D. quadriceps* venom are toxins that are highly likely to damage cell membranes and tissue, to cause neurotoxicity, and to induce allergic reactions, thus, expanding the knowledge about *D. quadriceps* venom composition and its potential biological effects on prey and victims.

Keywords: *Dinoponera quadriceps*; Formicidae; Hymenoptera venom; proteomics; venom allergens; ICK-like toxins

Key Contribution: This study describes the predominant toxin components expressed and found in the venom of *Dinoponera quadriceps*, as well as demonstrates the presence of other venom polypeptides that together make up the toxic cocktail of this giant ant species, endemic of the tropical forests of South America.

1. Introduction

Ants (Vespoidea, Formicidae) belong to the class Insecta and the order Hymenoptera, which include the families Formicidae (ants), Apidae (bees), and Vespidae (wasps) among others [1]. The family Formicidae comprises more than 13,000 species of ants, most of which have an intricate social organization, form colonies with thousands of individuals, and are often distributed in every type of ecosystems on Earth [2]. The majority of ant species have a specialized venom apparatus to sting prey and victims, inoculating a cocktail of biological and pharmacological active substances for predation and defense [3]. The structure of the venom systems of ants share similar ontogenetic and evolutive relationship with the venom systems of wasps, which are characterized by free secretory tubules, a convoluted gland, and a venom gland reservoir [4]. The venom composition of several ant species has been investigated more recently at molecular and pharmacological levels, revealing unique repertories of toxins and venom-related polypeptides that differ considerably from the toxic components of other venomous animals. To mention a few examples, the venom polypeptide contents of the giant red bull ant *Myrmecia gulosa* [5], the bullet ant *Paraponera clavata* [6] and the fire ant *Solenopsis invicta* [7,8]. Ant venoms are rich in organic compounds (e.g., alkaloids and amines), short linear peptides, allergens, and hydrolases, with a very few representatives of cysteine-stabilized peptides [9,10]. In this respect, the peptide composition profile of ant venom is intriguing and a rare exception within the field of venomics, given that most animal venoms contain distinct families of toxins with variable number (from 1 to 5) of internal disulfide bonds that contribute to polypeptide stability and potency [11,12].

The study of venom composition of certain group of animals is advantageous, since it advances (*i*) the overall understanding of the outcome of the pathophysiological process of envenomation, (*ii*) the isolation of a given group of toxins for determining structure-activity relationship and (*iii*) the development of lead compounds for clinical application from particular structures with intrinsic biological and pharmacological activities, among other factors of interest to biomedicine and pharmaceutical biotechnology. For instance, from the venom of the Israeli scorpion *Leiurus quinquestriatus*, a chloride-channel peptide inhibitor with insecticidal and cell-penetrating properties, has been investigated to treat glioma and other types of cancer [13]; from the Chinese red-headed centipede *Scolopendra subspinipes mutilans*, a novel selective peptide inhibitor of voltage-gated sodium channel (subtype 1.7), which could be converted into a lead compound for the development of analgesics, was characterized [14]. Considering that arthropods, particularly ants, are the predominant venomous species on Earth and the large majority of venomous species and their venoms have been comparatively scarcely investigated, a considerable diversity of venom-derived polypeptide structures and their intrinsic biological activities remain to be potentially discovered and characterized.

Among all known subfamilies of ants, the *Ponerinae* subfamily comprises a group of primitive, venomous and one of the largest species (~3 cm) of ants in the world found in tropical regions of the Earth and distributed mainly in the Amazon basin. The genus *Dinoponera* groups together eight described carnivorous species, collectively referred as "false tocandiras", in contrast to the bullet ant *P. clavata* ("tocandiras"). Like most ant species, the predatory *Dinoponera* giant ants utilize their venom, delivered by a sting, to hunt prey (insects, small birds, and mammals) and defend themselves against aggressors (microbials and predators) [2,15]. Accidental and fortuitous encounters with humans occur, but in such circumstance the extremely violent sting, aside from causing long-lasting local pain, provokes systemic symptoms, like fever, involuntary shaking, cold sweating, nausea, vomiting, lymphadenopathy, and cardiac arrhythmias [16]. The giant ant *D. quadriceps* (Santschi, 1921; Kempf, 1971) is distributed and found in the remains of the Atlantic forest, upland humid forests, and the Cerrado and Caatinga biomes in the northeastern region of Brazil, where xerophytic vegetation and low pluviometry regime prevails [15]. Previous studies have described numerous biological and pharmacological activities of the *D. quadriceps* crude venom, such as anti-coagulant, anti-inflammatory and anti-platelet activities and induction of allergic reactions and possible anaphylaxis [17]. The antinociception, anticonvulsant, neurotoxic and/or neuroprotection [18,19], as well as antimicrobial and anti-parasitic affects, have also been reported [20,21]. It is interesting to note that traditional knowledge advocates the use of these ants (and venom) in the treatment of asthma, rheumatism, ear pain, and back pain [22]. In fact, poneratoxin-like peptides obtained from the parental species *P. clavata* were shown to slowly induce the activation of ion currents in response to small depolarization steps and sustain currents due to inactivation blockage of the Nav1.7 channel [6], consequently serving to modulate neurotransmission.

In one of our recent works, a complete analysis of the venom gland transcriptome from *D. quadriceps* was reported [23]. The venom-derived polypeptide and toxin precursors were categorized in two main core components: a major core of predicted toxins that comprises venom allergens (homologous to Sol i 1/PLA1B, Sol i 2/4, and Sol i 3/Ag 5), lethal-like proteins, and esterases (phospholipases A and B, acid phosphatases, and carboxylesterase) and dinoponeratoxins; a minor group of components, which include conserved inhibitory cysteine knot (ICK)-like toxins and comprise, to date, one of the rare examples of this class of cysteine-stabilized toxin in the venom from ants, together with an ICK-like peptide from the venom of the Asian ant *Strumigenys kumadori* (Myrmicinae) [9]. Some of these toxin precursors, like dinoponeratoxins, are homologous to the peptide toxins present in the venom of other *D. quadriceps* populations [24] and in other giant ant species, such as *D. australis* [25]. Allergens are also conserved venom components retrieved from the *D. quadriceps* transcriptome that had been observed only in ant species outside the *Dinoponera* group, mainly in the fire ant *S. invicta* (Myrmicinae), from which the allergen nomenclature is derived (e.g., Sol 1, 2, 3, 4) [26].

The bottom-up proteomics approach involves the chemical or enzymatic cleavage of intact proteins into small peptides that are subsequently backtracked to their original structure and/or set of proteins (proteome). In this proteomic approach, proteins are resolved by one- or two-dimensional gel electrophoresis, after which the bands or spots are excised, in-gel digestion is achieved, and the resulting proteolytic (tryptic) peptides are analyzed by liquid chromatography–mass spectrometry (LC–MS). Additionally, the in-solution digestion of the total protein content in a homogeneous sample, like crude venom, is performed, and the resulting tryptic peptides are analyzed by LC–MS; this is a direct, associated approach [27].

Based on these facts and considering that the transcriptome of *D. quadriceps* venom gland predicted a predominant venom component not completely and functionally characterized yet, the aim of this work was to examine the polypeptide toxins of *D. quadriceps* expressed in the venom, by means of a bottom-up proteomic analysis, including in gel- and in-solution venom proteomics and comparison of toxin identifiers with products encoded by the transcripts expressed in *D. quadriceps* venom gland.

2. Results

2.1. Bottom-Up Proteomics of *Dinoponera quadriceps* Venom

We studied the protein content of *D. quadriceps* venom using two proteomic strategies: (1) in-gel digestion and (2) in-solution digestion, followed by analysis with two different mass spectrometers. Initiating with the first strategy, as shown in Figure 1, 12 major clear protein bands were observed in the denaturing sodium dodecyl sulfate-polyacrylamide gel electrophoresis (SDS-PAGE). These bands were excised from the polyacrylamide gel, submitted to an in-gel digestion procedure, and analyzed by liquid chromatography coupled to a mass/mass spectrometer (LC–MS/MS). The output data were compared with the transcriptomic database of the *D. quadriceps* venom gland. The list of venom proteins identified as toxins is presented in Table S1.

Our gel-based proteomics analysis resulted in the unequivocal identification of nine major venom components that match perfectly with their respective transcripts (contigs) expressed in the *D. quadriceps* venom gland (Table S1). After performing a homology search of databases, using the basic local alignment search tool (BLASTx), these main venom components were matched with the following polypeptides resolved by SDS-PAGE: gel band 1: venom dipeptidyl peptidase 4 (XP_014479089.1); gel bands 3 and 4: glucose dehydrogenase flavin adenine dinucleotide (FAD) (XP_014475855.1); gel band 5: protein yellow-like (XP_014473983.1); gel bands 6, 7, 8, 10, and 11: phospholipase A1 2-like

(XP_014477282.1); gel band 7: hyaluronidase-like (XP_014477391.1); gel band 9: venom allergen 3-like (XP_014469499.1). In addition, we found three uncharacterized components: (i) gel bands 10, 11, and 12 corresponding to an uncharacterized protein LOC106750875 (XP_014486970.1); (ii) gel band 11 representing an uncharacterized protein LOC106751228 (XP_014487552.1); (iii) gel bands 11 and 12 representing an uncharacterized protein LOC105189919 (XP_011150625.1). Peptide fragments from these three uncharacterized proteins revealed a toxin with a Sol_i_2 (pheromone-binding protein/odorant-binding protein, OBP/PBP) domain (Table S1). Only in gel band 2, the giant ant venom-protein was not accurately identified. The complete list of venom polypeptides and their correspondent transcriptomic contigs that were identified through gel-based proteomics approach is shown, as aforementioned, in Table S1.

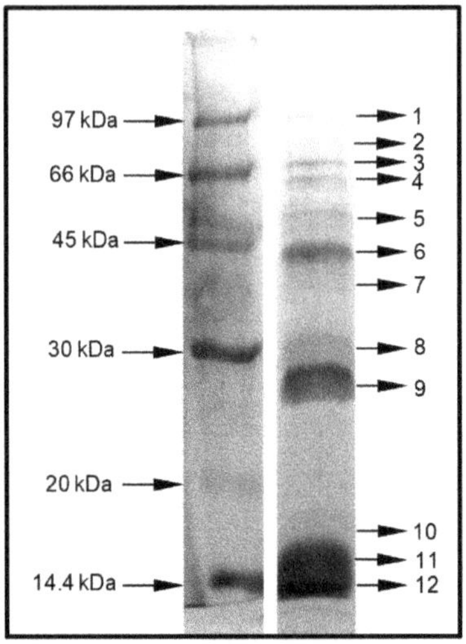

Figure 1. Resolution of *D. quadriceps* venom by denaturing sodium dodecyl sulfate -polyacrylamide gel electrophoresis (SDS-PAGE). Dried venom (30 μg) was solubilized in SDS-PAGE sample buffer and separated in 12.5% T/2.6% C SDS-PAGE, under reducing conditions. The Coomassie stained SDS-PAGE revealed the presence of 12 major, predominant bands in the crude venom. These bands were excised and submitted to an in-gel digestion protocol. The tryptic peptides (obtained for each band) were analyzed by liquid chromatography–electrospray ionization–mass spectrometry (LC-ESI-MS/MS) and the output data were analyzed against a transcriptomic database of *D. quadriceps* venom gland. The digitalized image was converted to black and white. Relative molecular mass is indicated in the left side. Bands of resolved venom toxins are numbered in the right side.

The second strategy employed to study the *D. quadriceps* venom was the solution-based proteomics approach, followed by analysis in two different mass spectrometers. This approach resulted in the identification of peptides corresponding to 61 venom-related transcript products in "analysis #1" (realized with the LTQ-Orbitrap Velos mass spectrometer) and 87 transcript products in "analysis #2" (realized with the Q Exactive Plus mass spectrometer) (Table S2). Both in-solution analyses led to the identification of 44 transcripts, of which seven were also identified in the in-gel analysis. These seven transcripts were venom dipeptidyl peptidase 4, glucose dehydrogenase FAD, protein yellow-like, phospholipase A1 2-like, hyaluronidase-like, venom allergen 3-like, and uncharacterized protein LOC106750875. These results reinforce the gel-based proteomics strategy, and also indicate the presence and expression of several protein components in the venom in quantities that is out of the dynamic range of Coomassie brilliant blue (CBB)-staining of venom proteins separated by denaturing SDS-PAGE. For example, the results from these in-solution proteomic analyses showed the presence of less abundant polypeptides visible in the CBB-stained SDS-PAGE, such as hydrolases (acidic phospholipase A2 PA4, arylsulfatase J, carboxypeptidase Q-like, cathepsin L1, lysozyme c-1-like, putative cysteine proteinase CG12163, venom acid phosphatase Acph-1-like, venom serine protease-like), oxydoreductases (superoxide dismutase [Cu-Zn]), protease inhibitor (serpin B3-like, Kunitz-type serine protease inhibitor ki-VN-like) or proteins related to lipid metabolism (apolipophorin-III, prosaposin, protein NPC2 homolog). A list of venom polypeptides and their corresponding transcriptomic contigs that were identified through solution-based proteomics are present in Table S2.

2.2. *Comparison of Identified Venom-Derived Polypeptides*

All proteins identified in the *D. quadriceps* venom were classified according to their typical functional and/or structural domains (structural protein units) (Tables S1 and S2), based on our previous transcriptome analysis, gene and genome databanks, and the Pfam library database. In the following sections a description of each of the predominant polypeptide component of the *D. quadriceps* crude venom is presented.

2.2.1. Venom Dipeptidyl Peptidase-4 (vDPP-4)

This protein was identified from gel band 1 (with peptide fragments covering 1% of the full sequence) and from the in-solution proteomic analysis protein 10 (with peptide fragments covering 44% and 54% of the full sequence). This venom-protein corresponds to the transcript contig164_B2-2 of the *D. quadriceps* venom gland transcriptome previously reported [23]. This transcript encodes a precursor of which the protein product, in the venom, is homologous to human dipeptidyl peptidase 4 (vDPP-4) or CD26. Such venom enzyme is also known as allergen C (Api m 5) in the honey bee *Apis mellifera* and Ves v 3 in common wasp *Vespula vulgaris* [28]. The organization of the cDNA precursor and the alignment of the *D. quadriceps* vDPP-4 (Venom allergen C) with its homologues from bee and wasp venoms are shown, respectively, in Figure S1 and Figure 2. Here, in *D. quadriceps*, the precursor consists of a signal peptide with 21 amino acid (aa) residues and a mature protein with 752 aa with a theoretical molecular mass of 85842.88 Da (Figure S1 and Figure 3). The vDDP-4 encoded by Contig164_B2-2 of the *D. quadriceps* transcriptome [23] has predictive glycosylation sites at the same positions of the best studied sequences of bee and wasp vDPPs, which cause an apparent distinct electrophoretic mobility on SDS-PAGE of approximately 100 kDa (Figure 1). A list of vDPPs in the Hymenoptera database can be found in the Peptidase S9B family and DPP-4 subfamily.

2.2.2. Glucose Dehydrogenase [FAD, Quinone]

This protein was identified from the SDS-PAGE gel bands 3 and 4 (with peptide fragments covering 6% and 3% of the full sequence), from the in-solution proteomic analysis protein 13 (with peptide fragments covering 34% and 45% of the full sequence), and from the protein precursor encoded in the *D. quadriceps* transcript contig75_B2-2, a venom polypeptide of the FAD family of flavoprotein oxidoreductases. Its sequence is structurally similar to other hymenopteran proteins, such as the *glucose dehydrogenase* [FAD, quinone] of the jumping (or Jerdon's) ant *Harpegnathos saltator* ant (XP_011140071.2) and fruit fly *Drosophila pseudoobscura* (DHGL_DROPS). These venom polypeptide sequences exhibit highly conserved sites for binding nucleotides and enzymatic catalysis (Figure 3). The protein identified in this band is also highly similar to the N-terminal (580 aa) of a duplicated genome-encoded sequence of *D. quadriceps* (XP_014475855) that predicts a polypeptide of 1271 aa. The organization of the *D. quadriceps* precursor of venom glucose dehydrogenase (GDH) [FAD, quinone] is shown in Figure S2. Owing to the presence of glycosylation sites, proteins bands (3 and 4) appear to migrate in SDS-PAGE with an apparent molecular mass of 55 to 65 kDa, instead of the theoretical molecular mass of 65379.84 Da. A list of similar polypeptides in the Hymenoptera database can be accessed in the entry family of glucose-methanol-choline (GMC) oxidoreductases.

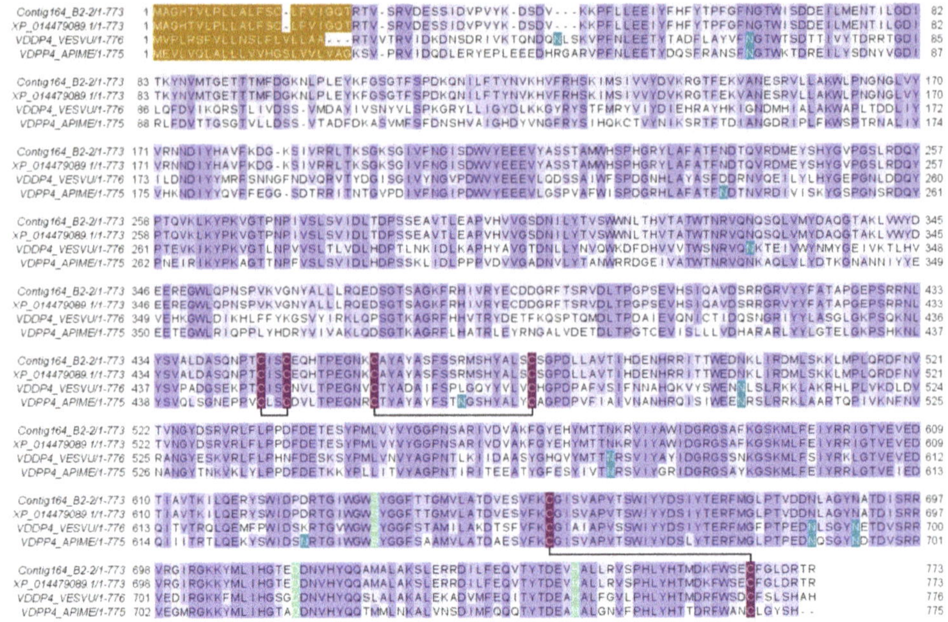

Figure 2. Alignment of the *D. quadriceps* dipeptidyl peptidase-4 (vDPP-4) encoded in the transcript Contig164_B2-2 and sequences of homologous proteins from common wasp and honey bee. The *D. quadriceps* vDPP-4 was aligned with its homologues from common wasp *V. vulgaris* (VDDP4_VESVU), honey bee *A. mellifera* (VDPP4_APIME) and a predicted sequence from the genome of *D. quadriceps* (XP_014479089.1). Asparagine residues (N), marked in emerald green, indicate glycosylation sites. The light green tagged amino acids indicate residues located at the enzyme active site. The cysteine residues that are involved in the formation of disulfide bridges are indicated in purple and the connectivity pattern is indicated by solid black lines. The peptide signals are labeled in brown and were predicted using SignalP 5. The conservation is indicated by BLOSUM62 matrix using the Jalview program.

2.2.3. Yellow Royal Jelly Protein Domain

This protein was identified from the SDS-PAGE gel band 5 (with peptide fragments covering 8% of the full sequence) and from the in-solution proteomic analysis protein 10 (with peptide fragments covering 56% and 70% of the full sequence). It was identified as the major royal jelly protein domain [MRJP domain], a 215-aa venom polypeptide corresponding to the transcript contig98_B2-2 (Figure 4 and Figure S3). This transcript (1614 bp) encodes a 430-aa long MRJP precursor, which has a signal peptide (16 aa) and a mature venom protein (414 aa) (Figure S3), with a theoretical molecular mass of 47616.06 Da and an apparent electrophoretic mobility of 45 kDa on SDS-PAGE (Figure 1, gel band 5). A list of proteins from this family in the Hymenoptera database can be found under the entry "major royal jelly protein family". The transcribed yellow protein-like protein of *D. quadriceps* (Figure 4) shares 27% similarity with the *A. mellifera* MRJP-1 protein and 40% identity with the *D. melanogaster* yellow protein. The honey bee-like glycoprotein MRJP-1 is a 55 kDa monomer, but forms oligomers of 420 kDa [29]. The MRJP-1 from honey bee has three pairs of cysteine bonds, whereas the MRJP-like protein from *D. quadriceps* venom contains only five residues of cysteine, possibly forming only two disulfide bonds.

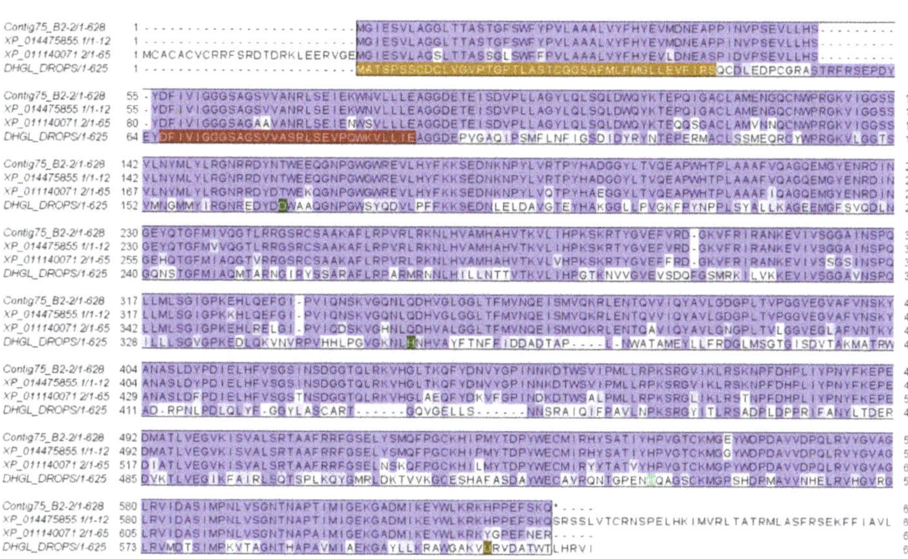

Figure 3. Alignment of *D quadriceps* venom glucose dehydrogenase [FAD, quinone] with homologous proteins from hymenopterans. This venom component identified by proteomic analysis of band 3 and 4, resolved in the SDS-PAGE, is encoded in the *D. quadriceps* venom gland transcript contig75_B2-2 was aligned to the N-terminal (the first 612 residues) of the predicted sequence generated by automatic annotation of *D. quadriceps* genome (XP_014475855), the Indian jumping ant *H. saltator* (XP_011140071) and the Glucose dehydrogenase [FAD, quinone] from fruit fly *D. pseudoobscura* (DHGL_DROPS). The *Drosophila* protein (DHGL_DROPS) comprises a peptide signal of 42 amino acids (experimental). The nucleotide binding site is indicated in red. The amino acids that are indicated in green are divergent or conflictive residues. Selenocysteine is indicated by "U".

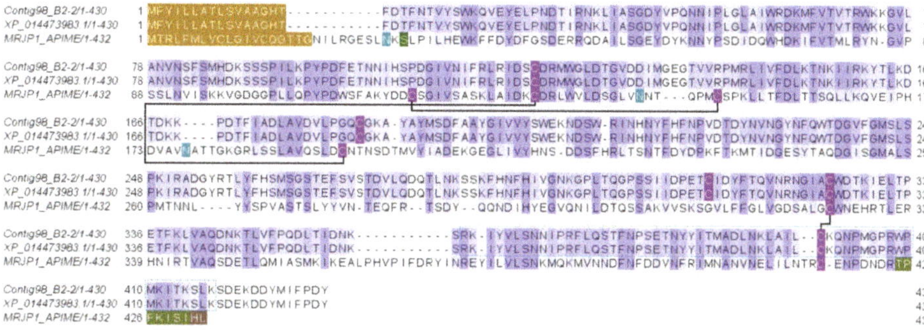

Figure 4. Alignment of *D. quadriceps* major royal jelly protein (MRJP)-like precursor to predicted and known similar sequences. MRJP-like protein identified initially in the *D. quadriceps* venom gland transcriptome, confirmed by the proteomic analysis of the crude venom (this study), was aligned to its counterparts in *D. melanogaster* [XP_014473983] and honey bee *A. mellifera* [MRJP1_APIME]. Pattern of conservation is indicated using the JalView program with the BLOSUM62 matrix. The signal peptides of MRJP-sequences are indicated in brown. The amino acid marked in green are divergent or conflictive residues. Asparagine residues are marked in light green and they indicate glycosylation sites. The MRJP-1 regions which generate the antimicrobial peptides Jelelin-1 to -4 are indicated in dark green. The cysteine residues are highlighted in purple and the pattern of MRJP-1 disulfide bonds is indicated by connecting lines.

2.2.4. Phospholipases A1 (PLA1)

These proteins were identified from gel bands 6, 7, 8, 10, and 11 (with peptide fragments covering 19% of the full sequence) and from the in-solution proteomic analysis protein 7 (with peptide fragments covering 51% and 65% of the full sequence). They correspond to the phospholipase A1 homologues, the polypeptide products of the *D. quadriceps* venom gland transcript contig27_B2-2. These peptides and transcript products also correspond to a predicted partial sequence transcribed and translated from the *D. quadriceps* genome segment (XP_014477282). The polypeptide is similar to the venom allergen 1 of *S. invicta,* sharing 51% identity. The *D. quadriceps* PLA1 homologue, encoded by contig27_B2-2 (1656 bp), is a preprotein of 379 residues and a mature polypeptide with 356 aa residues (theoretical molecular mass 38715.85). The structural organization of transcript contig27_B2-2 and its polypeptide product can be seen in Figure S4. As observed in the SDS-PAGE gel (Figure 1) and peptide mass fingerprinting (PMF) from the in-gel digestion of corresponding bands (Table S1), the *D. quadriceps* PLA1 has several post-translational modifications (PTMs) that interfere with the electrophoretic migration on SDS-PAGE. The identified venom PLA1 of *D. quadriceps*, aligned with other hymenopteran sequences, is shown in Figure 5. A list of Hymenoptera phospholipases that belong to the alpha/beta (AB) hydrolase superfamily (lipase family) can be found in the Hymenoptera database.

2.2.5. Hyaluronidase

This protein was identified from gel band 7 (with peptide fragments covering 3% of the full sequence) and from the in-solution proteomic analysis protein 16 (with peptide fragments covering 16% of the full sequence). The peptides detected in the venom proteome corresponded to the translated protein product of the *D. quadriceps* venom gland transcript contig385_B2-2 (1882 bp, Figure S5), which codes for the venom hyaluronidase that belongs to the family of glycosyl hydrolases 56 in the Hymenoptera database. Such sequence is identical to the predicted product of the gene segment of *D. quadriceps* genome [XP_014477391]. The protein precursor of *D. quadriceps* hyaluronidase is 368 aa long, with a signal peptide of 25 residues and a mature protein of 343 aa (theoretical molecular mass 38844.96 Da), but the glycosylation-specific sites, which could cause the apparent distinct pattern of electrophoretic migration to diverge from the theoretical molecular mass, are identifiable (Figure 1, Table S1). The *D. quadriceps* venom hyaluronidases share high similarity (99%) with homologous sequences from the venoms of common wasp and honey bee (Figure 6).

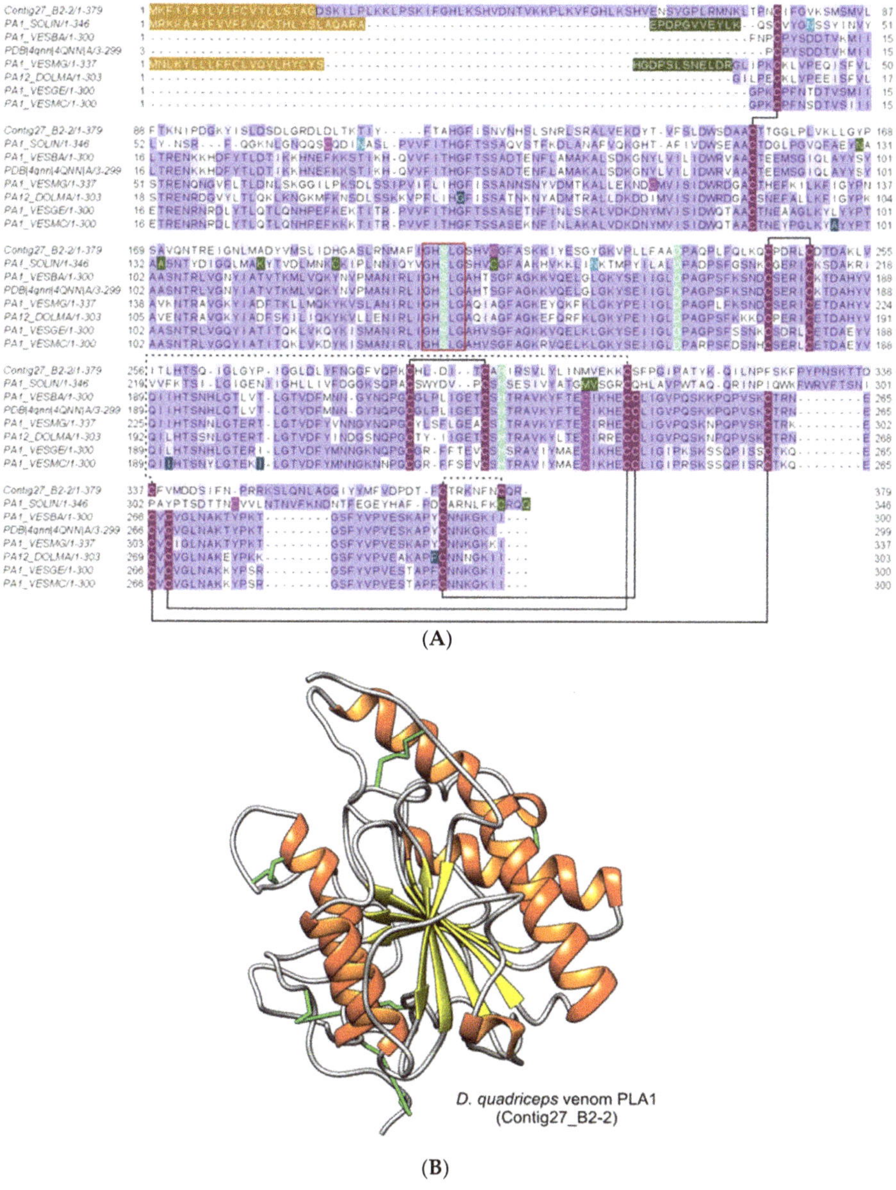

Figure 5. Alignment and structural model of *D. quadriceps* venom phospholipase A1. (**A**) *D. quadriceps* venom phospholipase A1 was aligned to some hymenopteran homologues: [PA1_SOLIN], PLA1 (Allergen Sol i 1) from *S. invicta*; [PA1_VESBA], Phospholipase A1 from black-bellied hornet *Vespa basalis* and [PDB | 4QNN | A], sequence that generated the crystal structure of the A chain by X-ray diffraction; [PA1_VESMG], hornet wasp *Vespa magnifica* phospholipase A1 magnifin; [PA12_DOLMA] phospholipase A1-2 (Allergen Dol m 1) from bald-faced hornet *Dolichovespula maculata*; [PA1_VESGE] phospholipase A1 (Allergen Ves g 1) form European wasp (German yellowjacket) *Vespula germanica*; [PA1_VESMC], phospholipase A1 (Allergen Ves m 1) from Eastern yellow jacket *Vespula maculifrons*. Glycosylated asparagine residues are indicated in emerald green. Dark green amino acids indicate natural variants. The amino acids from the enzymatic active site are indicated in light green and the consensus Gly-X-Ser-X-Gly motif, characteristic of the active serine hydrolases, is boxed in red. Moss

green indicated divergent or conflictive residues. The signal peptide is indicated in brown and the pro-peptide in military green. Conserved cysteine residues that participate in the formation of disulfide bridges are indicated by purple boxes and connected by solid black lines, as determined for wasps' PLA1s. Unpaired cysteines are indicated in light purple and the connecting lines indicate the possible connectivity based on homology model of the mature PLA1 sequence of *D. quadriceps*. The conservation was estimated with the BLOSUM62 matrix. (**B**) Structural model of *D. quadriceps* PLA1 predicted by homology modeling from venom gland transcript Contig27_B2-2 and the venom phospholipase A1 from hornet wasp *Vespa basalis* (PDB 4QNN), as template. This giant ant venom component was detected in-gel analysis (gel bands 6 and 7). Similarly, predicted from the transcripts consensus_20 Phospholipase A1-like 1_B04_E7_DVC2, that corresponds to gel bands 10 and 11. Also detected in-solution proteomic analysis: protein 7 (Contig27_B2-2); protein 17 (1_B04_E7_DVC2); Based on the structural analysis, this giant ant toxin is presumably a platelet activator, like in Vespidae venoms. Note: protein 12, from in-solution analysis, is a PLA2.

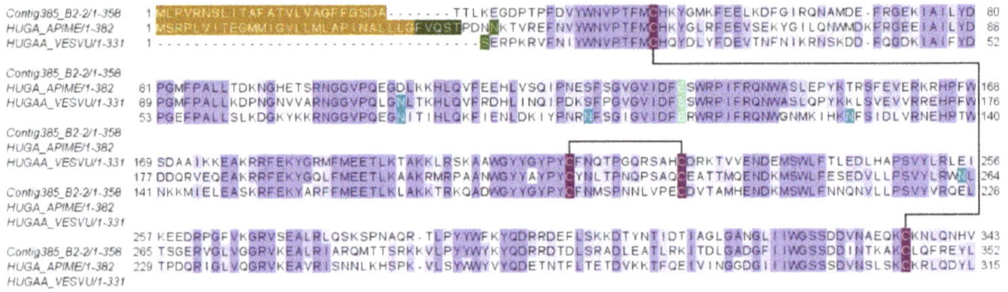

Figure 6. Alignment of the venom *D. quadriceps* hyaluronidase and homologous enzymes from hymenopterans. *D. quadriceps* venom hyaluronidase, encoded in the venom gland transcript contig385_B2-2 and identified by in-gel and in-solution proteomics analysis, is compared with similar proteins from honey bee *A. mellifera* [HUGA_APIME] and common wasp *V. vulgaris* [PHUGAA_VESVU]. Signal peptide is boxed in brown color and the prepropeptide in dark green. Glycosylation residues (N) are in blue. Conserved cysteine residues are indicated in purple color and the disulfide bonds by connecting solid black lines.

2.2.6. Major Venom Allergen 3, Cysteine-Rich Venom Protein Superfamily; Cysteine-Rich Secretary Protein (CRISP) Family

This protein was identified from the SDS-PAGE gel band 9 (with peptide fragments covering 23% of the full sequence) and from the in-solution proteomic analysis protein 16 (with peptide fragments covering 52% and 47% of the full sequence). It corresponded with the major venom allergen 3, a cysteine-rich venom protein precursor encoded by the *D. quadriceps* venom gland Contig12_B2-2 (Table S1). This protein belongs to the sperm-coating glycoprotein (SCP)/cysteine-rich secretory proteins (CRISP), antigen 5, and pathogenesis-related 1 proteins (CAP) superfamily that also includes cysteine-rich venom proteins that together make up 9 subfamilies of proteins. The 210-aa long mature protein product of the *D. quadriceps* transcript (molecular mass 23660.77 Da) could be glycosylated (Figure S6), as shown by the change in its electrophoretic mobility. Similar sequences in hymenopteran venom share high level of similarity, for example, venom allergen 3 [P35778] from *S. invicta* (Antigen Sol i 3) with 57% identity and major antigen of wasps (Vespid venom allergen V5) (Figure 7).

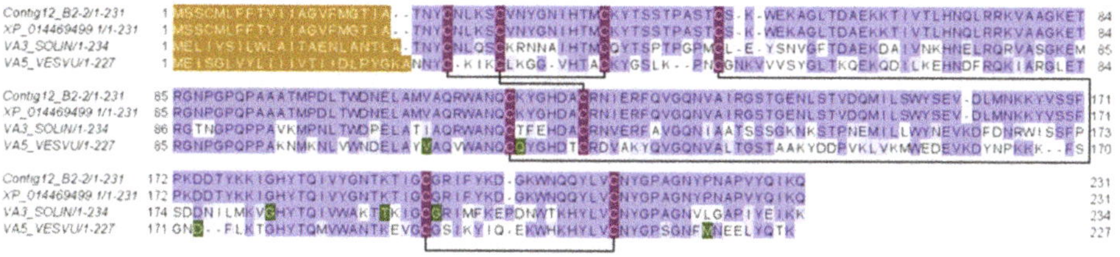

(A)

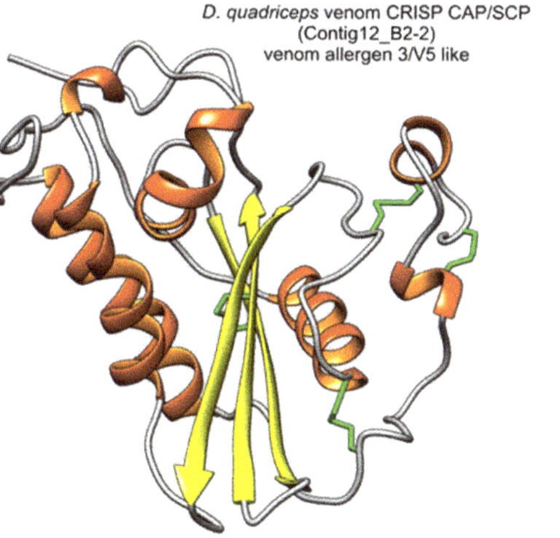

(B)

Figure 7. Alignment and structural model of cysteine-rich venom protein/major venom allergen 3 from *D. quadriceps* venom. (**A**) the *D quadriceps* venom CRISP-, CAP/SCP-like protein was aligned to its hymenopteran homologues. In this alignment, proteins were compared with the predicted protein from the gene segment of *D. quadriceps* genome [XP_014469499.1] (venom allergen 3-like), venom allergen 3 of *S. invicta* [VA3_SOLIN] and venom allergen 5 of *V. vulis* [VA5_VESVU]. (**B**) Structure of *D quadriceps* venom CRISP-, CAP/SCP-like protein that was modelled from the sequence predicted from *D. quadriceps* venom gland transcript Contig12_B2-2, using as template the crystal structure of the major allergen Sol i 3 from fire ant venom *Solenopsis invicta* (PDB 2VZN). The *D. quadriceps* CRISP-, CAP/SCP-like venom protein was identified by in-gel proteomics (gel band 9), and in-solution proteomics, proteins numbered 1, 8 and 67, which correspond to venom gland transcripts 1_A09_D9_DVA2-1; 1_A09_D9_DVA2; 1_C05_C6_3_DVB1; Consensus TX03; 1_E07_H11_DVC2-1; 1_E07_H11_DVC2; 1_B07_E6_DVC2-1; 1_A09_D9_DVA2-1; 1_A09_D9_DVA2; 1_E06_B4_DVC2-1; 1_E06_B4_DVC2; 1_B03_C4_2_DVC2; 1_C01_H9_3_DVC2. By comparative analysis with the major venom allergen 5 from vespoid wasps, the venom allergen 3 from fire ants and the scoloptoxins from the Thai centipede *Scolopendra dehaani*, which cause allergic reactions after stinging, this venom-protein in *D. quadriceps* is presumed to be a potent allergen.

2.2.7. Major Ant Venom Allergen 2/4-Like (Odorant/Pheromone-Binding Protein-Like)

This protein was identified from the SDS-PAGE gel bands 10, 11, and 12 (with peptide fragments covering 18% of the full sequence) and from the in-solution proteomic analysis protein 3 (with peptide fragments covering 32% and 31% of the full sequence). It corresponded to the protein product of the *D. quadriceps* venom gland transcript Contig8_B2-2, Figure S7) that codes for the major ant venom allergen 2/4-like (Odorant/pheromone-binding protein-, OBP/PBP-like). This identified toxin also corresponds to the predicted gene product of a gene segment of the *D. quadriceps* genome

[XP_014486970.1]. The theoretical molecular mass predicted for the mature sequence of this 119-aa long peptide is 12,984.28 Da. In Figure 8, the alignment of Venom Allergen 2/4-like (OBP/PBP-like) from the *D. quadriceps* venom and the venom proteins Sol i 2 and Sol i 4 from *S. invicta* is shown.

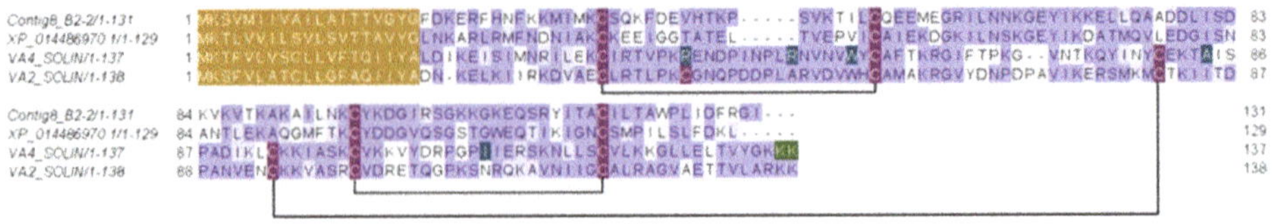

(A)

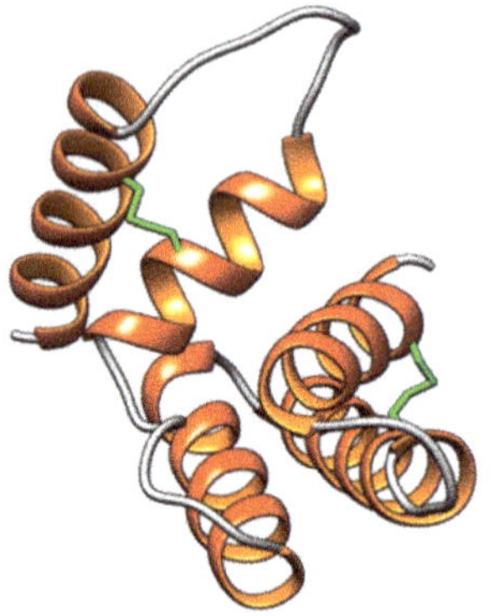

(B)

Figure 8. Structural analysis of *D. quadriceps* ant venom allergen 2/4, pheromone/odorant binding protein-like (OBP/PBP). (**A**) Alignment of *D. quadriceps* OBP/PBP-like and venom proteins Sol i 2 and Sol i 4 from fire ant *S. invicta*. The protein product of *D. quadriceps* transcript (Contig8_B2-2) expressed ion the venom gland, confirmed by proteomic analysis of the crude venom and the predicted amino acid sequence from the genomic annotation of *D. quadriceps*, XP_014486970.1, as well as the venom allergen 2 (Sol i 2) [VA2_SOLIN] and venom allergen 4 (Sol i 4) [VA4_SOLIN] from *S. invicta* were aligned. In brown, the leader sequences are shown as predicted by SignalP 5.0. In dark green, natural variants, conflictive or divergent residues are indicated and in light green. In purple, the conserved cysteine residues are highlighted. The solid black lines indicate the pattern of disulfide bonds, as determined for Sol i 2 [VA2_SOLIN]. Amino acid conservation are estimated with the BLOSUM62 matrix. (**B**) Structural model of *D. quadriceps* venom allergen 2/4, OBP/PBP-like venom protein. The predicted structure was homology modelled from *D. quadriceps* contig8_B2-2, based on the crystal structure of the venom allergen Sol i 2 from fire ant *S. invicta* (PDB 2YGU), as template. This *D. quadriceps* venom component was detected by in-gel analysis (gel bands 10, 11 and 12) and by in-solution proteomic analysis (protein 3 that corresponds to transcript Contig8_B2-2) and similar sequences, like protein 2 (1_B07_F8_2_DVB1); protein 4 (1_C11_G4_3_DVB1.2); protein 5 (1_D08_A8_4_DVB1); protein 6 (1_H10_F10_DVA2-1); protein 15 (1_G01_E8_3_DVB2); protein 45 (Consensus_41); protein 66 (1_G11_B10_3_PM). Based on similarity with known toxins in the structural family, the presumed biological function of in *D. quadriceps* venom OBP/PBP-like protein, appears to be of an extremely potent allergy-inducing agent, that causes IgE antibody production.

2.2.8. *Dinoponera quadriceps* Bovine Pancreatic Trypsin Inhibitor (BPTI)/Kunitz-Like Serine Protease Inhibitor

From the in-solution-based proteomics analysis, this *D. quadriceps* venom component corresponding to the protein product of the transcript contig511_B2-2 (protein 39) was identified (Table S2), and its structural organization can be seen in Figure S8. The mature protein, a bovine pancreatic trypsin inhibitor (BPTI) /Kunitz-like toxin, is stabilized by three disulfide bonds, as shown by the alignment of *D. quadriceps* BPTI/Kunitz-like toxin with its homologue in wasp and with another sequence predicted from the giant ant genome segment (Figure 9).

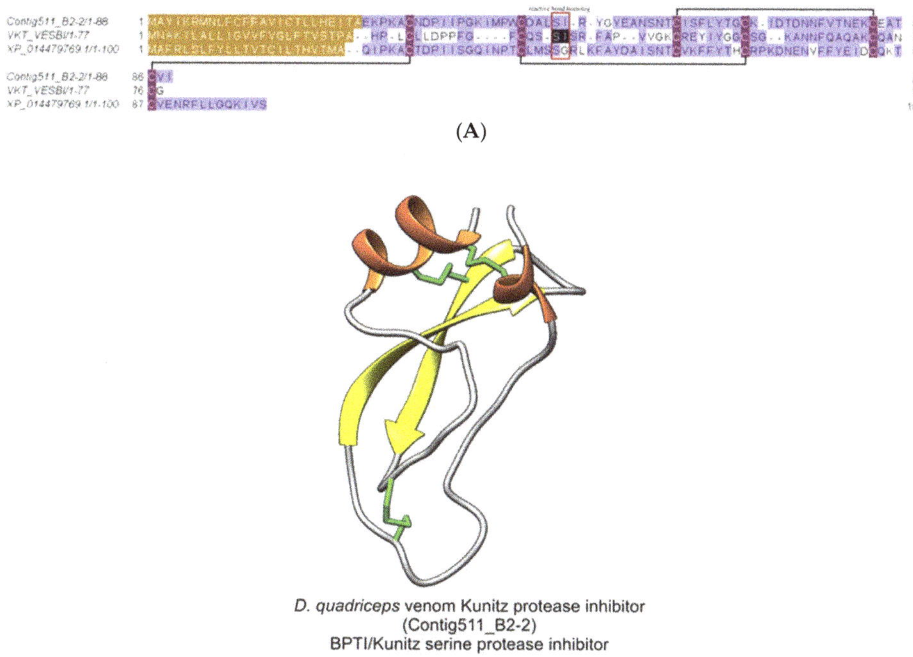

(B)

Figure 9. Structural analysis of *D. quadriceps* BPTI/Kunitz-type peptide toxin. (**A**) *D quadriceps* venom BPTI/Kunitz-type peptide was aligned with the bicolin peptide (Kunitz-type serine protease inhibitor bicolin) from black shield wasp *V. bicolor* venom (VKT_VESB) and with a predicted sequence identified in gene segment of *D. quadriceps* genome, the Kunitz-type serine protease inhibitor ki-VN-like (XP_014479769.1). The amino acid residues that located at the inhibitory active site, in bicolin peptide, are indicated by red box and are shown in black, for comparison. The connectivity pattern of the three disulfide bonds are indicated by solid black lines. The signal peptide is shown in brown. Sequence similarity was determined using BLOSUM62. (**B**) the structural model of *D. quadriceps* Kunitz-type toxin predicted from the venom gland transcript Contig511_B2-2, identified by in-solution proteomics (e.g., protein 39, Table S2) was elaborated by homology using as template the mambaquaretin-1 toxin (PDB 5M4V), a selective antagonist of the vasopressin type 2 receptor (V2R) from the green mamba *Dendroaspis angusticeps* venom. Mambaquaretin-1 is an efficient antagonist of the V2R activation pathways that involve cAMP production, beta-arrestin interaction, and MAP kinase activity [30], thus the presumed biological function of *D. quadriceps* Kunitz-type peptide in the venom. The typical structure is characterized by an α/β protein with few secondary structures that is constrained by 3 disulfide bonds.

2.2.9. Pilosulin- and Ponericin-Like Peptides

From the in-solution-based proteomics analysis, four dinoponeratoxins (DNTxs) corresponding to contigs 1_A12_G5_1_DVC1 (protein 26), 1_F07_C7_2_DVB1 (protein 22), consensus 34 (protein 21), and 1_F12_E3_DVA2 (protein 46) in the *D. quadriceps* venom gland transcriptome were identified (Table S2). The transcript precursors of these DNTxs, with their respective peptide products, are shown in Figure S9A–D. In Figure 10, the complete amino acid sequences are shown as aligned with their recognized homologues from the *Dinoponera* genus and other species of hymenopterans.

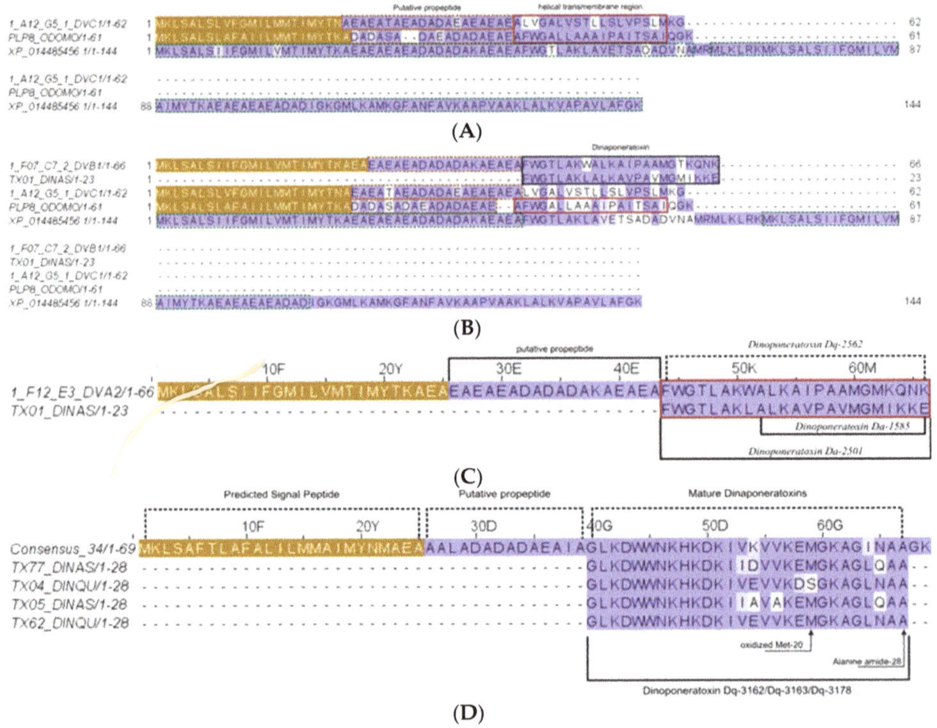

Figure 10. Dinoponeratoxins (DNTxs), pilosulin- and ponerecin- like peptides found by proteomic and transcriptomic analysis as part of the major components of *D. quadriceps* venom. (**A**) Sequence that corresponds to mature peptide encoded in the transcript contig 1_A12_G5_1_DVC1, a pilosulin-like precursor peptide [Dq-1969]; (**B**) Contig 1_F07_C7_2_DVB1, a pilosulin-like precursor peptide [Dq-2532]; (**C**) product from transcript Contig Consensus 34, a pilosulin-like precursor peptide; (**D**) product from transcript contig 1_F12_E3_DVA2, a pilosulin-like precursor peptide [Dq-2562]. The peptide signal in each case is colored in gold, the prepropeptide in magenta. The mature, processed peptide and fragments are boxed in red and black and the experimental molecular mass indicated. Note. the *D. quadriceps* dinoponeratoxins, pilosulin- and ponerecin- like peptides detected in the venom proteome are listed in Table S2.

2.2.10. Inhibitor Cysteine Knot (ICK)-Like Venom-Peptides

From the in-solution proteomics analysis, three types of knottins (1_D07_A11_4_DVB1-protein 88; Contig516_B2-2 gi|578895399| - protein 77; XM_014620749.1 - protein 99), referred to as ICK-like toxins, were found in the venom of *D. quadriceps* (Figure 11). The experimental data are presented in summarized information in Table S2. The transcript precursors for two of them are shown in Figure S10A,B. These ICK-like toxins (Figure 11A,B) expressed in the giant ant venom are consistent with similar structures that are known neurotoxins in other venoms, like spider huwentoxins and anemone ICKs (e.g., BcsTx3 and κ-actitoxin-Bcs4a), while the third ICK-like toxin is structurally similar to defensin-like-2 of insects (hymenopteran canonical invertebrate defensin-like-2 peptides). In Figure 11A, the *D. quadriceps* ICK-like toxins that share high level of similarity (~60–90%) with honey bee and spider homologues are compared by amino acid sequence alignment. In Figure 11B, the giant ant knottin-like peptides that are highly similar (>90%) to conotoxin-like neurotoxins from *A. mellifera* and *Conus* sea snail are presented. The defensin-like venom peptides from *A. mellifera* and *Odontomachus monticola*, with antimicrobial activity associated to their structures, are shown in C, and are compared with similar (~50% identical) sequence found in the venom of *D. quadriceps*.

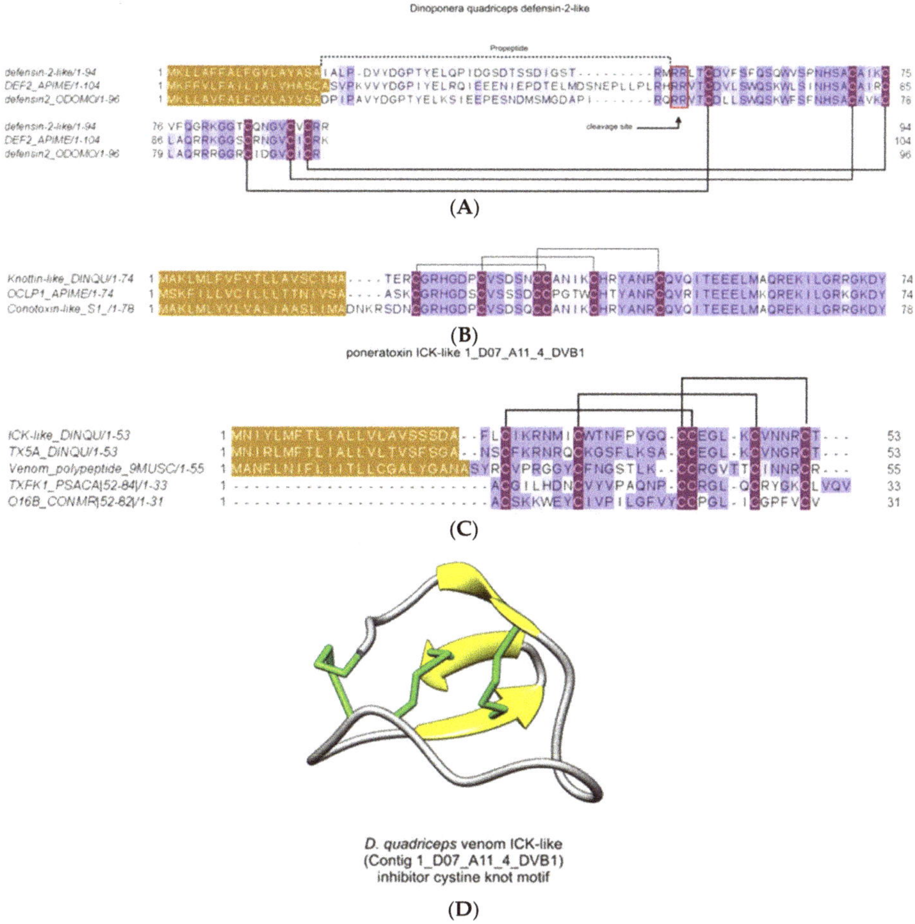

Figure 11. Knottins, ICK-like toxins, found in the crude venom of the giant ant *D. quadriceps*. (**A**) Defensin-like-2 venom-peptides that corresponds to the gene product of the nucleotide sequence XM_014620749.1 from *D. quadriceps*. (**B**) Knottin-like toxin found as the product from the venom gland transcript contig516_B2-2 gi|578895399|. (**C**) Sequence that corresponds to mature homologous peptide encoded in the transcript clone 1_D07_A11_4_DVB1 (U1-poneritoxin-Dq5a) from *D. quadriceps* transcriptome. The peptide signal in each case is colored in gold, the prepropeptide is indicated by a dashed line (in A). Disulfide bonds are represented by connecting solid lines, as known from the S-S patterns of homologous sequences. The mature, processed toxins are seen downstream the cleavage site, in the prepropeptide (in A) or downstream the signal peptides (in B and C). The gene and protein

database access codes are as follow: DEF2_APIME [Q5MQL3], defensin-2 from the honey bee *A. mellifera;* A0A348G5W3; Conotoxin-like_S1 from the ponerine ant *O. monticola;* A0A348G6A9_ODOMO, defensin2_ODOMO: defensin 2 from *O. monticola;* OCLP1_APIME [H9KQJ7], omega-conotoxin-like protein 1 de *A. mellifera;* A0A3G5BID7_9MUSC, venom polypeptide from the giant assassin fly *Dolopus genitalis;* O16B_CONMR [Q26443], Na^+-sodium channel gating-modifier toxin ω-conotoxin MrVIB from the sea snail *Conus marmoreus;* TXFK1_PSACA U1-theraphotoxin-Pc1a [P0C201] from the spider *Psalmopoeus cambridgei;* (**D**). Structural model of *D. quadriceps* ICK-like venom peptide predicted from the venom gland transcript contig1_D07_A11_4_DVB1. The structural model was predicted by homology modelling, using as template the toxin U5- scytotoxin-Sth1a (PDB 5FZX) from the venom of the Spitting Spider *Scytodes thoracica.* The function is still elusive, despite the potentiality to modulate ion-channel activity and neural receptors. This structure displays the classical short triple-stranded antiparallel beta-sheet of knottins, short peptides.

3. Discussion

Bottom-up proteomics strategies have been applied to study the venom protein profiles of several animals, such as cnidarians [31], mollusks [32], snakes [33], and ants. In fact, the compositional differences of the bullet ant *P. clavata* crude venoms that were collected by manual gland dissection and electrical stimulation were thus elucidated [34]. In another study, the venom protein content of the ponerine ant *Pachycondyla striata* was determined employing both in-gel (2-D electrophoresis) and in-solution digestion proteomics, resulting in the identification of 42 spots and 5 proteins [35]. Recently, several proteins were identified from the venom of the trap jaw ant *O. monticola* by in-solution digestion venom proteomics [36].

In the present study, the experimental data of our venomic analysis, which was performed using both in-gel and in-solution-based proteomics approaches, was compared with two transcriptomic datasets of the *D. quadriceps* venom glands, namely, (1) the predicted peptide products of 496 contigs from 800 Applied Biosystems (ABI) Prism files from the Sanger sequencing of venom gland cDNA library and (2) 18,546 assembled transcripts from more than 2,500,000 raw reads obtained from Ion Torrent RNA sequencing [23]. The majority of proteins identified by gel-based proteomics confirmed the transcriptional repertories expressed in the *D. quadriceps* venom gland and counterparts found in the venoms of not only other ant species, but also of wasps and honey bee, despite of their species-specific composition. For instance, in the *D. quadriceps* venom proteome, there are toxins that shared similarity with the venom dipeptidyl peptidase-4 from the parasitic ant *Ectatomma tuberculatum* [37]; the odorant-binding protein and venom allergen 2 from the fire ant *S. invicta* [7]; the phospholipase A1 2, hyaluronidase, venom allergen 3, and glucose dehydrogenase FAD from the stinging ant *P. striata* [35]; and the hyaluronidase and venom allergen 2 from the ponerine ant *O. monticola* were identfied [36]. Moreover, the intra- and interspecific variation of venom components is a known biological phenomenon observed from arthropods to snakes [38–40] herein observed.

The limit of detection for proteins in the Coomassie-stained polyacrylamide gels is approximately 50 ng with a dynamic range of up to 500 ng. Based on this, the resolution of the giant ant crude venom with one-dimensional SDS-PAGE allowed the visualization of the predominant venom polypeptide components of *D. quadriceps* (Figure 1, Table S1). Accordingly, the venom of the giant ant *D. quadriceps* is predominantly composed of venom allergens (major venom allergen 3 and 2/4-like), hydrolases (dipeptidyl peptidase-4, hyaluronidase, GDH, and PLA1), major royal jelly-like protein, and Kunitz-type toxin. However, considering the data from the in-solution proteomics, two additional classes of toxins of lower molecular mass should be included in the giant ant venom composition: pilosulin- and ponericin-like peptides (dinoponeratoxins) and cysteine-stabilized knottins (ICK-like). These experimental data are summarized in Tables S1 and S2.

In the venom cocktail, these polypeptide components can act in combination to efficaciously exert their effect in interfering with victim and/or prey homeostasis. For instance, the venom dipeptidyl peptidase-4-like can modulate the chemotactic activity of immune cells after the sting and trigger immunoglobulin E (IgE)-mediated allergic reactions produced by basophils. Such venom enzyme is also known as allergen C (Api m 5) in the honey bee *A. mellifera* and Ves v 3 in the common wasp *V. vulgaris*. It is also known as the major allergen of the European paper wasp *Polistes dominula* venom [28,41]. However, the role of glucose dehydrogenase [FAD, quinone] in the venom and venom gland of *D. quadriceps* remains unknown. In fruit fly *D. melanogaster*, similar enzyme, UniProtKB–P18173 (DHGL_DROME), is responsible for cuticular modification during morphogenesis. Notably, the homologues of glucose dehydrogenase [FAD, quinone] have being identified in the venom proteome of the parasitic ant *E. tuberculatum* [42], although it was not described as a genuine insect antigen or venom component.

The MRJPs sequence identified in the transcriptome and venom proteome of *D. quadriceps* might represent a new member of the same family, but with distinct function from its counterparts in bee and fruit fly. The MRJPs is known to have anti-apoptotic activity and act in similar way that the nerve growth factor (NGF) does in hepatocyte culture, interacting with mitogen-activated protein kinase and protein kinase B, controlling the pattern of adult fly cuticle pigmentation and larval buccal parts [43]. It is important to note that the MRJP-like protein of *D. quadriceps* shares only 27% of similarity with the *A. mellifera* MRJP-1 and 40% with the *D. melanogaster* yellow protein, which controls the pattern of pigmentation of the fly cuticle and larvae. The yellow proteins (MRJPs) are involved in the enzymatic conversion processes of the melanization pathways [44]. It is interesting note that the C-terminal end of the bee MRJP-1 can be cleaved in jellein-2, which is subsequently cleaved in jellein-1 and jellein-4, which in turn show antimicrobial activity [45]. The jellein-related peptides were not observed in the *D. quadriceps* venom either because the *D. quadriceps* MRJP-1 was not cleaved or because a molecular weight cut-off of 10 kDa was defined for polypeptide analysis in this study. Indeed, it would be necessary to verify if the C-terminus of the *D. quadriceps* MRJP-1 could be cleaved into smaller peptides, similar to jellein antimicrobial peptides, since the *D. quadriceps* MRJP-like venom protein displays a C-terminal segment that has alternating hydrophilic and hydrophobic residues and is rich in proline residues (see green box in Figure 5), close to the lysine residues, the likely site of proteolytic cleavage.

The phospholipases A2 are the main components of bee venoms, while PLA1s are found as the main allergens in wasp venom (e.g., Sol i1, Api m1, Bom p1, Bom t1, Ves v1, Ves m2, Ves s1, Vez c1, Pol a1 and Pol e1). Based on the structural similarity and conservation, the *D. quadriceps* venom PLA1 could cause hemorrhagic disorders and exacerbate envenoming response as a result of its expression in the venom and catalytic activity that generates pharmacologically active lipids. The wasp PLA1 catalyzes the hydrolysis of emulsified phospholipids exclusively at the sn-1 position, releasing free fatty acids and lysophospholipids. Lysophospholipis are multifunctional mediators and second messengers involved in diverse cellular processes, including platelet activity and blood coagulation, as well as in the physiopathology of a number of human diseases [46]. The phospholipase A1 from the black-bellied hornet wasp (*Vespa basalis*) was shown to display a potent hemolytic activity that is responsible for their lethal effects [47,48]. The roles of wasp venom PLAs in platelet activation and allergic response have been reported [49,50]. The roles of PLA1 and PLA2 in the envenomation and allergic response caused by wasps, as well as the involvement of venom PLA1 in allergy caused by ant stings, is reviewed elsewhere and further information can be taken [26,51]. In this context, the PLA1 from giant ant venom is not only an enzymatic component (hydrolase), but also appears as a potential allergen that contributes to trigger a late immune response in the victim.

In the venom of *D. quadriceps*, enzymes are one of the main components that apart from their role in catalytic destruction of tissues that can contribute to allergic responses. Among these venom-enzymes, the hyaluronidase-type found in the *D. quadriceps* crude venom shares structural characteristics with the wasp hyaluronidase; for example, two intra-molecular disulfide bridges formed between four cysteine residues located in conserved positions in contrast to the mammalian hyaluronidases that have four disulfide bonds. The wasp and honey bee hyaluronidases are known allergens found in the hymenopteran venoms (e.g., Ves v2 and Api m2) and, in their catalytically active forms, additionally appear to contribute, together with phospholipases, to the facilitation of venom dissemination [52,53]. In this respect, the venom of the giant ant *D. quadriceps* is comparatively more similar to the venom of wasps and other unrelated ants, like the red fire ant *S. invicta*.

It is well known that allergy is one of the main systemic symptoms in humans injected with hymenopteran venoms. Two other classes of allergens detected in the *D. quadriceps* venom are polypeptides highly similar to the major venom allergen 3 and major ant allergen 2/4-like that we will discuss in the following lines. The venom allergen 3 is the homologue of the red fire ant *S. invicta* Sol i 3 (major venom allergen 3/cysteine-rich venom protein–CAP/SCP superfamily; cysteine-rich secretary protein (CRISP) family). Proteins of this family are characterized by high structural conservation, especially in the arrangement of their disulfide bridges in the CRISP domain, but with high diversity beyond this central region that dramatically alters the target specificity and, therefore, the range of biological activities. Some proteins of the SCP/CAP family have a small CRISP domain, which is found in mammalian proteins and snake toxins, by which they were shown to regulate calcium signaling via the ryanodine receptor [54]. The Sol i 3 antigen is the most common venom polypeptide responsible for allergic hypersensitivity caused by insects in the southeastern United States [55]; therefore, the major venom allergen 3/cysteine-rich protein-like venom component in *D. quadriceps* could play a critical role to trigger allergy. Interestingly, in humans, the CRISP family proteins are most often secreted and have an extracellular endocrine or paracrine function; are involved in processes that include the regulation of matrix morphogenesis and extracellular branching, inhibition of proteases, ion-channel regulation and cell-cell adhesion in fertilization; and act as tumor suppressor or promoters in tissues, including the prostate.

The other venom allergen found preponderantly in the *D. quadriceps* venom belongs to a family of carrier proteins similar to insect pheromone/odorant-binding proteins that is homologous to the main antigen in the fire ant *S. invicta* (Sol i 2) venom (ant venom allergen 2/4 family). Sol i 2 and the related Sol i 4 are potent antigens of the red fire ant venom capable of triggering anaphylaxis [8,56]. The antigen Sol i 2 causes the production of IgE antibodies in approximately one-third of the individuals stung by fire ants. Based on the structural characteristics of Sol i 2 and Sol i 4, they can form homo and/or heterodimers. The recombinant dimeric Sol i 2 produced in baculovirus was crystallized as a native and seleno-methionylated derivative protein, and its structure was determined at 2.6 Å resolution. Its structure is stabilized by three intramolecular and one intermolecular disulfide bridges [57]. Conceivably, Sol i 2 might play a biological role in capturing and/or transport small hydrophobic ligands, such as pheromone, odorant molecules, fatty acids, or short-lived hydrophobic messengers. The venom allergen 2/4-like protein in *D. quadriceps*, herein identified and encoded in the venom gland transcript contig8_B2-2, has one less disulfide bridge in contrast to the *S. invicta* counterpart, which might be considered and grouped with *D. quadriceps* venom allergen 2/4-like polypeptide as a new member of the family of insect pheromone/odorant-binding proteins in hymenopterans. Moreover, based on the fragments detected from the in-gel proteomics analysis, at least three isoforms of similar proteins belonging to the ant venom allergen 2/4 family are expressed in the *D. quadriceps* venom. Altogether, the diverse classes of venom allergens comprise a significant part of venom components in *D. quadriceps* that could effectively cause local and systemic hypersensitivity and immuno-reaction in human and small mammals, being useful to avoid aggressors and predators.

Another important group of toxins in the *D. quadriceps* venom are DNTxs, which are pilosulin- and ponerecin-like peptides that could be classified into short- and long-DNTxs, ranging in size from 11 to 28 residues. They are present in large proportion in the venom gland transcriptome and venom proteome and display membranolytic, cytolytic, antimicrobial, and antiparasitic activities [10,24,25,58]. Given that DNTxs comprise a predominant fraction of transcripts expressed in the *D. quadriceps* venom gland, long and short DNTxs were synthesized and evaluated for their anti-infective activity. Against trypanosomatid parasites (i.e., *Trypanosoma cruzi*), they displayed variable levels of effect, but good profiles of anti-trypanosome activity, better than the drug-of-choice [58]. The *D. quadriceps* DNTxs share structural similarities with antimicrobial peptides, such as ponericins G2/G3 from ponerine and poneromorph ants, and frog temporins Brevinin-1PTa and Gaegurin-5, in case of short-DNTxs, and frog dermaseptin-H65 (and ant ponericins W3/W5, Q49/Q50), in case of long-DNTxs, from vertebrates [10,23–25]. In the present study, four types of DNTxs were found in the in-solution, but not the in-gel proteomics analysis, because of the exclusion size and cut-off value of each technique that selected peptide fragments for analysis. Despite of this fact, DNTxs are the components that contribute to the potency of the venom and, in combination with allergens, play a role in defense and predation.

Last but not the least, cysteine-stabilized peptides, like inhibitor cystine-knot (knottin, ICK-like) peptides are relatively rare in ant venoms, with few examples reported to date [9]. One of these examples is the ICK-like toxins (knottins) annotated from the venom gland transcriptome of *D. quadriceps*. Here, in the *D. quadriceps* crude venom proteomics, three homologous (two of which correspond to the expressed transcript products) were identified through the analytical procedure #2 of peptides generated by in-solution digestion. Found in low abundance, as compared with other venom toxin components, the ICK-like toxins in the *D. quadriceps* venom contrast with the predominance of this class of toxins in spider venom, where dozens of peptides with insecticidal roles are found and grouped in diverse families [59]. Spider ICK-like toxins act mainly on the voltage-gated sodium channels that usually involve three different mechanisms: inhibition of channel opening, prevention of fast inactivation, and facilitation of channel opening, but the final pharmacological effect is the disruption of normal neurotransmission [60]. The other knottin (ICK)-like peptide found in the venom of *D. quadriceps* shares similarity with defensin-2 of insects (Figure 11). Invertebrate (insect) defensins comprise a family of cysteine-stabilized antimicrobial peptides, primarily active against the Gram-positive bacteria. These defensins have been found in arthropods (insects, ticks, spiders, and scorpions), in bivalve mollusks, and even in fungi, but are unrelated to mammalian defensins [61]. The low predominance of the ICK-like toxins in the venom of *D. quadriceps* and in ants, in general, might be the result of the evolutionary pressure and the efficiency of linear and cytolytic peptides, as well as hydrolases (e.g., phospholipases), in prey paralysis and (2) the potency of ICK-like neurotoxins that might be sufficiently high to achieve an efficacious paralyzing effect. Interestingly, the venoms of ancient marine organisms, like cnidarians, are rich in cytolysins and phospholipases that constitute numerous neurotoxins that cause paralysis for prey hunting [62,63]. Taking these facts into account, the biological activity of the ICK-like toxins in *D. quadriceps* should be further investigated, given that they are potentially highly selective ion-channel disruptors, and consequently presumable, insecticidal and germicidal.

Based on our proteomic data, the combined effect of paralysis to hunt prey and induction of allergenicity, to avoid aggressors and predators, seem to be consistent with the compositional content of the *D. quadriceps* venom. Moreover, the cytolytic and membranolytic predicted properties of giant ant toxins to disrupt cell membranes and tissues, presumably contribute to toxin diffusion by increasing blood vessel permeability, thereby facilitating the spread of neurotoxins and allergens and, thus, provoking allergic reaction and hypersensitivity. It is interesting to note that in wasps, the predominance of venom allergens and (hydrolytic) enzymes as components of a toxin cocktail or the high content of neurotoxic peptides and disruptors of primary metabolism in other kind of venom mixture is associated with the behavior pattern of a given wasp species, that is, if a given wasp species is social or solitary. Solitary wasps are eminent hunters that immobilize prey with neurotoxins and metabolic disruptors for oviposition, while social wasps defend their colonies for eventual threats with allergens. Thus, the solitary wasp venom contains toxins that cause paralysis and restrain the metabolism for a very basal status, while the social wasp venom recruits toxins that cause pain and strong allergic reactions for defense [52]. In this view, based on our study, *D. quadriceps* appears to have both paralyzing toxins for hunting and allergens to defer attacks by virtue of their small colonies, with no more than hundreds of individuals [64]. Thus, the composition of the *D. quadriceps* venom, as seen here, seems to reflect a dual role: a toxin cocktail for defense and attack, from the ecological point of view, and a composition of venom polypeptides that cause long-lasting pain and systemic symptoms, from the medical aspects of human envenoming and accidents with ("false") tucandiras.

4. Conclusions

Using the bottom-up proteomic approach, we investigated the protein content of the giant ant *D. quadriceps* crude venom. We identified predominant components that are venom enzymes, allergens, and cytolytic and accessory polypeptides that together appear to potentially promote the diffusion of toxins and trigger allergic responses in prey and victims. Moreover, the less abundant ICK-like toxins could contribute to the paralyzing effect of this predatory giant ant species (*D. quadriceps*). Overall, the present work, shed light on the description of the venom composition of one of the thousands of species of ants and hymenopterans that inhabit Earth.

5. Materials and Methods

5.1. Ant Sampling and Venom Extraction

Adult *D. quadriceps* individuals (~100) were collected as described in one of our previous report [23] and maintained in a terrarium. For venom extraction, these 100 individuals were individually immobilized with a flexible clamp, and venom was collected using a capillary tube that was positioned in the back of an ant's gaster. After extraction, the venom was immediately transferred to ice and pooled. The pool of crude venom was then frozen in liquid nitrogen, lyophilized and stored at −20°C until required for proteomic analysis. This procedure was repeated every two weeks. The access for sampling and studying the venom content of *D. quadriceps* was registered under the numeric codes 28794-1 and A1D1ACF in the System of Management of Genetic Heritage and Associated Traditional Knowledge (SISGEN), Ministry of Environment, Federal Government of Brazil.

5.2. Proteomic Analysis

5.2.1. Separation of Venom Protein by Denaturing Polyacrylamide Gel Electrophoresis (PAGE)

The *D. quadriceps* crude venom was resolved by protein electrophoresis according to Laemmli [65]. The dried venom (30 µg) was solubilized in sample buffer and separated by sodium dodecyl sulfate-polyacrylamide gel electrophoresis (SDS-PAGE, 12.5% T, 2.8% C), under reducing conditions. Protein bands were visualized with Coomassie blue, using a rapid gel staining protocol. A low-molecular mass protein calibration kit for electrophoresis (Amersham, GE Healthcare, Chicago-IL, USA) was employed in this study.

5.2.2. In Gel Digestion and Mass Spectrometry Analyze

The in-gel digestion was conducted according to Westermeier, Naven, and Höpker [66] with small modifications. Firstly, the gel bands were selected, excised, and transferred to a 1.5-mL micro tube. Subsequently, a solution of 75 mM ammonium bicarbonate (in 40% ethanol) was added to destain the bands. Thereafter, the supernatant was removed, 5 mM dithiothreitol (in 25 mM ammonium bicarbonate) was added, and all samples were incubated at 60 °C for 30 min (reduction step); next, we added 55 mM iodoacetamide (in 25 mM ammonium bicarbonate) and incubated all samples at room temperature for 30 min in the absence of light. The supernatant of all individual samples was again removed, and the gel pieces dehydrated by adding acetonitrile (ACN). Subsequently, to each sample, 10 µL of proteomic grade trypsin solution (10 ng/µL in 50 mM ammonium bicarbonate) was added, and digestion was allowed for 45 min on ice. Thereafter, supernatants were removed, gel pieces were covered with 50 mM ammonium bicarbonate and incubated overnight at 30 °C. Finally, each sample was suspended in 20 µL of ACN/5% trifluoroacetic acid (TFA) (1:1, *v/v*) and sonicated for 10 min. The supernatant was again removed and dispensed in a separate tube. We repeated this step three times and combined the supernatants of the same samples. Lastly, we repeated the process using ACN instead of ACN/5% TFA. The obtained supernatant was combined with the previously obtained supernatants.

The tryptic peptides were analyzed by liquid chromatography–mass spectrometry (LC–MS) using an electrospray-ion trap-time of flight (ESI-IT-TOF) system coupled to a binary ultra-fast liquid chromatography system (UFLC) (20A Prominence, ShimadzuKyoto, Japan).. Briefly, samples were dried, resuspended in 0.1% acetic acid, and loaded onto a C18 column (Discovery C18, 5 µm, 50 × 2.1 mm) operating with a binary solvent system: (A) water:acetic acid (999:1, *v*/*v*) and (B) ACN:water:acetic acid (900:99:1, *v*/*v*/*v*). The column was eluted at a constant flow rate of 0.2 mL/min with a 0 to 40% linear gradient of solvent B for 40 min. The eluates were monitored by a Shimadzu SPD-M20A PDA detector before introduction into the mass spectrometer. The interface voltage was set to 4.5 KV, the capillary voltage used was 1.8 KV at 200 °C, and the fragmentation was induced by argon collision at 50% 'energy'. The MS spectra were acquired under the positive mode and collected in the range of 350 to 1400 *m*/*z*. The MS/MS spectra were collected in the range of 50 to 1950 *m*/*z*.

5.2.3. In-Solution Digestion and Mass Spectrometry Analysis

Analysis #1

One milligram of the *D. quadriceps* venom was solubilized in 1.0 mL of 0.1% formic acid, and a-250 µL aliquot was concentrated using a 10-kDa cut-off centrifugal filter (Amicon® Ultra-4 Centrifugal Filter Unit, Sigma-Aldrich, St. Louis-MO, USA). The retentate (peptide fraction >10 kDa) was dried and submitted to in-solution digestion according to Beraldo Neto and colleagues [67]. Briefly, the venom protein samples in 8 M urea were reduced using TCEP-HCl (20 mM Tris(2-carboxyethyl)phosphine hydrochloride, TCEP) at room temperature (RT) for 1 h and then alkylated (10 mM iodoacetamide, IAA) at RT for 1 h in the absence of light. Thereafter, the samples were diluted to a urea concentration of <2 M (with 100 mM Tris-HCl, pH 8.5), followed by the addition of 10 µL proteomic-grade trypsin (10 ng/µL in 100 mM Tris-HCl, pH 8.5). The incubation was performed at 30 °C overnight, and the enzymatic reaction was stopped by adding 50% ACN/5% TFA. The sample was lyophilized, desalted, and concentrated using a ZipTip® C-18 pipette tips (Millipore Co., Burlington, MA, USA). We repeated this step twice, pooling the material of the same samples and drying.

Finally, we resuspended the dried material in 5 µL of 0.1% formic acid, and 1 µL was automatically injected in the EASY Nano LCII system (Thermo Fisher Scientific) into the top 5 cm of a 10-µm Jupiter C-18 trap column (100 µm I.D. × 360 µm O.D.) coupled to an LTQ-Orbitrap Velos mass spectrometer (Thermo Fisher Scientific, Waltham,-MA, USA). The chromatographic separation was performed on a 15-cm long column (75 µm I.D. × 360 µm O.D.) packed in-house with 3-µm ReproSil-Pur C-18 beads (Dr. Maisch GmbH, Ammerbuch-Entringen, Germany) in a binary system: (A) water:formic acid (999:1, *v*/*v*) and (B) ACN:formic acid (999:1, *v*/*v*). The column was eluted at a constant flow rate of 300 nL min^{-1} with a 5% to 35% linear gradient of solvent B for 75 min. The spray voltage was set at 2.2 kV, and the mass spectrometer was operated in the data-dependent mode, in which one full MS scan was acquired in the *m*/*z* range of 300–1,600, followed by an MS/MS acquisition using the collision-induced dissociation of the ten most intense ions from the MS scan. The MS spectra were acquired in the Orbitrap analyzer at 30,000 resolution (at 400 *m*/*z*), whereas the MS/MS scans were acquired in the linear ion trap. The minimum signal threshold to trigger the fragmentation event, isolation window, activation time, and normalized collision energy were set to 1000 cps, 2 *m*/*z*, 10 ms, and 35%, respectively. We applied a dynamic peak exclusion list to avoid the same *m*/*z* of being selected for the next 20 s.

Analysis #2

One hundred micrograms of the *D. quadriceps* venom was analyzed by in-solution digestion, as described in the previous section. The solution of tryptic-digested venom polypeptides was lyophilized, desalted, and concentrated using a ZipTip® C-18 pipette tips (Millipore, Co., Burlington, MA, USA). This step was repeated twice, and the resulting peptide solutions were pooled and dried. Finally, the dried tryptic peptides were solubilized with 5 µL of 0.1% formic acid, and 1 µL was automatically injected into a 15 cm × 50 μm Acclaim PepMap™ C-18 column (Thermo Fisher Scientific, Waltham,-MA, USA) assembled in a nano chromatographer (EASY-nLC 1200 system, Thermo Fisher Scientific, Waltham,-MA, USA) coupled to a Q Exactive Plus mass spectrometer (Thermo Fisher Scientific, Waltham,-MA, USA). A binary solvent system was used: (A) water:formic acid (999:1, *v*/*v*) and (B) ACN:water:formic acid (800:199:1, *v*/*v*/*v*). The peptides were eluted at a constant flow rate of 300 nL/min with a 4% to 40% linear gradient of solvent B for 100 min. Spray voltage was set at 2.5 kV, and the mass spectrometer was operated in the data-dependent mode, in which one full MS scan was acquired in the *m*/*z* range of 300–1,500 followed by MS/MS acquisition using the higher-energy collision dissociation (HCD) of the 10 most intense ions from the MS scan. The MS and MS/MS spectra were acquired in the Orbitrap analyzer at 70,000 and 17,500 resolutions (at 200 *m*/*z*), respectively. The maximum injection time and automatic gain control (AGC) target were set to 25 ms and 3×10^6 for a full MS, and 40 ms and 105 for MS/MS, respectively. The minimum signal threshold to trigger fragmentation event, isolation window, and normalized collision energy (NCE) were set to 2.5×10^4 cps, 1.4 *m*/*z* and 28, respectively. A dynamic peak exclusion was applied to avoid the same *m*/*z* of being selected for the next 30 s.

5.3. Data Processing and Data Analysis

5.3.1. In-Gel Digestion

The LCD Shimadzu raw data were converted to the mascot generic format (MGF) files with the software LCMS Protein Postrun (Shimadzu, Kyoto, Japan) and loaded in the software Peaks Studio V7.0 (Bioinformatics Solutions Inc, BSI, Waterloo-ON, Canada) [68]. Proteomic identification was performed according to the following parameters: error mass (MS and MS/MS) set to 0.1 Da; methionine oxidation and carbamidomethylation were set as variable and fixed modifications, respectively; trypsin as proteolytic enzyme for cleavage; maximum missed cleavages (3), maximum variable PTMs per peptide (3), and non-specific cleavage (one); the false discovery rate was adjusted to ≤1% and only the proteins with score ≥30 and containing at least 1 unique peptide were considered in this study. All data were analyzed against a *D. quadriceps* transcriptomic database (6510 entries; National Center for Biotechnological Information (NCBI) BioProject: PRJNA217939) [23], compiled in 17 April 2016.

5.3.2. In-Solution Digestion

RAW files were directly loaded in the software Peaks Studio V7.0. The following parameters were specifically adjusted; for analysis #1, the MS and MS/MS error mass were set to 15 ppm and 0.5 Da, respectively and for analysis #2, the MS and MS/MS error mass were set to 10 ppm and 0.01 Da, respectively. The following parameters were used in both analyses: methionine oxidation and carbamidomethylation were set as variable and fixed modifications, respectively; trypsin as cleavage enzyme; maximum missed cleavages (3), maximum variable PTMs per peptide (3), and non-specific cleavage (both); the false discovery rate was adjusted to ≤0.1%; only the proteins with score ≥50 were considered in this study. We analyzed all data against a *D. quadriceps* transcriptomic database (29909 entries; built by downloading and merging two transcriptome databases: NCBI BioProjectsPRJNA301625 [69] and PRJNA217939 [23], compiled in 6 August 2018.

After analysis with the Peaks software, the in-gel and in-solution proteomics data were interpreted according to the following rationale:

(a) only one protein for each group (each group containing the proteins identified by a common set of peptides was maintained—Peaks software classification);
(b) If one group contained more than one identified protein, the first protein was maintained and the other protein hits were considered redundant and, thus, were removed;
(c) Despite the item b, additional 9 groups were left aside because they contained redundant sequences (three groups from the "in-solution analysis (i)" data and 6 groups from the "in-solution analysis (ii)" data);

(d) both in-solution datasets and highlighted proteins containing the same contig names were compared;

Based on this workflow, a basic local alignment search for proteins (BLASTx) was performed with all identified sequences, limiting the search for the Hymenoptera order (taxid: 7399). Thus, an alignment with a higher score was achieved in this study.

5.4. Structural Models of Selected Dinoponera Quadriceps Venom Toxin

The homology models of selected toxins were elaborated by means of the Swiss-model server [70]. Molecular graphics and analyses were performed with the UCSF Chimera package, developed by the Resource for Biocomputing, Visualization, and Informatics at the University of California, San Francisco (supported by NIGMS P41-GM103311). In all secondary structure models in this study the α-helix is highlighted in red, β-sheets in yellow, coil/turns in gray, and disulfide bounds in green.

Supplementary Materials: The following are available online at http://www.mdpi.com/2072-6651/11/8/448/s1: Figures S1–S10: Structural organization of toxin precursor transcripts that matched identifiers in proteomic analysis. Tables S1 and S2: Lists of peptide toxins found in the venom of giant ant *D. quadriceps* identified by in-gel and in-solution proteomic analysis, respectively.

Author Contributions: All authors participated in this project. For instance: conceptualization, G.R.-B., Á.R.d.B.P.-d.-S. and D.C.P.; methodology, D.O.C.M., Á.R.d.B.P.-d.-S. and D.C.P. software, D.O.C.M., Á.R.d.B.P.-d.-S., Ú.C.d.O. and D.C.P..; validation D.O.C.M., Á.R.d.B.P.-d.-S. and D.C.P.; formal analysis, D.O.C.M., Á.R.d.B.P.-d.-S., D.C.P. and G.R-B.; investigation, D.O.C.M., A.J.Z. and Á.R.d.B.P.-d.-S.; resources, D.C.P., Á.R.d.B.P.-d.-S. and G.R.-B.; data curation, D.O.C.M. and Á.R.d.B.P.-d.-S.; writing—original draft preparation, D.O.C.M., Á.R.d.B.P.-d.-S., D.C.P. and G.R.-B.; writing—review and editing, D.O.C.M., Á.R.d.B.P.-d.-S., D.C.P. and G.R-B.; visualization, Á.R.d.B.P.-d.-S., D.C.P. and G.R-B.; supervision, Á.R.d.B.P.-d.-S., D.C.P. and G.R.-B.; project administration, D.C.P., Á.R.d.B.P.-d.-S. and G.R.-B.; funding acquisition, Á.R.d.B.P.-d.-S., D.C.P. and G.R.-B.

Funding: Research grants were from São Paulo Research Foundation—FAPESP (#13/07467-1, Á.R.d.B.P.-d.-S.) and the Coordination for the Improvement of Higher Education Personnel (CAPES). Ministry of Education and Culture, federal Government of Brazil (Toxinology Program, Á.R.d.B.P.-d.-S. and G.R.-B.). This research was also funded by the National Council of Research and Development, (CNPq), the Ministry of Science, Technology, Innovation and Communication (MCTI-C), grant numbers 303792/2016 and 1406385/2018-1 (D.C.P.) and numbers 307733/2016-5 and 431077/2016-9 (G.R.-B.). D.C.P. and G.R-B. are senior researchers from CNPq/MCTI-C.

Acknowledgments: The authors are thankful to Katsuhiro Konno, Institute of Natural Medicine, University of Toyama, Toyama, Japan for the intellectual and scientific support to this study. The authors are also grateful to Alba Fabiola Costa Torres and Alice Maria Costa Martins, Faculty of Pharmacy, University Federal of Ceara, CE-Brazil for providing us with the crude venom of the giant ant used in this study.

Conflicts of Interest: The authors declare no conflict of interest. The funders had no role in the design of the study.

Abbreviations

BPTI	Bovine Pancreatic Trypsin Inhibitor
CRISP	Cysteine-rich secretory proteins
ICK	Inhibitor Cysteine Knott (Knottin)
LC-ESI-MS	Liquid chromatography-electrospray ionization mass spectrometry
MRJP	Major royal jelly protein
PDB	Protein Data Bank
PLA1	Phospholipase 1
PLA2	Phospholipase 2
SCP	SCP-like extracellular protein domain
CAP	Cysteine-rich secretory proteins, antigen 5, and pathogenesis-related 1 proteins
SDS-PAGE	Sodium dodecyl sulfate-polyacrylamide gel electrophoresis
Sol i 1	Venom Allergen 1, phospholipase A1, from the fire ant *Solenopsis invicta*
Sol i 2	Venom Allergen 2 from the fire ant *S. invicta*
Sol i 3	Venom Allergen 3, SCP/CRISP-like protein, from the fire ant *S. invicta*
Sol i 4	Venom Allergen 4 from the fire ant *S. invicta*

References

1. Wilson, R.; Gullan, P.J.; Cranston, P.S. *The Insects: An Outline of Entomology*, 4th ed.; Wiley: Hoboken, NJ, USA, 2010; Volume 14.
2. Fernández, F.; Ospina, M. *Sinopsis de las Hormigas de la Región Neotropical*; Instituto de Investigación de Recursos Biológicos Alexander Von Humbolt: Bogotá, Colombia, 2003.
3. Touchard, A.; Aili, S.R.; Fox, E.G.; Escoubas, P.; Orivel, J.; Nicholson, G.M.; Dejean, A. The Biochemical Toxin Arsenal from Ant Venoms. *Toxins (Basel)* **2016**, *8*, 30. [CrossRef] [PubMed]
4. Schoeters, E.; Billen, J. Morphology and ultrastructure of the convoluted gland in the ant *Dinoponera australis* (Hymenoptera: Formicidae). *Int. J. Insect Morphol. Embryol.* **1995**, *24*, 323–332. [CrossRef]
5. Robinson, S.D.; Mueller, A.; Clayton, D.; Starobova, H.; Hamilton, B.R.; Payne, R.J.; Vetter, I.; King, G.F.; Undheim, E.A.B. A comprehensive portrait of the venom of the giant red bull ant, *Myrmecia gulosa*, reveals a hyperdiverse hymenopteran toxin gene family. *Sci. Adv.* **2018**, *4*, eaau4640. [CrossRef] [PubMed]
6. Johnson, S.R.; Rikli, H.G.; Schmidt, J.O.; Evans, M.S. A reexamination of poneratoxin from the venom of the bullet ant *Paraponera clavata*. *Peptides* **2017**, *98*, 51–62. [CrossRef] [PubMed]
7. Dos Santos Pinto, J.R.; Fox, E.G.; Saidemberg, D.M.; Santos, L.D.; da Silva Menegasso, A.R.; Costa-Manso, E.; Machado, E.A.; Bueno, O.C.; Palma, M.S. Proteomic view of the venom from the fire ant *Solenopsis invicta* Buren. *J. Proteome Res.* **2012**, *11*, 4643–4653. [CrossRef] [PubMed]
8. Lockwood, S.A.; Haghipour-Peasley, J.; Hoffman, D.R.; Deslippe, R.J. Identification, expression, and immuno-reactivity of Sol i 2 & Sol i 4 venom proteins of queen red imported fire ants, *Solenopsis invicta* Buren (Hymenoptera: Formicidae). *Toxicon* **2012**, *60*, 752–759. [CrossRef]
9. Aili, S.R.; Touchard, A.; Escoubas, P.; Padula, M.P.; Orivel, J.; Dejean, A.; Nicholson, G.M. Diversity of peptide toxins from stinging ant venoms. *Toxicon* **2014**, *92*, 166–178. [CrossRef]
10. Pluzhnikov, K.A.; Kozlov, S.A.; Vassilevski, A.A.; Vorontsova, O.V.; Feofanov, A.V.; Grishin, E.V. Linear antimicrobial peptides from *Ectatomma quadridens* ant venom. *Biochimie* **2014**, *107 Pt B*, 211–215. [CrossRef]
11. Kikuchi, K.; Sugiura, M.; Kimura, T. High Proteolytic Resistance of Spider-Derived Inhibitor Cystine Knots. *Int. J. Pept.* **2015**, *2015*, 8. [CrossRef]
12. Kobayashi, Y.; Takashima, H.; Tamaoki, H.; Kyogoku, Y.; Lambert, P.; Kuroda, H.; Chino, N.; Watanabe, T.X.; Kimura, T.; Sakakibara, S.; et al. The cystine-stabilized alpha-helix: A common structural motif of ion-channel blocking neurotoxic peptides. *Biopolymers* **1991**, *31*, 1213–1220. [CrossRef]
13. Ojeda, P.G.; Wang, C.K.; Craik, D.J. Chlorotoxin: Structure, activity, and potential uses in cancer therapy. *Biopolymers* **2016**, *106*, 25–36. [CrossRef] [PubMed]
14. Yang, S.; Xiao, Y.; Kang, D.; Liu, J.; Li, Y.; Undheim, E.A.B.; Klint, J.K.; Rong, M.; Lai, R.; King, G.F. Discovery of a selective NaV1.7 inhibitor from centipede venom with analgesic efficacy exceeding morphine in rodent pain models. *Proc. Natl. Acad. Sci. USA* **2013**, *110*, 17534. [CrossRef] [PubMed]
15. Lenhart, P.A.; Dash, S.T.; Mackay, W.P. A revision of the giant Amazonian ants of the genus Dinoponera (Hymenoptera, Formicidae). *J. Hymenopt. Res.* **2013**, *31*, 119–164. [CrossRef]
16. Haddad Junior, V.; Cardoso, J.L.; Moraes, R.H. Description of an injury in a human caused by a false tocandira (*Dinoponera gigantea*, Perty, 1833) with a revision on folkloric, pharmacological and clinical aspects of the giant ants of the genera Paraponera and Dinoponera (sub-family Ponerinae). *Rev. Inst. Med. Trop. Sao Paulo* **2005**, *47*, 235–238. [CrossRef] [PubMed]
17. Madeira Jda, C.; Quinet, Y.P.; Nonato, D.T.; Sousa, P.L.; Chaves, E.M.; Jose Eduardo Ribeiro Honorio, J.; Pereira, M.G.; Assreuy, A.M. Novel Pharmacological Properties of *Dinoponera quadriceps* Giant Ant Venom. *Nat. Prod. Commun.* **2015**, *10*, 1607–1609. [CrossRef] [PubMed]
18. Lopes, K.S.; Rios, E.R.; Lima, C.N.; Linhares, M.I.; Torres, A.F.; Havt, A.; Quinet, Y.P.; Fonteles, M.M.; Martins, A.M. The effects of the Brazilian ant *Dinoponera quadriceps* venom on chemically induced seizure models. *Neurochem. Int.* **2013**, *63*, 141–145. [CrossRef] [PubMed]
19. Noga, D.A.; Brandao, L.E.; Cagni, F.C.; Silva, D.; de Azevedo, D.L.; Araujo, A.; Dos Santos, W.F.; Miranda, A.; da Silva, R.H.; Ribeiro, A.M. Anticonvulsant Effects of Fractions Isolated from *Dinoponera quadriceps* (Kempt) Ant Venom (Formicidae: Ponerinae). *Toxins (Basel)* **2016**, *9*, 5. [CrossRef]
20. Lima, D.B.; Torres, A.F.; Mello, C.P.; de Menezes, R.R.; Sampaio, T.L.; Canuto, J.A.; da Silva, J.J.; Freire, V.N.; Quinet, Y.P.; Havt, A.; et al. Antimicrobial effect of *Dinoponera quadriceps* (Hymenoptera: Formicidae) venom against *Staphylococcus aureus* strains. *J. Appl. Microbiol.* **2014**, *117*, 390–396. [CrossRef]

21. Lima, D.B.; Sousa, P.L.; Torres, A.F.; Rodrigues, K.A.; Mello, C.P.; Menezes, R.R.; Tessarolo, L.D.; Quinet, Y.P.; de Oliveira, M.R.; Martins, A.M. Antiparasitic effect of *Dinoponera quadriceps* giant ant venom. *Toxicon* **2016**, *120*, 128–132. [CrossRef]
22. Sousa, P.L.; Quinet, Y.; Ponte, E.L.; do Vale, J.F.; Torres, A.F.; Pereira, M.G.; Assreuy, A.M. Venom's antinociceptive property in the primitive ant *Dinoponera quadriceps*. *J. Ethnopharmacol.* **2012**, *144*, 213–216. [CrossRef]
23. Torres, A.F.; Huang, C.; Chong, C.M.; Leung, S.W.; Prieto-da-Silva, A.R.; Havt, A.; Quinet, Y.P.; Martins, A.M.; Lee, S.M.; Radis-Baptista, G. Transcriptome analysis in venom gland of the predatory giant ant *Dinoponera quadriceps*: Insights into the polypeptide toxin arsenal of hymenopterans. *PLoS ONE* **2014**, *9*, e87556. [CrossRef]
24. Cologna, C.T.; Cardoso Jdos, S.; Jourdan, E.; Degueldre, M.; Upert, G.; Gilles, N.; Uetanabaro, A.P.; Costa Neto, E.M.; Thonart, P.; de Pauw, E.; et al. Peptidomic comparison and characterization of the major components of the venom of the giant ant *Dinoponera quadriceps* collected in four different areas of Brazil. *J. Proteomics* **2013**, *94*, 413–422. [CrossRef]
25. Johnson, S.R.; Copello, J.A.; Evans, M.S.; Suarez, A.V. A biochemical characterization of the major peptides from the Venom of the giant Neotropical hunting ant *Dinoponera australis*. *Toxicon* **2010**, *55*, 702–710. [CrossRef]
26. Hoffman, D.R. Ant venoms. *Curr. Opin. Allergy Clin. Immunol.* **2010**, *10*, 342–346. [CrossRef]
27. Tholey, A.; Becker, A. Top-down proteomics for the analysis of proteolytic events—Methods, applications and perspectives. *Biochim. Biophys. Acta Mol. Cell Res.* **2017**, *1864*, 2191–2199. [CrossRef]
28. Blank, S.; Seismann, H.; Bockisch, B.; Braren, I.; Cifuentes, L.; McIntyre, M.; Ruhl, D.; Ring, J.; Bredehorst, R.; Ollert, M.W.; et al. Identification, recombinant expression, and characterization of the 100 kDa high molecular weight Hymenoptera venom allergens Api m 5 and Ves v 3. *J. Immunol.* **2010**, *184*, 5403–5413. [CrossRef]
29. Tian, W.; Li, M.; Guo, H.; Peng, W.; Xue, X.; Hu, Y.; Liu, Y.; Zhao, Y.; Fang, X.; Wang, K.; et al. Architecture of the native major royal jelly protein 1 oligomer. *Nat. Commun.* **2018**, *9*, 3373. [CrossRef]
30. Ciolek, J.; Reinfrank, H.; Quinton, L.; Viengchareun, S.; Stura, E.A.; Vera, L.; Sigismeau, S.; Mouillac, B.; Orcel, H.; Peigneur, S.; et al. Green mamba peptide targets type-2 vasopressin receptor against polycystic kidney disease. *Proc. Natl. Acad. Sci. USA* **2017**, *114*, 7154–7159. [CrossRef]
31. Li, R.; Yu, H.; Yue, Y.; Liu, S.; Xing, R.; Chen, X.; Li, P. Combined proteomics and transcriptomics identifies sting-related toxins of jellyfish *Cyanea nozakii*. *J. Proteomics* **2016**, *148*, 57–64. [CrossRef]
32. Leonardi, A.; Biass, D.; Kordis, D.; Stocklin, R.; Favreau, P.; Krizaj, I. *Conus consors* snail venom proteomics proposes functions, pathways, and novel families involved in its venomic system. *J. Proteome Res.* **2012**, *11*, 5046–5058. [CrossRef]
33. Tasoulis, T.; Isbister, G.K. A Review and Database of Snake Venom Proteomes. *Toxins (Basel)* **2017**, *9*, 290. [CrossRef]
34. Aili, S.R.; Touchard, A.; Petitclerc, F.; Dejean, A.; Orivel, J.; Padula, M.P.; Escoubas, P.; Nicholson, G.M. Combined Peptidomic and Proteomic Analysis of Electrically Stimulated and Manually Dissected Venom from the South American Bullet Ant *Paraponera clavata*. *J. Proteome Res.* **2017**, *16*, 1339–1351. [CrossRef]
35. Santos, P.P.; Games, P.D.; Azevedo, D.O.; Barros, E.; de Oliveira, L.L.; de Oliveira Ramos, H.J.; Baracat-Pereira, M.C.; Serrao, J.E. Proteomic analysis of the venom of the predatory ant *Pachycondyla striata* (Hymenoptera: Formicidae). *Arch. Insect Biochem. Physiol.* **2017**, *96*. [CrossRef]
36. Tani, N.; Kazuma, K.; Ohtsuka, Y.; Shigeri, Y.; Masuko, K.; Konno, K.; Inagaki, H. Mass Spectrometry Analysis and Biological Characterization of the Predatory Ant *Odontomachus monticola* Venom and Venom Sac Components. *Toxins (Basel)* **2019**, *11*, 50. [CrossRef]
37. Aili, S.R.; Touchard, A.; Koh, J.M.; Dejean, A.; Orivel, J.; Padula, M.P.; Escoubas, P.; Nicholson, G.M. Comparisons of Protein and Peptide Complexity in Poneroid and Formicoid Ant Venoms. *J. Proteome Res.* **2016**, *15*, 3039–3054. [CrossRef]
38. Zancolli, G.; Calvete, J.J.; Cardwell, M.D.; Greene, H.W.; Hayes, W.K.; Hegarty, M.J.; Herrmann, H.W.; Holycross, A.T.; Lannutti, D.I.; Mulley, J.F.; et al. When one phenotype is not enough: Divergent evolutionary trajectories govern venom variation in a widespread rattlesnake species. *Proc. Biol. Sci.* **2019**, *286*, 20182735. [CrossRef]

39. Carcamo-Noriega, E.N.; Olamendi-Portugal, T.; Restano-Cassulini, R.; Rowe, A.; Uribe-Romero, S.J.; Becerril, B.; Possani, L.D. Intraspecific variation of *Centruroides sculpturatus* scorpion venom from two regions of Arizona. *Arch. Biochem. Biophys.* **2018**, *638*, 52–57. [CrossRef]
40. Schaffrath, S.; Prendini, L.; Predel, R. Intraspecific venom variation in southern African scorpion species of the genera Parabuthus, Uroplectes and Opistophthalmus (Scorpiones: Buthidae, Scorpionidae). *Toxicon* **2018**, *144*, 83–90. [CrossRef]
41. Schiener, M.; Hilger, C.; Eberlein, B.; Pascal, M.; Kuehn, A.; Revets, D.; Planchon, S.; Pietsch, G.; Serrano, P.; Moreno-Aguilar, C.; et al. The high molecular weight dipeptidyl peptidase IV Pol d 3 is a major allergen of *Polistes dominula* venom. *Sci. Rep.* **2018**, *8*, 1318. [CrossRef]
42. Da Silva, J.R.; De Souza, A.Z.; Pirovani, C.P.; Costa, H.; Silva, A.; Dias, J.C.T.; Delabie, J.H.C.; Fontana, R. Assessing the Proteomic Activity of the Venom of the Ant *Ectatomma tuberculatum* (Hymenoptera: Formicidae: Ectatomminae). *Psyche* **2018**, *2018*, 11. [CrossRef]
43. Kamakura, M.; Sakaki, T. A hypopharyngeal gland protein of the worker honeybee *Apis mellifera* L. enhances proliferation of primary-cultured rat hepatocytes and suppresses apoptosis in the absence of serum. *Protein Expr. Purif.* **2006**, *45*, 307–314. [CrossRef]
44. Han, Q.; Fang, J.; Ding, H.; Johnson, J.K.; Christensen, B.M.; Li, J. Identification of *Drosophila melanogaster* yellow-f and yellow-f2 proteins as dopachrome-conversion enzymes. *Biochem. J.* **2002**, *368*, 333–340. [CrossRef]
45. Fontana, R.; Mendes, M.; Souza, B.; Konno, K.; Marcondes César, L.M.; Malaspina, O.; Palma, M. Jelleines: A Family of Antimicrobial Peptides from the Royal Jelly of Honeybees (*Apis mellifera*). *Peptides* **2004**, *25*, 919–928. [CrossRef]
46. Bolen, A.L.; Naren, A.P.; Yarlagadda, S.; Beranova-Giorgianni, S.; Chen, L.; Norman, D.; Baker, D.L.; Rowland, M.M.; Best, M.D.; Sano, T.; et al. The phospholipase A1 activity of lysophospholipase A-I links platelet activation to LPA production during blood coagulation. *J. Lipid Res.* **2011**, *52*, 958–970. [CrossRef]
47. Hou, M.H.; Chuang, C.Y.; Ko, T.P.; Hu, N.J.; Chou, C.C.; Shih, Y.P.; Ho, C.L.; Wang, A.H. Crystal structure of vespid phospholipase A(1) reveals insights into the mechanism for cause of membrane dysfunction. *Insect Biochem. Mol. Biol.* **2016**, *68*, 79–88. [CrossRef]
48. Rivera, R.; Chun, J. Biological effects of lysophospholipids. *Rev. Physiol. Biochem. Pharmacol.* **2008**, *160*, 25–46. [CrossRef]
49. King, T.P.; Kochoumian, L.; Joslyn, A. Wasp venom proteins: Phospholipase A1 and B. *Arch. Biochem. Biophys.* **1984**, *230*, 1–12. [CrossRef]
50. Yang, H.; Xu, X.; Ma, D.; Zhang, K.; Lai, R. A phospholipase A1 platelet activator from the wasp venom of *Vespa magnifica* (Smith). *Toxicon* **2008**, *51*, 289–296. [CrossRef]
51. Perez-Riverol, A.; Lasa, A.M.; Dos Santos-Pinto, J.R.A.; Palma, M.S. Insect venom phospholipases A1 and A2: Roles in the envenoming process and allergy. *Insect Biochem. Mol. Biol.* **2019**, *105*, 10–24. [CrossRef]
52. Lee, S.H.; Baek, J.H.; Yoon, K.A. Differential Properties of Venom Peptides and Proteins in Solitary vs. Social Hunting Wasps. *Toxins* **2016**, *8*, 32. [CrossRef]
53. Kemeny, D.M.; Dalton, N.; Lawrence, A.J.; Pearce, F.L.; Vernon, C.A. The purification and characterisation of hyaluronidase from the venom of the honey bee, *Apis mellifera*. *Eur. J. Biochem.* **1984**, *139*, 217–223. [CrossRef]
54. Gibbs, G.M.; Roelants, K.; O'Bryan, M.K. The CAP superfamily: cysteine-rich secretory proteins, antigen 5, and pathogenesis-related 1 proteins—Roles in reproduction, cancer, and immune defense. *Endocr. Rev.* **2008**, *29*, 865–897. [CrossRef]
55. Padavattan, S.; Schmidt, M.; Hoffman, D.; Marković-Housley, Z. Crystal Structure of the Major Allergen from Fire Ant Venom, Sol i 3. *J. Mol. Biol.* **2008**, *383*, 178–185. [CrossRef]
56. Potiwat, R.; Sitcharungsi, R. Ant allergens and hypersensitivity reactions in response to ant stings. *Asian Pac. J. Allergy Immunol.* **2015**, *33*, 267–275.
57. Borer, A.S.; Wassmann, P.; Schmidt, M.; Hoffman, D.R.; Zhou, J.J.; Wright, C.; Schirmer, T.; Markovic-Housley, Z. Crystal structure of Sol I 2: A major allergen from fire ant venom. *J. Mol. Biol.* **2012**, *415*, 635–648. [CrossRef]
58. Lima, D.B.; Mello, C.P.; Bandeira, I.C.J.; Pessoa Bezerra de Menezes, R.R.P.; Sampaio, T.L.; Falcao, C.B.; Morlighem, J.R.L.; Radis-Baptista, G.; Martins, A.M.C. The dinoponeratoxin peptides from the giant ant *Dinoponera quadriceps* display in vitro antitrypanosomal activity. *Biol. Chem.* **2018**, *399*, 187–196. [CrossRef]

59. Oldrati, V.; Koua, D.; Allard, P.M.; Hulo, N.; Arrell, M.; Nentwig, W.; Lisacek, F.; Wolfender, J.L.; Kuhn-Nentwig, L.; Stocklin, R. Peptidomic and transcriptomic profiling of four distinct spider venoms. *PLoS ONE* **2017**, *12*, e0172966. [CrossRef]
60. Kalia, J.; Milescu, M.; Salvatierra, J.; Wagner, J.; Klint, J.K.; King, G.F.; Olivera, B.M.; Bosmans, F. From foe to friend: Using animal toxins to investigate ion channel function. *J. Mol. Biol.* **2015**, *427*, 158–175. [CrossRef]
61. Koehbach, J. Structure-Activity Relationships of Insect Defensins. *Front. Chem.* **2017**, *5*, 45. [CrossRef]
62. Zhang, M.; Fishman, Y.; Sher, D.; Zlotkin, E. Hydralysin, a novel animal group-selective paralytic and cytolytic protein from a noncnidocystic origin in hydra. *Biochemistry* **2003**, *42*, 8939–8944. [CrossRef]
63. Sher, D.; Fishman, Y.; Zhang, M.; Lebendiker, M.; Gaathon, A.; Mancheno, J.M.; Zlotkin, E. Hydralysins, a new category of beta-pore-forming toxins in cnidaria. *J. Biol. Chem.* **2005**, *280*, 22847–22855. [CrossRef]
64. Monnin, T.; Peeters, C. Monogyny and regulation of worker mating in the queenless ant *Dinoponera quadriceps*. *Anim. Behav.* **1998**, *55*, 299–306. [CrossRef]
65. Laemmli, U.K. Cleavage of structural proteins during the assembly of the head of bacteriophage T4. *Nature* **1970**, *227*, 680–685. [CrossRef]
66. Westermeier, R.; Naven, T.; Höpker, H.-R. *Proteomics in Practice: A Guide to Successful Experimental Design*, 2nd ed.; Wiley-VCH Verlag GmbH & Co.: Weinheim, Germany, 2008. [CrossRef]
67. Beraldo Neto, E.; Mariano, D.O.C.; Freitas, L.A.; Dorce, A.L.C.; Martins, A.N.; Pimenta, D.C.; Portaro, F.C.V.; Cajado-Carvalho, D.; Dorce, V.A.C.; Nencioni, A.L.A. Tb II-I, a Fraction Isolated from *Tityus bahiensis* Scorpion Venom, Alters Cytokines': Level and Induces Seizures When Intrahippocampally Injected in Rats. *Toxins (Basel)* **2018**, *10*, 250. [CrossRef]
68. Ma, B.; Zhang, K.; Hendrie, C.; Liang, C.; Li, M.; Doherty-Kirby, A.; Lajoie, G. PEAKS: Powerful software for peptide de novo sequencing by tandem mass spectrometry. *Rapid Commun. Mass Spectrom.* **2003**, *17*, 2337–2342. [CrossRef]
69. Patalano, S.; Vlasova, A.; Wyatt, C.; Ewels, P.; Camara, F.; Ferreira, P.G.; Asher, C.L.; Jurkowski, T.P.; Segonds-Pichon, A.; Bachman, M.; et al. Molecular signatures of plastic phenotypes in two eusocial insect species with simple societies. *Proc. Natl. Acad. Sci. USA* **2015**, *112*, 13970–13975. [CrossRef]
70. Waterhouse, A.; Bertoni, M.; Bienert, S.; Studer, G.; Tauriello, G.; Gumienny, R.; Heer, F.T.; de Beer, T.A.P.; Rempfer, C.; Bordoli, L.; et al. SWISS-MODEL: Homology modelling of protein structures and complexes. *Nucleic Acids Res.* **2018**, *46*, W296–W303. [CrossRef]

toxins

MDPI

Article

Mass Spectrometry Analysis and Biological Characterization of the Predatory Ant *Odontomachus monticola* Venom and Venom Sac Components

Naoki Tani [1], Kohei Kazuma [2], Yukio Ohtsuka [3], Yasushi Shigeri [4], Keiichi Masuko [5], Katsuhiro Konno [6] and Hidetoshi Inagaki [3,*]

1 Liaison Laboratory Research Promotion Center, Institute of Molecular Embryology and Genetics, Kumamoto University, 2-2-1 Honjo, Chuo-ku, Kumamoto 860-0811, Japan; naotani@kumamoto-u.ac.jp
2 Eco-Frontier Center of Medicinal Resources, School of Pharmacy, Kumamoto University, 5-1 Oe, Chuo-ku, Kumamoto 862-0973, Japan; cokazuma@kumamoto-u.ac.jp
3 Biomedical Research Institute, National Institute of Advanced Industrial Science and Technology (AIST), 1-1-1 Higashi, Tsukuba, Ibaraki 305-8566, Japan; y-ohtsuka@aist.go.jp
4 Department of Chemistry, Wakayama Medical University, 580 Mikazura, Wakayama 641-0011, Japan; yshigeri@wakayama-med.ac.jp
5 School of Business Administration, Senshu University, 2-1-1 Higashimita, Tama-ku, Kawasaki 214-8580, Japan; kmasuko@isc.senshu-u.ac.jp
6 Institute of Natural Medicine, University of Toyama, 2630 Sugitani, Toyama, Toyama 930-0194, Japan; kkgon@inm.u-toyama.ac.jp
* Correspondence: h-inagaki@aist.go.jp; Tel./Fax: +81-29-861-6452

Received: 5 December 2018; Accepted: 12 January 2019; Published: 17 January 2019

check for updates

Abstract: We previously identified 92 toxin-like peptides and proteins, including pilosulin-like peptides 1–6 from the predatory ant *Odontomachus monticola*, by transcriptome analysis. Here, to further characterize venom components, we analyzed the venom and venom sac extract by ESI-MS/MS with or without trypsin digestion and reducing agent. As the low-molecular-mass components, we found amino acids (leucine/isoleucine, phenylalanine, and tryptophan) and biogenic amines (histamine and tyramine) in the venom and venom sac extract. As the higher molecular mass components, we found peptides and proteins such as pilosulin-like peptides, phospholipase A_2s, hyaluronidase, venom dipeptidyl peptidases, conotoxin-like peptide, and icarapin-like peptide. In addition to pilosulin-like peptides 1–6, we found three novel pilosulin-like peptides that were overlooked by transcriptome analysis. Moreover, pilosulin-like peptides 1–6 were chemically synthesized, and some of them displayed antimicrobial, hemolytic, and histamine-releasing activities.

Keywords: ant; venom; mass spectrometry analysis; pilosulin-like peptide

Key Contribution: Overview the venom compositions and bioactivities of the predatory ant *Odontomachus monticola*.

1. Introduction

Ants (Hymenoptera: Formicidae) have been believed to share the same ancestor with bees and wasps, and have many traits in common with them. Since most ant species have a sting with venoms including formic acid, hydrocarbons, amines, peptides, and proteins, for predatory purpose [1], the venom components have been attractive as potential lead compounds for drug development. One of the peptide components in the ant venom is the pilosulin-like peptide. Since Donovan et al. isolated pilosulin 1 cDNA from a *Myrmecia pilosula* cDNA library in 1993 [2], many pilosulin and pilosulin-like peptides have been identified from various ant species [3–5]. Some of the pilosulins and pilosulin-like peptides formed homo- or heterodimers by single or double disulfide bridges, and displayed various bioactivities [2,6,7].

Odontomachus monticola, a predatory ant species in the subfamily Ponerinae, is about 10 mm long, red-brown in color, and has long mandibles [8]. They prey on other insects using their venomous stings, which cause intense pain and prolonged itching in humans. In 2016, Aili et al. reported 528 molecular masses, including 27 disulfide-bonded, without information on their primary structures or biological activities, in the venom of *O. hastatus* by LC-MS analysis [9]. On the other hand, we identified 92 toxin-like peptides and proteins including pilosulin-like peptides 1–6 from *O. monticola* by transcriptome and peptidome analysis [10]. Despite the transcriptome and limited peptidome analysis, the venom components of the ant genus *Odontomachus* have not been fully understood.

In this study, we further analyzed the venom and venom sac extract by ESI-MS/MS with or without trypsin digestion and reducing agent. Our results uncovered 1244 molecular masses, including toxin-like peptides and toxin-like proteins in the venom and venom sac extract of *O. monticola* by ESI-MS/MS without trypsin digestion, and also confirmed the amino acid sequences, amidation, processing, and dimerization with a single disulfide bridge of pilosulin-like peptides. Furthermore, we characterized the physicochemical and biological properties of pilosulin-like peptides. Some of the pilosulin-like peptides have a cationic amphiphilic region and displayed antimicrobial, hemolytic, and histamine-releasing activities.

2. Results and Discussion

2.1. Low-Molecular-Mass Components in O. monticola Venom and Venom Sac Extract

Among the low-mass components, we found two biogenic amines (histamine and tyramine) and three amino acids (leucine/isoleucine, phenylalanine, and tryptophan) in the venom and venom sac extract of *O. monticola* by retention time comparison and elemental analysis (Figure 1).

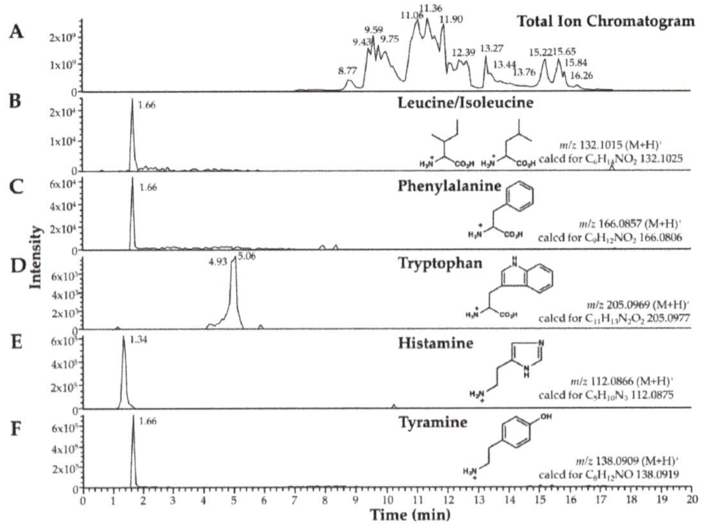

Figure 1. Low-molecular-mass components of *O. monticola* venom and venom sac extract as analyzed by LC-ESI-MS. (**A**) Selected ion chromatograms of total ion chromatogram, (**B**) leucine/isoleucine, (**C**) phenylalanine, (**D**) tryptophan, (**E**) histamine, and (**F**) tyramine. The observed and calculated *m/z* values are shown with the corresponding structural formulae.

Histamine and tyramine interact with their specific receptors and activate specific neurons, being major neurotransmitters in insects, to regulate physiology and behavior. In addition, histamine is partly involved in pain-producing and itching reactions [11]. According to the early studies about ant venoms, histamine has been detected in several ant species [12]. In *Myrmecia pyriformis*, histamine accounted for approximately 2% of venom dry weight [13]. Histamine might be a major and common biogenic amine in ant venoms. Glutamic acid, a neurotransmitter and neurotoxin, was a major and common component in the venoms of five ant species, *Myrmica ruginodis*, *Pogonomyrmex badins*, *Solenopsis saevissima*, *Tetramorium guineense*, and *T. caespitum* L [12], but did not exist in the venom and venom sac extract of *O. monticola*. Most of the ant species might have biogenic amines and amino acids in various combinations. Although social and solitary wasps often have nucleosides (e.g., adenosine and guanosine) and nucleotides (e.g., AMP and ADP), this ant species lacks these compounds in its venom [14].

2.2. Overview of High-Molecular-Mass Components in Venom and Venom Sac Extract

We determined the amino acid sequences from ESI-MS/MS data and searched the amino acid sequences using PEAKS 8.5 against the major 192 components from *O. monticola* venom gland transcriptome data (Table S1). These components were selected from the transcripts which have high relative expression level in the transcriptome analysis or have some similarities with the transcripts of well-known toxins. MS/MS analysis under reducing and nonreducing conditions without trypsin digestion yielded 973 and 517 amino acid sequences (247 overwrapped sequences), respectively. Overall, 545 sequences from a total of 1244 sequences were derived from pilosulin-like peptides.

From the 1244 sequences, 193 were mapped to 50 high-molecular-mass components other than pilosulin-like peptides. The amino acid sequences from MS/MS data without trypsin digestion suggests that some of the proteins might be partially degraded before or after the extraction step. Due to the limited number of sequences in the reference database of the PEAKS 8.5 software, we considered that many of the de novo amino acid sequences were not assigned. Next, we searched the de novo amino acid sequences against 41,764 contig sequences of transcriptome analysis [10] with the tbalstn program to prevent oversight. In this way, 109 sequences were additionally mapped to 70 high-molecular-mass components other than pilosulin-like peptides (Table S2), and 397 sequences were unassigned. Including the MS/MS data with trypsin digestion with the data without trypsin digestion, the amino acid sequences were mapped to 104 components other than pilosulin-like peptides in the venom and venom sac extract by PEAKS 8.5 (Table 1). The total number of components identified from mass spectrometry analysis (183) is much smaller than that of contigs yielded from transcriptome analysis (41,764).

Collecting the venom by electrostimulation has been successful in some large ant species [5]. Since most ant species are too small to apply electrostimulation for collecting venom, a method of dissecting and extracting the venom sac has been applied to collect venoms in many ant species. Because we collected the venom from dissected venom sacs, membrane proteins, cytoskeleton proteins, DNA-binding proteins, translation-related proteins, and replication-related proteins are not believed to represent venom components and are most likely contaminants from venom sac tissue.

The rest of the components were roughly classified into three groups: toxin-like components, non-toxin-like components, and uncharacterized components. Among the toxin-like components we found pilosulin-like peptides, phospholipase A_2s, hyaluronidase, and venom dipeptidyl peptidases of which amino acid sequences have some similarities to those of *Apis mellifera* orthologues in our previous study [10]. These proteins might function in tissue damage, venom diffusion, and venom maturation. Nontoxin-like components included cytochrome P450s and pheromone-binding proteins.

According to the classification of the venom components in *Solenopsis invicta* [15], these proteins might be classified into the groups of self-venom protection and chemical communication for alarm. Among uncharacterized components, we found uncharacterized proteins 1, 3, and 4. Uncharacterized protein 3 has nine cysteine residues, like some of the well-characterized toxins which are rich in cysteine residues, allowing them form unique conformations [16,17].

Table 1. High-molecular-mass components in the venom and venom sac extract detected by LC-ESI-MS.

Peptide/Protein	Accession Number	Coverage (%) [a]			
		TR [b] −, DTT [b] −	TR−, DTT+	TR+, DTT−	TR+, DTT+
acetylcholine esterase	FX985608			1	
apolipophorin 1	FX985561	2	4	8	7
apolipophorin 2	FX985562		10	61	29
calcium-independent phospholipase A_2 gamma	FX985510	12		7	7
carboxypeptidase D	FX985540		5	4	4
carboxypeptidase Q	FX985538			67	26
CDV3 homolog	FX986049		8		
chymotrypsin inhibitor 1	FX986026				11
cytochrome P450 1	FX985568	10		5	4
cytochrome P450 3	FX985570			11	
cytochrome P450 4	FX985571			4	
cytochrome P450 5	FX985572		9	6	9
cytochrome P450 6	FX985573		5		2
cytosolic carboxypeptidase-like protein 5	FX985541			4	7
dishevelled homolog 3	FX986050			3	4
hyaluronidase	FX985505		5	68	47
lysosomal ProX carboxypeptidase	FX985539			3	7
matrix metalloproteinase 14	FX985528			20	18
NADPH cytochrome P450 reductase	FX985574	5		6	5
neuroblastoma suppressor of tumorigenicity 1	FX986056			7	
neuropeptide-like 1	FX986015			7	7
peptidyl-prolyl cis-trans isomerase 1	FX986028			22	17
peptidyl-prolyl cis-trans isomerase 2	FX986029			4	
peptidyl-prolyl cis-trans isomerase 3	FX986030			3	8
peptidyl-prolyl cis-trans isomerase 4	FX986031			7	8
peptidyl-prolyl cis-trans isomerase 5	FX986032			6	7
peptidyl-prolyl cis-trans isomerase 7	FX986034			1	
peptidyl-prolyl cis-trans isomerase 8	FX986035	38			
pheromone binding protein 1	FX985594				14
pheromone binding protein 2	FX985595			11	
pheromone binding protein 3	FX985596			20	
pheromone binding protein 4	FX985597			16	
pheromone binding protein 6	FX985599		4		
phospholipase A_2 isozyme 2	FX985507		11	36	40
protein disulfide isomerase 1	FX985548		8	14	8
protein disulfide isomerase 2	FX985549	19		8	
royal jelly protein	FX986021				9
UDP glucuronosyltransferase 2C1	FX986048			14	4
uncharacterized protein 1	FX985636	4	5	3	6
uncharacterized protein 3	FX986042			19	64
uncharacterized protein 4	FX986043			54	64
UPF0518 protein	FX986054	4	3	3	2
VEGF ^{C}-like protein	FX985521			6	
venom allergen 1	FX985511		7		
venom allergen 2	FX985512			5	
venom allergen 3	FX985513			21	5
venom dipeptidyl peptidase 1	FX985542			4	12
venom dipeptidyl peptidase 2	FX985543			4	4
venom dipeptidyl peptidase 3	FX985544		10	3	5
venom serine carboxypeptidase	FX985537			3	
venom serine protease 2	FX985523		5		
venom serine protease 3	FX985524			6	
very high density protein 1	FX985566	3	3	3	4
very high density protein 2	FX985567		3	5	
vitellogenin 1	FX985563	3	5	5	2
vitellogenin 2	FX985564			10	
waprin 1	FX985515			22	
waprin 2	FX985516			7	11

Table 1. *Cont.*

Peptide/Protein	Accession Number	Coverage (%) [a]			
		TR [b]−, DTT [b]−	TR−, DTT+	TR+, DTT−	TR+, DTT+
40S ribosomal protein SA *	FX985616	8			8
60S acidic ribosomal protein P0 *	FX985621	22	6		3
60S ribosomal protein L10 *	FX985634				11
60S ribosomal protein L3 *	FX985633		10		7
60S ribosomal protein L34 *	FX985627			16	
60S ribosomal protein L36 *	FX985629			15	
60S ribosomal protein L4 *	FX985618			5	8
60S ribosomal protein L6 *	FX985625			5	11
60S ribosomal protein L7 *	FX985622				12
60S ribosomal protein L7a *	FX985617				13
60S ribosomal protein L9 *	FX985635				10
actin, muscle *	FX985587		13	7	7
ATPase WRNIP1 *	FX986047			13	
elongation factor 1-alpha *	FX985554	10		6	
elongation factor 1-beta *	FX985557		5		
elongation factor 1-delta *	FX985559			8	29
elongation factor 1-gamma *	FX985555	20		8	2
elongation factor 2 *	FX985553	4	4	2	8
elongation factor G, mitochondrial *	FX985558		2	11	
elongation factor Tu, mitochondrial *	FX985556		10		3
histone H2A *	FX985611			21	
histone H3 *	FX985610				15
laminin subunit alpha 1 *	FX985614	4	6	5	8
laminin subunit beta 1 *	FX985613		3	3	9
laminin subunit gamma 1 *	FX985612			3	3
myosin heavy chain, muscle *	FX985575	4	3	11	8
myosin heavy chain, nonmuscle *	FX985578		2	1	4
myosin IB *	FX985586			11	13
myosin Ie *	FX985583	5	7	5	9
myosin regulatory light chain *	FX985576				5
myosin Va *	FX985582	2	5	4	8
myosin VIIa *	FX985580		5	6	5
myosin XV *	FX985581	5	5	3	6
myosin XVIIIa *	FX985584	2	5	4	3
resistance to inhibitors of cholinesterase 3 *	FX986036			5	
transcription factor A, mitochondrial *	FX985588				12
transmembrane protein 214A *	FX986055		10	4	4
TRPA channel [d], *	FX985591	5			
TRPM channel [d], *	FX985592	10	2	5	5
TRPV channel [d], *	FX985593				3
voltage-gated potassium channel Shaker *	FX985601		9		
voltage-gated sodium channel beta subunit TipE *	FX985590	9		4	2
voltage-gated sodium channel Para *	FX985589			2	10

[a] The coverages were calculated by combining the peptide fragments with the same amino acid sequences and the same molecular masses by Peaks 8.5; [b] TR and DTT indicate MS/MS data with or without trypsin digestion and DTT treatment, respectively; [c] VEGF: Vascular Endothelial Growth Factor; [d] TRPA, TRPM, and TRPV channels are members of the transient receptor potential (TRP) channel superfamily; * The proteins might be derived from the venom sac.

2.3. Novel Pilosulin-Like Peptides

MS/MS analysis under reducing and nonreducing conditions without trypsin digestion showed that 545 sequences of 1244 total sequences were derived from pilosulin-like peptides; pilosulin-like peptides 1, 2, 3, 4, 5, and 6 have 47, 124, 98, 82, 34, and 101 derivatives, respectively. They included the precursors and degradation products (Table 2; Figure 2B; Figures S1–S6). Because pilosulin-like peptides 2 and 3 have closely related amino acid sequences, they share five common derivatives (Table 2; Figures S2 and S3). Furthermore, we found three novel pilosulin-like peptides in the de novo amino acid sequences, which we termed pilosulin-like peptides 7, 8, and 9 (Figure 2A). To isolate pilosulin-like peptides 7 and 8 cDNAs, we revised raw reads of the transcriptome data in our previous study and found several reads corresponding to pilosulin-like peptides 7 and 8. cDNA clones of pilosulin-like peptides 7 and 8 were isolated by RT-PCR (Figures S10 and S11), indicating that pilosulin-like peptides 4 and 7 and pilosulin-like peptides 5 and 8 each have related nucleotide sequences. Accordingly, four nucleotide sequences (pilosulin-like peptides 4, 5, 7, and 8) were integrated into two sequences (pilosulin-like peptides 4 and 5) by the cd-hit-est software during the assembly process of transcriptome analysis [10]. Pilosulin-like peptides 7 and 8 have 83 and 27 derivatives in the 1244 sequences, respectively. Pilosulin-like peptides 4 and 7 and pilosulin-like peptides 5 and 8 share 41 and 5 common derivatives, respectively (Table 2; Figure 2B; Figures S7 and S8).

We found pilosulin-like peptide 9 in the annotation of de novo amino acid sequences. The unassigned de novo amino acid sequences of MS/MS analysis with trypsin digestion were compared against 41,764 contig sequences of transcriptome analysis [10] by the tblastn program. One of the amino acid sequences (Met-Tyr-Gln-Gly-Leu-Gly-Glu-Lys) (Figure S9) was matched to the contig Om11177_c0_g1_i2, which was annotated to aspartyl/glutamyl tRNA in our previous study [10]. Although tRNAs must be eliminated during the extraction step of total RNA and must not be transcribed by reverse transcriptase, the relative expression level of Om11177_c0_g1_i2 was high and accounted for 1.3% of all reads; so, we considered the contig Om11177_c0_g1_i2 as being a misassembled product of the Trinity software.

We selected the raw reads that encoded the amino acid sequence Met-Tyr-Gln-Gly-Leu-Gly-Glu-Lys and manually assembled the selected reads. The assembled nucleotide sequence encoded a similar leader sequence with pilosulin-like peptides 1–8, and we considered the manually assembled contig as encoding a novel member of the pilosulin-like peptide family. Using the contig sequence, we designed oligonucleotide primers and isolated a DNA fragment encoding the entire open reading frame (ORF) of pilosulin-like peptide 9 by RT-PCR (Figure S12).

Interestingly, the cDNA of pilosulin-like peptide 9 had a structure in which a nucleotide sequence (5′-ATGTACCAAG-3′) was inserted between the nucleotide positions 214 and 215 of the pilosulin-like peptide 1 cDNA. As the result of insertion and frame shifting, the downstream amino acid sequence of pilosulin-like peptide 9 is far different from that of pilosulin-like peptide 1. This may indicate the process of diversification of pilosulin-like peptides. Although we predicted an amino acid sequence of the mature peptide from the nucleotide sequence, only a partial amino acid sequence of pilosulin-like peptide 9 has been confirmed by MS/MS analysis.

Table 2. Amino acid sequences of pilosulin-like peptide derivatives analyzed from MS/MS spectra.

Toxin	Sequence	Molecular Mass	Length	Precursor Ion	RT	Intensity
PLP1	GILDWGKKVMDWIKDKMGK	2247.1907	19	750.0702	37.15	3.67×10^8
	GILDWGKKVMDWIKDKMG	2119.0957	18	707.3729	38.28	9.58×10^9
	GILDWGKKVMDWIKDKM-NH_2	2061.0903	17	1031.5520	39.15	1.34×10^{10}
	GILDWGKKVMDWIKDKM	2062.0742	17	516.5270	38.35	5.74×10^8
	LDWGKKVMDWIKDKMGK	2077.0852	17	520.2803	34.11	2.65×10^8
	GILDWGKKVMDWIKDK	1931.0338	16	483.7657	33.21	1.64×10^8
	LDWGKKVMDWIKDKM-NH_2	1890.9849	15	631.3347	38.44	1.79×10^8
PLP2	EAGWGSIFKTVGKMIAKAAVKAAPEAISAMASQNE	3561.8323	35	891.4648	36.4	6.36×10^8
	GWGSIFKTVGKMIAKAAVKAAPEAISAMASQNE	3361.7527	33	1121.5916	34.85	6.41×10^9
	SIFKTVGKMIAKAAVKAAPEAISAMASQNE	3061.6304	30	766.4222	27.81	1.12×10^9
	GWGSIFKTVGKMIAKAAVKAAPEAISAM	2832.5393	28	709.1410	34.52	4.53×10^8
	GWGSIFKTVGKMIAKAAVKAAPEAISA	2701.4988	27	676.3826	33.09	6.43×10^8
	KMIAKAAVKAAPEAISAMASQNE	2329.2134	23	777.4113	17.04	4.98×10^8
	KAAVKAAPEAISAMASQNE	1885.9567	19	943.9856	15.44	9.06×10^8
PLP3	KIKWGKIFKKGGKLIGKTALEAAANAAASEAISAMASQNE	4101.2407	40	1026.3179	25.25	4.47×10^9
	KIFKKGGKLIGKTALEAAANAAASEAISAMASQNE	3488.8660	35	873.2313	25.16	1.83×10^9
	KIKWGKIFKKGGKLIGKTALEAAANAAASEAISAM	3572.0276	35	894.0147	24.79	2.65×10^8
	KKGGKLIGKTALEAAANAAASEAISAMASQNE	3100.6187	32	776.1608	25.63	2.51×10^8
	KGGKLIGKTALEAAANAAASEAISAMASQNE	2972.5237	31	744.1398	27.22	2.09×10^8
	GGKLIGKTALEAAANAAASEAISAMASQNE	2844.4287	30	949.1498	28.73	5.85×10^8
	KTALEAAANAAASEAISAMASQNE	2319.1011	24	1160.5585	28.03	1.63×10^9
PLP4	GVKELFGKAWGLVKKHLPKAC*GLLGYVKQ	3223.8418	29	806.9683	28.76	1.14×10^{10}
	GVKELFGKAWGLVKKHLPKAC*GLL	2648.5352	24	663.1436	30.27	2.98×10^9
	FGKAWGLVKKHLPKAC*GLLGYVKQ	2697.5305	24	675.3940	20.53	5.56×10^8
	GKAWGLVKKHLPKAC*GLLGYVKQ	2550.4619	23	638.6231	18.8	4.34×10^9
	AWGLVKKHLPKAC*GLLGYVKQ	2365.3457	21	789.4556	19.93	6.44×10^8
	GKAWGLVKKHLPKAC*GLL	1975.1553	18	659.3927	17.99	6.76×10^8
	KHLPKAC*GLLGYVKQ	1710.9603	15	428.7475	16	1.13×10^9
PLP5	IWGALLGTLIPAITSAIQG	1894.0928	19	948.0541	43.31	3.50×10^8
	IWGALLGTLIPAITSAIQ-NH_2	1836.0873	18	919.0532	44.83	7.46×10^9
	IWGALLGTLIPAITSAIQ	1837.0713	18	919.5428	42.58	3.75×10^7
	ALLGTLIPAITSAIQ-NH_2	1479.9025	15	740.9585	36.38	2.25×10^8
	LLGTLIPAITSAIQ-NH_2	1408.8654	14	705.4390	34.1	1.45×10^8
	LLGTLIPAITSA	1168.7067	12	585.3602	30.26	5.15×10^6
	IWGALLGTLIP	1152.6907	11	577.3530	38.86	1.34×10^7
PLP6	IKGKKIMKNMGKAMKIAGKVAKAMAPIVVPLIVSAA-NH_2	3704.2307	36	927.0673	28.61	1.58×10^9
	KIMKNMGKAMKIAGKVAKAMAPIVVPLIVSAA-NH_2	3277.9353	32	820.4910	30.81	8.46×10^7
	IKGKKIMKNMGKAMKIAGKVAKAMAPIVVPL	3263.9561	31	816.9973	23.56	6.27×10^8
	KNMGKAMKIAGKVAKAMAPIVVPLIVSAA-NH_2	2905.7158	29	727.4368	30	2.21×10^8
	GKAMKIAGKVAKAMAPIVVPLIVSAA-NH_2	2532.5376	26	845.1871	29.7	1.46×10^8
	AMKIAGKVAKAMAPIVVPLIVSAA-NH_2	2347.4211	24	587.8628	31.32	1.60×10^8
	KAMAPIVVPLIVSAA-NH_2	1477.9054	15	739.9600	31.65	1.18×10^8
PLP7	GVKELFGKAWGLVKKHLPKAC*GLMGYVKQ	3241.7983	29	811.4578	28.54	4.63×10^9
	GVKELFGKAWGLVKKHLPKAC*GLMGY	2886.5764	26	722.6530	29.82	5.00×10^8
	FGKAWGLVKKHLPKAC*GLMGYVKQ	2715.4868	24	679.8821	19.52	5.42×10^8
	GVKELFGKAWGLVKKHLPKAC*GLM	2666.4917	24	667.6287	29.1	2.48×10^9
	GKAWGLVKKHLPKAC*GLMGYVKQ	2568.4185	23	643.1163	17.44	4.67×10^9
	LVKKHLPKAC*GLMGYVKQ	2069.1641	18	518.2991	13.87	2.37×10^7
	HLPKAC*GLMGYVKQ	1600.8218	14	534.6163	16.8	9.41×10^8
PLP8	FWGALLAAAIPAITSAIQG	1870.0352	19	936.0242	42.69	2.01×10^8
	FWGALLAAAIPAITSAIQ-NH_2	1812.0298	18	907.0258	44.13	2.77×10^9
	GALLAAAIPAITSAIQ-NH_2	1478.8820	16	740.4485	44.09	2.20×10^7
	FWGALLAAAIPAITS	1500.8340	15	751.4250	37.82	1.60×10^7
	ALLAAAIPAITSAIQ-NH_2	1421.8606	15	711.9372	32.08	7.32×10^7
	LAAAIPAITSAIQ-NH_2	1237.7394	13	619.8778	25.83	8.77×10^7
	AAAIPAITSAIQ-NH_2	1124.6553	12	563.3350	23.08	2.19×10^9

C* = S-(carbamoylmethyl)-L-cysteine. The amino acid sequences of the highest and second-highest intensities are highlighted by red and yellow, respectively.

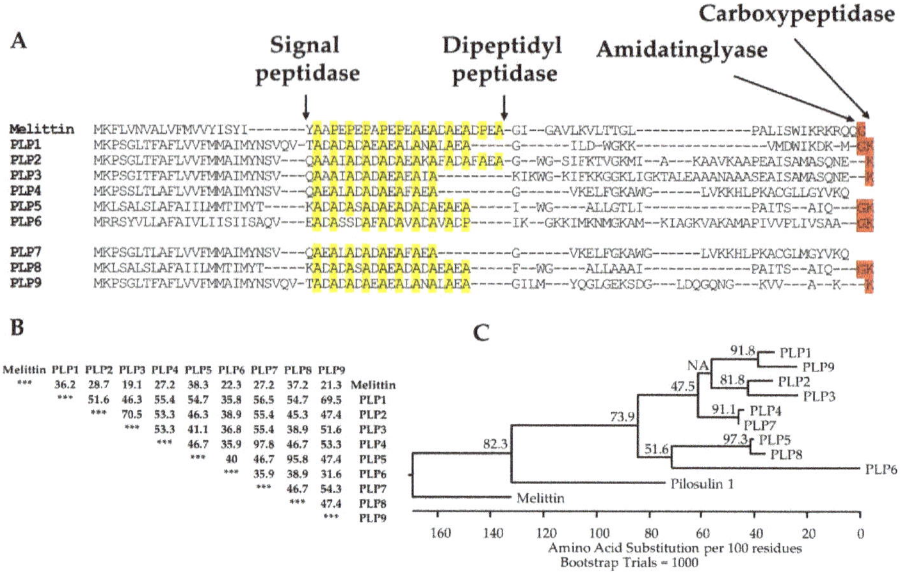

Figure 2. Multiple alignment, identity matrix, and phylogenic analysis of pilosulin-like peptides. (**A**) The amino acid sequences of melittin and pilosulin-like peptides were aligned with ClustalW in Lasergene 12 (DNASTAR, Madison, WI, USA) and manually modified. Arrows indicate the putative processing and modification sites for signal peptidase, dipeptidyl peptidase, amidatinglyase, and carboxypeptidase. Proline and alanine residues in the spacer region between the signal and mature peptides of pilosulin-related peptides are highlighted in yellow. Nucleotide sequences for pilosulin-like peptides 7, 8, and 9 were assigned DDBJ/EMBL/GenBank Accession Numbers LC416796–LC416798, respectively. (**B**) Percentage amino acid sequence identities between melittin and pilosulin-like peptides are shown. (**C**) The alignment of pilosulin-like peptides, pilosulin 1, and melittin precursors by ClustalV in Lasergene 12 was used to construct a phylogenic tree using the neighbor-joining (NJ) method. The phylogenic tree rooted with the amino acid sequence of melittin. The numbers above the branches indicate the percentage of 1000 bootstrap replicates.

2.4. Mature Forms of Pilosulin-Like Peptides

In our previous study, we predicted the N-termini of every mature pilosulin-like peptide, the elimination of Lys residues at the C-termini, and the amidation at the C-termini of some of the mature pilosulin-like peptides [10]. Signal peptidase, dipeptidyl peptidase, amidatinglyase, and carboxypeptidase, some of which are detected by ESI-MS/MS analysis (Tables 1 and S2), might be involved in the processing and modification of pilosulin-like peptides (Figure 2A). The peptides of highest or second-highest signal intensity corresponded to the predicted mature peptides by nucleotide sequences. Since the signal intensity is affected by the abundance of the peptide in the venom and venom sac extract, the peptides of highest or second-highest signal intensity might be the major components in the venom. In addition to the mature peptides, we found the precursors of pilosulin-like peptides that have Gly or Gly–Lys residues at the C-termini and the degradation products of pilosulin-like peptides (Table 2). We compared the LC-ESI-MS profile of the crude venom and venom sac extract under reducing and nonreducing conditions. A broad peak (retention time around 31.58 min), which consisted of three masses (6331.6249, 6349.6355, and 6367.6460) under the nonreducing condition, was divided into two peaks (retention time 28.14 and 28.80 min), which consisted of two masses (3223.8418 and 3241.7983) under the reducing condition (Figure 3). These observed molecular masses were identical to the theoretical masses of mature pilosulin-like peptides 4 and 7 monomers, respectively. Consequently, we confirmed that pilosulin-like peptides 4 and 7 formed a homo- or heterodimer by a disulfide bridge (Figure 4).

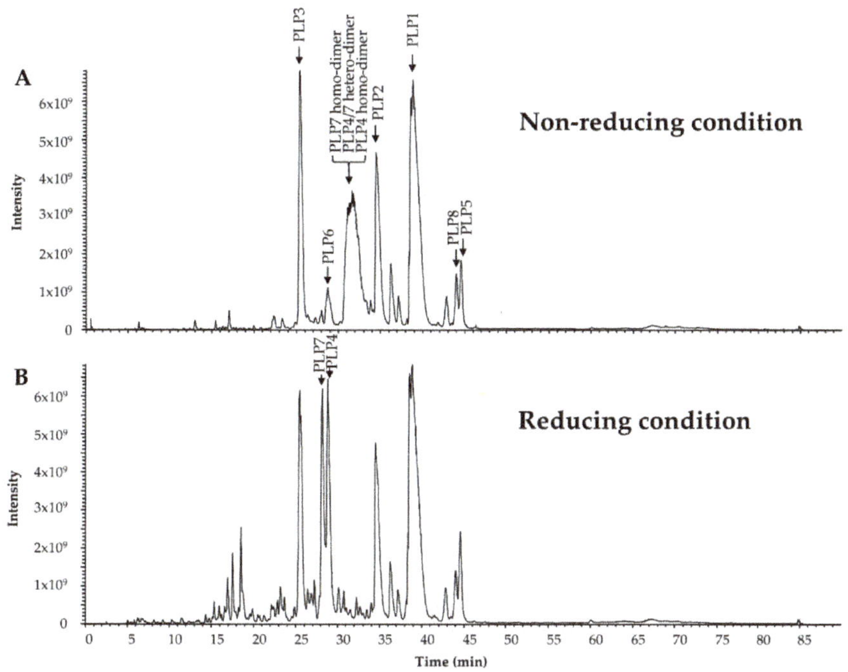

Figure 3. High-molecular-mass components of *O. monticola* venom and venom sac extract as analyzed by LC-ESI-MS. (**A**) The patterns of the total ion current of *O. monticola* venom and venom sac extract under nonreducing and (**B**) reducing conditions are shown. Peaks containing pilosulin-like peptides are labeled by arrows.

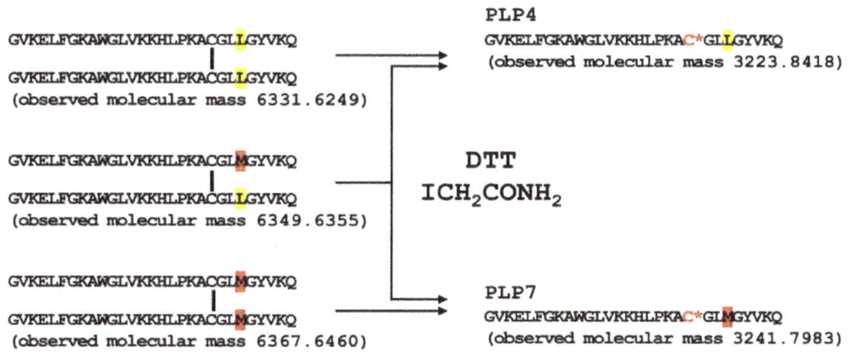

Figure 4. Dimer formation of pilosulin-like peptides 4 and 7. Monomers of pilosulin-like peptides 4 and 7 were connected by a disulfide bridge at the amino acid position 21. Unique amino acid residues in pilosulin-like peptides 4 and 7 are highlighted in yellow and red, respectively. C* indicates S-(carbamoylmethyl)-L-cysteine.

2.5. Structural and Physicochemical Properties of Pilosulin-Like Peptides

Pilosulins are α-helical cationic antimicrobial peptides [2,6,7]. We examined the secondary structure of pilosulin-like peptides using Proteus [18]. Proteus showed that mature regions of pilosulin-like peptides 1–8 are α-helical structures, but pilosulin-like peptide 9 is a coiled-coil structure. The pI of the mature pilosulin-like peptides, without consideration of amidation at C-termini, was calculated with IPC [19]. IPC demonstrated that the mature pilosulin-like peptides 5 and 8 are acidic peptides (calculated pI = 5.98) and the others are basic peptides. The calculated pIs of the mature pilosulin-like peptides 1, 2, 3, 4, 6, 7, and 9 are 8.46, 8.89, 9.06, 9.18, 9.96, 9.18, and 8.46, respectively. Taken together, pilosulin-like peptides 1–4, 6, and 7 may function as α-helical cationic antimicrobial peptides. To test whether pilosulin-like peptides have a cationic, amphiphilic helical conformation, the net charge and hydrophobic indexes of pilosulin-like peptides were examined using HeliQuest [20]. Parameters to search cationic amphipathic α-helix regions of pilosulin-like peptides were determined based on a well-known cationic amphipathic antimicrobial peptide, cecropin A (GenBank accession No. AAA29185): hydrophobicity 0–0.6, hydrophobic moment 0.1–1.0, and net charge 3–10. HeliQuest found cationic amphipathic α-helix sequences in pilosulin-like peptides 2–4, 6, and 7 (Figure 5A). Furthermore, helical wheel projections demonstrated that they are typical cationic α-helical amphiphilic peptides, in which hydrophobic amino acids are located on one side and basic amino acids are on the other side (Figure 5B). However, HeliQuest could not find an α-helical region that showed a typical cationic amphiphilic peptide in pilosulin-like peptide 1, since the mature form of pilosulin-like peptide 1 is shorter than the default setting (18 amino acids) of HeliQuest and the net charge is less than two.

A

PLP2	GWGSIFKTVGKMIAKAAVKAAPEAISAMASQNE
PLP3	KIKWGKIFKKGGKLIGKTALEAAANAAASEAISAMASQNE
PLP4, 7	GVKELFGKAWGLVKKHLPKACGL(L/M)GYVKQ
PLP6	IKGKKIMKNMGKAMKIAGKVAKAMAPIVVPLIVSAA

B

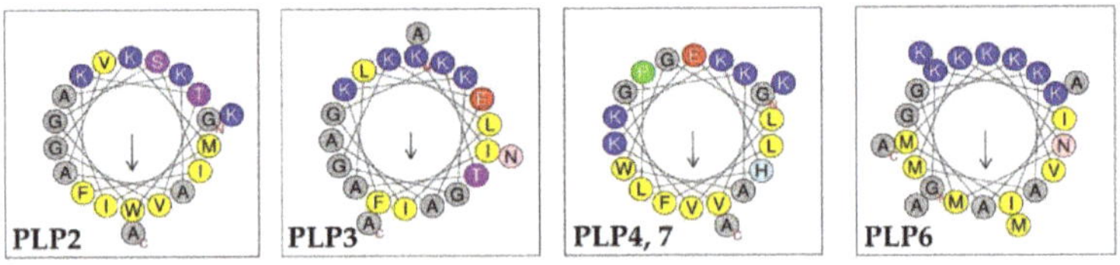

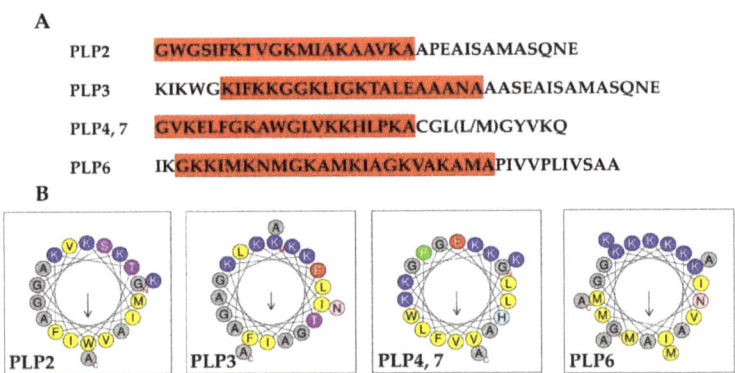

Figure 5. Amino acid sequences and helical wheel projection of pilosulin-like peptides 2, 3, 4, 6, and 7. (**A**) Amino acid sequences of mature pilosulin-like peptides. The cationic amphipathic helix regions in pilosulin-like peptides (PLP) 2, 3, 4, 6, and 7 predicted by HeliQuest are highlighted in red. (**B**) Helical wheel projections of pilosulin-like peptides 2, 3, 4, 6, and 7 drawn by HeliQuest. Nonpolar amino acids (F, I, L, M, V, and W), basic amino acids (K), acidic amino acids (D), small polar amino acids (A and G), aromatic polar amino acids (H), hydroxyl-containing polar amino acids (S and T), amide-containing polar amino acids (N), and proline (P) are highlighted by yellow, blue, red, gray, sky-blue, purple, pink, and green color, respectively.

2.6. Biological Activities of Pilosulin-Like Peptides

Pilosulin-like peptides 1–6 were chemically synthesized by the 9-fluorenylmethyloxycarbonyl (Fmoc) method, and we examined their biological activities (Table 3). We synthesized homodimeric pilosulin-like peptide 4, which was linked by a single disulfide bond. Pilosulin-like peptides 1–4 and 6 with a cationic α-helix displayed antimicrobial activities against *Escherichia coli* and *Staphylococcus aureus*. These activities were higher than those of magainin, a well-known *Xenopus laevis* antimicrobial peptide [21]. Interestingly, pilosulin-like peptide 4 also had high antimicrobial activities against *Saccharomyces cerevisiae*. In support of these experimental results, the antifungal peptide prediction server Antifp predicted that pilosulin-like peptide 4, but not other pilosulin-like peptides, was an antifungal peptide [22]. Virtual alanine scanning of pilosulin-like peptide 4 by Antifp revealed that the replacement of a cysteine residue remarkably reduced the index of antifungal activity. Cysteine residues are known to be abundant in antifungal peptides in general [22], and the replacement of cysteine with serine in brevinin-1B Ya, a frog antimicrobial peptide, reduced the antifungal activity [23]. The cysteine residue of pilosulin-like peptide 4 may be important for antifungal activity.

Table 3. Biological properties of *O. monticola* pilosulin-like peptides.

Peptide	**MIC [a] (μM)**			**Hemolytic Activity (%)**		**Histamine-Releasing Activity at 10 μM (%)**
	E. coli **(NBRC 14237)**	***S. aureus*** **(NBRC 12732)**	***S. cerevisiae*** **(NBRC 10217)**	**at 10 μM**	**at 50 μM**	
PLP1	<3.1	<3.1	<50	Negative		32.9
PLP2	<6.2	<6.2	<50	Negative	10.4	30.1
PLP3	<3.1	<25	<50	Negative		37.5
PLP4	<3.1	<3.1	<3.1	Negative	10.5	66.4
PLP5	<50	Negative	Negative	6.9	94.8	28.3
PLP6	<3.1	<3.1	Negative	Negative		33.6
Magainin	<12.5	<25	Negative	-		-
Mastoparan	-	-	-	13.5 [b]	-	31.1 [b]
Melittin	-	-	-	100.0 [b]	-	64.3 [b]

[a] MIC: minimum inhibitory concentration; [b] The activities indicate from Shigeri et al. [24]; -: not determined.

Pilosulin-like peptide 5 with an acidic α-helix had no or low antimicrobial activities against all the microbes tested in this study, but had the highest hemolytic activity among pilosulin-like peptides 1–6. This hemolytic activity may depend on higher hydrophobicity. Previous studies suggested a correlation between peptide hydrophobicity and hemolytic activity [25]. For example, melittin, a honey bee hemolytic peptide, shows a higher hydrophobicity (0.45–0.88). Hydrophobicity of pilosulin-like peptide 5 is 0.914, which is the highest among pilosulin-like peptides.

Pilosulin-like peptides are major components of *O. monticola* venom sac extract. The first step in the antimicrobial mechanism has been suggested to be these peptides binding to the anionic phospholipids that are abundant in bacterial membranes, which is then followed by pore formation by α-helical cationic peptides as the second step [26]. The variations of antimicrobial activities might reflect on the difference of the physicochemical properties among pilosulin-like peptides.

Pilosulin-like peptide 4 had histamine-releasing activity against rat mast cells comparable to that of melittin, which displays histamine-releasing activity.

3. Conclusions

In this study, we have analyzed the venom and venom sac extract of *O. monticola* by mass spectrometry analysis. Because of the high sensitivity of the analysis, the extract accounting for just one fifth of a venom sac was enough for a single MS/MS analysis. We determined 1244 amino acid sequences by ESI-MS/MS analysis without trypsin digestion. In total, 545 of them were derived from pilosulin-like peptides 1–8, and 302 amino acid sequences corresponded to the high molecular mass components that were identified from our previous transcriptome analysis. This MS/MS analysis suggests that the majority of the venom components might be 2–6.5-kDa peptides.

Synthetic pilosulin-like peptides 1–4 and 6 displayed antimicrobial and histamine-releasing activities. Moreover, pilosulin-like peptide 5 showed the highest hemolytic activity among pilosulin-like peptides. Some of the ant toxins show various biological activities, such as neurotoxic [27,28] and enzymatic activity [29]. In future studies, we will further explore the multiple activities of pilosulin-like peptides.

4. Materials and Methods

4.1. *Ants*

One *O. monticola* colony was collected in Musashimurayama, Tokyo, Japan, on 1 July 2016. The species was morphologically identified.

4.2. *Liquid Chromatography-Mass Spectrometry (LC-MS) Analysis for Low-Molecular-Weight Components*

Twenty *O. monticola* venom sacs were collected and extracted with 50% acetonitrile containing 0.1% (*v*/*v*) trifluoroacetic acid (50 μL) for 2 h at 4 °C. A single venom sac contains 50–150 nL of venom. The extract was passed through a 0.45-μm filter and successively diluted with the extraction solvent to a final concentration of 0.04 sacs/μL. This dilution was used for the LC-MS analysis. The LC conditions were: solvent A, 0.1% (*v*/*v*) aqueous formic acid; solvent B, 0.1% (*v*/*v*) formic acid in acetonitrile; 5–65% linear gradient of solvent B in solvent A at a flow rate of 200 μL/min; column, Capcell Pak C18 UG 120 (1.5 × 150 mm, Shiseido, Tokyo, Japan); column temperature, 25 °C. The molecular weights of the ant peptides were verified by LTQ Orbitrap XL-ETD (Thermo Fisher Scientific, Waltham, MA, USA). The MS conditions were: ionization, electrospray in positive mode; ion spray voltage, 4.6 kV; capillary temperature, 350 °C; capillary and tube lens voltages, 19 V and 35 V, respectively; detector, an Orbitrap at a resolution of 60,000 at m/z 400. MS scan range was m/z 100–2000. The mass spectrometer was calibrated with polytyrosine, and the resolution was usually 1–3 ppm after measurement.

4.3. *Liquid Chromatography-Mass Spectrometry (LC-MS) Analysis for Peptide and Protein Components*

After filtration of the venom sac extract, the extract was diluted 10 times with 50 mM ammonium bicarbonate, pH 8.0, to improve separation and prevent peak tailing in HPLC. The diluted extract was reduced with DTT at a concentration of 10 mM (Thermo Fisher Scientific), alkylated with iodoacetamide at a concentration of 20 mM (Thermo Fisher Scientific), or digested by trypsin at a concentration of ca. 30 μg/mL (Promega, Madison, WI, USA) overnight at 37 °C. Separation was achieved by Zaplous α pep C18 analytical column (3 μm 120A, 1.5 × 150 mm, AMR, Tokyo, Japan) with L-Trap column (5 μm, 0.3 × 5 mm, AMR, Tokyo, Japan) at a flow rate of 500 μL/min using two mobile phases, 0.1% (*v*/*v*) aqueous formic acid (solvent A) and 0.1% (*v*/*v*) formic acid in acetonitrile (solvent B). The following gradient was used: 0–60 min, 5–65% solvent B; 60–70 min, 65–95% solvent B; 70–80 min, 95% solvent B.

The molecular weights of the ant peptides were verified by Q Exactive (Thermo Fisher Scientific, Waltham, MA, USA). The MS conditions were: ionization, nanoelectrospray (CaptiveSpray Ionization: CSI) in positive mode; ion spray voltage, 1.4 kV; capillary temperature, 250 °C; S-lens level, 50; detector, an Orbitrap at a resolution of 70,000 from m/z 350–2000. The mass spectrometer was calibrated with a calibrant of LTQ Velos ESI Positive Ion Calibration Solution (Thermo Fisher Scientific), and the mass accuracy was usually 1–3 ppm after measurement. The raw mass spectrum was processed by using Xcalibur (Thermo Fisher Scientific). Peptide sequences were determined from MS/MS spectra by PEAKS 8.5 (Bioinformatics Solutions, Waterloo, Canada; parent mass error tolerance 10.0 ppm, fragment mass error tolerance 0.02 Da, score threshold 15.0) and manually checked. We selected 192 amino acid sequences derived from major transcripts in the venom gland transcriptome analysis and the 116 amino acid sequences of common external contaminants from cRAP (Global Proteome Machine Organization). After construction of a FASTA format file including 308 amino acid sequences, the file was incorporated into PEAKS 8.5 software as the reference database.

To assign the de novo amino acid sequences, tblastn (parameters: *E*-value 0.1, matrix PAM40, word size 3) was performed using 41,764 contig sequences of transcriptome analysis.

4.4. *Pilosulin-Like Peptides 7–9 cDNA Cloning and Sequencing*

Total RNA isolated from the ant venom glands with sacs was reverse-transcribed to cDNA and amplified by PCR with KOD-Plus-Neo (Toyobo, Osaka, Japan). The oligonucleotide primers used for pilosulin-like peptide 7 were Pilo U1 (5′-ATGAAACCGTCGGGTATCAC-3′), corresponding to nucleotides (nt) 9–28 of pilosulin-like peptide 2; 41CPas (5′-TTGCTTTACGTATCCCAT-3′); 41CP (5′-CCAAAGCGTGTGGACTGA-3′); and Oligo-dT (5′-GAGTCGACTCGAGAA(T)17-3′). 41CP and 41CPas primers were designed from transcriptome analysis data and the amino acid sequences: Met-Gly-Tyr-Val-Lys-Gln; Lys-Ala-Cys-Gly-Leu-Met. The oligonucleotide primers used for pilosulin-like peptide 8 were 51S (5′-TATGTGTGAAAGCTCTTC-3′) and 51AS (5′-CCAATGTAATGCCAATCG-3′), designed based on the 5′ and 3′ untranslated regions predicted by transcriptome analysis. The oligonucleotide primers used for pilosulin-like peptide 9 were Pilo U1, 9CPas (5′-CCCCAGTCCTTGGTACAT-3′), 9CP (5′-ATGTACCAAGGACTGGGG-3′), and Oligo-dT. 9CP and 9CPas primers were designed from the transcriptome analysis data and the amino acid sequence: Met-Tyr-Gln-Gly-Leu-Gly-Glu-Lys. The amplified products of the cDNAs were cloned into the EcoRI site of pBluescript II SK(-) (Agilent Technologies, La Jolla, CA, USA). All inserts were sequenced using a Model 3500 Genetic Analyzer (Thermo Fisher Scientific, Waltham, MA, USA).

4.5. Synthesis and Biological Activities of Pilosulin-Like Peptides

Pilosulin-like peptides 1–6 were prepared using Fmoc chemistry by GenScript (Nanjing, Jiangsu, China). The peptides were purified by RP-HPLC with a preparative C18 column. The purity and molecular weight of the final peptides were verified by HPLC and MS. Antimicrobial, hemolytic, and histamine-releasing activities were measured as described previously [6].

4.6. WEB Server Used to Analyze the Physiochemical Properties

Secondary structure prediction was performed by Proteus (http://www.proteus2.ca/proteus/). The pI of peptides was calculated with IPC (http://isoelectric.org/index.html). The physicochemical properties were examined using HeliQuest (http://heliquest.ipmc.cnrs.fr/). The antifungal peptide prediction was carried out using the Antifp server (http://webs.iiitd.edu.in/raghava/antifp/index.html).

Supplementary Materials: The following are available online at http://www.mdpi.com/2072-6651/11/1/50/s1, Figures S1–S9 (MS spectra of pilosulin-like peptides 1–9), Figures S9–S12 (Nucleotide and deduced amino acid sequences of pilosulin-like peptides 7–9), Table S1 (Major 192 components of *O. monticola* venom), and Table S2 (Protein assignment of the de novo amino acid sequences).

Author Contributions: N.T., K.K. (Kazuma), and K.K. (Konno) performed the ESI-MS; K.M. corrected and classified the ant species; H.I. examined the biological activities; Y.O. checked physicochemical properties; Y.S. and K.K. (Konno) prepared pilosulin-like peptides; Y.O., Y.S., and H.I. wrote the paper.

Funding: This work was supported by JSPS KAKENHI (Grant Nos. 15K07805 and 15K01814) and the program of the Joint Usage/Research Center for Developmental Medicine, Institute of Molecular Embryology and Genetics, Kumamoto University.

Acknowledgments: We thank Toshiyuki Sato (Tokyo University of Agriculture and Technology), Mamoru Terayama (University of Tokyo), Katsuyuki Eguchi (Tokyo Metropolitan University), Rijal Satria (Tokyo Metropolitan University) for their assistance in the field survey, and Masaki Okano for the arrangement of ESI-MS/MS usage. We are also grateful to Leslie Sargent Jones (Appalachian State University, Retired) for her careful reading of our manuscript.

Conflicts of Interest: The authors declare no conflict of interest.

References

1. Aili, S.R.; Touchard, A.; Escoubas, P.; Padula, M.P.; Orivel, J.; Dejean, A.; Nicholson, G.M. Diversity of peptide toxins from stinging ant venoms. *Toxicon* **2014**, *92*, 166–178. [CrossRef] [PubMed]
2. Donovan, G.R.; Baldo, B.A.; Sutherland, S. Molecular cloning and characterization of a major allergen (Myr p I) from the venom of the Australian jumper ant, *Myrmecia pilosula*. *Biochim. Biophys. Acta* **1993**, *1171*, 272–280. [CrossRef]

3. Torres, A.F.; Huang, C.; Chong, C.M.; Leung, S.W.; Prieto-da-Silva, A.R.; Havt, A.; Quinet, Y.P.; Martins, A.M.; Lee, S.M.; Radis-Baptista, G. Transcriptome analysis in venom gland of the predatory giant ant *Dinoponera quadriceps*: Insights into the polypeptide toxin arsenal of hymenopterans. *PLoS ONE* **2014**, *9*, e87556. [CrossRef] [PubMed]
4. Touchard, A.; Tene, N.; Song, P.C.T.; Lefranc, B.; Leprince, J.; Treilhou, M.; Bonnafe, E. Deciphering the molecular diversity of an ant venom peptidome through a venomics approach. *J. Proteome Res.* **2018**, *17*, 3503–3516. [CrossRef]
5. Robinson, S.D.; Mueller, A.; Clayton, D.; Starobova, H.; Hamilton, B.R.; Payne, R.J.; Vetter, I.; King, G.F.; Undheim, E.A.B. A comprehensive portrait of the venom of the giant red bull ant, *Myrmecia gulosa*, reveals a hyperdiverse hymenopteran toxin gene family. *Sci. Adv.* **2018**, *4*, eaau4640. [CrossRef]
6. Inagaki, H.; Akagi, M.; Imai, H.T.; Taylor, R.W.; Kubo, T. Molecular cloning and biological characterization of novel antimicrobial peptides, pilosulin 3 and pilosulin 4, from a species of the Australian ant genus *Myrmecia*. *Arch. Biochem. Biophys.* **2004**, *428*, 170–178. [CrossRef]
7. Inagaki, H.; Akagi, M.; Imai, H.T.; Taylor, R.W.; Wiese, M.D.; Davies, N.W.; Kubo, T. Pilosulin 5, a novel histamine-releasing peptide of the Australian ant, *Myrmecia pilosula* (Jack Jumper Ant). *Arch. Biochem. Biophys.* **2008**, *477*, 411–416. [CrossRef]
8. Kubota, M.; Imai, H.T.; Kondo, M.; Onoyama, K.; Ogata, K.; Terayama, M.; Yoshimura, M. Japanese Ant Image Database. Available online: http://ant.miyakyo-u.ac.jp/ (accessed on 21 November 2018).
9. Aili, S.R.; Touchard, A.; Koh, J.M.; Dejean, A.; Orivel, J.; Padula, M.P.; Escoubas, P.; Nicholson, G.M. Comparisons of protein and peptide complexity in poneroid and formicoid ant venoms. *J. Proteome Res.* **2016**, *15*, 3039–3054. [CrossRef]
10. Kazuma, K.; Masuko, K.; Konno, K.; Inagaki, H. Combined venom gland transcriptomic and venom peptidomic analysis of the predatory ant *Odontomachus monticola*. *Toxins* **2017**, *9*, 323. [CrossRef]
11. Davidson, S.; Giesler, G.J. The multiple pathways for itch and their interactions with pain. *Trends Neurosci.* **2010**, *33*, 550–558. [CrossRef]
12. Vonsicard, N.A.E.; Candy, D.J.; Anderson, M. The biochemical-composition of venom from the pavement ant (*Tetramorium-Caespitum* L.). *Toxicon* **1989**, *27*, 1127–1133. [CrossRef]
13. De la Lande, I.S.; Lewis, J.C. Constituents of the venom of the Australlian bull ant, *Myrmecia pyriformis*. *Memorias do Instituto Butantan* **1966**, *33*, 951–955. [PubMed]
14. Hisada, M.; Satake, H.; Masuda, K.; Aoyama, M.; Murata, K.; Shinada, T.; Iwashita, T.; Ohfune, Y.; Nakajima, T. Molecular components and toxicity of the venom of the solitary wasp, *Anoplius samariensis*. *Biochem. Biophys. Res. Commun.* **2005**, *330*, 1048–1054. [CrossRef] [PubMed]
15. dos Santos Pinto, J.R.; Fox, E.G.; Saidemberg, D.M.; Santos, L.D.; da Silva Menegasso, A.R.; Costa-Manso, E.; Machado, E.A.; Bueno, O.C.; Palma, M.S. Proteomic view of the venom from the fire ant *Solenopsis invicta* Buren. *J. Proteome Res.* **2012**, *11*, 4643–4653. [CrossRef] [PubMed]
16. Escoubas, P.; Diochot, S.; Corzo, G. Structure and pharmacology of spider venom neurotoxins. *Biochimie* **2000**, *82*, 893–907. [CrossRef]
17. Goudet, C.; Chi, C.W.; Tytgat, J. An overview of toxins and genes from the venom of the Asian scorpion *Buthus martensi Karsch*. *Toxicon* **2002**, *40*, 1239–1258. [CrossRef]
18. Montgomerie, S.; Cruz, J.A.; Shrivastava, S.; Arndt, D.; Berjanskii, M.; Wishart, D.S. PROTEUS2: A web server for comprehensive protein structure prediction and structure-based annotation. *Nucleic Acids Res.* **2008**, *36*, W202–W209. [CrossRef]
19. Kozlowski, L.P. IPC—Isoelectric point calculator. *Biol. Direct* **2016**, *11*, 55. [CrossRef]
20. Gautier, R.; Douguet, D.; Antonny, B.; Drin, G. HELIQUEST: A web server to screen sequences with specific alpha-helical properties. *Bioinformatics* **2008**, *24*, 2101–2102. [CrossRef]
21. Zasloff, M.; Martin, B.; Chen, H.C. Antimicrobial activity of synthetic magainin peptides and several analogues. *Proc. Natl. Acad. Sci. USA* **1988**, *85*, 910–913. [CrossRef]
22. Agrawal, P.; Bhalla, S.; Chaudhary, K.; Kumar, R.; Sharma, M.; Raghava, G.P.S. In silico approach for prediction of antifungal peptides. *Front. Microbiol.* **2018**, *9*, 323. [CrossRef] [PubMed]
23. Pal, T.; Abraham, B.; Sonnevend, A.; Jumaa, P.; Conlon, J.M. Brevinin-1BYa: A naturally occurring peptide from frog skin with broad-spectrum antibacterial and antifungal properties. *Int. J. Antimicrob. Agents* **2006**, *27*, 525–529. [CrossRef] [PubMed]

24. Shigeri, Y.; Horie, M.; Yoshida, T.; Hagihara, Y.; Imura, T.; Inagaki, H.; Haramoto, Y.; Ito, Y.; Asashima, M. Physicochemical and biological characterizations of Pxt peptides from amphibian (*Xenopus tropicalis*) skin. *J. Biochem.* **2016**, *159*, 619–629. [CrossRef] [PubMed]
25. Chen, Y.; Guarnieri, M.T.; Vasil, A.I.; Vasil, M.L.; Mant, C.T.; Hodges, R.S. Role of peptide hydrophobicity in the mechanism of action of alpha-helical antimicrobial peptides. *Antimicrob. Agents Chemother.* **2007**, *51*, 1398–1406. [CrossRef] [PubMed]
26. Powers, J.P.; Hancock, R.E. The relationship between peptide structure and antibacterial activity. *Peptides* **2003**, *24*, 1681–1691. [CrossRef] [PubMed]
27. Touchard, A.; Brust, A.; Cardoso, F.C.; Chin, Y.K.; Herzig, V.; Jin, A.H.; Dejean, A.; Alewood, P.F.; King, G.F.; Orivel, J.; et al. Isolation and characterization of a structurally unique beta-hairpin venom peptide from the predatory ant *Anochetus emarginatus*. *Biochim. Biophys. Acta* **2016**, *1860*, 2553–2562. [CrossRef]
28. Johnson, S.R.; Rikli, H.G.; Schmidt, J.O.; Evans, M.S. A reexamination of poneratoxin from the venom of the bullet ant *Paraponera clavata*. *Peptides* **2017**, *98*, 51–62. [CrossRef]
29. Schmidt, J.O.; Blum, M.S.; Overal, W.L. Comparative enzymology of venoms from stinging Hymenoptera. *Toxicon* **1986**, *24*, 907–921. [CrossRef]

toxins

MDPI

Article

Antimicrobial and Antibiofilm Effects of Peptides from Venom of Social Wasp and Scorpion on Multidrug-Resistant *Acinetobacter baumannii*

Rogério Coutinho das Neves [1], Márcia Renata Mortari [2], Elisabeth Ferroni Schwartz [2], André Kipnis [1] and Ana Paula Junqueira-Kipnis [1,*]

1 Laboratory of Immunopathology of infectious diseases, Department of Immunology, Institute of Tropical Pathology and Public Health, Federal University of Goiás, Rua 235, Goiania, 74605-050 Goiás, Brazil; rogeriocdasneves@hotmail.com (R.C.d.N.); andre.kipnis@gmail.com (A.K.)

2 Laboratory of Neuropharmacology, Department of Physiological Sciences, Institute of Biological Sciences, University of Brasília, 70910-900 Brasilia, Brazil; mamortari@gmail.com (M.R.M.); beth.ferroni@gmail.com (E.F.S.)

* Correspondence: ana_kipnis@ufg.br; Tel.: +55-062-3209-6174

Received: 13 March 2019; Accepted: 4 April 2019; Published: 10 April 2019

check for updates

Abstract: Intravascular stent infection is a rare complication with a high morbidity and high mortality; bacteria from the hospital environment form biofilms and are often multidrug-resistant (MDR). Antimicrobial peptides (AMPs) have been considered as alternatives to bacterial infection treatment. We analyzed the formation of the bacterial biofilm on the vascular stents and also tested the inhibition of this biofilm by AMPs to be used as treatment or coating. Antimicrobial activity and antibiofilm were tested with wasp (Agelaia-MPI, Polybia-MPII, Polydim-I) and scorpion (Con10 and NDBP5.8) AMPs against *Acinetobacter baumannii* clinical strains. *A. baumannii* formed a biofilm on the vascular stent. Agelaia-MPI and Polybia-MPII inhibited biofilm formation with bacterial cell wall degradation. Coating biofilms with polyethylene glycol (PEG 400) and Agelaia-MPI reduced 90% of *A. baumannii* adhesion on stents. The wasp AMPs Agelaia-MPI and Polybia-MPII had better action against MDR *A. baumannii* adherence and biofilm formation on vascular stents, preventing its formation and treating mature biofilm when compared to the other tested peptides.

Keywords: AMP; mastoparan; *Acinetobacter baumannii*; stent

Key Contribution: The peptide Agelaia-MPI acts against the different stages of *A. baumannii* biofilm formation and could be used as a coating of vascular stents.

1. Introduction

The use of synthetic materials, such as ureter catheters and urinary stents for temporary or permanent insertion in the body may result in bacterial infections associated with colonization, which is important in the cases of morbidity and can lead to systemic dissemination [1,2]. Treatment with conventional antibiotics against bacterial biofilms formed on implants is inefficient to eradicate the infecting microorganism due to its low bacterial metabolic activity and biofilm protective matrix [3], resulting in a chronic infection of difficult treatment that requires the implant to be removed. Cases of vascular stent infections are rare complications, but associated with high mortality rates; according to current data, mortality may reach 40%, despite antibiotic treatment and/or surgical removal [4,5]. The most likely cause of stent infections is equipment reuse, such as balloons, catheters, and guide-wire, or poor ascetical techniques during the procedure [6]. These bacteria from the hospital environment and human skin are the most frequently found in stent infections: *Staphylococcus* spp. [6–8], *Streptococcus* spp. [9], *Pseudomonas* spp. [10,11], Fungi [12], and, in rare cases, rapidly growing mycobacteria (RGM) have also been reported [13]. Different case reports have been published showing cases of patients with stent infection, however, the relationship between the implantation of vascular stent with the development of nosocomial infection and the formation of bacterial biofilm is still not clear. Bacterial adhesion on the surface of the vascular stent material as well as the formation of bacterial biofilm has not been studied.

Vascular stents are used to increase the luminal diameter of the coronary arteries. The use of drugs to coat stents drastically reduces the process of re-stenosis [14,15]. Its expandable metal composition, whether coated with any drug or not, has a structure comprising a metal core of cobalt–chromium alloy or stainless steel and on the outside may have a coating of two polymers, lactic acid-co-glycolic acid (PLGA) or polylactic acid (PLA) that, in turn, can be manipulated to have additional drugs or antibodies integrated [16–18]. Some of the most commonly used drugs in stents are immunosuppressants, such as sirulimus, to reduce the risk of stent thrombosis caused by cell rejection [17]. In addition to implant intervention, patients still use anticoagulants or antiplatelet agents, which prevents the formation of thrombi on the stent [19].

The use of drug-eluting stents (DES) has increased recently, in comparison to the use of bare metal stents, however, DES have been shown to be more susceptible to infections [20]. Stent implantation may result in inflammation that could favor the formation of a conditioning film such as that shown for ureter stents [21]. This conditioning film facilitates bacterial adhesion and biofilm formation [22]. The metallic structure of the stent acts as a nest for bacterial colonization, increasing the risk of dissemination to the arterial wall, causing inflammation, necrosis, and ultimately vessel rupture [23]. Together with the fact that stents are implanted in a hospital setting, with a high prevalence of multidrug-resistant (MDR) bacteria, the risk of biofilm formation by MDR bacteria on biofilm poses an additional realistic threat.

One of the main bacteria responsible for nosocomial infections is *Acinetobacter baumannii* [24]. This Gram-negative coccobacillus commonly found on skin, in the respiratory tract, and in hospital environments has increased survival rates and the ability to produce biofilm [25,26]. *Acinetobacter* spp. are more frequently found in the intensive care units (ICU) than *Staphylococcus aureus* and *Pseudomonas* spp. [27]. Additionally, 80% of *A. baumannii* clinical isolates were shown to have some type of carbapenem resistance associated with high mortality rates [28]. However, although there are works showing *A. baumannii* biofilm formation in ureters [29] and vascular catheters [30], as well as treatment with different antibiotics against those biofilms, to our knowledge, no study has been done on the ability of *A. baumannii* to form biofilms on cobalt–chromium stents.

Biofilms made of MDR strains makes the treatment using conventional antibiotics more challenging. New therapeutic alternatives are necessary for these types of cases and antimicrobial peptides (AMP) are promising choices. AMPs are typically less than 100 amino acids in length that exhibit antimicrobial activity and can be obtained from the poisons of various animals, such as wasps [31], ants [32], bees [33], spiders [34], and scorpions [35]. Mastoparan (MP) peptides, which are the most commonly isolated peptide class from the *Vespidae* venom [31], present 10–14 amino acids that include distinct hydrophobic amino acids and an amphipathic helix conformation, which confers broad-spectrum antimicrobial activity against Gram-positive and Gram-negative bacteria [36], fungi [37], and mycobacteria [31,38]. Many AMPs are also present in the scorpion venom, which are classified as AMPs presenting disulfide bridges and AMPs that do not [39]. AMPs have a broad antimicrobial spectrum and are not affected by classical mechanisms of resistance to conventional antibiotics. AMPs interact primarily with the lipids of cytoplasmic membranes or cell walls leading to membrane permeabilization, cell lysis, and death [40]. AMP interaction with the lipid monolayer as described by Brogden (2005) can cause peptide aggregation forming pores, lipid and peptide combination forming a toroidal pore, or direct membrane disruption [41]. This unique mechanism of action allows AMPs to act on bacteria at different biofilm stages such as attachment, structure, and dispersion [42].

Therefore, our objectives were to analyze MDR *A. baumannii* biofilm formation on cobalt–chromium coronary stents and to evaluate the action of several antimicrobial peptides from wasp and scorpion venoms against those biofilms.

2. Results

2.1. Biofilm Formation by A. baumannii Clinical Isolates

In this work, three *A. baumannii* isolates previously described by Castilho et al. that were isolated from patients with hospital-acquired infections were used [43]. Isolates AB 02 and AB 72 were resistant to ampicillin, amikacin, and ciprofloxacin. AB 53 isolate only presented resistance to ampicillin. All isolates showed intermediate susceptibility to tetracycline, while all isolates were susceptible to meropenem [43]. Thus, AB 02 and AB 72 were considered as MDR strains. The ability to form biofilms by *A. baumannii* isolates AB 02, AB 53 and AB 72 was determined by crystal violet staining of cultures in 96 polystyrene well plates. Figure 1A shows that bacterial growth in the plates were similar between all isolates and *Escherichia coli*, but biofilm formation occurred only with *A. baumannii* isolates (Figure 1B). The AB 72 isolate produced more biofilm than the other isolates. Considering that isolate AB 72 presented resistance to three antimicrobial drugs and showed the highest capacity to form biofilm, we decided to test its ability to adhere to the cobalt chromium vascular stent.

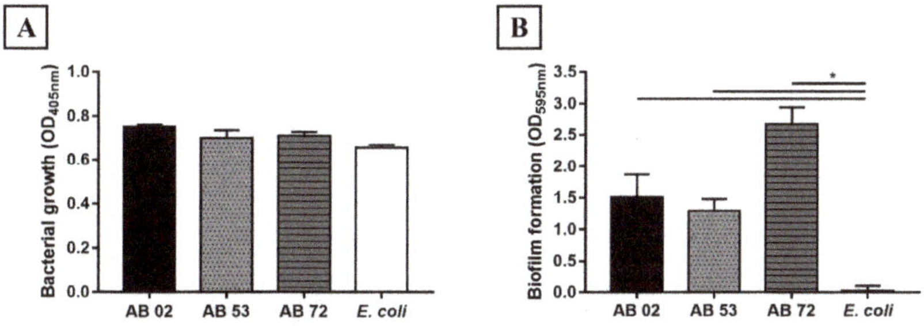

Figure 1. *Acinetobacter baumannii* biofilm formation. (**A**) The bacterial growth of *Acinetobacter baumannii* AB 02, AB 53, AB 72, and *Escherichia coli* (control) were incubated with LB + Glu for 24 h at 29 °C and the growth was determined by OD readings at 405 nm. (**B**) After this period, the presence of biofilms was evaluated using crystal violet dye staining. The bars represent the mean and standard deviations of triplicates. * Significant difference between biofilm formations by *A. baumannii* clinical isolates compared to *E. coli* ($p < 0.05$).

2.2. Adhesion and Early Formation of Biofilm on Cobalt–Chromium Vascular Stent

In order to determine if *A. baumannii* was able to adhere to stents, a cobalt–chromium stent was incubated with AB 72 isolate for 24 h. Figure 2 shows the results of scanning electronic microscopy (SEM) and the colony forming units (CFU) of bacteria recovered from the stents. The first image (Figure 2A) reveals the framework and the configuration of the coronary stent used. Fragments with five cells were used for the analyses. In the SEM analyses (Figure 2C,D) the bacteria adhered to the stent and secreted substances that also adhered to the stent and to the bacterial colonies indicating biofilm formation (Figure 2E). Determination of the bacterial load attached to the stents resulted in 1.3×10^6 CFU per used stent. These results represent one of three independent experiments.

2.3. Determination of Minimum Inhibitory Concentration of Antimicrobial Peptides against Isolates of A. baumannii

Since *A. baumannii* was shown to form biofilm on stents, we first investigated if AMPs derived from arthropod venom were active against these bacteria. Agelaia-MPI, Polybia-MPII, and Polydim-I derived from wasp venom and Con10 or NBDP-5.8 derived from scorpion venom were used.

The hydrophobicity evaluation of the peptides showed a range of 0.435 to 0.795 (Con10 < NDBP-5.8 < Polybia-MPII < Agelaia-MPI < Polydim-I) (Table 1). Agelaia-MPI and Polybia-MPII peptides were similar peptides differing by two amino acids. In the 9th position an alanine present in Agelaia-MPI is substituted by a methionine in Polybia-MPII and an isoleucine is substituted by a valine in the 10th position in Polybia-MPII, but their hydrophobicities were maintained (Table 1).

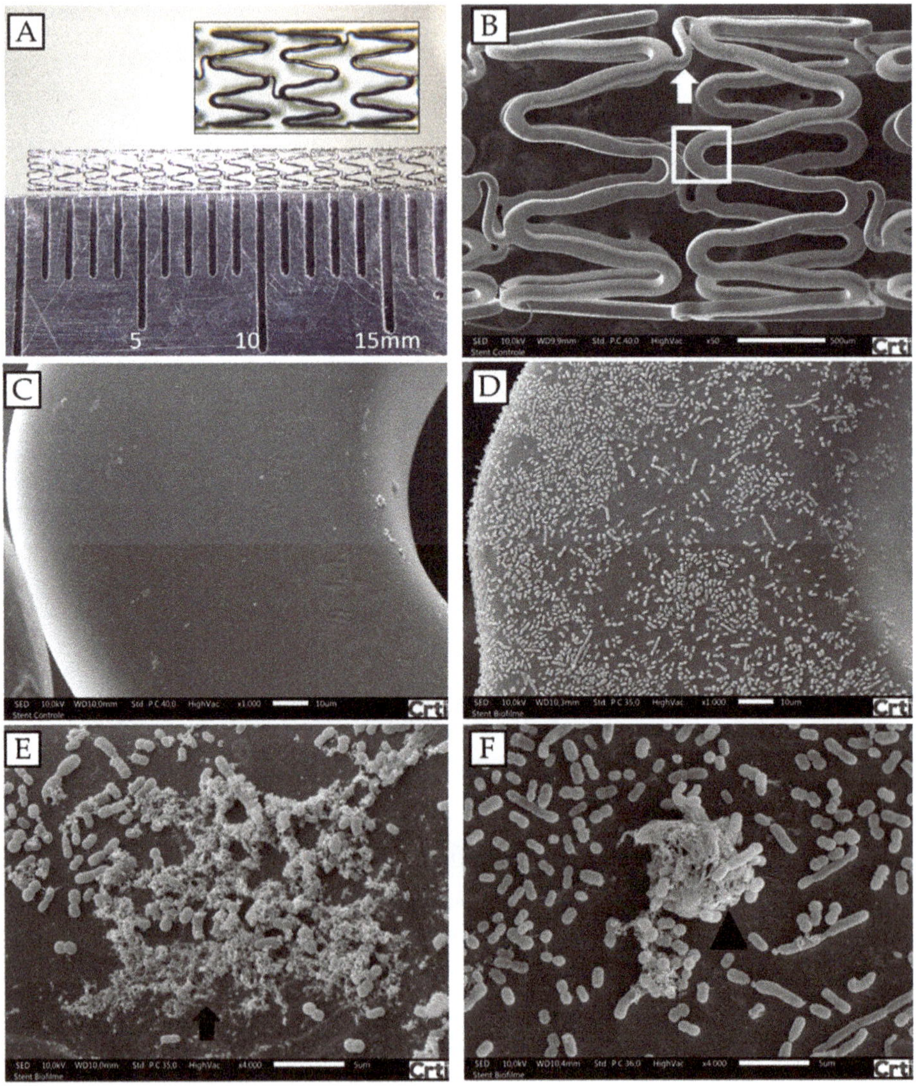

Figure 2. *A. baumannii* biofilm formations on fragments of cobalt–chromium vascular stents analyzed by SEM. (**A**) Coronary stent photography; the fragments used in the experiments were 6 mm long. (**B**) Architecture of the cobalt–chromium vascular stent, presenting two cells, connected by a link (arrow). (**C**) Stent structure enlargement of box in B. (**D** and **E**) Stent after incubation with *A. baumannii* AB 72 for 24 h under conditions for biofilm formation (arrow). (**F**) Protuberant bacterial accumulation, suggestive of initial biofilm formation (arrow head). Magnifications: (**B**) 40×; (**C**) and (**D**) 1000×; (**E**) and (**F**) 4000×.

Table 1. Description of the sequence, source, and publication of the antimicrobial peptides used in this study.

Peptide	Sequence	Venom source	Hydrophobicity	First Description
Agelaia-MPI	INWLKLGKAIIDAL	*Agelaia pallipes pallipes*	0.781	[44]
Polybia-MPII	INWLKLGKMVIDAL	*Pseudopolybia vespiceps testacea*	0.740	[45]
Polydim-I	AVAGEKLWLLPHLLKMLLTPTP	*Polybia dimorpha*	0.791	[38]
Con10	FWSFLVKAASKILPSLIGGGDDNKSSS	*Opisthacanthus cayaporum*	0.435	[46]
NDBP-5.8	GILGKIWEGVKSLI	*Opisthacanthus cayaporum*	0.686	[46]

The ability of AMPs (Agelaia-MPI, Polybia-MPII and Polydim-I, Con10 and NBDP-5.8) to inhibit the bacteria growth by incubating them with three different MDR *A. baumannii* isolates for 24 h was analyzed (Figure 3). The MIC for Agelaia-MPI peptide against AB 02 and AB 72 isolates was 6.25 µM and against AB 53 was 3.12 µM (Figure 3A). Polybia-MPII presented an MIC of 12.5 µM for AB 02 and 6.25 µM for both AB 53 and AB 72 isolates (Figure 3B). Polydim-1 did not completely inhibit the growth of any isolate at the tested concentrations (Figure 3C). The Con10 AMP presented an MIC of 12.5 µM for the AB 02 isolate and 6.25 µM for both AB 53 and AB 72 isolates (Figure 3D). NBDP 5.8 showed a MIC of 25 µM for all isolates analyzed (Figure 3E).

2.4. *Impact of Antimicrobial Peptides on Bacterial Biofilm Formation*

Since the AMPs were shown to act against *A. baumannii* isolates, we then investigated if they could avoid the formation of biofilm in 96-well plates, calculating the minimum biofilm eradication concentration (MBEC). Agelaia-MPI showed adhesion inhibition for isolates AB 02 at a concentration of 25 µM while isolates AB 53 and AB 72 were inhibited at a concentration of 6.25 and 12.5 µM, respectively (Table 2). Polybia-MPII inhibited at the minimum concentration of 25 µM for AB 02 and AB 72 and 12.5 µM for AB 53 (Table 2). Polydim-I showed low adhesion inhibition—50% for the AB 53 isolate at a concentration greater than 25 µM (Table 2). The Con10 scorpion peptide inhibited the biofilm formation at the concentration of 12.5 µM for the AB 53 and 72 isolates and for the AB 02 isolate the minimum concentration was 25 µM (Table 2). For NBDP 5.8 peptide, it was able to inhibit the biofilm (>95%) of the three isolates at a minimum concentration of 25 µM (Table 2). Therefore, Agelaia-MPI e Polybia-MPII peptides that presented best activities against biofilm formation were selected.

2.5. *Effect of the Agelaia-MPI and Polybia-MPII Peptides on Mature Biofilm and on the Dispersion of Adherent Cells*

Agelaia-MPI and Polybia-MPII wasp peptides were analyzed for their ability to inhibit mature biofilm formed after 24 h of culture (Figure 4). Agelaia-MPI at 12.5 and 25 µM decreased 50% and 60% of the mature biofilm previously formed in the plates, respectively. Additionally, Agelaia-MPI and Polybia-MPII peptides were able to inhibit cells that were dispersed from the formed biofilm (Figure 5). Agelaia-MPI inhibited the dispersed cells at the minimum concentration of 12.5 µM for the AB 72 isolate and 6.25 µM for the other two (Figure 5A). Polybia-MPII inhibited the dispersed cells of all isolates at the same concentration of 6.25 µM (Figure 5B).

2.6. *SEM Analysis of the Activity of the Agelaia-MPI and Polybia-MPII Wasp Peptides against AB 72 Isolate Biofilm adhered to the Vascular Stent*

After incubating AB 72 isolate for 24 h with one fragment of vascular stent, the stents were treated with Agelaia-MPI or Polybia-MPII for 24 h (Figure 6). AMP treatment reduced the bacillary load adhered to the material and the bacteria that remained present on the stent showed morphological modifications on the bacterial surface with cellular debris accumulation (Figure 6D,F).

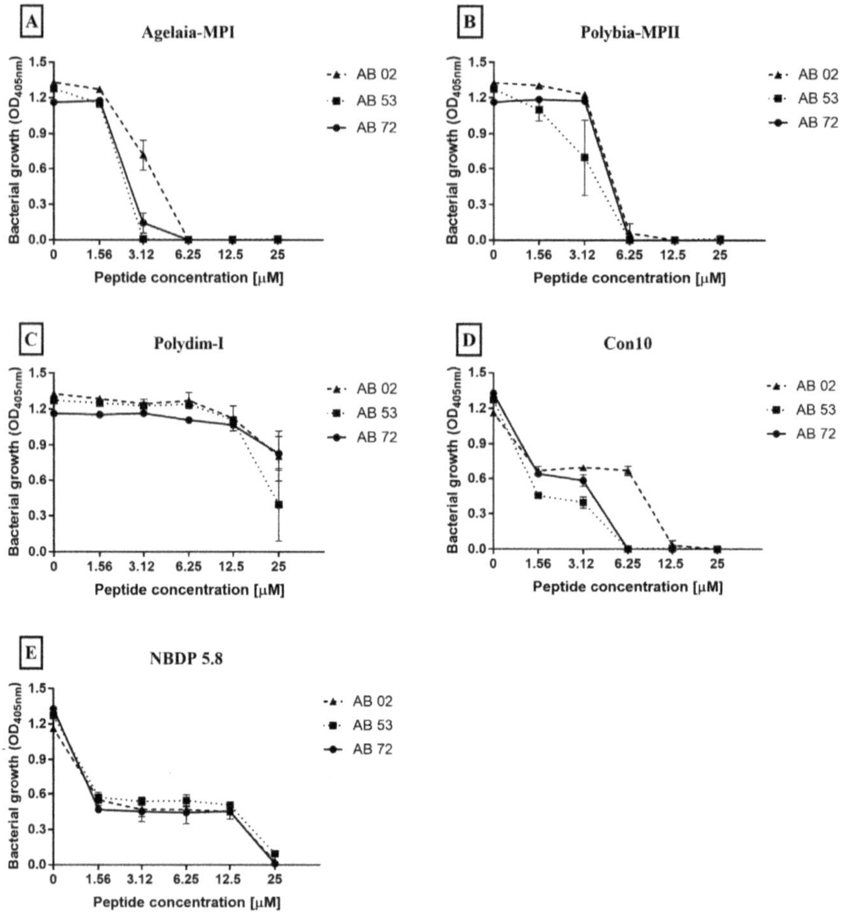

Figure 3. Effect of the antimicrobial peptides (**A**) Agelaia-MPI, (**B**) Polybia-MPII, (**C**) Polydim-I, (**D**) Con10, and (**E**) NBDP 5.8 on the inhibition of adhesion of *A. baumannii* to 96-well polystyrene plates. The curves represent the bacterial growth of adhered cells on polystyrene plate by reading OD in the range of 405 nm. Results are reported as mean and standard deviations of triplicates. These results represent one of three independent experiments.

Table 2. Minimal inhibitory concentration of antimicrobial peptides against the formation of *A. baumannii* biofilm on polystyrene plates.

Peptide	Isolate AB 02 [1]	Isolate AB 53	Isolate AB 72
Agelaia-MPI	25	6.25	12.5
Polybia-MPII	25	12.5	25
Polydim-I	>25	>25	>25
Con 10	25	12.5	12.5
NDBP 5.8	>25	>25	>25

[1] Values are presented as concentration in μM that inhibited biofilm formation after violet crystal staining of the biofilm adhered to polystyrene plate by reading OD in the range of 595 nm.

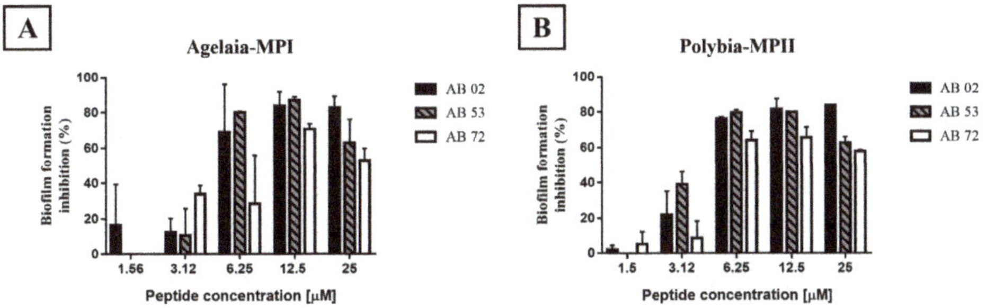

Figure 4. Effect of the antimicrobial peptides Agelaia-MPI and Polybia-MPII on the mature biofilm of *A. baumannii* on polystyrene plates. (**A**) Agelaia-MPI and (**B**) Polybia-MPII significantly inhibited mature biofilm at the lowest concentration of 6.25 µM. Results are reported as mean and standard deviations of triplicates. These results represent one of three independent experiments.

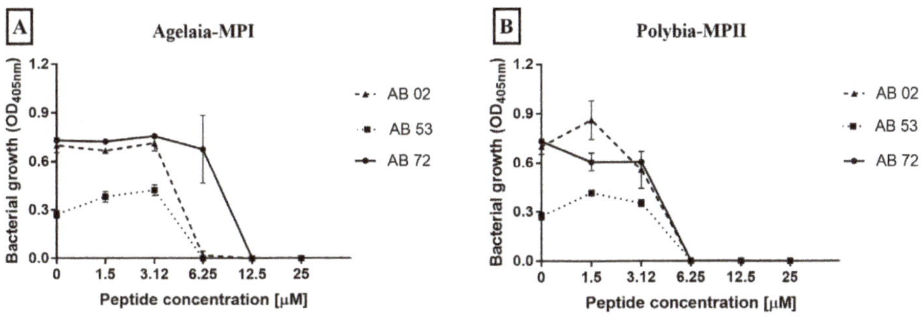

Figure 5. Effect of the antimicrobial peptides (**A**) Agelaia-MPI and (**B**) Polybia-MPII on *A. baumannii*-dispersed cells from biofilms on polystyrene wells. After washing the wells where biofilms had been previously formed and removing the non-adherent or poorly adhered bacteria, more culture medium was added with antimicrobial peptides and, 24 h later, bacteria present in the supernatant was measured. Results are reported as mean and standard deviations of triplicates. These results represent one of three independent experiments.

2.7. Inhibition of Bacterial adherence on the Cobalt–hromium Stent Coated with PEG Mixed with Agelaia-MPI

Stents were assembled using PEG 400 solution with Agelaia-MPI (25 µM), PEG 400 alone, or uncoated as control. Then all stents were incubated with 1.5×10^8 CFU of AB 72. After 24 h, approximately 4.8×10^6 CFU remained unattached to the vascular stent. Coating the stent with PEG 400 alone resulted in a slight reduction of biofilm formation (30%; ~3.25×10^6 CFU). When the stent was coated with Agelaia-MPI plus PEG, a 91% reduction (~4.8×10^5 CFU) was observed when compared to non-treated stents (uncoated; Figure 7).

2.8. Effect of Antimicrobial Peptides on Staphylococcus Biofilm Formation

The species of *Staphylococcus* are the most common agent that causes coronary infections [4,47], thus we decided to test the microbicidal efficiency of Agelaia-MPI and Polybia-MPII peptides against *S. epidermidis* and methicillin-resistant *S. aureus* (MRSA) species. We also evaluated if the selected AMPs could avoid the formation of biofilm. Agelaia-MPI and Polybia-MPII AMPs showed similar growth inhibition at 12.5 µM for both *Staphylococcus* species (Figure 8A,C). When evaluating the biofilm formation by these bacteria, the peptides inhibited 85% of biofilm formation at 12.5 µM (Figure 8C,D). Thus, Polybia-MPII and Agelaia-MPI were microbicidal and avoided biofilm formation by *A. baumannii* and *Staphylococcus* spp. bacteria.

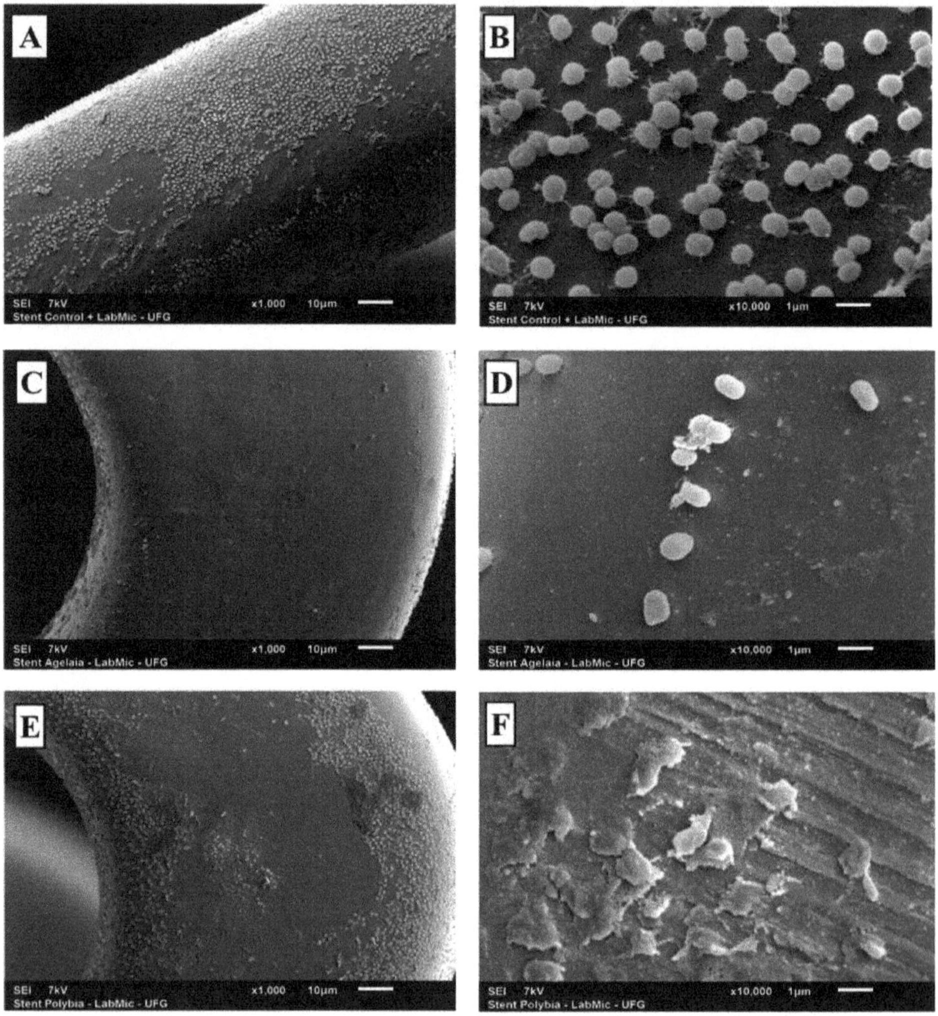

Figure 6. Role of the peptides Agelaia-MPI and Polybia-MPII on the inhibition of biofilm formation by *A. baumannii* on stents. (**A** and **B**) SEM evaluation of *A. baumannii* biofilms formed on stents. (**C** and **D**) Biofilm formation on stents by *A. baumannii* treated with Agelaia-MPI for 24 h. (**E** and **F**) Biofilm formation on stents by *A. baumannii* treated with Polybia-MPII for 24 h. Magnification of ×1000 (**A**, **C** and **E**); ×10,000 (**B**, **D** and **F**).

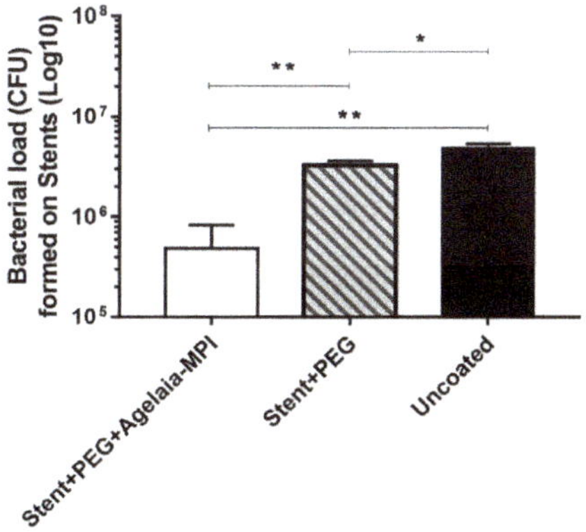

Figure 7. Coating of the vascular stent with Agelaia-MPI plus PEG prevented the adherence of *A. baumannii.* The vascular stent was left for 3 h in a PEG 400 solution containing 25 µM of Agelaia-MPI (stent + PEG + Agelaia−MPI) or not (stent + PEG). Coated stents were transferred to a new well containing fresh medium and then *A. baummanii* was added and incubated for 24 h. Uncoated stent was used as a control. At the end of incubation, wells were rinsed with fresh media and the stents were sonicated and the bacterial load adhered in each situation was determined. Results are reported as means and standard deviations of triplicates from one of three independent experiments. These results in all three independent experiments were similar, * $p < 0.05$ and ** $p < 0.0001$.

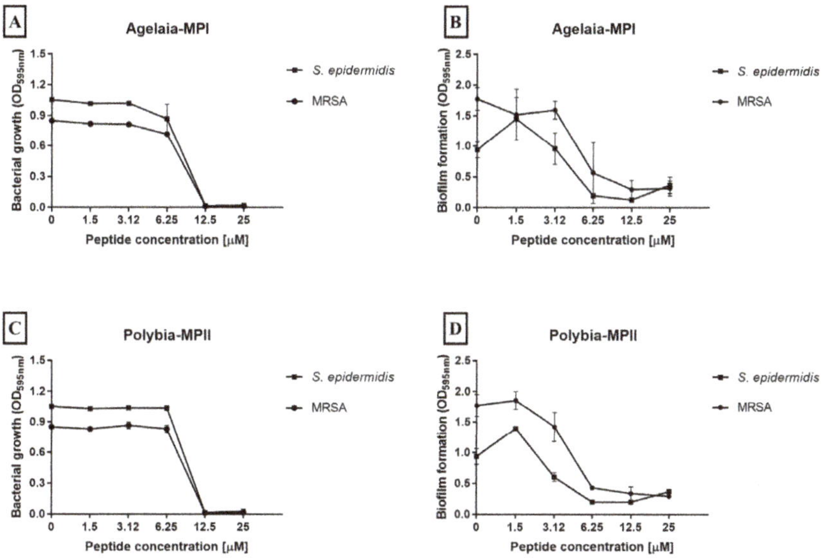

Figure 8. Effect of Agelaia-MPI and Polybia-MPII AMPs on the adherence and biofilm formation of *Staphylococcus* strains. (**A**) Agelaia-MPI activity against adhesion and (**B**) biofilm. Polybia-MPII activity against (**C**) adhesion and (**D**) biofilm. Results are expressed as means and standard deviations of triplicates. These results represent one of three independent experiments.

3. Discussion

Infections caused by MDR *Acinetobacter baumannii* are found in patients in hospitals due to contamination and biofilm formation of clinical materials and instruments [27]. In this work we used three *A. baumannii* clinical isolates, AB 02, AB 53, and AB 72 with resistance to different classes of antibiotics and potential biofilm formation in plates as described by Castilho et al. [43]. Here, we showed the bacterial adherence in a coronary stent with the formation of biofilm. We showed that three peptides from wasps and scorpions presented antimicrobial and antibiofilm activities. Additionally, the peptides had activity against different stages of biofilm formation: Adhesion, maturation, and dispersion. Agelia-MPI + PEG coating was used to prevent adherence of bacteria on the coronary stents and this coating reduced 90% of bacteria adhered to them. Thus, we propose that Agelaia-MPI could be an alternative therapeutic against MDR *A. baumannii* deposition and biofilm formation in clinical materials.

Two of the clinical isolates used in this study presented resistance to the beta-lactam antibiotic ampicillin and carbapenems, the aminoglycoside amikacin, and the quinolone ciprofloxacin, therefore presenting several mechanisms of drug resistance, representing a challenge to treat infections by these bacteria [43]. In recent years, there has been an increase in the number of cases of infection by MDR *A. baumannii* strains [27]. *Acinetobacter* spp. are more frequently found on inanimate objects and hands of staff in the ICU than *Staphylococcus aureus* and *Pseudomonas* spp. [27]. Another problem is the increased use of prophylactic antibiotics, which decreases the risk of infection, but increase the selection of resistant strains, such as emergent MDR *A. baumannii.* Analysis of isolates of *A. baumannii* reveal that those producing biofilms are more frequently associated with genes of antibiotic resistance compared to the weak biofilm producers [48]. In combination with different genetic profiles responsible for antimicrobial resistance, biofilm formation increases the chances of pathogen survival. Because biofilm formation may occur in medical materials, prospecting new molecules that could avoid antibiotic resistance might contribute to the treatment of such bacteria.

The strains of *A. baumannii* used in this study were capable of adherence to the cobalt–chromium structure of the vascular stent. Also, the presence of structures that resemble exopolisaccharides that support adherence to the stent were observed, which were shown be important for the beginning of biofilm formation [49]. The initial agglomeration of bacteria on surfaces might improve their resistance to desiccation and antimicrobial solutions [50]. *A. baumannii* can survive for long periods in hospital environments; many reservoirs have been identified, including mattresses, metal tables, door handles, and air vents [51]. *A. baumannii* is a cause of primarily hospital-acquired infection associated with septicemia, bacteremia, ventilator-associated pneumonia, sepsis, endocarditis, meningitis, and urinary tract infections [27]. Although contaminated stents reviewed by Bosma et al. [4] did not show the presence of *A. baumannii*, we believe that more studies should be done since *A. baumannii* can easily infect hospitalized immunosuppressed individuals and *A. baumannii* bacteremia could induce biofilm formation on the implanted stents. Very often the diagnosis of an infected stent is missed in the first phase, with a subsequent delay in definitive treatment, yet in up to 50.0% of cases it has a fatal outcome [4]. Also, wrong practices of coronary stent manipulation can lead to contamination, even when antibiotics are used preventively [52–54]. Our hypothesis is that there is an underestimation of cases of coronary stent infection by *A. baumannii.*

Antimicrobial peptides (AMPs) derived from wasps (Agelaia-MPI, Polybia-MPII, and Polydim-I) and scorpions (Con10 and NBDP-5.8) were tested for their ability to inhibit the growth of *A. baumannii* isolates. Among all AMPs, the Agelaia-MPI had the best MIC and MBEC values when compared to the other peptides. AMPs derived from wasp and scorpion venom have been widely tested against different microorganisms and have a microbicidal function on bacteria and fungi, besides having antiviral action [33]. Although the bactericidal activity of Agelaia-MPI against Gram-negative bacteria was not tested before, we believe that it could involve the interaction of the peptide with negatively-charged molecules on the surface of bacteria that would cause disruption of bacterial membranes [31,55]. Because AMPs acts on the lipid portion of cellular membranes, it is believed that they could avoid the development of resistance mechanisms such as those commonly induced by antibiotics, i.e., *A. baumannii* bacterial resistance mechanisms to conventional antibiotics comprises multidrug efflux pumps, aminoglycoside-modifying enzymes, selective membrane permeability, alteration of target sites, and hydrolytic enzymes like carbapenemase [56–58].

Agelaia-MPI presented the MIC of 6.25 μM for the AB 02 isolate and 3.12 μM for the AB 53 and AB 72 isolates. Such MIC variation could be due to the particular characteristics of each clinical isolate, such as membrane composition, protease secretion, etc. [59] and has been also described for antimicrobial testings [60]. The acquired antimicrobial drug resistance attributed to the biofilm formation was also observed for the isolates studied here. A reduction of 50%–60% of the bacterial load on the mature biofilms only occurred using higher AMP concentrations (12.5 and 25 μM). The *A. baumannii* reduction observed here could prevent the formation of the biofilm by killing planktonic bacteria, which reduces/eradicates mature biofilm or induce the detachment of the bacteria. In this case, Agelaia-MPI probably acts in a "classic" manner against biofilm, according to Batoni et al. [39]. When MBEC is higher than the MIC, AMP acts in a microbicidal way, preventing the biofilm by the death of the planktonic bacteria, reducing/eradicating the bacteria in the mature biofilm and finally killing those who detach from the biofilm [42]. Despite the direct correlation between AMPs concentration and bacterial death, a transient and slight bacterial growth was observed at concentrations lower than MIC (sub-MIC). Although not statistically significant, this behavior has been shown previously and explained as bacterial detachment from the biofilm that cannot be killed by sub-MIC of AMPs [61].

Agelaia-MPI and Polybia-MPII modified the bacterial surface and reduced the bacterial load on the stents (Figure 6). These peptides differ from each other by two amino acids; an alanine in Agelaia-MPI by a methionine in Polybia-MPII and an isoleucine by a valine, in the 9th and 10th position, respectively. These amino acid differences apparently did not interfere with their ability to cause membrane lesions. Polybia-MPII was shown before to present microbicidal functions against fungi (*Candida albicans* and *Cryptococcus neoformans*), *Mycobacterium abscessus* subsp. *massiliense* and *S. aureus* [31]. The ability of Polybia-MPII to avoid *A. baumannii* biofilm formation was also shown against *Staphylococcus* strains [31]. The probable mechanism of action on membrane/cell wall observed with *M. a. massiliense* SEM analyses were also observed for *A. baumannii* stent biofilms, thus indicating physical rather than metabolic alterations induced by the AMPs (i.e., general membrane alterations). In addition to the amino acid sequence of AMPs, some features may influence their binding to bacterial and eukaryotic membranes, i.e., hydrophobicity and the resulting charge. Increasing or diminishing hydrophobicity of AMPs has been shown to improve their bactericidal functions [62,63]. In the present work, this phenomena was not the case; Agelaia-MPI and Polybia-MPII presented similar hydrophobicity and bactericidal action, while Polydim-I, although having similar hydrophobicity, presented lower bactericidal function. Additionally, CON10 and NDBP-5.8 that presented the lowest hydrophobicity showed higher bactericidal function than Polydim-I. Thus, for the results presented here, the peptide hydrophobicity was not the only driving factor in the microbicidal activities.

Disadvantages of the use of peptides as an antimicrobial are the production costs and their low stability in human serum, due to the action of peptidases and proteases present in the human body, especially in the liver [64]; however, there is a way to optimize the amount of peptide used and increase its stability, i.e., by using it combined with other molecules or coating medical material. Polyethylene glycol (PEG) is hydrophilic and presents low toxicity and it has been shown before to assist the slow release of AMPs such as LL37 [65]. Thus, we decided to use PEG to coat the stent with Agelia-MPI. Coating stents with Agelaia-MPI + PEG reduced 90% of the biofilm formation. Different peptides have already been used to inhibit biofilm formation; in those cases, they were adhered to silicone catheters and titanium structures [64,66]. Similar to our results, Baghery et al. immobilized AMPs with PEG and showed an improvement in the antimicrobial efficiency of the AMPs against biofilm formation [67]. Analysis comparing the immobilization of AMP with and without PEGylated spacers demonstrated that some immobile AMPs are only bactericidal when PEGylated spacer was used [65,68]. Although the works done before did not use PEG alone as control, in our case of using PEG-coated stents, the biofilm formation was reduced 30%. This fact could indicate that PEG may alter the bacteria adherence to the stent and thus avoid the complete biofilm formation, but more studies should be done to prove this fact. Thus, surface coating composed of antimicrobial peptides offers additional advantages, such as decreased potential cytotoxicity associated with higher concentrations of soluble peptides and increased peptide life [69].

4. Conclusions

In summary, this work showed two peptides, Agelaia-MPI and Polybia-MPII, derived from wasps with bactericidal activity, as well as activity against different stages of biofilm-forming by MDR *A. baumannii*. We also showed that coating cobalt–chromium vascular stents with Agelaia-MPI together with PEG 400 prevented 90% of bacterial biofilm formation. This study revealed potential applications of Agelaia-MPI and Polybia-MPII peptides derived from wasp venom as antimicrobials to treat biofilm-resistant agents such as *A. baumannii* and *Staphylococcus* spp. coated on the surfaces of implanted medical devices.

5. Materials and Methods

5.1. Bacterial Strains and Growth Conditions

Clinical isolates of MDR *A. baumannii* described by Castilho et al. [43] identified as AB 02, AB 53, and AB 72 cryopreserved at −80 °C were reactivated in Luria Bertani (LB) agar medium (HiMedia) and grown at 37 °C for 24 h. A colony isolated from each strain was inoculated into 5 mL of LB broth medium (HiMedia, Pennsylvania, USA) until growth corresponded to 0.5 of the MacFarland scale. Some growth conditions were modified for each experiment to evaluate the different stages of biofilm formation described below.

5.2. Analysis of Bacterial Biofilm Formation by A. baumannii Isolates by Colorimetric Dyes in 96-Well Polystyrene Culture Plates

The estimated quantification of bacterial biofilm formation in a 96-well polystyrene culture plate was done according to methodology described by Castilho et al. [43], with minor modifications. After growth of the strains in LB broth medium to a concentration corresponding to 0.5 of MacFarland scale, the culture concentration was adjusted to 1.5×10^8 CFU/mL and 30 μL of that suspension was added to 170 μL of LB broth at 1/4 of its concentration with an additional 0.2% of glucose (Ecibra) (LB$\frac{1}{4}$-Glu). The bacterial culture was incubated in a 96-well plate for 24 h at a temperature of 29 °C. Bacterial growth was measured at an absorbance of 405 nm in a Thermo Scientific™ Multiskan™ FC Microplate Photometer. The supernatant was removed and the well was washed with phosphate buffered saline (PBS). The attached biofilm was stained with 0.2% (w/v) crystal violet (Vetec) and solubilized with ethanol/acetone (80/20 v/v) to quantify at 595 nm. A common laboratory *Escherichia coli* strain (XL1blue) known not to form biofilm was used as a negative control.

5.3. Adhesion of A. baumannii to Abiotic Surfaces

A. baumannii strains form bacterial biofilm on a polystyrene plate under incubation conditions (LB$\frac{1}{4}$-Glu 29 °C). Biofilm formation on stents was evaluated by placing a sterile fragment of the cobalt–chromium alloy vascular stent into a well containing strain AB 72 at a concentration of 1.5×10^8 CFU/mL in LB$\frac{1}{4}$-Glu. As a control, a fragment of the vascular stent was incubated with culture medium alone. After 24 h of incubation, the stents were rinsed with sterile PBs and analyzed by Scanning Electron Microscopy (SEM) and CFU counting. The SEM was performed using a methodology from das Neves et al. [36], with minor modifications. The fragments were washed with PBS to remove the unbound bacteria, then fixed with Karnovsky's solution (1% paraformaldehyde and 3% glutaraldehyde) in 0.07M cacodilide buffer (pH 7.2) for 30 min at 4 °C. The fixative solution was removed and serial dehydration was performed, followed by ethanol washes (30%, 50%, 70%, 90%, and 100%) for 10 min, followed by acetone and hexamethyldisilazane (HMDS) (v/v) for a further

Author Contributions: R.C.d.N., A.K. and A.P.J.-K. conceived and designed the experiments; R.C.d.N. performed the experiments; M.R.M. and E.F.S. reviewed the manuscript and analyzed the data; R.C.d.N., A.K. and A.P.J.-K. analyzed the data; R.C.d.N. wrote the manuscript draft.

Funding: This research was funded by FAPEG, CNPq and CAPES.

Acknowledgments: We would like to thank LabMic UFG for assistance with scanning electron microscopy.

Conflicts of Interest: The authors declare no conflict of interest.

References

1. Minardi, D.; Ghiselli, R.; Cirioni, O.; Giacometti, A.; Kamysz, W.; Orlando, F.; Silvestri, C.; Parri, G.; Kamysz, E.; Scalise, G.; et al. The antimicrobial peptide Tachyplesin III coated alone and in combination with intraperitoneal piperacillin-tazobactam prevents ureteral stent Pseudomonas infection in a rat subcutaneous pouch model. *Peptides* **2007**, *28*, 2293–2298. [CrossRef] [PubMed]
2. De Breij, A.; Riool, M.; Kwakman, P.H.S.; de Boer, L.; Cordfunke, R.A.; Drijfhout, J.W.; Cohen, O.; Emanuel, N.; Zaat, S.A.J.; Nibbering, P.H.; et al. Prevention of Staphylococcus aureus biomaterial-associated infections using a polymer-lipid coating containing the antimicrobial peptide OP-145. *J. Control. Release* **2016**, *222*, 1–8. [CrossRef]
3. Arciola, C.R.; Campoccia, D.; Montanaro, L. Implant infections: Adhesion, biofilm formation and immune evasion. *Nat. Rev. Microbiol.* **2018**, *16*, 397–409. [CrossRef]
4. Bosman, W.M.P.F.; Borger van der Burg, B.L.S.; Schuttevaer, H.M.; Thoma, S.; Hedeman Joosten, P.P. Infections of intravascular bare metal stents: A case report and review of literature. *Eur. J. Vasc. Endovasc. Surg.* **2014**, *47*, 87–99. [CrossRef]
5. Dalal, J.J.; Digrajkar, A.; Hastak, M.; Mulay, A.; Lad, V.; Wani, S. Coronary stent infection—A grave, avoidable complication. *IHJ Cardiovasc. Case Rep.* **2017**, *1*, 77–79. [CrossRef]
6. Reddy, K.V.C.; Sanzgiri, P.; Thanki, F.; Suratkal, V. Coronary stent infection: Interesting cases with varied presentation. *J. Cardiol. Cases* **2018**, *19*, 8–11. [CrossRef] [PubMed]
7. Elieson, M.; Mixon, T.; Carpenter, J. Coronary stent infections. *Tex. Heart Inst. J.* **2012**, *39*, 884–889.
8. Whitcher, G.H.; Bertges, D.J.; Shukla, M. Peripheral vascular stent infection: Case report and review of literature. *Ann. Vasc. Surg.* **2018**, *51*, 326.e9–326.e15. [CrossRef]
9. Desai, J.A.; Husain, S.F.; Islam, O.; Jin, A.Y. Carotid artery stent infection with Streptococcus agalactiae. *Neurology* **2010**, *74*, 344. [CrossRef]
10. Sekhar, S.; Vupputuri, A.; Nair, R.C.; Palaniswamy, S.S.; Natarajan, K.U. Coronary stent infection successfully diagnosed using 18F-flurodeoxyglucose positron emission tomography computed tomography. *Can. J. Cardiol.* **2016**, *32*, 1575.e1–1575.e3. [CrossRef]
11. Sudhakar, B.G.K. Pseudomonas aeruginosa septicemia resulting in coronary stent infection and coronary artery aneurysm and acute infective endocarditis of mitral valve causing severe mitral regurgitation—A case report. *IHJ Cardiovasc. Case Rep.* **2018**, *2*, 191–195. [CrossRef]
12. Raychaudhuri, R.; Yu, W.; Hatanpaa, K.; Cavuoti, D.; Pride, G.L.; White, J. Basilar artery dissection treated by Neuroform stenting: Fungal stent infection. *Surg. Neurol.* **2009**, *71*, 477–480. [CrossRef]
13. Soman, R.; Gupta, N.; Suthar, M.; Sunavala, A.; Shetty, A.; Rodrigues, C. Intravascular stent-related endocarditis due to rapidly growing mycobacteria: A new problem in the developing world. *J. Assoc. Phys. India* **2015**, *63*, 18–21.
14. Wu, X.; Yin, T.; Tian, J.; Tang, C.; Huang, J.; Zhao, Y.; Zhang, X.; Deng, X.; Fan, Y.; Yu, D.; et al. Distinctive effects of CD34- and CD133-specific antibody-coated stents on re-endothelialization and in-stent restenosis at the early phase of vascular injury. *Regen. Biomater.* **2015**, *2*, 87–96. [CrossRef]
15. DeCunha, J.; Janicki, C.; Enger, S.A. A retrospective analysis of catheter-based sources in intravascular brachytherapy. *Brachytherapy* **2017**, *16*, 586–596. [CrossRef]
16. Abhyankar, A.D.; Thakkar, A.S. In vivo assessment of stent recoil of biodegradable polymer-coated cobalt–chromium sirolimus-eluting coronary stent system. *Indian Heart J.* **2012**, *64*, 541–546. [CrossRef]
17. Buccheri, D.; Orrego, P.S.; Cortese, B. Drug-eluting stent treatment of left main coronary artery disease: The case for a sirolimus-eluting, autoexpandable alternative. An optical coherence tomography analysis. *Int. J. Cardiol.* **2015**, *199*, 119–120. [CrossRef]

18. Ito, S.; Saeki, T. Coronary angioscopic imaging of in-stent restenosis after biolimus-eluting coronary stent implantation. *J. Cardiol. Cases* **2015**, *12*, 145–149. [CrossRef]
19. Li, C.H.; Gao, B.L.; Wang, J.W.; Liu, J.F.; Li, H.; Yang, S.T.; Ren, C.F. Endovascular stent deployment in the management of lesions related to internal carotid artery redundancy. *World Neurosurg.* **2018**, *116*, e903–e912. [CrossRef]
20. Omar, A.; Pendyala, L.K.; Ormiston, J.A.; Waksman, R. Review: Stent fracture in the drug-eluting stent era. *Cardiovasc. Revasc. Med.* **2016**, *17*, 404–411. [CrossRef]
21. Zumstein, V.; Betschart, P.; Albrich, W.C.; Buhmann, M.T.; Ren, Q.; Schmid, H.P.; Abt, D. Biofilm formation on ureteral stents—Incidence, clinical impact and prevention. *Swiss Med. Wkly.* **2017**, *147*. [CrossRef]
22. Garrett, T.R.; Bhakoo, M.; Zhang, Z. Bacterial adhesion and biofilms on surfaces. *Prog. Nat. Sci.* **2008**, *18*, 1049–1056. [CrossRef]
23. Elbadawi, A.; Saad, M.; Elgendy, I.Y.; Zafar, A.; Chow, M.-Y. Multiple myocardial abscesses secondary to late stent infection. *Cardiovasc. Pathol.* **2017**, *28*, 1–2. [CrossRef]
24. Babapour, E.; Haddadi, A.; Mirnejad, R.; Angaji, S.-A.; Amirmozafari, N. Biofilm formation in clinical isolates of nosocomial Acinetobacter baumannii and its relationship with multidrug resistance. *Asian Pac. J. Trop. Biomed.* **2016**, *6*, 528–533. [CrossRef]
25. Longo, F.; Vuotto, C.; Donelli, G. Biofilm formation in Acinetobacter baumannii. *New Microbiol.* **2014**, *37*, 119–127.
26. Liu, C.P.; Shih, S.C.; Wang, N.Y.; Wu, A.Y.; Sun, F.J.; Chow, S.F.; Chen, T.L.; Yan, T.R. Risk factors of mortality in patients with carbapenem-resistant Acinetobacter baumannii bacteremia. *J. Microbiol. Immunol. Infect.* **2016**, *49*, 934–940. [CrossRef]
27. Almasaudi, S.B. *Acinetobacter* spp. as nosocomial pathogens: Epidemiology and resistance features. *Saudi J. Biol. Sci.* **2018**, *25*, 586–596. [CrossRef]
28. Deiham, B.; Douraghi, M.; Adibhesami, H.; Yaseri, M.; Rahbar, M. Screening of mutator phenotype in clinical strains of Acinetobacter baumannii. *Microb. Pathog.* **2017**, *104*, 175–179. [CrossRef]
29. Djeribi, R.; Bouchloukh, W.; Jouenne, T.; Menaa, B. Characterization of bacterial biofilms formed on urinary catheters. *Am. J. Infect. Control* **2012**, *40*, 854–859. [CrossRef]
30. Cobrado, L.; Silva-Dias, A.; Azevedo, M.M.; Pina-Vaz, C.; Rodrigues, A.G. In vivo antibiofilm effect of cerium, chitosan and hamamelitannin against usual agents of catheter-related bloodstream infections. *J. Antimicrob. Chemother.* **2013**, *68*, 126–130. [CrossRef]
31. Silva, J.C.; Neto, L.M.; Neves, R.C.; Gonçalves, J.C.; Trentini, M.M.; Mucury-Filho, R.; Smidt, K.S.; Fensterseifer, I.C.; Silva, O.N.; Lima, L.D.; et al. Evaluation of the antimicrobial activity of the mastoparan Polybia-MPII isolated from venom of the social wasp Pseudopolybia vespiceps testacea (Vespidae, Hymenoptera). *Int. J. Antimicrob. Agents* **2017**, *49*, 167–175. [CrossRef]
32. Pluzhnikov, K.A.; Kozlov, S.A.; Vassilevski, A.A.; Vorontsova, O.V.; Feofanov, A.V.; Grishin, E.V. Linear antimicrobial peptides from Ectatomma quadridens ant venom. *Biochimie* **2014**, *107*, 211–215. [CrossRef]
33. Perumal Samy, R.; Stiles, B.G.; Franco, O.L.; Sethi, G.; Lim, L.H.K. Animal venoms as antimicrobial agents. *Biochem. Pharmacol.* **2017**, *134*, 127–138. [CrossRef]
34. Garcia, F.; Villegas, E.; Espino-Solis, G.P.; Rodriguez, A.; Paniagua-Solis, J.F.; Sandoval-Lopez, G.; Possani, L.D.; Corzo, G. Antimicrobial peptides from arachnid venoms and their microbicidal activity in the presence of commercial antibiotics. *J. Antibiot.* **2013**, *66*, 3–10. [CrossRef]
35. Harrison, P.L.; Abdel-Rahman, M.A.; Miller, K.; Strong, P.N. Antimicrobial peptides from scorpion venoms. *Toxicon* **2014**, *88*, 115–137. [CrossRef]
36. Souza, B.M.D.; Cabrera, M.P.D.S.; Gomes, P.C.; Dias, N.B.; Stabeli, R.G.; Leite, N.B.; Neto, J.R.; Palma, M.S. Structure-activity relationship of mastoparan analogs: Effects of the number and positioning of Lys residues on secondary structure, interaction with membrane-mimetic systems and biological activity. *Peptides* **2015**, *72*, 164–174. [CrossRef]
37. Wang, K.; Yan, J.; Dang, W.; Xie, J.; Yan, B.; Yan, W.; Sun, M.; Zhang, B.; Ma, M.; Zhao, Y.; et al. Dual antifungal properties of cationic antimicrobial peptides polybia-MPI: Membrane integrity disruption and inhibition of biofilm formation. *Peptides* **2014**, *56*, 22–29. [CrossRef]
38. Das Neves, R.C.; Trentini, M.M.; de Castro e Silva, J.; Simon, K.S.; Bocca, A.L.; Silva, L.P.; Mortari, M.R.; Kipnis, A.; Junqueira-Kipnis, A.P. Antimycobacterial activity of a new peptide polydim-I isolated from neotropical social Wasp Polybia dimorpha. *PLoS ONE* **2016**, *11*, e0149729. [CrossRef]

39. Moerman, L.; Bosteels, S.; Noppe, W.; Willems, J.; Clynen, E.; Schoofs, L.; Thevissen, K.; Tytgat, J.; Van Eldere, J.; Van Der Walt, J.; et al. Antibacterial and antifungal properties of ??-helical, cationic peptides in the venom of scorpions from southern Africa. *Eur. J. Biochem.* **2002**, *269*, 4799–4810. [CrossRef]
40. O'Brien-Simpson, N.M.; Hoffmann, R.; Chia, C.S.B.S.B.; Wade, J.D.D.; Brien-Simpson, N.M.O.; Hoffmann, R.; Chia, C.S.B.S.B.; Wade, J.D.D. (Eds.) *Antimicrobial and Anticancer Peptides*; Frontiers Research Topics; Frontiers Media: Lausanne, Switzerland, 2018; Volume 6, ISBN 9782889454709.
41. Brogden, K.A. Antimicrobial peptides: Pore formers or metabolic inhibitors in bacteria? *Nat. Rev. Microbiol.* **2005**, *3*, 238–250. [CrossRef]
42. Batoni, G.; Maisetta, G.; Esin, S. Antimicrobial peptides and their interaction with biofilms of medically relevant bacteria. *Biochim. Biophys. Acta Biomembr.* **2016**, *1858*, 1044–1060. [CrossRef]
43. Castilho, S.R.A.; Godoy, C.S.D.M.; Guilarde, A.O.; Cardoso, J.L.; André, M.C.P.; Junqueira-Kipnis, A.P.; Kipnis, A. Acinetobacter baumannii strains isolated from patients in intensive care units in Goiânia, Brazil: Molecular and drug susceptibility profiles. *PLoS ONE* **2017**, *12*, e0176790. [CrossRef]
44. Mendes, M.A.; De Souza, B.M.; Marques, M.R.; Palma, M.S. Structural and biological characterization of two novel peptides from the venom of the neotropical social wasp Agelaia pallipes pallipes. *Toxicon* **2004**, *44*, 67–74. [CrossRef]
45. De Souza, B.M.; Marques, M.R.; Tomazela, D.M.; Eberlin, M.N.; Mendes, M.A.; Palma, M.S. Mass spectrometric characterization of two novel inflammatory peptides from the venom of the social waspPolybia paulista. *Rapid Commun. Mass Spectrom.* **2004**, *18*, 1095–1102. [CrossRef]
46. Silva, É.C.N.; Camargos, T.S.; Maranhão, A.Q.; Silva-Pereira, I.; Silva, L.P.; Possani, L.D.; Schwartz, E.F. Cloning and characterization of cDNA sequences encoding for new venom peptides of the Brazilian scorpion Opisthacanthus cayaporum. *Toxicon* **2009**. [CrossRef]
47. Kaufmann, B.A.; Kaiser, C.; Pfisterer, M.E.; Bonetti, P.O. Coronary stent infection: A rare but severe complication of percutaneous coronary intervention. *Swiss Med. Wkly.* **2005**, *135*, 483–487.
48. Sanchez, C.J.; Mende, K.; Beckius, M.L.; Akers, K.S.; Romano, D.R.; Wenke, J.C.; Murray, C.K. Biofilm formation by clinical isolates and the implications in chronic infections. *BMC Infect. Dis.* **2013**, *13*, 1. [CrossRef]
49. Espinal, P.; Martí, S.; Vila, J. Effect of biofilm formation on the survival of Acinetobacter baumannii on dry surfaces. *J. Hosp. Infect.* **2012**, *80*, 56–60. [CrossRef]
50. Bravo, Z.; Chapartegui-González, I.; Lázaro-Díez, M.; Ramos-Vivas, J. Acinetobacter pittii biofilm formation on inanimate surfaces after long-term desiccation. *J. Hosp. Infect.* **2018**, *98*, 74–82. [CrossRef]
51. Munier, A.-L.; Biard, L.; Rousseau, C.; Legrand, M.; Lafaurie, M.; Lomont, A.; Donay, J.-L.; de Beaugrenier, E.; Flicoteaux, R.; Mebazaa, A.; et al. Incidence, risk factors, and outcome of multidrug-resistant Acinetobacter baumannii acquisition during an outbreak in a burns unit. *J. Hosp. Infect.* **2017**, *97*, 226–233. [CrossRef]
52. Furtado, A.D.; Bhat, S.P.S.; Peer, S.M.; Chikkatur, R. Infected pseudoaneurysm involving a drug-eluting stent. *Interact. Cardiovasc. Thorac. Surg.* **2011**. [CrossRef]
53. Venkatesan, A.M.; Kundu, S.; Sacks, D.; Wallace, M.J.; Wojak, J.C.; Rose, S.C.; Clark, T.W.I.; D'Othee, B.J.; Itkin, M.; Jones, R.S.; et al. Practice guideline for adult antibiotic prophylaxis during vascular and interventional radiology procedures. *J. Vasc. Interv. Radiol.* **2010**, *21*, 1611–1630. [CrossRef]
54. Schoenkerman, A.B.; Lundstrom, R.J. Coronary stent infections: A case series. *Catheter. Cardiovasc. Interv.* **2009**, *73*, 74–76. [CrossRef]
55. Vila-Farrés, X.; López-Rojas, R.; Pachón-Ibáñez, M.E.; Teixidó, M.; Pachón, J.; Vila, J.; Giralt, E. Sequence-activity relationship, and mechanism of action of mastoparan analogues against extended-drug resistant Acinetobacter baumannii. *Eur. J. Med. Chem.* **2015**, *101*, 34–40. [CrossRef]
56. Huang, Y.; Wiradharma, N.; Xu, K.; Ji, Z.; Bi, S.; Li, L.; Yang, Y.Y.; Fan, W. Cationic amphiphilic alpha-helical peptides for the treatment of carbapenem-resistant Acinetobacter baumannii infection. *Biomaterials* **2012**, *33*, 8841–8847. [CrossRef]
57. Lin, C.H.; Lee, M.C.; Tzen, J.T.C.; Lee, H.M.; Chang, S.M.; Tu, W.C.; Lin, C.F. Efficacy of mastoparan-AF alone and in combination with clinically used antibiotics on nosocomial multidrug-resistant Acinetobacter baumannii. *Saudi J. Biol. Sci.* **2017**, *24*, 1023–1029. [CrossRef]
58. Lin, M.-F. Antimicrobial resistance in *Acinetobacter baumannii*: From bench to bedside. *World J. Clin. Cases* **2014**, *2*, 787. [CrossRef]

59. Wang, Y.C.; Kuo, S.C.; Yang, Y.S.; Lee, Y.T.; Chiu, C.H.; Chuang, M.F.; Lin, J.C.; Chang, F.Y.; Chen, T.L. Individual or combined effects of meropenem, imipenem, sulbactam, colistin, and tigecycline on biofilm-embedded Acinetobacter baumannii and biofilm architecture. *Antimicrob. Agents Chemother.* **2016**, *60*, 4670–4676. [CrossRef]
60. Andreassen, S.; Zalounina, A.; Paul, M.; Sanden, L.; Leibovici, L. Interpretative reading of the antibiogram—Semi-naïve Bayesian approach. *Artif. Intell. Med.* **2015**, *65*, 209–217. [CrossRef]
61. Ammann, C.G.; Neuhauser, D.; Eberl, C.; Nogler, M.; Coraça-Huber, D. Tolerance towards gentamicin is a function of nutrient concentration in biofilms of patient-isolated Staphylococcus epidermidis. *Folia Microbiol.* **2018**, *63*, 299–305. [CrossRef]
62. Saint Jean, K.D.; Henderson, K.D.; Chrom, C.L.; Abiuso, L.E.; Renn, L.M.; Caputo, G.A. Effects of hydrophobic amino acid substitutions on antimicrobial peptide behavior. *Probiotics Antimicrob. Proteins* **2018**, *10*, 408–419. [CrossRef]
63. Andreev, K.; Martynowycz, M.W.; Huang, M.L.; Kuzmenko, I.; Bu, W.; Kirshenbaum, K.; Gidalevitz, D. Hydrophobic interactions modulate antimicrobial peptoid selectivity towards anionic lipid membranes. *Biochim. Biophys. Acta Biomembr.* **2018**, *1860*, 1414–1423. [CrossRef]
64. Mishra, B.; Lushnikova, T.; Golla, R.M.; Wang, X.; Wang, G. Design and surface immobilization of short anti-biofilm peptides. *Acta Biomater.* **2017**, *49*, 316–328. [CrossRef]
65. Gabriel, M.; Nazmi, K.; Veerman, E.C.; Amerongen, A.V.N.; Zentner, A. Preparation of LL-37-grafted titanium surfaces with bactericidal activity. *Bioconjug. Chem.* **2006**. [CrossRef]
66. Mishra, B.; Basu, A.; Chua, R.R.Y.; Saravanan, R.; Tambyah, P.A.; Ho, B.; Chang, M.W.; Leong, S.S.J. Site specific immobilization of a potent antimicrobial peptide onto silicone catheters: Evaluation against urinary tract infection pathogens. *J. Mater. Chem. B* **2014**. [CrossRef]
67. Bagheri, M.; Beyermann, M.; Dathe, M. Immobilization reduces the activity of surface-bound cationic antimicrobial peptides with no influence upon the activity spectrum. *Antimicrob. Agents Chemother.* **2009**, *53*, 1132–1141. [CrossRef]
68. Costa, F.; Carvalho, I.F.; Montelaro, R.C.; Gomes, P.; Martins, M.C.L. Covalent immobilization of antimicrobial peptides (AMPs) onto biomaterial surfaces. *Acta Biomater.* **2011**, *7*, 1431–1440. [CrossRef]
69. Singha, P.; Locklin, J.; Handa, H. A review of the recent advances in antimicrobial coatings for urinary catheters. *Acta Biomater.* **2017**, *50*, 20–40. [CrossRef]
70. Wiegand, I.; Hilpert, K.; Hancock, R.E.W. Agar and broth dilution methods to determine the minimal inhibitory concentration (MIC) of antimicrobial substances. *Nat. Protoc.* **2008**, *3*, 163–175. [CrossRef]
71. Feng, X.; Sambanthamoorthy, K.; Palys, T.; Paranavitana, C. The human antimicrobial peptide LL-37 and its fragments possess both antimicrobial and antibiofilm activities against multidrug-resistant Acinetobacter baumannii. *Peptides* **2013**, *49*, 131–137. [CrossRef]
72. Kwasny, S.M.; Opperman, T.J. Static biofilm cultures of gram positive pathogens grown in a microtiter format used for anti-biofilm drug discovery. *Curr. Protoc. Pharmacol.* **2010**, *50*, 13A.8.1–13A.8.23. [CrossRef]

toxins

MDPI

Review

Chemical and Biological Characteristics of Antimicrobial α-Helical Peptides Found in Solitary Wasp Venoms and Their Interactions with Model Membranes

Marcia Perez dos Santos Cabrera [1], Marisa Rangel [2], João Ruggiero Neto [1] and Katsuhiro Konno [3,*]

[1] Department of Physics, IBILCE, São Paulo State University, São José do Rio Preto, SP 15054-000, Brazil; cabrera.marcia@gmail.com (M.P.d.S.C.); joao.ruggiero@unesp.br (J.R.N.)
[2] Immunopathology Laboratory, Butantan Institute, Sao Paulo, SP 05503-900, Brazil; marisarangel2112@gmail.com
[3] Institute of Natural Medicine, University of Toyama, 2630 Sugitani, Toyama, Toyama 930-0194, Japan
* Correspondence: kkgon@inm.u-toyama.ac.jp; Tel.: +81-76-434-7617; Fax: +81-76-434-5055

Received: 31 July 2019; Accepted: 16 September 2019; Published: 24 September 2019

check for updates

Abstract: Solitary wasps use their stinging venoms for paralyzing insect or spider prey and feeding them to their larvae. We have surveyed bioactive substances in solitary wasp venoms, and found antimicrobial peptides together with some other bioactive peptides. Eumenine mastoparan-AF (EMP-AF) was the first to be found from the venom of the solitary eumenine wasp *Anterhynchium flavomarginatum micado*, showing antimicrobial, histamine-releasing, and hemolytic activities, and adopting an α-helical secondary structure under appropriate conditions. Further survey of solitary wasp venom components revealed that eumenine wasp venoms contained such antimicrobial α-helical peptides as the major peptide component. This review summarizes the results obtained from the studies of these peptides in solitary wasp venoms and some analogs from the viewpoint of (1) chemical and biological characterization; (2) physicochemical properties and secondary structure; and (3) channel-like pore-forming properties.

Keywords: solitary wasp; venom; antimicrobial peptide; linear cationic α-helical peptide; amphipathic α-helix structure; channel-like pore-forming activity

Key Contribution: Antimicrobial and α-helical peptides were found in solitary wasp venoms, and their biological, physicochemical, and channel-like pore-forming properties were investigated.

1. Introduction

Antimicrobial peptides are widely found in plants, insects, amphibians, and mammals, playing an important role in innate immune systems and host defense mechanisms [1,2]. They have attracted much attention as a novel class of antibiotics, in particular for antibiotic-resistant pathogens, because of their action mechanism of non-selective interaction with cell surface membranes of microbes [3,4]. In some cases, antimicrobial peptides are produced when challenged by microbes, and they are also contained in arthropod venoms. They may play a role in preventing potential infection [5–7].

We have surveyed bioactive substances in solitary wasp venoms, in particular neurotoxins, because the venom is used for paralyzing their prey. Consequently, we indeed isolated novel peptide neurotoxins, but also found novel antimicrobial peptides. Eumenine mastoparan-AF (EMP-AF) was the first antimicrobial peptide to be found in solitary wasp venoms in the year 2000 [8]. Since then, several other antimicrobial peptides have been found, mostly in solitary eumenine wasp venoms [9–14]. These peptides are only 10–15 amino acids in length, are rich in hydrophobic and basic amino acids with no disulfide bond, and can adopt an α-helical amphipathic secondary structure under appropriate conditions. Besides the antimicrobial activity, they commonly show histamine-release from mast cells, as well as hemolytic and leishmanicidal activities. Physicochemical properties of these peptides, i.e., charge, hydrophobicity, and amphipathicity, have been investigated, and some of these properties were shown to be important to our understanding of the structure-function relationship and useful for the design of new sequences with improved biological properties [10–15]. The biological activities of these peptides may be due to the adoption of an amphipathic α-helical secondary structure that inserts into the lipids of biological membranes. Accordingly, these peptides were tested in artificial lipid bilayers, and the channel-like activity observed demonstrated that ion conduction through biological membranes must be important to their lytic activity against mammal cells, but more importantly, against microorganisms [10,12,14–16]. This review summarizes these results from the studies on antimicrobial α-helical peptides in solitary wasp venoms. An overview of peptide toxins in solitary wasp venoms was summarized previously [17].

2. Chemical and Biological Characterization

Chemical studies on solitary wasp venom components were not well documented until we started our own research on solitary wasp venoms in 1995. This may be a result of their solitary lifestyle: collecting a large number of wasp individuals and providing a sufficient amount of venom constituents required for chemical analysis is very difficult. Pioneering studies in 1980s, however, reported on neurotoxins: megascoliakinins in scoliid wasps [18] and philanthotoxins in digger wasps [19]. We collected 40 species of solitary wasps inhabiting Japan, and surveyed bioactive substances in their venoms focused on small molecules and peptides. The peptide neurotoxins, pompilidotoxins (PMTXs), blocking sodium channel inactivation were found first [20], and further survey led to finding antimicrobial peptides, mostly from eumenine wasp venoms. Table 1 summarizes the amino acid sequences of antimicrobial α-helical peptides hitherto found in solitary wasp venoms, and Table 2 shows selected biological activities shown by these peptides.

Table 1. Antimicrobial and α-helical peptides in solitary wasp venoms. EMP: eumenine mastoparan.

Peptide	Sequence	Peptide	Sequence
EMP-AF	INLLKIAKGIIKSL-NH_2	Eumenitin	LNLKGIFKKVKSLLT
EMP-EF	FDVMGIIKKIASAL-NH_2	Eumenitin-F	LNLKGLFKKVASLLT
EMP-ER	FDIMGLIKKVAGAL-NH_2	Eumenitin-R	LNLKGLIKKVASLLN
EMP-EM1	LKLMGIVKKVLGAL-NH_2	EpVP1	INLKGLIKKVASLLT
EMP-EM2	LKLLGIVKKVLGAI-NH_2	Decoralin	SLLSLIRKLIT
EpVP2a	FDLLGLVKKVASAL-NH_2	OdVP3	KDLHTVVSAILQAL-NH_2
EpVP2b	FDLLGLVKSVVSAL-NH_2	EMP-OD (OdVP1)	GRILSFIKGLAEHL-NH_2
Anoplin	GLLKRIKTLL-NH_2	Orancis-Protonectin (OdVP2)	ILGIITSLLKSL-NH_2

Table 2. Selected biological activities of antimicrobial and α-helical peptides in solitary wasp venoms.

Peptides	Antimicrobial Activity (MIC, μM)			Hemolysis (EC_{50}, μM)	Degranulation (EC_{50}, μM)	References
	S. aureus	*E. coli*	*C. albicans*			
EMP-AF	3	33	-	50	30	[8,14]
EMP-EF	30	30	7.5	181	60	[12]
EMP-ER	30	30	7.5	200	70	[12]
EMP-EM1	7	7	>60	na	70	[13]
EMP-EM2	3	3	>60	na	60	[13]
Eumenitin	6	6	-	na	70	[10]
Eumenitin-F	>60	30	7.5	353	na	[12]
Eumenitin-R	60	30	7.5	530	na	[12]
Decoralin	40	80	40	na	na	[11]
Anoplin	4	43	-	na	30	[9]

MIC: minimum inhibitory concentration; EC_{50}: effective concentration that produces 50% of the maximum effect; na: no activity or virtually no activity; *S. aureus*: *Staphylococcus aureus* ATCC 6538 or ATCC 25923 (Gram-positive bacteria; *E. coli*: *Escherichia coli* CCT 6538 or ATCC 25922 (Gram-negative bacteria); *C. albicans*: *Candida albicans* (UMP) (Yeast); Hemolysis: human or mouse erythrocytes; Degranulation: rat peritoneal mast cells or RBL-2H3 cells.

2.1. Mastoparans

Eumenine mastoparan-AF (EMP-AF) was the first antimicrobial α-helical peptide that we found in the venom of the solitary eumenine wasp *Anterhynchium flavomarginatum micado* in the year 2000 [8]. The HPLC profile of the crude venom extracts was rather simple, and accordingly, only one single fractionation led to the purification and isolation of this major peptide. The structure of EMP-AF is homologous to mastoparans found in social wasp venoms (hornets and paper wasps). Mastoparan was originally found in the venom of the social vespid wasp *Vespula lewisii* as a new mast cell degranulating peptide [21]. Since then, many similar peptides have been found in the vespid wasp venoms, and they are collectively called mastoparans or mastoparan peptides [22]. These peptides have common chemical features: they are 14 amino acids in length with C-terminal amidation, they are rich in hydrophobic and basic amino acids, and adapt an α-helical secondary structure under appropriate conditions. Mastoparans exhibit antimicrobial, hemolytic, and mast cell degranulation activities, which are based on this amphipathic chemical character associating with cell membranes [23]. EMP-AF has all the chemical and biological characteristics of mastoparans: in particular, this peptide showed high content of α-helical conformation in 2,2,2-trifluoroethanol (TFE) and sodium dodecylsulfate (SDS) micelles [14], and stimulated degranulation from rat peritoneal mast cells and RBL-2H3 cells to a similar extent as mastoparan [8]. The C-terminal amidation is very important for these chemical and biological properties. For example, a synthetic analog bearing a free-carboxyl terminus (not amidated) showed reduced α-helical content and antibacterial activity [14]. NMR analysis demonstrated that the C-terminal amide contributed to stabilizing the α-helical conformation [24].

Mastoparan-like peptides are commonly distributed in eumenine wasp venoms. EMP-OD (OdVP1) and OdVP3 were found in the venom of the eumenine wasp *Orancistrocerus drewseni drewseni* [25,26]. Despite poor sequence similarity to mastoparan, these peptides have typical chemical features of mastoparans: they are 14 amino acids in length, with an amidated C-terminus, and a possible α-helical secondary structure. EMP-OD exhibits more potent hemolytic activity than that of mastoparan, and OdVP3 shows potent antifungal activity rather than antibacterial activity. EMP-EF and EMP-ER from *Eumenes fraterculus* and *Eumenes rubrofemoratus*, respectively, contain an aspartic acid residue at the second position, which is characteristic for these peptide structures, and less usual for mastoparan peptides. Biological activities (mast cell degranulation, antimicrobial and hemolytic activity) of these peptides are significantly lower than found for mastoparan and EMP-AF [12]. EpVP2a and EpVP2b from *Eumenes pomiformis* are structurally quite similar to EMP-EF and EMP-ER. However, they were found by transcriptomic analysis, and the biological activities were not investigated [27]. EMP-EM1 and EMP-EM2 from *Eumenes micado* are the most recently found mastoparan peptides, and highly homologous to EMP-AF [13]. They show antimicrobial and mast cell degranulating activities at similar extent as EMP-AF, but virtually no hemolytic activity.

2.2. Eumenitins

Eumenitin, in the venom of the solitary eumenine wasp *Eumenes rubronotatus*, has basically the same chemical features as those of mastoparans, but an extra hydrophilic amino acid at the C-terminus without amide modification [10]. Accordingly, it rather belongs to linear cationic α-helical peptides. The biological properties are also similar to mastoparans, but the potencies are lower [10]. Three other eumenine wasp venoms contain eumenitin-type peptides: eumenitin-R from *Eumenes rubrofemoratus* [12], eumenitin-F from *Eumenes fraterculus* [12], and EpVP1 from *Eumenes pomiformis* [27]. In contrast to the case of mastoparans, eumenitin-type peptides have been found only in solitary wasp venoms, whereas social wasp venoms never contain this type of peptides.

2.3. Protonectin

Orancis-protonectin (OdVP2) from *Orancistrocerus drewseni drewseni* is a dodecapeptide with an amidated C-terminus [25], and is closely related to protonectin, which was originally found in Brazilian social wasp venom. Its analogs are distributed in some other social wasp venoms [22]. Protonectins are rich in hydrophobic amino acid residues and exhibit potent hemolytic activity. Orancis-protonectin is the first example of the protonectin analog isolated from a solitary wasp venom. This peptide shows more potent hemolytic activity than that of mastoparan and moderate antimicrobial activity [25,26].

2.4. Decoralin

Decoralin from *Oreumenes decoratus* is a smaller peptide, with a length of only 11 amino acids without C-terminal amidation [11]. This sequence has the characteristic features of linear cationic α-helical peptides, rich in hydrophobic and basic amino acids with no disulfide bond, and accordingly, it can be predicted to adopt an amphipathic α-helix secondary structure, as indicated by circular dichroism [11]. In fact, on biological evaluation, decoralin exhibited a significant broad-spectrum antimicrobial activity and moderate mast cell degranulation and leishmanicidal activities, but showed virtually no hemolytic activity. A synthetic analog with C-terminal amidation showed much more potent activity in all the biological assays [11], and NMR experiments demonstrated its amphipathic α-helix secondary structure [28].

2.5. Anoplin

Anoplin was purified from the venom of the solitary spider wasp *Anoplius samariensis* as a minor peptide component [9], while the major component of this venom is α-pompilidotoxin (α-PMTX), a neurotoxin blocking sodium channel inactivation [20,29]. Anoplin consists of only 10 amino acids, and has typical chemical and biological characteristics of antimicrobial α-helical peptides. This is among the smallest antimicrobial peptides with an α-helical structure found from natural sources, which can be advantageous for structural modification, structure-activity relationships studies, and therapeutic applications as a new and useful antimicrobial agent. There are many studies along this line [30–43].

The antimicrobial α-helical peptides in solitary wasp venoms may have a key role in preventing potential microbial infection of the paralyzed preys during consumption by their larvae [9]. When injected into lepidopteran larvae, the α-helical peptides caused feeding disorder, which indicated that the α-helical peptides might function as non-specific neurotoxins or myotoxins by inducing cell lysis and venom-spreading factors by increasing cell permeability [44].

3. Physicochemical Properties and Secondary Structure

Despite being produced by widely different organisms, antimicrobial peptides share similar structural patterns, which are known for their inter-dependency. The same applies for peptides found in solitary wasp venoms, which have been shown to be predominantly amphipathic, helical, and cationic at physiological pH. Some physicochemical properties have been investigated and shown to be important to understand structure-function relationships and to help designing new sequences with improved performance. Amongst solitary wasp venoms this tool has also been employed. Table 3 lists the physicochemical properties of antimicrobial peptides found in some solitary wasp venoms, which are briefly discussed below, and in Figure 1 helical wheel projections of these peptides are shown.

Table 3. Physicochemical parameters and α-helical content of antimicrobial peptides in solitary wasp venom in different environments.

Peptides	*N*	Q	C-Term	<H>	μ	f_H			References
						TFE	SDS	PC	
EMP-AF	14	+4	amide	0.051	0.342	0.55	0.72	0.16	[14]
EMP-EF	14	+2	amide	0.115	0.279	0.41	0.44	nd	[12]
EMP-ER	14	+2	amide	0.131	0.251	0.53	0.59	nd	[12]
EMP-EM1	14	+4	amide	0.104	0.258	0.31	0.33	0.11	[13]
EMP-EM2	14	+4	amide	0.138	0.278	0.37	0.41	< 0.03	[13]
Eumenitin	15	+3	carboxyl	0.002	0.265	0.43	0.50	0.07/0.11	[10]
Eumenitin-F	15	+3	carboxyl	-	0.256	0.34	0.44	nd	[12]
Eumenitin-R	15	+3	carboxyl	-	0.281	0.43	0.48	nd	[12]
Decoralin	11	+3	carboxyl	0.028	0.393	0.38	0.50	rc	[11]
Anoplin	10	+4	amide	-	0.366	0.24	0.26	rc	[9]

N: number of residues; **Q**: net charge; **C-term**: C-terminus; **<H>**: mean hydrophobicity; **μ**: hydrophobic moment; f_H: α-helix fraction, 40% TFE, 8 mM SDS, 380 μM PC; nd: non-determined; rc: random coil.

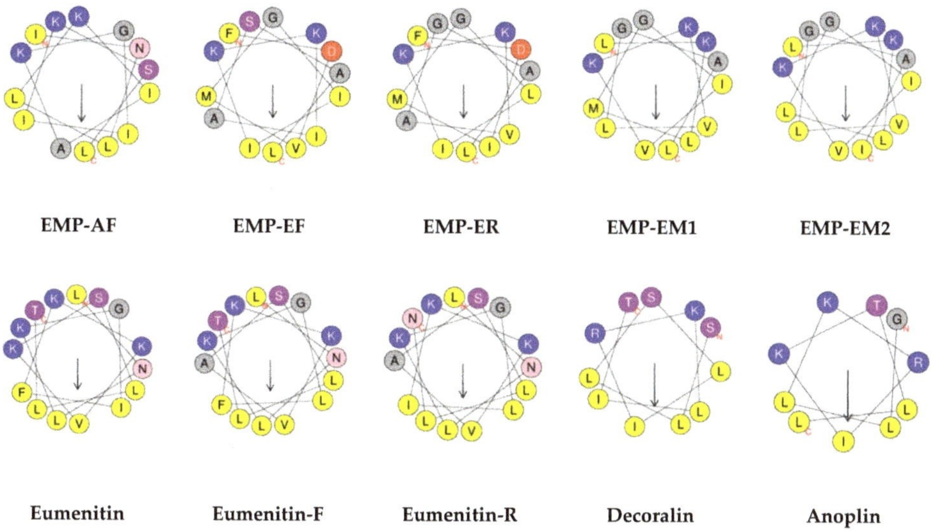

Figure 1. Helical wheel projection of antimicrobial α-helical peptides in solitary wasp venoms. In this view through the helix axis, the hydrophilic residues (D, N, K, S, T, R) are located on one side and the hydrophobic residues (F, I, L, M, V) on the other side of the helix. The arrow shows the hydrophobic moment (μ) vector. N: N-terminus; C: C-terminus.

3.1. Sequence and Chain Length

To date, antimicrobial peptides from solitary wasp venoms have been found to be built almost exclusively by naturally occurring amino acids with a chain length ranging from 10 to 15 residues. Truncation studies with anoplin, a decapeptide, resulted in partial loss of the antimicrobial activity [30], suggesting that this chain length is close to the minimum required for significant activity. Truncation of three N-terminal residues inn EMP-AF totally abolished the biological activities [14]. Taken together, these results with anoplin and EMP-AF suggest that specific residues are more important than chain length, and that in such short chain peptides, features of some amino acid residues have a major importance. In solitary wasp venom peptides, anionic residues seldom appear, and among the cationic residues, Lys is much more frequent than Arg or His. Some of the apolar residues such as Trp, Pro, and Met seldom appear and polar uncharged residues such as Cys and Tyr are rare. On the other hand, bulky aliphatic residues such as Ile, Leu, and Val are ubiquitous, and similarly to what has been found for antimicrobial peptides in general they form the hydrophobic face [45,46].

3.2. N- and C-Termini

End effects are especially important for the structure and performance of short chain peptides [47]. The most frequent modification found with solitary wasp venom peptides is the amidation of the C-terminus, probably the most common posttranslational modification that occurs in a wide variety of peptides. Amidation involves oxidative decarboxylation of an additional glycine residue at the C-terminus. It prevents cleavage by carboxypeptidases, enables the accommodation of the otherwise negatively charged C-terminus in a nonpolar environment [48,49], and provides an extra hydrogen bond for the formation of α-helices [24]. The correlation between amidation and biological activity has been found to be an important feature, with carboxylated peptides showing significantly impaired activity [11,12,14,15].

3.3. Charge and Helix Macro-Dipole

The cationicity due to the net positive charge of solitary wasp venom peptides ranges from +1 to +4 (Table 3) and this feature has been considered essential for the activity of antimicrobial peptides, although the number of positive charges required for activity is case sensitive [48,50]. The action of cationic peptides on negatively charged pathogen membranes starts with the electrostatic interaction between them; hence, an increase in positive charge of peptides should increase microbial activity [48,51,52]. The first most comprehensive structure-function study carried out with a solitary wasp venom peptide and analogs was that by Ifrah and co-workers [30]. This work was recently further developed [33]. Although the impact of increasing the number of charged residues has not been specifically investigated to date, in the first work they showed that decreasing the number of positively charged residues either decrease antimicrobial activity or the selectivity, showing also an increase in the hemolytic activity. Increasing the net charge, the effect is position-dependent and most of the tested analogs showed increased hemolytic activity. In a more recent investigation [33], it was confirmed that increasing the charge and/or hydrophobicity improves antimicrobial activity, but also increases the hemolytic activity. With a different approach [36], the antimicrobial activity of anoplin was improved without compromising the therapeutic index by increasing the net charge, introducing Trp residues at specific positions, slightly modifying the retention times and increasing amphiphilicity. These findings are in good accordance with those by Dathe and co-workers [53] that showed that increasing the number of positive charges is followed by an increase in antimicrobial activity of magainin 2 analogs within certain limits. Above them, antimicrobial activity decreases and hemolytic activity appears. A minimum of charge around +2 has been suggested as required for antimicrobial peptide selectivity [54], because it facilitates initial interaction with microbial membranes, transitions in orientation (pore formation) and translocation of peptides to the cytoplasmic membrane, and helps displacing membrane-bound cations [48,54,55]. More recently, series of decoralin derivatives were studied for anticancer, antimicrobial, and antiplasmodial activities [56–60]. In the anticancer studies, it was observed that increasing the positive net charge favored the activity, although the amidated form of decoralin was among those with higher activity [56,59]. Concerning the antimicrobial activity, the works by Torres et al. [57,58] achieved lower hemolytic activity of the designed analogs in relation to amidated decoralin at equipotent antimicrobial levels. However, in the study of the antiplasmodial activity, while amidated decoralin was deprived of activity, three analogs showed potent activity and revealed that, for this activity, the net charge variation was not as important as it showed to be for the antimicrobial and anticancer activities [60].

Each peptide unit has a dipole moment of 3.5 D (1.155×10^{-29} Cm); in an α-helix the sum of individual residue dipoles, which are aligned almost parallel to the helix axis, builds up the helix dipole. The significant electric field of an α-helix is thus generated by the macro-dipole that runs from the negative pole at the C-terminus to the positive pole at the N-terminus. The strength of the field of this macro-dipole increases up to 10 Å helix length, which roughly corresponds to eight folded residues, and further elongation does not contribute significantly [61], although this field will be dependent on the solvent dielectric constant [62]. Considering the short chain length of solitary wasp venom peptides, the effects of the helix field have a major importance and represent a useful tool in the designing of new peptides since it contributes to the interaction with charged substrates in the long-range attraction, in facilitating the binding, and the suitable orientation in relation these substrates [61]. Nevertheless, the above-mentioned studies did not show differences in the activities that could be attributed to the helix macrodipole of the peptides.

3.4. Helical Propensity and Helicity

The folding of an amino acid sequence into a helix is a cooperative process [63] characterized by the Zimm–Bragg parameters σ and s, respectively defined as nucleation factor and propagation constant [64,65]. Inner helical residues will form two hydrogen bonds, coil residues will form no hydrogen bonds, and end residues might form only one hydrogen bond to the third or fourth nearest neighboring residue. Each amino acid residue has its own conformational preferences, and in a sequence, the sum of these preferences leads to the stabilization or not of the α-helix [66], depending on chain length [65,67] and on the environment [68–70].

Helicity is a consequence of the primary sequence of amino acid residues [63,71] and of their interaction with the environment [68], which includes peptide hydrogen-bond formation and van der Waals and hydrophobic interactions, contributing to helix stabilization [66]. Helical structuring seems to be an important contributor to the antimicrobial action, since helical peptides are prevalent in the universe of antimicrobial peptides [45] and of solitary wasp venom peptides. Among factors that influence α-helix formation, there are (1) electrostatic interactions at the N-terminus, and at i, i +3 or i, i + 4 side chain interactions at the center of the chain [63] and (2) the hydrophobic interaction, as has been demonstrated by Blondelle and Houghten [72].

Amongst solitary wasp venom peptides and analogs, the helical content ranged from nearly 10 to 70%, more often around 50%, as determined in CD experiments (Table 3, Figure 2) in SDS micelles (8 mM). Although presenting preferential interaction with anionic media, in the presence of different membrane mimetic environments the helical fraction may vary, generally as a function of peptide hydrophobicity in electrically neutral media or as a function of peptide net charge in anionic environments. In aqueous or buffer media, solitary wasp venom peptides show random coil conformations [9–12,14,15]. Helical content influences peptide activity on negatively charged membranes, as is suggested by the examples in Table 3: there is a good correlation between the helical content and the antimicrobial activity among solitary wasp venom peptides. According to Dathe and Wieprecht [73] and Giangaspero and co-workers [46], higher helicity correlates with increased activity towards zwitterionic membranes. However, results obtained with model peptides suggested that helicity is more important to peptide activity on zwitterionic membranes than to permeabilization of the negatively charged ones [74]. Structural information on solitary wasp venom peptides is mainly based on CD data; to the best of our knowledge, NMR experiments were carried out just for EMP-AF [24] and decoralin [28]. Accumulating information obtained from the interaction of solitary wasp venom peptides with model membranes by NMR would help establishing a database with an increased confidence level.

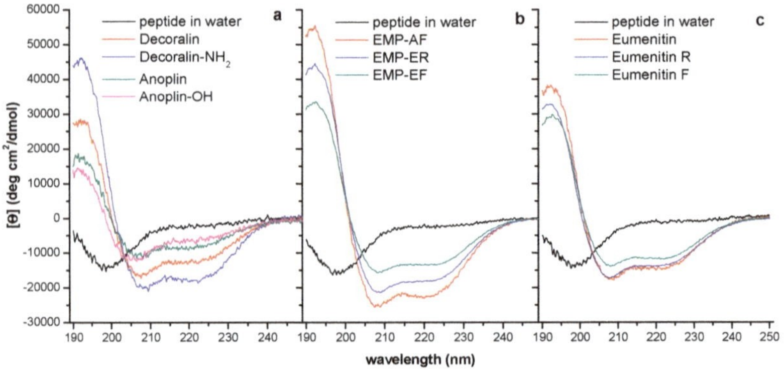

Figure 2. Examples of CD spectra obtained for solitary wasp venom peptides and analogs in 8-mM SDS solution. This micelle environment is frequently used as a mimetic of prokaryotic membranes due to its anionic character. (**a**) The shorter chain peptides, anoplin and decoralin, and their analogs: amidated forms display higher helical content. (**b**) The wild type amidated tetradecapeptides, EMP-AF, EMP-ER, and EMP-EF with +4 and +3 charges, respectively, share similar structural features with mastoparans and present higher helical content and higher hydrophobicity level. (**c**) The wild type carboxylated pentadecapeptides, eumenitin, eumenitin R, and eumenitin F with +3 charges and lower hydrophobicity level, show intermediate helicity level and correspond to the most selective solitary wasp venom peptides.

3.5. Amphipathicity and Hydrophobic Moment

The most common structure among antimicrobial peptides and solitary wasp venom peptides, including analogs, is the amphipathic helix, ideal for interacting with equally amphipathic biomembranes. Amphipathicity reflects the possibility that an amino acid sequence has to form well-structured hydrophobic and hydrophilic domains in opposite faces. The hydrophobic moment represents a quantitative measurement of amphipathicity [75]. However, it assumes that 100% of the side-chains protrude perpendicular to the helix axis at regular 100° intervals, i.e., as an ideal α-helix. It could be more accurate for the short solitary wasp venom peptides if it were calculated based on NMR structural data. Nevertheless, a search among antimicrobial peptides showed that the hydrophobic moment ranges from 0.45 to 0.6 [45,46], while for solitary wasp venom peptides we found values ranging from around 0.2 to 0.4. Increasing the hydrophobic moment results in a significant increase in the permeabilizing and hemolytic activities of model peptide and magainin [52,76]. Pathak and co-workers [77] suggested that amphipathicity was more important than hydrophobicity or α-helical content in governing antimicrobial peptide activity. However, Dathe and co-workers, working with KLA model peptides designed to have individual parameter modifications, showed that increasing hydrophobic moment appears to have only modest effects on anionic bilayer permeabilizing efficiency, but for zwitterionic bilayers, where electrostatic peptide–lipid interactions are minimized, a higher hydrophobic moment results in a significant increase in permeabilizing activity [76]. It was suggested that an imperfect segregation of hydrophilic and hydrophobic groups of the peptide chain contributes to the bilayer disturbing abilities and thus to the antimicrobial activity, according to the proposed model of interfacial activity [78]. In this case, also an accumulation of NMR structural data would contribute to our knowledge of the real amphipaticity of peptides when bound to membranes or their models.

3.6. Hydrophobicity

In aqueous media hydrophobic units do not make hydrogen bond to water; this creates excluded volume regions where the absence of water enables attraction among apolar groups, originating hydrophobic interactions [79]. Hydrophobicity measures the peptide affinity for the membrane interior and is calculated as the average value of all peptide residues in the chain, according to different scales, but in the present work, according to the Eisenberg consensus scale [75]. Mean hydrophobicity levels among solitary wasp venom peptides range from as low as −0.11 to +0.14 and show selectivity for bacterial membranes (Table 3). Hydrophobicity is necessary for effective membrane permeabilization, however, increased levels favor interactions with acidic and zwitterionic vesicles, impairing the selectivity to bacterial membranes [45,54,80]. Blondelle and Houghten established good correlations between decreased hydrophobicity and increased antimicrobial activity and between decreased hydrophobicity and decreased hemolytic activity, working with de novo designed peptides [72].

From the physicochemical properties that influence the biological activities of antimicrobial peptides and solitary wasp venom peptides, mean hydrophobicity and charge have proved to be important modulating factors [81]. Dathe and co-workers showed that hydrophobicity at very low levels abolishes activity, at high levels enhances hemolysis, at too high levels cause aggregation or precipitation, and at reasonable low levels enhances Gram-negative bacterial specificity [52,73]. Besides discriminating lipid head groups [82] and the importance on the peptides adsorption to the lipid membrane, charged residues are shown by all atoms or coarse graining molecular dynamics simulations to play key role on the pore formation [83,84]. Simulations have also shown that hydrophobicity is important for peptide aggregation before pore formation [83,84] and, reinforced by X-ray experiments [85,86], hydrophobicity was demonstrated to influence the peptides embedding into the membrane core. The combination of higher charge (+4) and positive hydrophobicity (+0.051), as in the case of EMP-AF, increased the hemolytic activity, while anoplin and eumenitin R are good examples of the opposite effect. One of the great contributions of the structure-function studies with solitary wasp venom peptides is the fact that they highlight many possibilities of designing active antimicrobials considering short chains with lower toxicity.

4. Channel-Like Pore-Forming Properties

Substances that are hemolytic or cytotoxic due to pore formation in membranes generally form non-selective pores that conduct ions, toxins, and metabolites that may produce progressive membrane depolarization and prevent both eukaryotic and prokaryotic cells to keep homeostasis [87,88]. The biological activities of solitary wasp venom peptides (antimicrobial, fungicidal, mast cell degranulating, hemolytic, and antiprotozoal activities) are often due to the adoption of an amphipathic α-helical secondary structure that inserts into the lipids of biological membranes. The membrane permeation induced by amphipathic α-helical peptides may occur by one of two general mechanisms: "barrel-stave", that is, the formation of transmembrane pores; and the "carpet" mechanism, which causes membrane destruction or solubilization [89]. So far, anoplin, eumenitin, eumenitin-F, eumenitin-R, EMP-EF, and EMP-ER have been tested in artificial lipid bilayers, and the channel-like activity observed demonstrated that ion conduction through biological membranes must be important to their lytic activity against mammalian cells, but more importantly, against microorganisms.

4.1. Anoplin

Anoplin is the shortest known pore-forming peptide from a solitary wasp [9]. In experiments with planar lipid bilayers of asolectin, anoplin, which has an amidated C-terminus (ANP-NH_2), formed pores in the artificial lipid bilayers, with channel-like activity [15].

The channel activity of ANP-NH_2 starts 20–30 min after addition, under applied voltages preferentially above +100 mV. ANP-NH_2 channels showed fluctuations of similar amplitudes (unitary currents) and occasionally, integer multiples of the unitary value [15]. Mean open times ranged from 39 to 45 ms, and open probabilities were higher at +100 mV, reaching 66%, with an average conductance of 50 pS (Table 4). The pores are essentially selective to cation, and the diameter of a pore was estimated to be 0.5–0.6 nm, considering KCl as conductive solution.

The single channel conductance measurements with the carboxylated form of the peptide (ANP-OH) showed only small and rare transitions with maximum bilayer conductance of 40 pS at

100 mV potential. Under higher or lower holding potentials, transitions are even rarer and insignificant, showing that the amidation of the peptide C-terminus was crucial for channel-like activity in the anionic lipid bilayers of asolectin [15].

Table 4. Conductances of pores induced by solitary wasp venom peptides in anionic (asolectin) or zwitterionic (DPhPC and DPhPC-cholesterol) bilayers, according to the V_{hold} (mean and standard error of mean, minimum of three different experiments).

Peptides	Lipid	V_{hold} (mV)	Conductance (pS)	SEM	References
Eumenitin	asolectin	−50	118.0/160.0	3.67/7.07	[16]
	asolectin	+50	118.0/160.0	3.67/7.07	[16]
	DPhPC	+50	61.13	7.57	[16]
	DPhPC-cholesterol	−100	None	-	[16]
	DPhPC-cholesterol	+100	None	-	[16]
Eumenitin-R	asolectin	−100	82.5	17.1	[12]
	asolectin	+100	118.8	44	[12]
Eumenitin-F	asolectin	−100	298.6	51	[12]
	asolectin	+100	187.1	67.7	[12]
EMP-ER	asolectin	−100	68.2	4	[12]
	asolectin	+100	61.4	3.7	[12]
EMP-EF	asolectin	−100	33.6	8.9	[12]
	asolectin	+100	32.2	6.9	[12]
Anoplin	asolectin	+100	50.7	3.8	[15]
	asolectin	+130	58.4	2.7	[15]
	asolectin	+150	66.8	6.7	[15]

DPhPC: 1,2-diphytanoyl-sn-glycero-3-phosphocholine; V_{hold}: clamping voltage in milivolts; pS: picosemens.

4.2. *Eumenitin*

The antimicrobial peptide eumenitin interacts preferentially with charged lipids, but incorporated channel-like pores in both charged (asolectin, negative) and zwitterionic (1,2-diphytanoyl-sn-glycero-3-phosphocholine or DPhPC) membranes. Interestingly, cholesterol addition to DPhPC membranes did not inhibit the binding of eumenitin to the membrane, as measured by the surface potential, but abolished the pore activity [16].

In asolectin bilayers, eumenitin at the concentration of 0.25 μM induced current fluctuations under a constant voltage pulse that corresponded to open (conducting) and closed (non-conducting) states. Under either +50 or −50 mV, the pore mean conductance was 118 pS (Table 4), and a second and less frequent conducting state was also observed, with conductance of 160 pS [16]. Using the same concentration of eumenitin in experiments with zwitterionic membranes (made of DPhPC), the observed pore activity was very different from the recordings in negatively charged membranes (asolectin). The mean conductance of single-channels in DPhPC bilayers at a +50 mV pulse was 61 pS, nearly half of asolectin's membrane pore conductance (Table 3). Cholesterol addition to the DPhPC membranes abolished channel-like activity induced by eumenitin, even with increased voltage pulses (up to +100 mV) [16].

The eumenitin-induced pores presented a higher selectivity for cations over anions when tested in asolectin membranes, using KCl as conducting solution. Taking all information about eumenitin pores, Arcisio-Miranda and co-workers suggested that the formation of toroidal pores in membranes was the most adequate model to explain the biological activities of this peptide [16]. Matsuzaki and co-workers proposed this model for magainin 2 pores [89]. In this model, the interfacial peptide interaction induces the lipid monolayers to bend continuously through the pore, so that the water-filled core is lined by both inserted peptide and the lipid head groups, together forming well-defined pores. The use of negatively charged lipids, such as asolectin, would reduce the repulsive force due to the positive charge of the peptide (eumenitin has three positive charges, see Table 3). Thus, the 'residual' negative lipid charge could determine the cation selectivity observed for eumenitin, mainly in asolectin membranes [74].

4.3. Eumenitin-F and Eumenitin-R

Recently, four new linear cationic α-helical peptides from solitary wasp venoms were described [12]. Their sequences, physicochemical properties, channel incorporation and biological activities were studied to give a full profile of these peptides. Two of them have sequences related to eumenitin, thus named eumenitin-F and eumenitin–R. The other two are related to mastoparan, a class of peptide that was first found in social wasps [21], but has also been found in solitary eumenine wasps, the first being named EMP-AF [8]: EMP-EF and EMP-ER [12].

The two eumenitin peptides, eumenitin-F and eumenitin-R, were studied in mimetic lipid bilayers of asolectin obtained from GUVs (giant unilamellar vesicles). Using a 150-mM HCl bathing solution, eumenitin-F and eumenitin-R induced channel-like activity within 10 min of incubation (0.5–2 μM concentration, added to the *cis* side). Pore formation was observed in the presence of both peptides under positive and negative voltage pulses, and single-channel conductances were calculated. Eumenitin-F showed higher conductance levels, of 298.6 and 187.1 pS (−100 and +100 mV, respectively), while eumenitin-R channels had conductances of 82.5 and 118.8 pS at the same holding potentials (Table 4). Different conductance levels were detected in the pores formed, and were not double or triple of single channels conductance. Pores with conductances higher than 500 pS were recorded, indicating that clusters could be formed, and several units of the peptides organize to form bigger pores. Rectification was observed only in the eumenitin-F channels [12]. The above-mentioned eumenitin and anoplin pores presented similar behavior, as well as a social wasp peptide, HR-1, that has some similarities to mastoparan [90].

4.4. EMP-EF and EMP-ER

The two eumenine-mastoparan peptides, EMP-EF and EMP-ER (Table 1), that have high homology to mastoparan [21], and EMP-AF [8] presented channel-like activity in asolectin bilayers under positive and negative voltage pulses at concentrations ranging from 0.5 to 2 μM, added at the *cis* side. Single channel conductances formed by EMP-EF were 33.6 and 32.2 pS (−100 and +100 mV, respectively) lower than for EMP-ER channels (68.2 and 61.4) at the same holding potentials (Table 4). Double conductance levels were recorded, equivalent to the aperture of two single channels simultaneously, but no rectification was detected [12]. The pore conductance levels for EMP-EF and EMP-ER were equivalent to those for mastoparan HR-1, although the double conductance levels were recorded only in presence of EMP-EF and EMP-ER [12], but not with HR-1 [90]. The higher hydrophobicities of EMP-EF and EMP-ER when compared to HR-1 could account for the presence of double conductance levels in the recordings with the eumenine mastoparan peptides.

According to Rangel and co-workers [12], the new eumenitins (eumenitin-F and eumenitin-R) and mastoparan peptides' (EMP-EF and EMP-ER) pore-like activity and other characteristics, such as the length (shorter than bilayer thickness) and bulky residues, favor the toroidal pore model. By this model, the pore is described as a complex made of lipid molecules, predominantly, and peptide molecules that insert into the bilayer, inducing its destabilization [91,92]. The toroidal pore model was also proposed for the pores induced by the peptide eumenitin [16], and due to the high homology of these peptides it is the best model to explain the electrophysiology results so far.

It is interesting to highlight that the conformational and pore-forming activity of the peptides above were investigated predominately in asolectin bilayers, which due to its anionic character mimic the cytoplasmic membrane of bacteria. This phospholipid mixture has an approximate composition of 23.5% phosphatidylcholine, 20% phosphatidylethanolamine, and 14% inositol phosphatides (other components are 39.5% other phospholipids, lipids, and carbohydrates, and 2% triglycerides, tocopherols, and sterols). It holds some similarities to the lipid composition of rat mast cells; the phospholipids amount roughly to 50% of the total lipids. From these, phosphatidylcholine represents 30%, phosphatidylethanolamine 27%, sphingomyelin 20%, and phosphatidylserine and phosphatidylinositol 16%. An important difference lies in cholesterol, which represents around 20% of the total lipid content in rat mast cell membranes, while in asolectin sterols represent less than 0.3% [93].

In relation to sterols and the general anionic character, this bilayer can also be considered a mimetic of microbial membranes. Thus, the behavior of the eumenine peptides can be reasonably well modeled and their mechanism of action understood with the use of asolectin bilayers. Furthermore, when other lipids such as DPhPC and DPhPC with cholesterol were used to form planar bilayers with zwitterionic character, the pore-forming activity of the eumenitin peptide was reduced or even abolished [16]. This may be due to the positive net charge of the peptides (Table 3), and the lipid charge that may favor or diminish the interactions and pore-forming capability of these cationic peptides. Furthermore, cholesterol, which is only present in eukaryotic cells, changes the interactions of cationic peptides with the membrane [94]. Cholesterol also affects the fluidity and the dipole potential of phospholipid membranes [95].

The amidated C-terminus was favorable to the hemolytic and mast cell degranulating properties of the peptides, as observed for EMP-AF [8], EMP-EF, and EMP-ER [12] when compared with eumenitins [10,12]. However, the high conductance pores in artificial bilayers were only recorded with peptides that have carboxylated C-terminus, eumenitin-F, and eumenitin-R (Figure 3) [12].

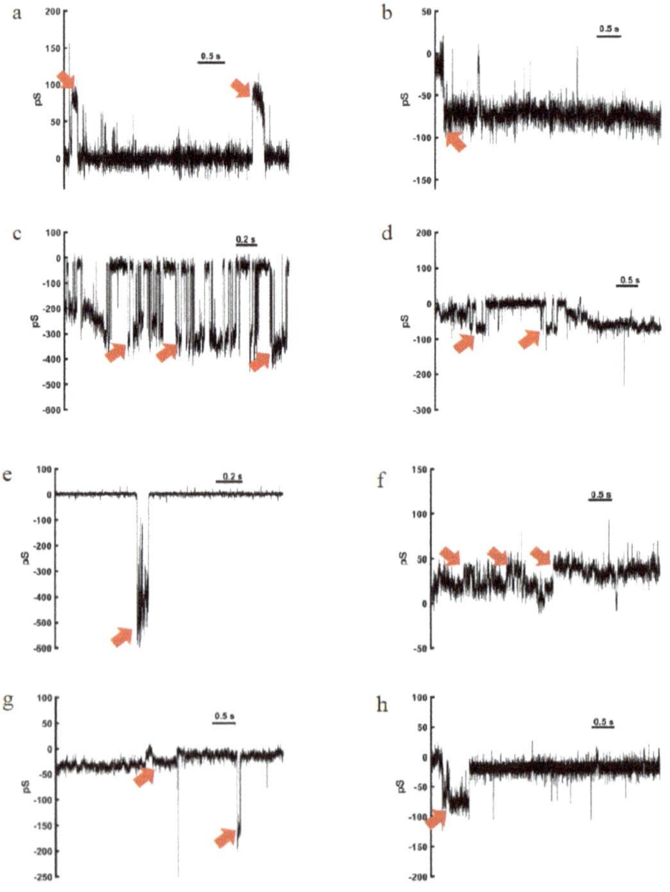

Figure 3. Representative recordings of single channel incorporation of solitary wasp venom peptides in asolectin bilayers. Eumetin-F (**a–c**) and eumenitin–R (**d**,**e**), both with carboxylated C-terminus, formed pores with low (<100 pS) and high conductance (>400 pS) levels. EMP-EF (**f**,**g**) and EMP-ER (**h**), however, presented higher hemolytic activity due to the amidated C-terminus, but incorporated channels of low conductance. Arrows indicate channel apertures.

5. Concluding Remarks

Our studies on solitary wasps surveying bioactive components in their venoms revealed that antimicrobial peptides are contained in many wasp venoms, mostly in eumenine wasp venoms. Their chemical and biological characteristics are typical for linear cationic α-helical peptides. Physicochemical properties and the pore-forming activity of these peptides were investigated in detail, and the results can be useful for investigation of the structure-activity relationship and mechanism of action.

Antimicrobial α-helical peptides are widely distributed in arthropod venoms e.g., scorpion and spider venoms. They may function not only in preventing the prey from microbial infection during long-time storage, but also in potentiating venom toxicity by disturbing excitable membranes [5–7]. Similarly, the solitary wasp venom peptides can act as antimicrobials against microbial infection [9] and as a venom toxicity potentiator [44].

The simple structure (consisting of only 10–15 amino acids without disulfide bonds) of the solitary wasp venom peptides is advantageous for chemical modification and structure-activity relationship studies. Furthermore, some of these peptides show only weak or virtually no hemolytic activity, which is another advantage especially for medical applications and development. In particular, anoplin and decoralin have lengths of only 10 and 11 amino acids, respectively, with virtually no hemolytic activity. There are many studies based on these peptides towards developing new antibiotic and anticancer agents [30–43,57–60].

Author Contributions: K.K., M.R., and M.P.d.S.C. conceived the contents. K.K., J.R.N. M.R., and M.P.d.S.C. analyzed the data. M.R., M.P.S.C., and K.K. wrote the paper.

Funding: A part of this work was financially supported by the JSPS KAKENHI (Grant Number 15K07805) Grant-in-Aid for Scientific Research from the Ministry of Education, Culture, Sports, Science and Technology (MEXT) of Japan.

Acknowledgments: Thanks are due to Sôichi Yamane (Ibaraki University) and Manabu Kato (Yamada Apiculture Center, Inc.) for collection and identification of solitary wasps and their invaluable discussions.

Conflicts of Interest: The authors declare no conflict of interest.

Abbreviations

EMP	eumenine mastoparan
PMTX	pompilidotoxin
HPLC	high performance liquid chromatography
CD	circular dichroism
TFE	2,2,2-trifluoroethanol
SDS	sodium dodecylsulfate
NMR	nuclear magnetic resonance
KLA	lysine-leucine-alanine (amino acid sequence)
DPhPC	1,2-diphytanoyl-sn-glycero-3-phosphocholine

References

1. Wang, G.; Li, X.; Wang, Z. APD3: The antimicrobial peptide database as a tool for research and education. *Nucleic Acids Res.* **2016**, *44*, D1087–D1093. [CrossRef] [PubMed]
2. Koehbach, J.; Craik, D.J. The vast structural diversity of antimicrobial peptides. *Trends Pharmacol. Sci.* **2019**, *40*, 517–528. [CrossRef] [PubMed]
3. Narayana, J.L.; Chen, J.-Y. Antimicrobial peptides: Possible anti-infective agents. *Peptides* **2015**, *72*, 88–94. [CrossRef] [PubMed]
4. Wang, J.; Dou, X.; Song, J.; Lyu, Y.; Zhu, X.; Xu, L.; Li, W.; Shan, A. Antimicrobial peptides: Promising alternatives in the post feeding antibiotic era. *Med. Res. Rev.* **2019**, *39*, 831–859. [CrossRef] [PubMed]
5. Kuhn-Nentwig, L. Antimicrobial and cytolytic peptides of venomous arthropods. *Cell. Mol. Life Sci.* **2003**, *60*, 2651–2668. [CrossRef] [PubMed]

6. Bulet, P.; Stöcklin, R.; Menin, L. Anti-microbial peptides: From invertebrates to vertebrates. *Immunol. Rev.* **2004**, *198*, 169–184. [CrossRef] [PubMed]
7. Fratini, F.; Cilia, G.; Turchi, B.; Felicioli, A. Insects, arachnids and centipedes venom: A powerful weapon against bacteria. A literature review. *Toxicon* **2017**, *130*, 91–103. [CrossRef]
8. Konno, K.; Hisada, M.; Naoki, H.; Itagaki, Y.; Kawai, N.; Miwa, A.; Yasuhara, T.; Morimoto, Y.; Nakata, Y. Structure and biological activities of eumenine mastoparan-AF (EMP-AF), a novel mast cell degranulating peptide in the venom of the solitary wasp (*Anterhynchium flavomarginatum micado*). *Toxicon* **2000**, *38*, 1505–1515. [CrossRef]
9. Konno, K.; Hisada, M.; Fontana, R.; Lorenzi, C.C.B.; Naoki, H.; Itagaki, Y.; Miwa, A.; Kawai, N.; Nakata, Y.; Yasuhara, T.; et al. Anoplin, a novel antimicrobial peptide from the venom of the solitary wasp *Anoplius samariensis*. *Biochim. Biophys. Acta* **2001**, *1550*, 70–80. [CrossRef]
10. Konno, K.; Hisada, M.; Naoki, H.; Itagaki, Y.; Fontana, R.; Rangel, M.; Oliveira, J.S.; Cabrera, M.P.; Ruggiero Neto, J.; Hide, I.; et al. Eumenitin, a novel antimicrobial peptide from the venom of the solitary eumenine wasp *Eumenes rubronotatus*. *Peptides* **2006**, *27*, 2624–2631. [CrossRef]
11. Konno, K.; Rangel, M.; Oliveira, J.S.; Cabrera, M.P.S.; Fontana, R.; Hirata, I.Y.; Nakata, Y.; Mori, K.; Kawano, M.; Fuchino, H.; et al. Decoralin, a novel linear cationic α-helical peptide from the venom of the solitary eumenine wasp *Oreumenes decoratus*. *Peptides* **2007**, *28*, 2320–2327. [CrossRef] [PubMed]
12. Rangel, M.; Cabrera, M.P.S.; Kazuma, K.; Ando, K.; Wang, X.; Kato, M.; Nihei, K.; Hirata, I.Y.; Cross, T.; Garcia, A.N.; et al. Chemical and biological characterization of four new antimicrobial and α-helical peptides from the venoms of two solitary eumenine wasps. *Toxicon* **2011**, *57*, 1081–1092. [CrossRef] [PubMed]
13. Konno, K.; Rangel, M.; de Oliveira, J.S.; Fontana, R.; Kawano, M.; Fuchino, H.; Hide, I.; Yasuhara, T.; Nakata, Y. New mastoparan peptides in the venom of the solitary eumenine wasp *Eumenes micado*. *Toxins* **2019**, *11*, 155. [CrossRef] [PubMed]
14. Cabrera, M.P.S.; Souza, B.M.; Fontana, R.; Konno, K.; Palma, M.S.; de Azevedo, W.F., Jr.; Ruggiero Neto, J. Conformation and lytic activity of eumenine mastoparan: A new antimicrobial peptide from wasp venom. *J. Pept. Res.* **2004**, *64*, 95–103. [CrossRef] [PubMed]
15. Cabrera, M.P.S.; Arcisio-Miranda, M.; Costa, S.T.B.; Konno, K.; Ruggiero, J.R.; Procopio, J.; Ruggiero Neto, J. Study of the mechanism of action of Anoplin, a helical antimicrobial decapeptide with ion channel-like activity, and the role of the amidated C-terminus. *J. Pept. Sci.* **2008**, *14*, 661–669. [CrossRef] [PubMed]
16. Arcisio-Miranda, M.; Cabrera, M.P.S.; Konno, K.; Rangel, M.; Procopio, J. Effects of the cationic antimicrobial peptide Eumenitin from the venom of solitary wasp *Eumenes rubronotatus* in planar lipid bilayers: Surface charge and pore formation activity. *Toxicon* **2008**, *51*, 736–745. [CrossRef] [PubMed]
17. Konno, K.; Kazuma, K.; Nihei, K. Peptide toxins in solitary wasp venoms. *Toxins* **2016**, *8*, 114. [CrossRef] [PubMed]
18. Piek, T. Neurotoxic kinins from wasp and ant venoms. *Toxicon* **1991**, *29*, 139–149. [CrossRef]
19. Nakanishi, K.; Goodnow, R.; Konno, K.; Niwa, M.; Bukownik, R.; Kalimopoulos, T.A.; Usherwood, P.N.R.; Eldefrawi, A.T.; Eldefrawi, M.E. Philanthotoxin-433 (PhTX-433), a non-competitive glutamate receptor inhibitor. *Pure Appl. Chem.* **1990**, *62*, 1223–1230. [CrossRef]
20. Konno, K.; Kawai, N. Pompilidotoxins: Novel peptide neurotoxins blocking sodium channel inactivation from solitary wasp venom. *Curr. Med. Chem. Cent. Nerv. Syst. Agents* **2004**, *4*, 139–146. [CrossRef]
21. Hirai, Y.; Yasuhara, T.; Yoshida, H.; Nakajima, T.; Fujino, M.; Kitada, C. A new mast cell degranulating peptide "mastoparan" in the venom of *Vespula lewisii*. *Chem. Pharm. Bull.* **1979**, *27*, 1942–1944. [CrossRef] [PubMed]
22. Murata, K.; Shinada, T.; Ohfune, Y.; Hisada, M.; Yasuda, A.; Naoki, H.; Nakajima, T. Novel biologically active peptides from the venom of *Polistes rothneyi Iwatai*. *Biol. Pharm. Bull.* **2006**, *29*, 2493–2497. [CrossRef] [PubMed]
23. Nakajima, T. Pharmacological biochemistry of vespid venoms. In *Venoms of the Hymenoptera: Biochemical, Pharmacological and Behavioural Aspects*; Piek, T., Ed.; Academic Press: London, UK, 1986; pp. 309–327, ISBN 0-12-554771-4.
24. Sforça, M.L.; Oyama, S., Jr.; Canduri, F.; Lorenzi, C.C.B.; Pertinez, T.A.; Konno, K.; Souza, B.M.; Palma, M.S.; Ruggiero Neto, J.; de Azevedo, W.F., Jr.; et al. How C-terminal carboxyamidation alters the mast cell degranulating activity of peptides from the venom of the eumenine solitary wasp. *Biochemistry* **2004**, *43*, 5608–5617. [CrossRef] [PubMed]

25. Murata, K.; Shinada, T.; Ohfune, Y.; Hisada, M.; Yasuda, A.; Naoki, H.; Nakajima, T. Novel mastoparan and protonectin analogs isolated from a solitary wasp, *Orancistrocerus drewseni drewseni*. *Amino Acids* **2009**, *37*, 389–394. [CrossRef] [PubMed]
26. Baek, J.H.; Lee, S.H. Isolation and molecular cloning of venom peptides from *Orancistrocerus drewseni* (Hymenoptera: Eumenidae). *Toxicon* **2010**, *55*, 711–718. [CrossRef] [PubMed]
27. Baek, J.H.; Lee, S.H. Differential gene expression profiles in the venom gland/sac of Eumenes pomiformis (Hymenoptera: Eumenidae). *Toxicon* **2010**, *55*, 1147–1156. [CrossRef] [PubMed]
28. Rodrigues Guerra, M.E.; Fadel, V.; Maltarollo, V.G.; Baldissera, G.; Honorio, K.M.; Ruggiero, J.R.; dos Santos Cabrera, M.P. MD simulations and multivariate studies for modeling the antileishmanial activity of peptides. *Chem. Biol. Drug Des.* **2017**, *90*, 501–510. [CrossRef] [PubMed]
29. Konno, K.; Hisada, M.; Itagaki, Y.; Naoki, H.; Kawai, N.; Miwa, A.; Yasuhara, T.; Takayama, H. Isolation and structure of pompilidotoxins (PMTXs), novel neurotoxins in solitary wasp venoms. *Biochem. Biophys. Res. Commun.* **1998**, *250*, 612–616. [CrossRef]
30. Ifrah, D.; Doisy, X.; Ryge, T.S.; Hansen, P.R. Structure-activity relationship study of anoplin. *J. Pept. Sci.* **2005**, *11*, 113–121. [CrossRef]
31. Won, A.; Khan, M.; Gustin, S.; Akpawu, A.; Seebun, D.; Avis, T.J.; Leung, B.O.; Hitchcock, A.P.; Ianoul, A. Investigating the effects of L- to D-amino acid substitution and deamidation on the activity and membrane interactions of antimicrobial peptide anoplin. *Biochim. Biophys. Acta* **2011**, *1808*, 1592–1600. [CrossRef]
32. Won, A.; Pripotnev, S.; Ruscito, A.; Ianoul, A. Effect of point mutations on the secondary structure and membrane interaction of antimicrobial peptide anoplin. *J. Phys. Chem. B* **2011**, *115*, 2371–2379. [CrossRef] [PubMed]
33. Munk, J.K.; Uggerhøj, L.E.; Poulsen, T.J.; Frimodt-Møller, N.; Wimmer, R.; Nyberg, N.T.; Hansen, P.R. Synthetic analogs of anoplin show improved antimicrobial activities. *J. Pept. Sci.* **2013**, *19*, 669–675. [CrossRef] [PubMed]
34. Slootweg, J.C.; van Schaik, T.B.; van Ufford, H.C.Q.; Breukink, E.; Liskamp, R.M.J.; Rijkers, D.T.S. Improving the biological activity of the antimicrobial peptide anoplin by membrane anchoring through a lipophilic amino acid derivative. *Bioorgan. Med. Chem. Lett.* **2013**, *23*, 3749–3752. [CrossRef] [PubMed]
35. Jindrichova, B.; Burketova, L.; Novotna, Z. Novel properties of antimicrobial peptide anoplin. *Biochem. Biophys. Res. Commun.* **2014**, *444*, 520–524. [CrossRef] [PubMed]
36. Wang, Y.; Chen, J.; Zheng, X.; Yang, X.; Ma, P.; Cai, Y.; Zhang, B.; Chen, Y. Design of novel analogues of short antimicrobial peptide anoplin with improved antimicrobial activity. *J. Pept. Sci.* **2014**, *20*, 945–951. [CrossRef] [PubMed]
37. Munk, J.K.; Ritz, C.; Fliedner, F.P.; Frimodt-Møller, N.; Hansen, P.R. Novel method to identify the optimal antimicrobial peptide in a combination matrix, using anoplin as an example. *Antimicrob. Agents Chemother.* **2014**, *58*, 1063–1070. [CrossRef] [PubMed]
38. Uggerhøj, L.E.; Poulsen, T.J.; Munk, J.K.; Fredborg, M.; Sondergaard, T.E.; Frimodt-Møller, N.; Hansen, P.R.; Wimmer, R. Rational design of alpha-helical antimicrobial peptides: do's and don'ts. *ChemBioChem* **2015**, *16*, 242–253. [CrossRef] [PubMed]
39. Aschi, M.; Luzi, C.; Fiorillo, A.; Bozzi, A. Folding propensity of anoplin: A molecular dynamics study of the native peptide and four mutated isoforms. *Biopolymers* **2015**, *103*, 692–701. [CrossRef] [PubMed]
40. Sahariah, P.; Sørensen, K.K.; HjáLlmarsdóttir, M.A.; Sigurjónsson, Ó.E.; Jensen, K.J.; Másson, M.; Thygesen, M.B. Antimicrobial peptide shows enhanced activity and reduced toxicity upon grafting to chitosan polymers. *Chem. Commun.* **2015**, *51*, 11611–11614. [CrossRef]
41. Daben, M.; Libardo, J.; Nagella, S.; Lugo, A.; Pierce, S.; Angeles-Boza, A.M. Copper-binding tripeptide motif increases potency of the antimicrobial peptide Anoplin via Reactive Oxygen Species generation. *Biochem. Biophys. Res. Commun.* **2015**, *456*, 446–451. [CrossRef]
42. Chionis, K.; Krikorian, D.; Koukkou, A.I.; Sakarellos-Daitsiotis, M.; Panou-Pomonis, E. Synthesis and biological activity of lipophilic analogs of the cationic antimicrobial active peptides anoplin. *J. Pept. Sci.* **2016**, *22*, 731–736. [CrossRef]
43. Salas, R.L.; Garcia, J.K.D.L.; Miranda, A.C.R.; Rivera, W.L.; Nellas, R.B.; Sabido, P.M.G. Effects of truncation of the peptide chain on the secondary structure and bioactivities of palmitoylated anoplin. *Peptides* **2018**, *104*, 7–14. [CrossRef] [PubMed]

44. Baek, J.H.; Ji, Y.; Shin, J.-S.; Lee, S.; Lee, S.H. Venom peptides from solitary hunting wasps induce feeding disorder in lepidopteran larvae. *Peptides* **2011**, *32*, 568–572. [CrossRef] [PubMed]
45. Tossi, A.; Sandri, L.; Giangaspero, A. Amphipathic, α-helical antimicrobial peptides. *Biopolymers* **2000**, *55*, 4–30. [CrossRef]
46. Giangaspero, A.; Sandri, L.; Tossi, A. Amphipathic α-helical antimicrobial peptides—A systematic study of the effects of structural and physical properties on biological activity. *Eur. J. Biochem.* **2001**, *268*, 5589–5600. [CrossRef] [PubMed]
47. Scholtz, J.M.; Qian, H.; York, E.J.; Stewart, J.M.; Baldwin, R.L. Parameters of helix-coil transition theory for alanine-based peptides of varying chain lengths in water. *Biopolymers* **1991**, *31*, 1463–1470. [CrossRef] [PubMed]
48. Andreu, D.; Rivas, L. Animal antimicrobial peptides: An overview. *Biopolymers* **1998**, *47*, 415–433. [CrossRef]
49. Schulz, G.E.; Schirmer, R.H. *Principles of Protein Structure*; Springer: New York, NY, USA, 1978; pp. 10–16.
50. Sitaram, N.; Nagaraj, R. Interaction of antimicrobial peptides with biological and model membranes: Structural and charge requirements for activity. *Biochim. Biophys. Acta* **1999**, *1462*, 29–54. [CrossRef]
51. Matsuzaki, K.; Sugishita, K.; Harada, M.; Fujii, N.; Miyajima, K. Interactions of an antimicrobial peptide, magainin 2, with outer and inner membranes of Gram-negative bacteria. *Biochim. Biophys. Acta* **1997**, *1327*, 119–130. [CrossRef]
52. Dathe, M.; Wieprecht, T.; Nikolenko, H.; Handel, L.; Maloy, W.L.; MacDonald, D.L.; Beyermann, M.; Bienert, M. Hydrophobicity, hydrophobic moment and angle subtended by charged residues modulate antibacterial and haemolytic activity of amphipathic helical peptides. *FEBS Lett.* **1997**, *403*, 208–212. [CrossRef]
53. Dathe, M.; Nikolenko, H.; Meyer, J.; Beyermann, M.; Bienert, M. Optimization of the antimicrobial activity of Magainin peptides by modification of charge. *FEBS Lett.* **2001**, *501*, 146–150. [CrossRef]
54. Yeaman, M.R.; Yount, N.Y. Mechanisms of antimicrobial peptide action and resistance. *Pharmacol. Rev.* **2003**, *55*, 27–55. [CrossRef] [PubMed]
55. Matsuzaki, K. Magainins as paradigm for the mode of action of pore forming polypeptides *Biochim. Biophys. Acta* **1998**, *1376*, 391–400. [CrossRef]
56. Lin, Y.-C.; Lim, Y.F.; Russo, E.; Schneider, P.; Bolliger, L.; Edenharter, A.; Altmann, K.H.; Halin, C.; Hiss, J.A.; Schneider, G. Multidimensional design of anticancer peptides. *Angew. Chem. Int. Ed.* **2015**, *54*, 10370–10374. [CrossRef] [PubMed]
57. Torres, M.D.T.; Pedron, C.N.; Araujo, I.; Silva, P.I., Jr.; Silva, F.D.; Oliveira, V.X. Decoralin analogs with increased resistance to degradation and lower hemolytic activity. *ChemistrySelect* **2017**, *2*, 18–23. [CrossRef]
58. Torres, M.D.T.; Pedron, C.N.; Silva Lima, J.A.; Silva, P.I., Jr.; Silva, F.D.; Oliveira, V.X. Antimicrobial activity of leucine-substituted decoralin analogs with lower hemolytic activity. *J. Pept. Sci.* **2017**, *23*, 818–823. [CrossRef] [PubMed]
59. Torres, M.D.T.; Andrade, G.T.; Sato, R.H.; Pedron, C.N.; Manieri, T.M.; Cerchiaro, G.; Ribeiro, A.O.; Fuente-Nunez, C.; Oliveira, V.X., Jr. Natural and redesigned wasp venom peptides with selective antitumoral activity. *Beilstein J. Org. Chem.* **2018**, *14*, 1693–1703. [CrossRef]
60. Torres, M.D.T.; Silva, F.D.; Pedron, C.N.; Capurro, M.L.; Fuente-Nunez, C.; Oliveira, V.X., Jr. Peptide design enables reengineering of an inactive wasp venom peptide into synthetic antiplasmodial agents. *ChemistrySelect* **2018**, *3*, 5859–5863. [CrossRef]
61. Hol, W.G.; van Duijnen, P.T.; Berendsen, H.J.C. The α-helix dipole and the properties of proteins. *Nature* **1978**, *273*, 443–446. [CrossRef]
62. Joshi, H.V.; Meier, M.S. The effect of a peptide helix macrodipole on the pK_a of an Asp side chain carboxylate. *J. Am. Chem. Soc.* **1996**, *118*, 12038–12044. [CrossRef]
63. Rohl, C.A.; Baldwin, R.L. Deciphering rules of helix stability in peptides. *Methods Enzymol.* **1998**, *295*, 1–26. [CrossRef] [PubMed]
64. Chou, P.Y.; Fasman, G.D. Conformational parameters for amino acids in helical, β-sheet, and random coil regions calculated from proteins. *Biochemistry* **1974**, *13*, 211–222. [CrossRef] [PubMed]
65. Gans, P.J.; Lyu, P.C.; Manning, M.C.; Woody, R.W. The helix-coil transition in heterogeneous peptides with specific side-chain interactions: Theory and comparison with CD spectral data. *Biopolymers* **1991**, *31*, 1605–1614. [CrossRef] [PubMed]
66. O'Neil, K.T.; DeGrado, W.F. A thermodynamic scale for the helix-forming tendencies of the commonly occurring amino acids. *Science* **1990**, *250*, 646–651. [CrossRef] [PubMed]

67. Marqusee, S.; Robbins, H.V.; Baldwin, R.L. Unusually stable helix formation in short alanine-based peptides. *Proc. Natl. Acad. Sci. USA* **1989**, *86*, 5286–5290. [CrossRef] [PubMed]
68. Blondelle, S.E.; Forood, B.; Houghten, R.A.; Pérez-Payá, E. Secondary structure induction in aqueous vs membrane-like environments. *Biopolymers* **1997**, *42*, 489–498. [CrossRef]
69. Waterhous, D.V.; Johnson, W.C., Jr. Importance of environment in determining secondary structure in proteins. *Biochemistry* **1994**, *33*, 2121–2128. [CrossRef] [PubMed]
70. Zhong, L.; Johnson, C., Jr. Environment affects amino acid preference for secondary structure. *Proc. Natl. Acad. Sci. USA* **1992**, *89*, 4462–4465. [CrossRef]
71. Deber, C.M.; Li, S.C. Peptides in membranes: Helicity and hydrophobicity. *Biopolymers* **1995**, *37*, 295–318. [CrossRef] [PubMed]
72. Blondelle, S.E.; Houghten, R.A. Design of model amphipathic peptides having potent antimicrobial activities. *Biochemistry* **1992**, *31*, 12688–12694. [CrossRef] [PubMed]
73. Dathe, M.; Wieprecht, T. Structural features of helical antimicrobial peptides: Their potential to modulate activity on model membranes and biological cells. *Biochim. Biophys. Acta* **1999**, *1462*, 71–87. [CrossRef]
74. Dathe, M.; Schümann, M.; Wieprecht, T.; Winkler, A.; Beyermann, M.; Krause, E.; Matsuzaki, K.; Murase, O.; Bienert, M. Peptide helicity and membrane surface charge modulate the balance of electrostatic and hydrophobic interactions with lipid bilayers and biological membranes. *Biochemistry* **1996**, *35*, 12612–12622. [CrossRef] [PubMed]
75. Eisenberg, D.; Schwarz, E.; Komaromy, M.; Wall, R. Analysis of membrane and surface protein sequences with the hydrophobic moment plot. *J. Mol. Biol.* **1984**, *179*, 125–142. [CrossRef]
76. Dathe, M.; Meyer, J.; Beyermann, M.; Maul, B.; Hoischen, C.; Bienert, M. General aspects of peptide selectivity towards lipid bilayers and cell membranes studied by variation of the structural parameters of amphipathic helical model peptides. *Biochim. Biophys. Acta* **2002**, *1558*, 171–186. [CrossRef]
77. Pathak, N.; Salas-Auvert, R.; Ruche, G.; Janna, M.H.; McCarthy, D.; Harrison, R.G. Comparison of the effects of hydrophobicity, amphiphilicity, and α-helicity on the activities of antimicrobial Peptides. *Proteins Struct. Funct. Bioinf.* **1995**, *22*, 182–186. [CrossRef] [PubMed]
78. Wimley, W.C. Describing the mechanism of antimicrobial peptide action with the interfacial activity model. *ACS Chem. Biol.* **2010**, *5*, 905–917. [CrossRef] [PubMed]
79. Lum, K.; Chandler, D.; Weeks, J.D. Hydrophobicity at small and large length scales. *J. Phys. Chem. B* **1999**, *103*, 4570–4577. [CrossRef]
80. Wieprecht, T.; Dathe, M.; Beyermann, M.; Krause, E.; Maloy, W.L.; MacDonald, D.L.; Bienert, M. Peptide hydrophobicity controls the activity and selectivity of Magainin 2 amide in interaction with membranes. *Biochemistry* **1997**, *36*, 6124–6132. [CrossRef]
81. Leite, N.B.; da Costa, L.C.; Dos Santos Alvares, D.; Dos Santos Cabrera, M.P.; De Souza, B.M.; Palma, M.S.; Ruggiero Neto, J. The effect of acidic residues and amphipathicity on the lytic activities of mastoparan peptides studied by fluorescence and CD spectroscopy. *Amino Acids* **2011**, *40*, 91–100. [CrossRef]
82. Neville, F.; Cahuzac, M.; Konovalov, O.; Ishitsuka, Y.; Lee, K.Y.C.; Kuzmenko, I.; Kale, G.M.; Gidalevitz, D. Lipid head group discrimination by antimicrobial peptide LL-37: Insight into mechanism of action. *Biophys. J.* **2006**, *90*, 1275–1287. [CrossRef]
83. Leontiadou, H.; Mark, A.E.; Marrink, S.J. Antimicrobial peptides an action. *J. Am. Chem. Soc.* **2006**, *128*, 12156–12161. [CrossRef]
84. Rzepiela, A.J.; Sengupta, D.; Goga, N.; Marrink, S.J. Membrane poration by antimicrobial peptides combining atomistic and coarse-grained descriptions. *Faraday Discuss.* **2010**, *144*, 431–443. [CrossRef]
85. Giladevitz, D.; Ishitzuka, Y.; Murean, A.S.; Konovalov, O.; Waring, A.L.; Lehrer, R.I.; Lee, K.Y.C. Interaction of antimicrobial peptide protegrin with biomembranes. *Proc. Natl. Acad. Sci. USA* **2003**, *100*, 6302–6307. [CrossRef]
86. Andreev, K.; Martynowycz, M.W.; Huang, M.L.; Kuzmenko, I.; Bu, W.; Kirshenbaum, K.; Gidalevitz, D. Hydrophobic interactions modulate antimicrobial peptoid selectivity toward anionic lipid membranes. *Biochim. Biophys. Acta* **2018**, *1860*, 1414–1423. [CrossRef]
87. Rangel, M.; Konno, K.; Brunaldi, K.; Procopio, J.; Freitas, J.C. Neurotoxic activity induced by a haemolytic substance in the extract of the marine sponge *Geodia corticostylifera*. *Comp. Biochem. Physiol. C Toxicol. Pharmacol.* **2005**, *141*, 207–215. [CrossRef]

88. Boland, M.P.; Separovic, F. Membrane interactions of antimicrobial peptides from Australian tree frogs. *Biochim. Biophys. Acta* **2006**, *1758*, 1178–1183. [CrossRef]
89. Shai, Y. Mechanism of the binding, insertion and destabilization of phospholipid bilayer membranes by α-helical antimicrobial and cell non-selective membrane-lytic peptides. *Biochim. Biophys. Acta* **1999**, *1462*, 55–70. [CrossRef]
90. Dos Santos Cabrera, M.P.; Arcisio-Miranda, M.; da Costa, L.C.; De Souza, B.M.; Broggio Costa, S.T.; Palma, M.S.; Ruggiero Neto, J.; Procopio, J. Interactions of mast cell degranulating peptides with model membranes: A comparative biophysical study. *Arch. Biochem Biophys.* **2009**, *486*, 1–11. [CrossRef]
91. Matsuzaki, K.; Murase, O.; Fujii, N.; Miyajima, K. An antimicrobial peptide, magainin 2, induced rapid flip-flop of phospholipids coupled with pore formation and peptide translocation. *Biochemistry* **1996**, *35*, 11361–11368. [CrossRef]
92. Yang, L.; Harroun, T.A.; Weiss, T.M.; Ding, L.; Huang, H.W. Barrel-stave model or toroidal model? A case study on melittin pores. *Biophys. J.* **2001**, *81*, 1475–1485. [CrossRef]
93. Strandberg, K.; Westerberg, S. Composition of phospholipids and phospholipid fatty acids in rat mast cells. *Mol. Cell. Biochem.* **1976**, *11*, 103–107. [CrossRef] [PubMed]
94. Christensen, B.; Fink, J.; Merrifield, R.B.; Mauzerall, D. Channel-forming properties of cecropins and related model compounds incorporated into planar lipid membranes. *Proc. Natl. Acad. Sci. USA* **1988**, *85*, 5072–5076. [CrossRef] [PubMed]
95. Bechinger, B.; Lohner, K. Detergent-like actions of linear amphipathic cationic antimicrobial peptides. *Biochim. Biophys. Acta* **2006**, *1758*, 1529–1539. [CrossRef] [PubMed]

toxins

MDPI

Article

A New Topical Eye Drop Containing LyeTxI-b, A Synthetic Peptide Designed from A *Lycosa erithrognata* Venom Toxin, Was Effective to Treat Resistant Bacterial Keratitis

Carolina Nunes da Silva [1,*], Flavia Rodrigues da Silva [2], Lays Fernanda Nunes Dourado [1], Pablo Victor Mendes dos Reis [3], Rummenigge Oliveira Silva [1], Bruna Lopes da Costa [1], Paula Santos Nunes [2], Flávio Almeida Amaral [3], Vera Lúcia dos Santos [4], Maria Elena de Lima [5] and Armando da Silva Cunha Júnior [1]

1 Faculdade de Farmácia, Universidade Federal de Minas Gerais, Belo Horizonte 31270-901 MG, Brazil; laysndourado@gmail.com (L.F.N.D.); rummeniggeita@gmail.com (R.O.S.); brunalc1991@gmail.com (B.L.d.C.); armando@farmacia.ufmg.br (A.d.S.C.J.)

2 Programa de Pós-Graduação em Ciências Aplicadas à Saúde-PPGCAS, Universidade Federal de Sergipe, Lagarto 49400-000 SE, Brazil; dra.flaviarodrigues@hotmail.com (F.R.d.S.); paulanunes_se@yahoo.com.br (P.S.N.)

3 Departamento de Bioquímica e Imunologia, Instituto de Ciências Biológicas, Universidade Federal de Minas Gerais, Belo Horizonte 31270-901 MG, Brazil; reispvm@gmail.com (P.V.M.d.R.); dr.famaral@gmail.com (F.A.A.)

4 Departamento de Microbiologia, Instituto de Ciências Biológicas, Universidade Federal de Minas Gerais, Belo Horizonte 31270-901 MG, Brazil; verabio@gmail.com

5 Programa de Pós-graduação em Ciências da Saúde, Biomedicina e Medicina, Ensino e Pesquisa da Santa Casa de Belo Horizonte, Grupo Santa Casa de Belo Horizonte, Belo Horizonte 30150-250, MG, Brazil; mariaelena@santacasabh.org.br

* Correspondence: carolinnanunes@yahoo.com.br; Tel.: +55-31-34096846

Received: 9 March 2019; Accepted: 2 April 2019; Published: 4 April 2019

check for updates

Abstract: Bacterial keratitis is an ocular infection that can lead to severe visual disability. *Staphylococcus aureus* is a major pathogen of the eye. We recently demonstrated the strong antimicrobial activity of LyeTxI-b, a synthetic peptide derived from a *Lycosa erithrognatha* toxin. Herein, we evaluated a topical formulation (eye drops) containing LyeTxI-b to treat resistant bacterial keratitis. Keratitis was induced with intrastromal injection of 4×10^5 cells (4 µL) in New Zealand female white rabbits. Minimum inhibitory concentration (MIC) and biofilm viability were determined. LyeTxI-b ocular toxicity was evaluated through chorioallantoic membrane and Draize tests. One drop of the formulation (LyeTxI-b 28.9 µmol/L +0.5% CMC in 0.9% NaCl) was instilled into each eye four times a day, for a week. Slit-lamp biomicroscopy analysis, corneal histopathological studies and cellular infiltrate quantification through myeloperoxidase (MPO) and N-acetylglucosaminidase (NAG) detection were performed. LyeTxI-b was very effective in the treatment of keratitis, with no signs of ocular toxicity. Planktonic bacteria MIC was 3.6 µmol/L and LyeTxI-b treatment reduced biofilm viability in 90%. LyeTxI-b eliminated bacteria and reduced inflammatory cellular activity in the eyes. Healthy and treated animals showed similar NAG and MPO levels. LyeTxI-b is a potent new drug to treat resistant bacterial keratitis, showing effective antimicrobial and anti-inflammatory activity.

Keywords: LyeTxI-b; *Staphylococcus aureus*; keratitis

Key Contribution: The spider toxin derivative LyeTxI-b eliminates bacteria and reduces inflammatory cellular activity in the eyes, with no signs of ocular toxicity. Our data highlight the possible use of LyeTxI-b for the development of new drugs as candidates for the treatment of resistant bacterial keratitis.

1. Introduction

The eye is relatively resistant to microorganisms and most pathogens cannot cross the intact cornea, because the eye provides a diverse collection of antimicrobial factors, especially in the tear film, which protects the cornea from infection [1]. However, if there is any structural damage or failure in the defense mechanisms that maintain its entire surface, opportunistic infections can easily develop, resulting in microbial keratitis [1–3].

Microbial keratitis is characterized by a defect in the corneal epithelium with stromal inflammation caused by microorganisms. The onset of symptoms is acute, causing pain and risking loss or reduction of vision, which requires rapid diagnosis and treatment. Ocular trauma, incorrect use of contact lenses, ocular surface diseases, and ocular surgeries are some factors that can trigger the disease [4,5]. Bacterial keratitis is considered one of the most serious ocular conditions in the world and may cause partial or total loss of visual acuity [4–6]. Bacterial infections are still predominant and are found in 80% of patients with ulcerative keratitis [3]. *Staphylococcus aureus* is a major pathogen of the eye, being a natural inhabitant of the ocular surface, skin, nostrils, and environment [7]. *S. aureus* is able to infect the tear duct, eyelid, conjunctiva, cornea, and the anterior, posterior and vitreous chambers.

Although the incidence of *S. aureus* eye infections varies worldwide, the growing trend of resistance to antibiotics makes this condition an important global healthcare issue. The therapeutic arsenal against bacterial infections is rapidly shrinking and the development of novel antibiotics overcoming antimicrobial resistance is therefore urgent and in great demand. Antimicrobial peptides (AMPs), which act as protective agents against microbes, have been recognized as powerful novel weapons against pathogenic organisms that are resistant to customary antibiotics, because of their unique action mechanisms and broad-spectrum activities [8–10]. Today, new drugs are necessary to combat the emergence of antibiotic-resistant germs [11].

Spider venoms contain diverse bioactive peptides and toxins, which have attracted great attention, making them a valuable resource for drug discovery, and excellent candidates for developing novel antibiotics against drug-resistant bacteria [10,12].

LyeTxI is an antimicrobial peptide purified from *Lycosa erythrognatha* spider venom. This peptide was characterized and chemically synthesized [12]. LyeTxI was able to inhibit the proliferation of periodontal bacteria and epithelial cells, and was not cytotoxic to osteoblasts [13]. It can be used to prevent biofilm development and was active against periodontopathic bacteria, showing rapid bactericidal effect [14].

Considering that LyeTxI presents great antimicrobial potential, its structure was used as a template to develop new drugs against bacteria. Its derivative synthetic peptide LyeTxI-b has a well-defined helical segment and is 10-fold more effective against gram-positive and gram-negative planktonic bacteria if compared with the natural peptide LyeTxI. The derivative LyeTxI-b differs from LyeTxI only by a lacking histidine residue. It was very effective in treating in vivo septic arthritis in a mouse model [15]. In addition, this synthetic peptide was not toxic to rabbits' eyes after intravitreal injection and was able to prevent neovascularization in the chorioallantoic membrane, at Bevacizumab levels [16]. Thus, the main goal of this work was to check the effectiveness of LyeTxI-b to the treat in vivo resistant *S. aureus* keratitis by topical application.

2. Results

2.1. Antimicrobial Activity in Planktonic and Biofilm Culture

To evaluate the minimum inhibitory concentration (MIC) and to determine the minimum biofilm eradication concentrations (MBEC), the formulation (LyeTxI-b +0.5% CMC in 0.9% NaCl) was serially diluted, from 927.7 to 1.8 μmol/L, as previously described in [15] and incubated for MIC test with 5×10^4 CFU/well for 24 h at 37 °C. For MBEC test, the bacterial suspensions had this same densityfor 24 h at 37 °C. Positive (without LyeTxI-b) and negative (without bacteria) controls were submitted to the same procedures as described in methods.

LyeTxI-b showed potent antimicrobial activity against gram-positive planktonic cells and *S. aureus* established biofilms, reducing their viability under aerobic conditions (Figure 1A,B). The MIC values were 3.6 μmol/L and MBEC was 57.9 μmol/L for LyeTxI-b formulation.

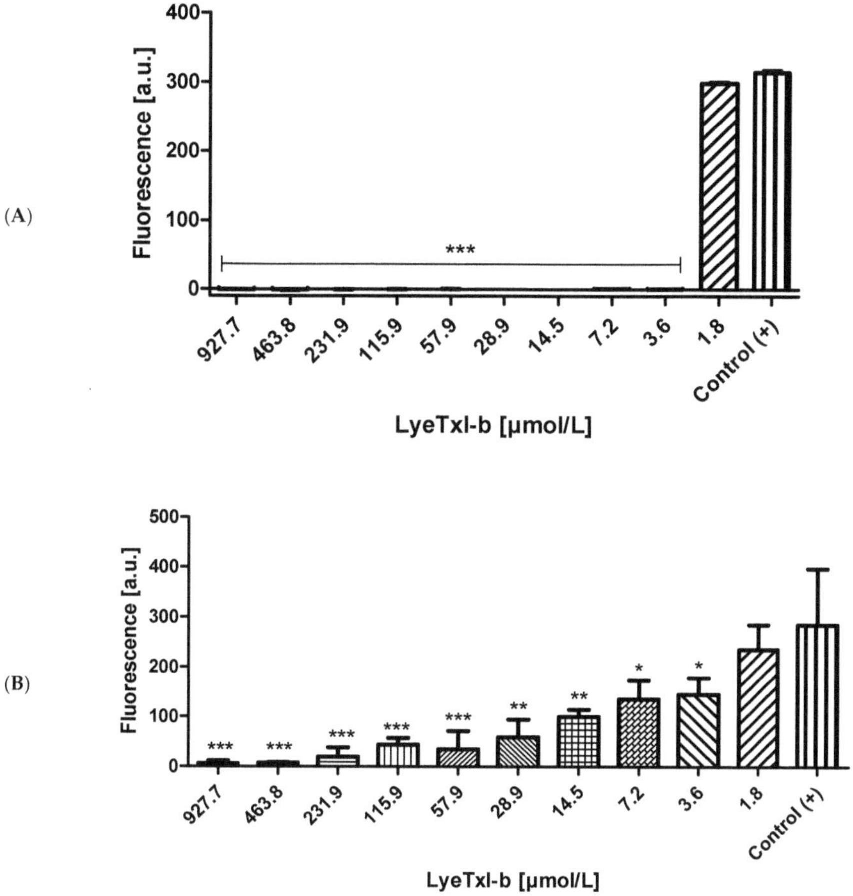

Figure 1. LyeTxI-b action on *S. aureus* planktonic bacteria (**A**) and biofilm (**B**) with different concentrations of the peptide: 1.8–927.7 μmol/L. The viable mass was fluorometrically measured with resazurin (λex 570 nm and λem 590 nm). a.u., arbitrary units. Data are expressed as the mean ± SD. Asterisk indicates LyeTxI-b vs. Control (+) one-way ANOVA plus Bonferroni post-test * $p < 0.05$; ** $p < 0.01$; *** $p < 0.001$.

2.2. Ocular Toxicity of the LyeTxI-b by HET-CAM Assay

In the HET-CAM test, embryonated eggs were used to test the toxicity of LyeTxI-b formulation. In vitro tests indicated that the MBEC was 57.9 µmol/L. Based on these data, we performed a toxicity curve. For this, we chose two points below and one point above the MBEC, thus the four test concentrations of LyeTxI-b were: 14.5 µmol /L, 28.9 µmol/L, 57.9 µmol/L and 115.9 µmol/L. Note that 0.5% CMC in 0.9% NaCl was used as the negative control and 0.1 M sodium hydroxide as the positive control. The ocular irritation index (OII) was calculated according to the expression described in methods.

The results showed that, in the positive control, initial injuries were observed in the first 30 s, as hemorrhage and rosette-like coagulation, which further increased within 5 min (Figure 2). The average cumulative score of the positive control of 0.1 M NaOH was 21.11 ± 0.32 (Figure 2A and Table 1). In the negative control, no modifications were observed after 5 min, and the OII was ≤0.9 ± 0.0 (Figure 2B and Table 1). LyeTxI-b formulation, at the four tested concentrations, showed no signs of vascular response (Figure 2C–F), and the average cumulative scores were ≤0.9 ± 0.0, which categorized this formulation as non-irritant when applied on CAM surface (Table 1).

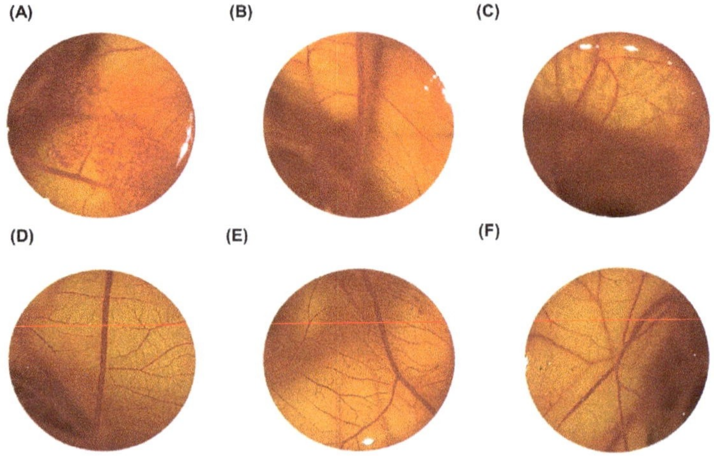

Figure 2. Images of HET-CAM after 5 min exposure to: (**A**) 0.1M NaOH (positive control); (**B**) 0.5% CMC in 0.9% NaCl (negative control); and treatment with LyeTxI-b eye drop at the following concentrations: (**C**) 14.5 µmol/L; (**D**) 28.9 µmol/L; (**E**) 57.9 µmol/L; and (**F**) 115.9 µmol/L.

Table 1. Ocular irritation index (OII) scores for the tested LyeTxI-b eye drops.

Tested Solution/Dispersion	OII ± SEM	Irritancy Classification
0.1 M NaOH (Positive control)	21.11 ± 0.32	SI
0.9% NaCl +CMC 5% (Negative control)	≤0.9 ± 0.0	NI
LyeTxI-b—14.5 µmol/L	≤0.9 ± 0.0	NI
LyeTxI-b—28.9 µmol/L	≤0.9 ± 0.0	NI
LyeTxI-b—57.9 µmol/L	≤0.9 ± 0.0	NI
LyeTxI-b—115.9 µmol/L	≤0.9 ± 0.0	NI

NI, Non-irritant or slightly irritant; SI, Severely irritant. The results are expressed as mean ± SD (n = 10).

2.3. LyeTxI-b Was Not Irritant for Topical Administration

The total scores for all concentrations of LyeTxI-b were validated between 0 and 3 in long-term eye irritation test. The results show that the formulation with LyeTxI-b did not stimulate irritation on rabbit eye tissues. The corneal and iris scores were zero (Table 2). Although conjunctival hyperemia was observed in the group treated with 115.9 μmol/L, no acute reactions by the rabbits and no prolonged or delayed toxicity were observed.

Table 2. Draize test demonstrating the maximum mean total scores of rabbit eyes treated with several concentrations of LyeTxI-b eye drop.

Location	Concentrations (μmol/L)			
	14.5	28.9	57.9	115.9
Cornea opacity	0	0	0	0
Iris inflammation degree	0	0	0	0
Conjunctival congestion	0	0	0	0.6
Conjunctival swelling	0	0	0	0
Conjunctival discharge	0	0	0	0
Total score	0	0	0	0.6

2.4. *LyeTxI-b Reduces Bacterial Growth in Ocular Keratitis*

Considering our positive results regarding LyeTxI-b activity in the MIC trial, its ability to reduce biofilm viability and its behavior on ocular tolerance test, we evaluated the in vivo efficacy of this peptide on *S. aureus*-induced keratitis model in rabbits. For these tests, the dose selected was 28.9 μmol/L, which was eight times higher than the MIC and was able to reduce around 50% of the biofilm formation.

The results show that LyeTxI-b was able to significantly reduce bacterial growth. Rabbit eyes were examined for changes through slit lamp examination (SLE) every 24 h. The ocular parameters (according to methods, Table 3) was graded on a scale of 0 (none) to 4 (severe). Figure 3 shows gross pathological signs of infection and significant increases in SLE scores in the control, and these signs significantly reduced after treatment with LyeTxI-b. Corneas infected with bacteria showed a visible increase in haze and clinical deterioration if compared with treated corneas (Figure 4).

Table 3. Grading of observable ocular disease in infected rabbits.

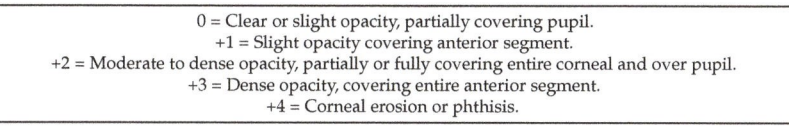

0 = Clear or slight opacity, partially covering pupil.
+1 = Slight opacity covering anterior segment.
+2 = Moderate to dense opacity, partially or fully covering entire corneal and over pupil.
+3 = Dense opacity, covering entire anterior segment.
+4 = Corneal erosion or phthisis.

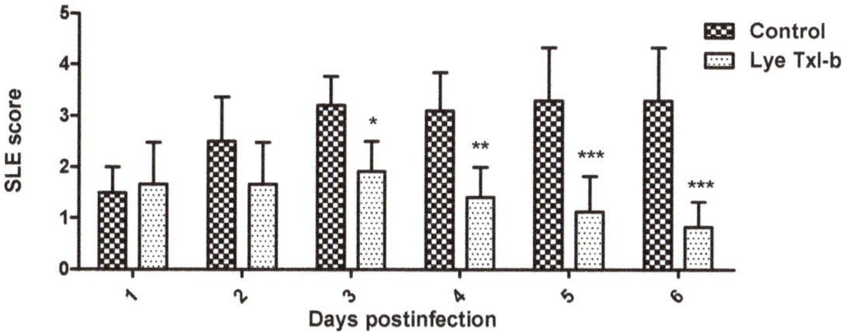

Figure 3. Slit lamp examination (SLE) of ocular disease after infection with *S. aureus*. The ocular disease was graded, and mean SLE scores were calculated by summing the scores for each group (n = 6) of rabbits divided by the total number of rabbits graded at each time point. Control: vehicle; Lye TxI-b: LyeTxI-b eye drop. Data are expressed as the mean ± SD. Asterisk indicates LyeTxI-b vs. Control (+) two-way ANOVA plus Bonferroni post-test * $p < 0.05$; ** $p < 0.01$; *** $p < 0.001$.

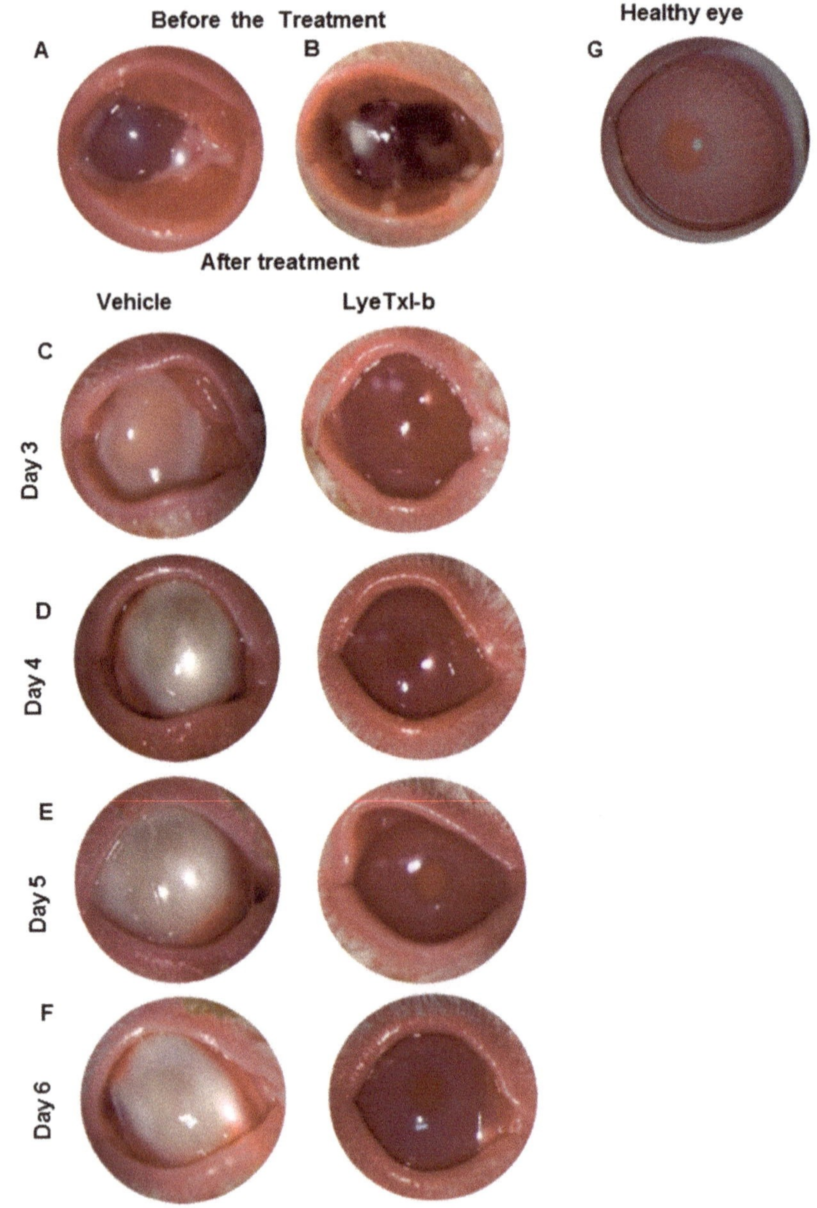

Figure 4. Photomicrographs of the ocular disease in rabbits at post infection (PI) with *S. aureus*. (**A**) Eye control: infected with *S. aureus* before receiving the vehicle. (**B**) Eye infected with *S. aureus* before receiving the LyeTxI-b eye drop. (**C**) Vehicle: three days PI with *S. aureus* treatment with vehicle; and LyeTxI-b: three days PI with *S. aureus* treatment with LyeTxI-b. (**D**) Vehicle: four days PI with *S. aureus* treatment with vehicle; and LyeTxI-b: four days PI with *S. aureus* treatment with LyeTxI-b. (**E**) Vehicle: five days PI with *S. aureus* treatment with vehicle; and LyeTxI-b: five days PI with *S. aureus* treatment with LyeTxI-b. (**F**) Vehicle: six days PI with *S. aureus* treatment with vehicle; and LyeTxI-b: six days PI with *S. aureus* treatment with LyeTxI-b. (**G**) Healthy eye.

The observed pathological changes in rabbits' eyes included severe iritis, corneal infiltrates and erosions. At Post-Infection (PI) Day 1 with treatments, some corneal opacity was observed in both control and LyeTxI-b eye-drop-treated (+1.5 to +2.0) rabbits (Figure 3). Dense corneal opacity was observed in infected rabbits' eyes after PI Day 2 with vehicle (+2.5 to +3) (Figure 3). The animals that received the eye drop treatment showed inhibited disease progression and a significant reduction in corneal opacity density after PI Day 4 (+1.0 to +1.5) (Figures 3 and 4). The disease did not progress beyond (+2.5 to +3.5) after PI Day 6 in controls (Figures 3 and 4). In addition, dense opacities that covered the entire corneal surface and corneal erosions were observed in control on PI Day 6 (Figures 3 and 4). The same was not observed in the animals that received the eye drop with LyeTxI-b (Figures 3 and 4).

To further characterize the course of infection and the treatment with LyeTxI-b eye drop, we quantified the number of viable *S. aureus* (CFU) recovered from infected rabbits' eyes on PI Day 6. The number of CFU recovered from infected eyes without treatment (Control) was significantly higher when compared to treated eyes (LyeTxI-b) (Figure 5).

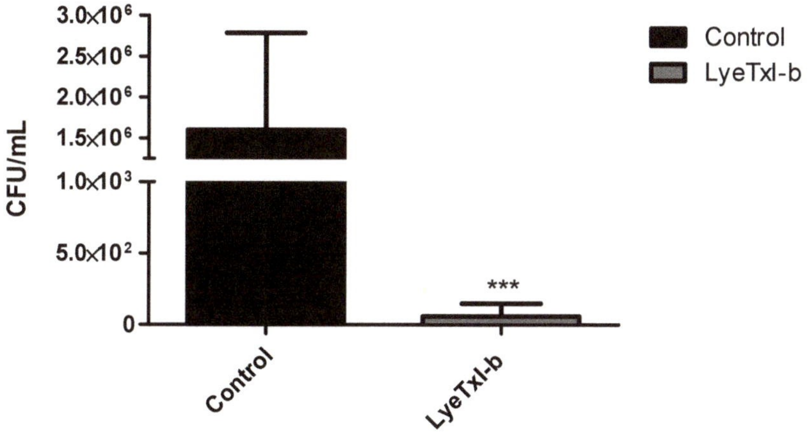

Figure 5. Quantification of viable *S. aureus* in infected rabbit eyes. CFU per infected rabbits eye (Control and LyeTxI-b (28.9 μmol/L), $n = 6$/group) after topical inoculation of *S. aureus* (1×10^8 CFU). Data are expressed as the mean ± SD. Asterisk indicates Control vs. LyeTxI-b treatment unpaired *t*-Student test, *** $p < 0.001$.

2.5. *Eyes after LyeTxI-b Treatment Show Tissue Repair*

Histopathologic analysis of the infected eyes demonstrated congestion of the vascularized tissue of the anterior chamber (Figure 6B,C) and severe edema (Figure 6C). In addition, there was an increase in the corneal epithelium, stroma infiltrate with polymorphonuclear cells, erythrocyte diapedesis, serous exudate accumulation between the collagenous fibers, and destruction of the Bowman's membrane (Figure 6B,C) on PI Day 6.

In contrast, eyes treated with LyeTxI-b eye drops showed intact anterior epithelium and Bowman's membrane demonstrated few polymorphonuclear infiltrations of the stroma and anterior limiting membrane, minor edema and minor change of collagenous fibers in the stroma (Figure 6D).

2.6. *PMN Infiltration was Lower After Treatment with LyeTxI-b Eye Drops*

We assessed the leukocyte recruitment by measuring the activity of myeloperoxidase (MPO) and N-acetylglucosaminidase (NAG) in the rabbits' eye. The results show that, after treatment with LyeTxI-b, there was a significant reduction in the activity of MPO and NAG ($p < 0.001$), being close to the values of healthy animals (Figure 7).

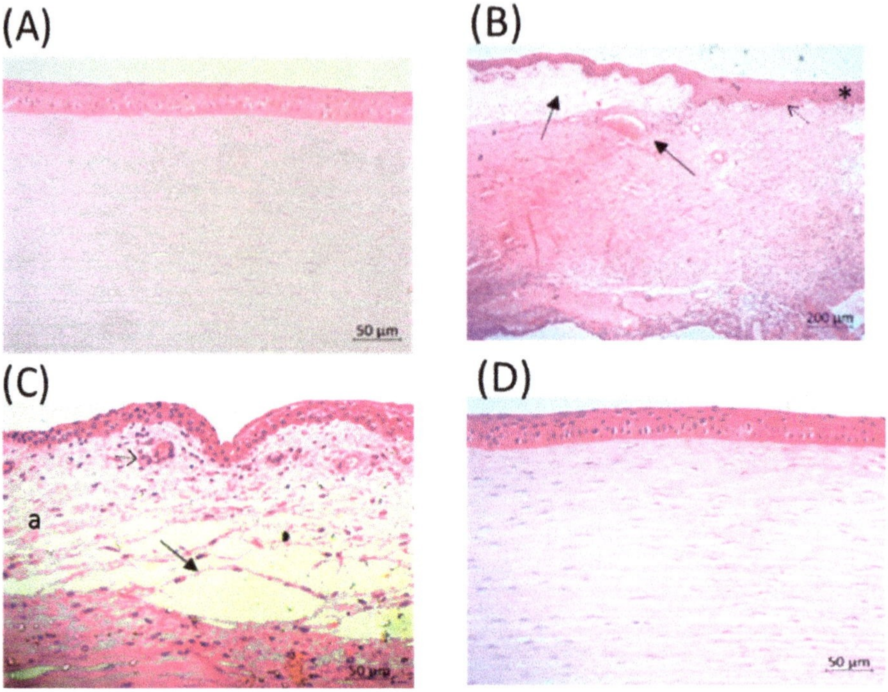

Figure 6. Histopathology of rabbit corneas. (**A**) Healthy cornea. (**B**,**C**) Cross section of a cornea infected with *S. aureus* on PI Day 6. (**B**) Corneal stroma showing vascular congestion, severe edema (arrows), an increase in the corneal epithelium (asterisk) and destruction of the Bowman's membrane (dotted arrow). (**C**) Severe corneal edema (arrow), stroma infiltrate with polymorphonuclear cells (dotted arrow) and serous exudate accumulation between the collagenous fibers (a). (**D**) Cornea infected with *S. aureus* treated with LyeTx1-b on PI Day 6. (**A**,**C**,**D**) 20× objective; and (**B**) 5× objective.

(**A**)

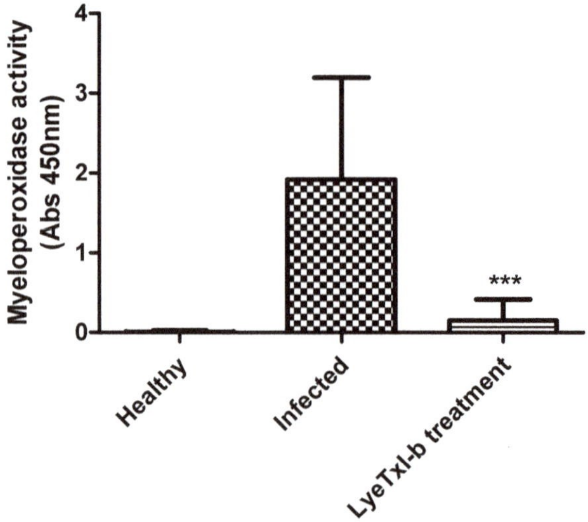

Figure 7. *Cont.*

(B)

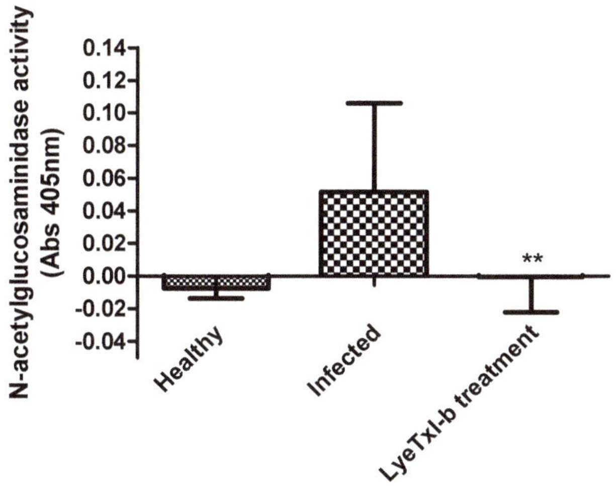

Figure 7. Evaluation of PMN infiltrates by the activity of Myeloperoxidase (MPO) and N-acetylglucosaminidase (NAG) enzymes in the cornea of infected animals: (**A**) MPO activity; and (**B**) NAG activity. $n = 6$, results expressed as mean ± SD. Asterisk indicates LyeTxI-b (28.9 μmol/L) treatment vs. Infected one-way ANOVA plus Bonferroni post-test ** $p < 0.01$; *** $p < 0.001$.

3. Discussion

The main finding of this study was the effectiveness of LyeTxI-b eye drops in the treatment of resistant *S. aureus* keratitis in rabbits and its ability to reduce the inflammatory process in consequence of this infection, which shows LyeTxI-b as a promising antimicrobial agent, corroborating the previous results [15]. Nowadays, there has been an alarming evolution of antimicrobial resistance. Antibiotics are powerful drugs that disrupt or change the composition of the infectious agent and are used to combat severe diseases. As with any powerful medication, the appropriate use of such agents has a highly beneficial effect. However, when improperly used, it leads to bacterial adaptation or mutations and, in turn, to new strains that are resistant to the current antibiotic regiment. In the United States, antibiotic resistance kills around 23,000 patients a year [17].

Novel drugs for gram-positive multidrug-resistant bacteria, such as *Staphylococcus aureus*, may contribute in the reduction of bacterial spread and the rate of treatment failure. *S. aureus* is able to form biofilms when colonizing tissues by an aggregation of bacterial cells immobilized in an adhesive extracellular polymeric matrix [18,19]. This hampers its eradication, mainly due to the barrier preventing drug entry or host clearance mechanisms [20–22]. Furthermore, an excessive and harmful inflammatory response can be triggered, since the toxins released by the bacteria contribute to the recruitment of immune cells.

Several organisms have developed an arsenal of host-defense molecules, aiming at controlling microbial proliferation and other biological or physical insults, including antimicrobial peptides (AMPs). Spider venoms represent a rich source of AMPs against infectious pathogens. An example is LyeTxI, a peptide isolated from *Lycosa erithrognata* venom that is active against fungi (*Candida krusei* and *Cryptococcus neoformans*) and bacteria (*Escherichia coli* and *S. aureus*) and was able to alter the permeabilization of α-phosphatidylcholine-liposomes in a dose-dependent manner [12]. Its derivative, LyeTxI-b peptide, if compared with LyeTxI, has a deletion of a His residue and is acetylated in its N-terminal portion. These modifications altered its structure and improved its antimicrobial activity in vitro and in vivo. In addition, LyeTxI-b produces lethal pores and membrane-damaging effects on bacteria, besides being effective to treat septic arthritis in mouse [15].

To check the efficiency of this peptide as an antibacterial agent in the ophthalmic system, we formulated an eye drop containing LyeTxI-b using carboxymethylcellulose (0.5%) polymer, which was chosen for its physical properties, such as viscosity and mucoadhesiveness, which contribute to its prolonged retention time in the ocular surface [23].

In this work, LyeTxI-b eye drops showed potent antimicrobial inhibition activity against planktonic *S. aureus* (Figure 1A) and were able to eradicate the *S. aureus* biofilm (Figure 1B) only at the highest concentrations tested (463.8 and 927.7 μmol/L). However, at concentrations above 3.6 μmol/L, the peptide potently reduced biofilm when compared with the control group.

It has been reported that, in a biofilm environment, bacteria could increase the production and excretion of molecules, such as polysaccharides and DNA, in the biofilm matrix, and these molecules, which are negatively charged, would interact with cationic peptides, preventing their binding to the bacterial membrane [24,25]. This could explain the reduction of LyeTxI-b activity in biofilms.

Considering the positive results regarding LyeTxI-b activity in the in vitro assay, we evaluated its possible toxic effects as a consequence of the instillation, aimed at treating keratitis infection. Our results report, for the first time, that LyeTxI-b formulation, at all tested concentrations, was non-irritant when applied on CAM (Figure 2). In contrast, the positive control (NaOH) was adequate for quality control because it was severely irritant, showing a high score in OII (Table 1). The HET-CAM test, as a model for the study of the precision and safety, can provide information about the conjunctiva ocular effects that formulations may develop. The chorioallantoic membrane is analogous to human retina and its vasculature. Therefore, the irritation with a risk of vascular damage such as hemorrhage, lysis and coagulation can be evaluated for ocular formulations [26,27].

Despite the non-irritancy of LyeTxI-b formulation in the HET-CAM test, Draize test was also performed for the full understanding of ocular tolerance. No signs of ocular inflammation, corneal opacity, conjunctival congestion, swelling or discharge were observed for the doses of 14.5, 28.9 and 57.9 μmol/L of LyeTxI-b during the time of analysis (seven days). However, conjunctival congestion was observed at 115.9 μmol/L of the peptide and this reaction disappeared after one day (Table 2).

Convinced that the peptide was safe for ocular use, we induced the bacterial keratitis in rabbits and evaluated the efficiency of the LyeTxI-b formulation to treat the infection. The results obtained in this work (Figures 3 and 4) turn clear the potential use of LyeTxI-b to treat bacterial keratitis. LyeTxI-b, at a low dose (28.9 μmol/mL), could eliminate penicillin-, erythromycin- and ampicillin-resistant *S. aureus* if compared to ciprofloxacin (1.5 mMol/mL), although, at first, they present different mechanisms of action. O'Callaghan [1] showed that ciprofloxacin was more effective than vancomycin or cefazolin in the early stages of cornea infection with methicillin-resistant *S. aureus*. The concentration of LyeTxI-b eye drop was near to one hundred times lower if compared to ciprofloxacin, which indicates its higher potency. A similar effect was observed when LyeTxI-b was used for the treatment of septic arthritis: the peptide decreased the bacterial load to the same level as clindamycin, but LyeTxI-b concentration was two hundred times lower [15].

Several pathological changes could be observed in infected control eyes, but the same was not observed in the eyes treated with LyeTxI-b eye drops. Keratitis resulting from intrastromal injection is characterized by bacterial replication and severe ocular changes, including edema, corneal epithelial cell destruction, iritis, as well as the migration of polymorphonuclear neutrophils (PMNs) from the eyelid to the tear film [28,29]. All these changes were observed in the animals that received vehicle (Control). Gross signs of infection appeared within 24 h in the infected rabbit eye and progressed in control group beyond +2.5 to +3.5 SLE score. In contrast, the formulation with LyeTxI-b reduced the disease progression almost reaching the morphology of healthy eyes.

The CFU results highlight the potential of this peptide to treat this disease, as shown in Figure 5. Corroborating these results, the histopathological analysis evidenced the alterations caused by *S. aureus* cornea infection and showed significant improvement after treatment with LyeTxI-b eye drops, including the reduction of cellular infiltrate (Figure 6).

Myeloperoxidase enzyme (MPO) is mainly found in cytoplasmic granules of neutrophils, but also in monocytes. MPO is a protein of the heme group secreted by activated leukocytes. It promotes the conversion of hydrogen peroxide to hypochlorous acid and halides in hypoallergenic acids, leading to the formation of highly reactive intermediates, which in turn contributes to lipid peroxidation [30,31]. NAG, on the other hand, is a lysosomal enzyme highly present in activated macrophages. Together, MPO and NAG serve as good markers of neutrophil and macrophage infiltration in tissues and inflammation, respectively [32]. Our study shows that LyeTxI-b eye drops were able to significantly reduce neutrophil and macrophage activity after topical keratitis induction (Figure 7).

LyeTxI-b eye drops were safe for ocular use and were able to treat topical and resistant bacterial keratitis in rabbits. In addition, this formulation was able to reduce the inflammatory process triggered by the disease, since there was a significant reduction in the cellular infiltrate or a reduction in the activity of these cells. In conclusion, our results show that LyeTxI-b is an excellent candidate as an alternative drug to treat keratitis.

4. Materials and Methods

4.1. Materials

The following were used: Mueller–Hinton (MH) broth (Himedia, Mumbai, Índia), brain heart infusion (BHI) (Kasvi, São José do Pinhais, Brazil), mannitol salt agar (Kasvi, São José do Pinhais, Brazil), resazurin, carboxymethylcellulose (CMC) and Dimethyl sulfoxide (DMSO) were purchased from Sigma-Aldrich (Darmstadt, Germany); Ketamin® (Cristália, São Paulo, Brazil); xylazine hydrochloride (Copanize®, Schering-Plough Coopers, São Paulo, Brazil); proxymetacaine hydrochloride (Anestalcon; Alcon, São Paulo, Brazil); 3,3′,5,5′-Tetramethylbenzidine (TMB, Sigma-aldrich, Germany); and 4-Nitrophenyl N-acetyl-β-D-glucosaminide (NAG, Sigma-aldrich, Darmstadt, Germany).

The peptide LyeTxI-b (CH3CO-IWLTALKFLGKNLGKLAKQQLAKL-NH2) was synthesized by GenOne Biotechnologies (Rio de Janeiro, Brazil).

4.2. Methods

4.2.1. In Vitro Antimicrobial Test

A strain of *Staphylococcus aureus* resistant to penicillin, erythromycin and ampicillin was isolated from ocular samples of a 22-year-old female patient, in a private clinical analysis laboratory in Belo Horizonte-MG, Brazil. This strain was employed in both planktonic and biofilm forms in this study. BHI broth was used to culture planktonic in aerobic conditions. The MIC using the microdilution method was performed. Samples containing the formulation (LyeTxI-b +0.5% CMC in 0.9% NaCl) were serially diluted from 927.7 to 1.8 μmol/L in MH broth and incubated with 5×10^4 CFU/well for 24 h at 37 °C. The lowest concentration of the peptide formulation that prevented the visible growth of the microorganism was defined as the MIC.

The determination of minimum biofilm eradication concentrations (MBEC)was performed as previously described [33], with modifications. Bacterial suspensions (10 μL), with the same densityof MIC, were added to 96-well plates with MH medium supplemented with glucose 1% and incubated on a horizontal shaking plate at 37 °C, for 24 h, for biofilm formation. The growth medium was discarded and biofilms were washed with sterile saline. Formulations of LyeTxI-b were added at decreasing concentrations (927.7–1.8 μmol/L). After incubation at 37 °C for 24 h, *S. aureus* biofilms were resuspended, resazurin solution (0.1 g/L) was added and the plates were incubated at 37 °C for 20 min in the absence of light. Then, the plates were read in VarioskanTM (λ ex 570 nm e λ em 590 nm) and MBEC was determined as the lowest concentration of peptide formulation that prevented biofilm formation. Resazurin is an indicator of oxidation-reduction used for the evaluation of cell growth [34]. It is a non-fluorescent blue and non-toxic dye. When reduced to resorufin by oxidoreductases within viable cells, it becomes pink and fluorescent. The level of reduction can be quantified by spectrophotometer.

Positive and negative controls were submitted to the same procedures. In the positive control, there was no addition of any peptide or inhibitory drug, just the formulation (0.5% CMC in 0.9% NaCl). The negative control did not have any bacteria and the value was normalized to zero in all analyses. MIC and MBEC assays were performed in triplicate.

4.2.2. Evaluation of LyeTxI-b Toxicity by Chorioallantoic Membrane Test (HET-CAM)

HET-CAM is described in [35] and adapted in [36,37]. Ten fertilized chicken eggs were selected for each concentration tested. The eggs were incubated at 37 ± 1 °C and 60 ± 1% relative humidity for 10 days. On the tenth day, the eggshell was opened and the inner membrane of the egg was carefully removed to avoid any damage to the thin vessels of the chorioallantoic membrane. The concentrations of 14.5, 28.9, 57.9 and 115.9 µmol/L of LyeTxI-b +0.5% CMC in 0.9% NaCl (300 µL) were applied to CAM. Note that 0.5% CMC in 0.9% NaCl was used as negative control and 0.1M sodium hydroxide as positive control. The intensity of the reactions was semi-quantitatively evaluated, on a scale from 0 (no reaction) to 3 (strong reaction). The appearance and intensity of all reactions, if any, were observed at 0 s, 30 s, 2 min and 5 min. The ocular irritation index (OII) was then calculated by the following expression, where h is the time (in seconds) of the onset of hemorrhage, l lysis, and c coagulation, over a period of 300 s (5 min). The separate ratio was multiplied by a factor indicating the impact on vascular damage by the observed effect. Thus, coagulation has the highest impact indicated by factor 9 [35,36].

$$\mathbf{OII} = \frac{(301 - h)}{300} + \frac{(301 - l)}{300} + \frac{(301 - c)\ x\ 9}{300} \tag{1}$$

4.2.3. Ocular Tolerability of LyeTxI-b

Sixteen female New Zealand white rabbits were used. Ocular irritation in the rabbits was evaluated according to the Draize test [38,39] at 1 h, 24 h, 48 h, 72 h and 7 days after the instillation with 4 concentrations 14.5, 28.9, 57.9 or 115.9 µmol/L of LyeTxI-b formulated in 0.5% CMC in 0.9% NaCl, $n = 4$. The method provides an overall scoring system for grading the severity of ocular lesions involving the cornea (opacity), iris (inflammation degree), and conjunctiva (congestion, swelling, and discharge). The Draize score was determined by visual assessment of changes in these ocular structures. Maximum mean total scores (MMTS) were calculated and eye irritation was classified.

4.2.4. Induction of Bacterial Keratitis and Treatment with LyeTxI-b

Twelve female New Zealand white rabbits, aged approximately three months and weighing 2 kg were purchased from the Experimental Farm Professor Hélio Barbosa (Igarapé, MG, Brazil). The animals remained in individual cages throughout the period of adaptation (1 week) and experimentation (7 days) at 25 °C and brightness varying according to sunlight. There was no restriction of water or food during the experiment. The animals were divided into two groups: control (received vehicle) and treated (received LyeTxI-b eye drop).

The study was approved by the Ethics Committee in Experimentation Animal of the Federal University of Minas Gerais (CEUA, Belo Horizonte, Brazil, Protocol No. 298/2017, date of approval: 11 January 2017). All experiments were conducted in accordance with the Association for Research in Vision and Ophthalmology (ARVO).

The rabbits were anesthetized with intramuscular combination injection of ketamine hydrochloride (30 mg/kg) and xylazine hydrochloride (4 mg/kg) and the eyes were topically anesthetized with 0.5% proxymetacaine hydrochloride. Before injection with bacteria, the eyes were wiped with 5% povidone-iodine.

To induce unilateral keratitis, 4×10^5 colony-forming units/mL (4 µL) suspensions of clinical *Staphylococcus aureus* isolates in logarithmic growth phase were injected into the central corneal stroma in the eye. The injection was performed with a 30-gauge needle. Twenty-four hours after bacterial injection, the rabbits were randomly separated in two groups with six animals each and were submitted to the following treatments: (1) Formulation with Lye TxI-b (28.9 μmol/L); and (2) Control (vehicle 0.5% CMC in 0.9% NaCl). The LyeTxI-b eye drops (20 μL) and vehicle were instilled in rabbits' eyes into a space (fornix) created by gently pulling down the lower lid, every 6 h, for 6 days. Two hours after the last dose of LyeTxI-b or vehicle, the rabbits were euthanized using an overdose of sodium pentobarbital (81 mg/kg). Corneas were carefully and aseptically removed and cut in three parts. One part was cultured to enumerate viable bacteria, the other was used for histopathology and the third part was used for MPO and NAG quantification. The rabbit's corneas (20 mg) excised were immediately homogenized in phosphate buffered saline (PBS). The material was serially diluted and 0.1 mL aliquots were plated in triplicate on mannitol salt agar for enumeration of *S. aureus*. The specimens were incubated at 35 °C for 24 h.

4.2.5. Slit Lamp Examination (SLE)

The ocular disease was evaluated both macroscopically and microscopically using a slit lamp biomicroscope (Apramed HS5, São Carlos, Brazil) during the experiment, every 24 h by two masked observers. Observations of *S. aureus*-infected rabbits' eyes were graded with a modification of the scale previously described [40]. The corneal response was graded from 0 to +4 (Table 3).

4.2.6. Histological Analysis

Immediately after sacrifice, one part of the cornea was removed and fixed in Davidson solution [16]. Samples were included in paraffin and 4-μm-thick sections of the sagittal plane, to allow dorsal-to-ventral observation of the cornea and retina, were stained with hematoxylin and eosin and were analyzed in unmyelinated areas under light microscopy (Zeiss®, Model Axio Imager M2, San Diego, California, USA). Eyes that received LyeTxI-b eye drops were compared with the control.

4.2.7. Inflammatory Analysis: MPO and NAG Activity

Initially, 20 mg of cornea were homogenized in ice-cold Buffer 1 solution (0.1 M NaCl, 0.02 M Na_3PO_4 and 0.015 M Na_2EDTA) and centrifuged at 4 °C (5000 g, 10 min). The supernatant was discarded and the pellet was resuspended in 0.2% NaCl solution and 1.6% NaCl plus 5% glucose. The samples were homogenized and centrifuged at 4 °C (5000 g, 10 min). The supernatant was discarded and the pellet resuspended in buffer 2 (Na_3PO_4 and 0.5% HETAB *w/v*) solution. For the MPO assay, this homogenate was frozen in liquid nitrogen and unfrozen in water at room temperature for three consecutive times. The samples were then centrifuged at 4 °C (5000 g, 15 min). An aliquot of the supernatant was removed for dilution in buffer 2 and performance of the enzymatic assay. In the microplate, the sample was plated in triplicate. TMB substrate, previously diluted in DMSO, was added. The plate was placed in an oven at 37 °C for 5 min. Then hydrogen peroxide solution (0.002%) was added and the samples were again incubated at 37 °C for 5 min. After the incubation, the reaction was stopped with the addition of sulfuric acid (1M). The absorbance was read at 450 nm. The mean of the values obtained in each triplicate was used to determine the activity of the enzyme.

For indirect quantification of N-acetylglucosaminidase (NAG) activity in macrophages, 20 mg of cornea tissue were weighed and homogenized with Saline/Triton solution (Saline 0.9% and Triton x-100, 1%) and then centrifuged at 4 °C (1500 g, 10 min). The supernatant was collected and diluted in phosphate-citrate buffer (0.1 M citric acid and 0.1 M Na_2HPO_4) to perform the NAG assay. One hundred microliters of each diluted sample were plated in triplicate. The substrate p-nitrophenyl-N-acetyl-β-D-glucosaminide (2.2 mM), diluted in phosphate-citrate buffer, was added. Samples were incubated in an oven at 37 °C for 5 min. After the reaction, 0.2 M of glycine buffer was added to the samples to paralyze the reaction. The absorbance was read at 405 nm. The mean of the values obtained in each triplicate was used to determine the activity of the enzyme.

4.2.8. Statistical Analysis

Statistical analyses were performed using the GraphPad Prism™ software version 5.0 and data were expressed as mean ± standard deviation (SD), followed by single-variance analysis (ANOVA one-way) with Bonferroni post-test. Results were considered significant for values of $p < 0.05$.

Author Contributions: C.N.d.S., F.R.d.S., L.F.N.D., P.V.M.d.R., R.O.S., B.L.d.C., P.S.N., F.A.A., V.L.d.S., M.E.d.L. and A.d.S.C.J. Conceptualization; C.N.d.S., F.R.d.S., L.F.N.D., P.V.M.d.R., R.O.S. and B.L.d.C. Methodology and Validation and Investigation; C.N.d.S., F.R.d.S., L.F.N.D. and P.V.M.d.R. Formal Analysis; C.N.d.S., F.R.d.S., L.F.N.D., R.O.S., B.L.d.C., V.L.d.S., M.E.d.L. and A.d.S.C.J. Writing-Original Draft Preparation; C.N.d.S., F.R.d.S., M.E.d.L. and A.d.S.C.J. Writing-Review & Editing the article; P.S.N., F.A.A., V.L.d.S., M.E.d.L. and A.d.S.C.J. Supervision; M.E.d.L. and A.d.S.C.J. Project Administration and Funding Acquisition.

Funding: This study was part of the National Institute of Science and Technology in Pharmaceutical Nanotechnology: a transdisciplinary approach (INCT-NANOFARMA), which is supported by São Paulo Research Foundation (FAPESP, Brazil), Grant #2014/50928-2; by the National Council for Scientific and Technological Development (Conselho Nacional de Pesquisa, CNPq, Brazil), Grant #465687/2014-8 and 150010/2018-4; by Coordenação de Aperfeiçoamento de Pessoal de Nível Superior (CAPES), Grant# 23038.000776/2017O54 and Universidade Federal de Minas Gerais.

Acknowledgments: We would like to thank the fellowships and grants were awarded by the Brazilian University UFMG (Universidade Federal de Minas Gerais), CAPES (Coordenação de Aperfeiçoamento de Pessoal de Nível Superior), FAPEMIG (Fundação de Pesquisa do Estado de Minas Gerais) and CNPq (Conselho Nacional de Desenvolvimento Científico e Tecnológico).

Conflicts of Interest: The authors declare no conflict of interest.

References

1. O'Callaghan, R.J. The Pathogenesis of Staphylococcus aureus Eye Infections. *Pathogens* **2018**, *10*. [CrossRef] [PubMed]
2. Whitcher, J.P.; Srinivasan, M.; Upadhyay, M.P. Corneal blindness: A global perspective. *Bull. World Health Organ.* **2001**, *79*, 214–221. [PubMed]
3. Rachwalik, D.; Pleyer, U. Bacterial Keratitis. *Klinische Monatsblätter Augenheilkunde* **2015**, *232*, 738–744.
4. Keay, L.; Edwards, K.; Naduvilath, T.; Taylor, H.; Snibson, G.; Forde, K.; Stapleton, F. Microbial keratitis predisposing factors and morbidity. *Ophthalmology* **2006**, *113*, 109–116.
5. McGhee, C.N.J.; Niederer, R. Resisting susceptibility: Bacterial keratitis and generations of antibiotics. *Clin. Exp. Ophthalmol.* **2006**, *34*, 3–5. [PubMed]
6. De Oliveira Fulgêncio, G.; Viana, F.A.; Silva, R.O.; Lobato, F.C.; Ribeiro, R.R.; Fanca, J.R.; Byrro, R.M.; Faraco, A.A.; da Silva Cunha-Júnior, A. Mucoadhesive chitosan films as a potential ocular delivery system for ofloxacin: Preliminary in vitro studies. *Vet. Ophthalmol.* **2014**, *17*, 150–155. [CrossRef] [PubMed]
7. Dajcs, J.J.; Moreau, J.M.; Thibodeaux, B.A.; Traidej, M.; Austin, M.S.; Marquart, M.E.; Stroman, D.W.; O'callaghan, R.J. Effectiveness of Ciprofloxacin and Ofloxacin in a prophylaxis model of Staphylococcus Keratitis. *Cornea* **2001**, *20*, 878–880. [CrossRef] [PubMed]
8. Brogden, K.A.; Ackermann, M.; McCray, P.B., Jr.; Tack, B.F. Antimicrobial peptides in animals and their role in host defences. *Int. J. Antimicrob. Agents* **2003**, *22*, 465–478. [CrossRef]
9. Kang, S.J.; Park, S.J.; Mishig-Ochir, T.; Lee, B.J. Antimicrobial peptides: Therapeutic potentials. *Expert Rev. Ant. Infect. Ther.* **2014**, *12*, 1477–1486. [CrossRef] [PubMed]
10. Lakshmaiah, N.J.; Chen, J.Y. Antimicrobial peptides: Possible anti-infective agents. *Peptides* **2015**, *72*, 88–94. [CrossRef] [PubMed]
11. Atia, R.; Jouve, L.; Knoeri, J.; Georgeon, C.; Laroche, L.; Borderie, V.; Bouheraoua, N. Corneal collagen cross-linking to treat infectious keratitis. *J. Fr. Ophtalmol.* **2018**, *41*, 560–568. [CrossRef] [PubMed]
12. Santos, D.M.; Verly, R.M.; Pilo-Veloso, D.; De Maria, M.; De Carvalho, M.A.R.; Cisalpino, P.S.; Soares, B.M.; Diniz, C.G.; Farias, L.M.; Moreira, D.F.; et al. LyeTx I, a potent antimicrobial peptide from the venom of the spider *Lycosa erythrognatha*. *Amino Acids* **2010**, *39*, 135–144. [CrossRef] [PubMed]
13. Consuegra, J.; de Lima, M.E.; Santos, D.; Sinisterra, R.D.; Cortés, M.E. Peptides: B-cyclodextrin inclusion compounds as highly effective antimicrobial and anti-epithelial proliferation agents. *J. Periodontol.* **2013**, *84.*, 1858–1868. [CrossRef]

14. Cruz Olivo, E.A.; Santos, D.; de Lima, M.E.; Dos Santos, V.L.; Sinisterra, R.D.; Cortés, M.E. Antibacterial Effect of Synthetic Peptide LyeTxI and LyeTxI/β-Cyclodextrin Association Compound Against Planktonic and Multispecies Biofilms of Periodontal Pathogens. *J. Periodontol.* **2017**, *88*, 88–96. [CrossRef] [PubMed]
15. Reis, P.V.M.; Boff, D.; Verly, R.M.; Melo-Braga, M.N.; Cortés, M.E.; Santos, D.M.; Pimenta, A.M.D.C.; Amaral, F.A.; Resende, J.M.; de Lima, M.E. LyeTxI-b, a Synthetic Peptide Derived from *Lycosa erythrognatha* Spider Venom, Shows Potent Antibiotic Activity in Vitro and in Vivo. *Front. Microbiol.* **2018**, *9*, 667. [CrossRef] [PubMed]
16. Silva, F.R.; Paiva, M.R.B.; Dourado, L.F.N.; Silva, R.O.; da Silva, C.N.; da Costa, B.L.; Toledo, C.R.; de Lima, M.E.; da Silva-Cunha, A. Intravitreal injection of the synthetic peptide LyeTx I b, derived of a spider toxin, in rabbit's eye is safety and prevents neovascularization on Chorio-allantoic Membrane Model. *J. Venom. Anim. Toxins Include. Trop. Dis.* **2018**, *24*, 31. [CrossRef] [PubMed]
17. Habboush, Y.; Guzman, N. Antibiotic Resistance. SourceStatPearls [Internet]. 2018. Available online: https://www.ncbi.nlm.nih.gov/books/NBK513277/ (accessed on 3 March 2019).
18. Mancl, K.A.; Kirsner, R.S.; Ajdic, D. Wound biofilms: Lessons learned from oral biofilms. *Wound Repair Regen* **2013**, *21*, 352–362. [CrossRef] [PubMed]
19. Mangoni, M.L.; McDermott, A.M.; Zasloff, M. Antimicrobial peptides and wound healing: Biological and therapeutic considerations. *Exp. Dermatol.* **2016**, *25*, 167–173. [CrossRef]
20. Wolcott, R.D.; Rhoads, D.D.; Bennett, M.E.; Wolcott, B.M.; Gogokhia, L.; Costerton, J.W.; Dowd, S.E. Chronic wounds and the medical biofilm paradigm. *J. Wound Care* **2010**, *19*, 45–46. [CrossRef] [PubMed]
21. Breidenstein, E.B.; de la Fuente-Nunez, C.; Hancock, R.E. *Pseudomonas aeruginosa*: All roads lead to resistance. *Trends Microbiol.* **2011**, *19*, 419–426. [CrossRef] [PubMed]
22. Taylor, P.K.; Yeung, A.T.; Hancock, R.E. Antibiotic resistance in *Pseudomonas aeruginosa* biofilms: Towards the development of novel anti-biofilm therapies. *J. Biotechnol.* **2014**, *191*, 121–130. [CrossRef]
23. Garrett, Q.; Simmons, P.A.; Xu, S.; Vehige, J.; Zhao, Z.; Ehrmann, K.; Willcox, M. Carboxymethylcellulose binds to human corneal epithelial cells and is a modulator of cornealepithelial wound healing. *Investig. Ophthalmol. Vis. Sci.* **2007**, *48*, 1559–1567. [CrossRef] [PubMed]
24. Chan, C.; Burrows, L.L.; Deber, C.M. Helix induction in antimicrobial peptides by alginate in biofilms. *J. Biol. Chem.* **2004**, *279*, 38749–38754. [CrossRef] [PubMed]
25. Mulcahy, H.; Charron-Mazenod, L.; Lewenza, S. Extracellular DNA chelates cations and induces antibiotic resistance in *Pseudomonas aeruginosa* biofilms. *PLoS Pathog.* **2008**, *4*, e1000213. [CrossRef] [PubMed]
26. Abdelkader, H.; Ismail, S.; Hussein, A.; Wu, Z.; Al-Kassas, R.; Alany, R.G. Conjunctival and corneal tolerability assessment of ocular naltrexone niosomes and their ingredients on the hen's egg chorioallantoic membrane and excised bovine cornea models. *Int. J. Pharm.* **2012**, *432*, 1–10. [CrossRef]
27. Vargas, A.; Zeisser-Labouèbe, M.; Lange, N.; Gurny, R.; Delie, F. The chick embryo and its chorioallantoic membrane (CAM) for the in vivo evaluation of drug delivery systems. *Adv. Drug Deliv. Rev.* **2007**, *59*, 1162–1176. [CrossRef]
28. Sloop, G.D.; Moreau, J.M.; Conerly, L.L.; Dajcs, J.J.; O'Callaghan, R.J. Acute inflammation of the eyelid and cornea in Staphylococcus keratitis in the rabbit. *Investig. Ophthalmol. Vis. Sci.* **1999**, *40*, 385–391.
29. Hume, E.B.; Dajcs, J.J.; Moreau, J.M.; Sloop, G.D.; Willcox, M.D.; O'Callaghan, R.J. Staphylococcus corneal virulence in a new topical model of infection. *Investig. Ophthalmol. Vis. Sci.* **2001**, *42*, 2904–2908.
30. O'brien, P.J. Peroxidases. *Chemico-Biol. Interact.* **2000**, *129*, 113–139. [CrossRef]
31. Giovannini, S.; Onder, G.; Leeuwenburgh, C.; Carter, C.; Marzetti, E.; Russo, A.; Capoluongo, E.; Pahor, M.; Bernabei, R.; Landi, F.; et al. Myeloperoxidase levels and mortality in frail community-living elderly individuals. *J. Gerontol. Med. Sci.* **2010**, *65A*, 369–376. [CrossRef] [PubMed]
32. Oguido, A.P.M.T.; Hohmann, M.S.N.; Pinho-Ribeiro, F.A.; Crespigio, J.; Domiciano, T.P.; Verri, W.A.; Casella, A.M. Naringenin Eye Drops Inhibit Corneal Neovascularization by Anti-Inflammatory and Antioxidant Mechanisms. *Investig. Ophthalmol. Vis. Sci.* **2017**, *58*, 5764–5776. [CrossRef] [PubMed]
33. Toté, K.; Horemans, T.; Vanden Berghe, D.; Maes, L.; Cos, P. Inhibitory Effect of Biocides on the Viable Masses and Matrices of Staphylococcus aureus and Pseudomonas aeruginosa Biofilms. *Appl. Environ. Microbiol.* **2010**, *76*, 3135–3142. [CrossRef] [PubMed]
34. Sarker, S.D.; Nahar, L.; Kumarasamy, Y. Microtitre plate based antibacterial assay incorporating resazurin as an indicator of cell growth, and its application in the in vitro antibacterial screening of phytochemicals. *Methods* **2007**, *42*, 321–324. [CrossRef] [PubMed]

35. Gilleron, L.; Coecke, S.; Sysmans, M.; Hansen, E.; Van Oproy, S.; Marzin, D.; Van Cauteren, H.; Vanparys, P. Evaluation of a modified HET-CAM assay as a screening test for eye irritancy. *Toxicol. In Vitro* **1996**, *10*, 431–446. [CrossRef]
36. Fangueiro, J.F.; Calpena, A.C.; Clares, B.; Andreani, T.; Egea, M.A.; Veiga, F.J.; Garcia, M.L.; Silva, A.M.; Souto, E.B. Biopharmaceutical evaluation of epigallocatechin gallate-loaded cationic lipid nanoparticles(EGCG-LNs): In vivo, in vitro and ex vivo studies. *Int. J. Pharm.* **2016**, *502*, 161–169. [CrossRef]
37. Ferreira, A.E.; Castro, B.F.; Vieira, L.C.; Cassali, G.D.; Souza, C.M.; Fulgêncio, G.O.; Ayres, E.; Oréfice, R.L.; Jorge, R.; Silva-Cunha, A.; et al. Antiangiogenic activity of a bevacizumab-loaded polyurethane device in animal neovascularization models. *J. Fr. Ophtalmol.* **2017**, *40*, 202–208. [CrossRef] [PubMed]
38. Draize, J.H.; Woodward, G.; Calvery, H.O. Methods for the study of irritation and toxicity of articles applied topically to the skin and mucous membranes. *J. Pharmacol. Exp. Ther.* **1944**, *82*, 377–390.
39. Fialho, S.L.; da Silva-Cunha, A. New vehicle based on a microemulsion for topical ocular administration of dexamethasone. *Clin. Exp. Ophthalmol.* **2004**, *32*, 626–632. [CrossRef] [PubMed]
40. Hazlett, L.D.; Moon, M.M.; Strejc, M.; Berk, R.S. Evidence for N-acetylmannosamine as an ocular receptor for, *P. aeruginosa* adherence to scarified cornea. *Investig. Ophthalmol. Vis. Sci.* **1987**, *28*, 1978–1985.

toxins

MDPI

Review

Natural Occurrence in Venomous Arthropods of Antimicrobial Peptides Active against Protozoan Parasites

Elias Ferreira Sabiá Júnior, Luis Felipe Santos Menezes, Israel Flor Silva de Araújo and Elisabeth Ferroni Schwartz *

Departamento de Ciências Fisiológicas, Instituto de Ciências Biológicas, Universidade de Brasília, Brasília, DF 70910-900, Brazil; elias.fsabia@gmail.com (E.F.S.J.); luisfelipe_100@outlook.com (L.F.S.M.); israelfsaraujo@gmail.com (I.F.S.d.A.)

* Correspondence: efschwa@unb.br; Tel.: +55-6131073106

Received: 15 August 2019; Accepted: 10 September 2019; Published: 25 September 2019

check for updates

Abstract: Arthropoda is a phylum of invertebrates that has undergone remarkable evolutionary radiation, with a wide range of venomous animals. Arthropod venom is a complex mixture of molecules and a source of new compounds, including antimicrobial peptides (AMPs). Most AMPs affect membrane integrity and produce lethal pores in microorganisms, including protozoan pathogens, whereas others act on internal targets or by modulation of the host immune system. Protozoan parasites cause some serious life-threatening diseases among millions of people worldwide, mostly affecting the poorest in developing tropical regions. Humans can be infected with protozoan parasites belonging to the genera *Trypanosoma*, *Leishmania*, *Plasmodium*, and *Toxoplasma*, responsible for Chagas disease, human African trypanosomiasis, leishmaniasis, malaria, and toxoplasmosis. There is not yet any cure or vaccine for these illnesses, and the current antiprotozoal chemotherapeutic compounds are inefficient and toxic and have been in clinical use for decades, which increases drug resistance. In this review, we will present an overview of AMPs, the diverse modes of action of AMPs on protozoan targets, and the prospection of novel AMPs isolated from venomous arthropods with the potential to become novel clinical agents to treat protozoan-borne diseases.

Keywords: antimicrobial peptide; venom; arthropod; malaria; Chagas disease; human African trypanosomiasis; leishmaniasis; toxoplasmosis

Key Contribution: The breakthroughs or highlights of the manuscript. Authors can write one or two sentences to describe the most important part of the paper.

1. Introduction

Arthropoda is a phylum of invertebrate animals that have a rigid exoskeleton with several pairs of articulated appendages whose number varies according to the class [1]. It is a diverse and ancient group of invertebrate animals, which underwent spectacular evolutionary radiation [2], totaling more than 5 million different organisms, approximately 80% of all known species on Earth [3–6]. This vast radiation allowed the occupation of a broad range of ecological niches, with gigantic variations in their lifestyle and dietary preferences [7–12].

The colonization of new environments probably enforced novel evolutionary challenges and requirements, improving morphological, biochemical, and behavioral features, enabling the selection of a series of exceptional adaptations, making them one of the first animal groups adapted to occupying terrestrial habitats [13,14]. Alongside these adaptations, evolutionary pressures on genes allowed the development of a highly efficient and rare predatory tool, found in only a few arthropod taxa: venom.

New specialized organs or even whole venom delivery systems were evolutionarily selected (adapted) to actively inoculate venom inside the body of their victim, such as fangs or stings [15,16], resulting in a drastic increase in fitness, predatory success, and predator deterrence.

Venom apparatus is responsible for production of toxins, their storage and delivery through injection into prey [14,17,18]. Venom usage is so important in the animal kingdom that it evolved independently at least 19 times in arthropods [19]. Based on this vast radiation, the venom injection apparatus can be found in different arthropod body parts: in the distal end of the body, in the antennae, in the palpal chelae, present as modified legs, but most commonly in an adaptation of mouth parts [14,19]. Besides, venom has more specialized functions, such as preservation of prey for feeding parasitic larvae and aiding extra-oral digestion of prey [19,20]. The venom of the vast majority of arthropods is a complex mixture of peptides, proteins, and enzymes with a rich diversity of biological activities. Other minor components can be found in salt, inorganic ions, carbohydrates, glucose, and amino acids. [21–23]. Besides these, acypolyamines, biogenic amines, serotonin, histamine, protease inhibitors, mucopolysaccharides, proteases, hyaluronidase, phospholipases, and phosphoesterases can be found in the venom of scorpions and spiders [23–25].

Intriguingly, venomous animals belonging to the arthropod group are found in three major classes: Insecta, Arachnida, and Chilopoda. Recently, venom was described within the crustacean subphylum, the only species of venomous predator reported so far, the remipede *Xibalbanus tulumensis* [26]. Within the Insecta class, six orders have venomous representative species: Hemiptera, Neuroptera, Hymenoptera, Diptera, Lepidoptera, and Coleoptera. Together, these orders possess about 925,000 described species. The best studied order of venomous insects is Hymenoptera, comprising around 117,000 different species [27]. Regarding the Arachnida and Chilopoda classes, to date, the number of spiders, scorpions and chilopods described reached approximately 48,300, 2400, and 3200, respectively [28–30]. It has recently been suggested that ticks should be referred to as venomous ectoparasites, due to the composition and function of their saliva, and the clear differences between proteins present in tick saliva and other non-venomous animals. Tick saliva contains features of other venomous animals, such as proteins capable of inducing paralysis, interfering with normal host physiological processes [31].

Indeed, several drugs come from research on venomous animals. Captopril, Exenatide, and Ziconotide are some examples of biomolecules that have become drugs for the management and treatment of hypertension, diabetes and chronic pain, respectively [32–34]. In this context, venomous animals are a source of new compounds, arousing great interest from the biotechnology and pharmaceutical industries, making them apposite leading candidates for the development of new drugs.

2. AMPs

The majority of multicellular organisms are constantly vulnerable to dangerous pathogens, through contact and exposure in the environment. For their survival, they have created various mechanisms in a host defense network to combat this invasion [35–37]. AMPs represent the first-line host defense mechanism in all invertebrates; they were evolutionarily preserved as an essential component from the innate immune system, remaining an ancient (archaic), but powerful weapon throughout those years [38,39]. AMPs are usually small molecules (~10–50 residues long), gene-encoded, cationic, and amphipathic, with a miscellaneous composition of amino acids [40–43]. Despite their vast structural diversity, most AMPs kill pathogens microorganisms similarly, through membrane damage, protecting the host from bacteria, viruses, fungi, and parasites [44–46].

After microbial infection or even by means of stimuli such as stress, AMPs are synthesized in the fatty body of insects and hemocytes of invertebrates and, consequently, released into the hemolymph to combat infection [47]. Some genes encoding these peptides are intronless, suggesting that they are early response genes, facilitating post transcriptional modification and expression, working as a rapidly induced response to pathogens [48]. Furthermore, arthropod venom is also a vast source of AMPs, and it has been suggested that the presence of these biomolecules in venom works both in protecting the venom gland against microorganisms and in assisting the action of other toxins [49,50]. About 3000 antimicrobial peptides were described and isolated from six kingdoms (bacteria, archaea, protists, fungi, plants, and from animals) in recent years [51–54]. Antibacterial, antifungal, and antiparasitic peptides derived from these natural sequences have showed broad-spectrum and enhanced activity against target microorganisms [55–57].

Despite the vast diversity of sequences and sources of AMPs, they can be classified, according to structural features, into three main groups—α-Helical, β-sheet, and extended/flexible peptides [58–60]. The α-helical is the most common AMP structure, abundantly found in the extracellular fluids of insects, frogs, mammals, and other vertebrates. These molecules are free of cysteine residues and usually unstructured in aqueous solution but adopt the helical conformation upon contact with membranes [60,61]. β-sheet peptides are a diverse group of molecules, containing six to eight cysteine residues, responsible for formation of two or more disulfide bonds that will stabilize the β-sheet structure. They also present a well-defined number of β-strands, amphipathically organized, with distinguishable hydrophobic and hydrophilic surfaces [62–64]. The last subgroup of AMPs includes peptides that are linear without cysteine residues and possesses a unique extended coil structure. These AMPs have been less characterized, but they contain a high proportion of proline, arginine, tryptophan, glycine, and histidine [63,65–67].

Currently, over 10 AMPs have entered clinical trials or started the pre-clinical development stages [68,69]. The natural lipopeptide antibiotic approved by the Food and Drug Administration in 2003, named Daptomycin, and the glycopeptide Vancomycin are some examples of AMPs routinely used to treat drug-resistant Gram-positive bacteria. They are labeled "last resort" antibiotics, used only when clinical and commonly used drugs are not sufficient to stop the infection [70–73]. Additional efforts are necessary to extend these findings in the path to drug development and to prospect further the antiparasitic potential of AMPs from animal venoms.

3. Differences between Plasma Membranes of Protozoan and Mammalian Cells

The plasma membrane of mammalian cells contains over one hundred different lipids, carrying little net charge and possessing an even lower outer membrane charge, mainly because of the most common non-polar lipid cholesterol and the four major phospholipids present in this structure: zwitterionic phospholipids enriched with phosphatidylcholine and sphingomyelin, phosphatidylethanolamine, and phosphatidylserine [74–77]. These phospholipids are distributed irregularly between the inner and outer membrane bilayers. Negatively charged lipids are mostly confined to the inner leaflet of the mammalian cytoplasmatic membrane, and the charges are not exposed, which could explain why AMPs do not target mammalian cells. Added to this, possible electrostatic interaction between AMPs and mammalian membrane cells is not stable and, if it happens, it will not affect the integrity of the lipidic bilayer [62,76,78,79].

On the other hand, the surface of the protozoan membrane is very conserved among individuals of this group, including the presence of glycosylphosphatidylinositol (GPI)-anchored glycoproteins, a covering that surrounds the cell membranes and forms the glycocalyx, a boundary between the parasite and the external environment, which also helps to form a negative net charge membrane. The glycocalyx mediates cell attachment, protects against harmful molecular and cellular agents, like AMPs, preventing their action on the membrane and/or affecting other vital functions [80,81].

In *Leishmania*, some free GPIs are also phosphoglycosylated to form lipophosphoglycan, the most common surface glycoconjugate of promastigote forms and a highly anionic GPI anchored component that, together with ergosterol, constitutes the principal molecules responsible for the negatively charged membrane of this parasite. Enzymes such as the metalloprotease Gp63 decrease the charge of the membrane, displaying a protective effect against AMPs through peptide cleavage, and are found in all developmental forms of the parasite, especially the promastigote form [82–87]. The toxicity of bombinin H2 and H4 peptides when tested against *Leishmania* promastigotes was considerably higher than treated amastigotes. These contrasting results are probably connected with the differences in glycocalyx complexity of these two different developmental forms. Intracellular amastigotes present an elementary organization, where glycocalyx is almost nonexistent, surrounded only by an endocytic vacuole of the phagocyte cell [70,88–91].

The glycocalyx surface of *T. cruzi* is mostly covered by mucin-like glycoproteins attached by GPI-anchored proteins. Free GPIs aggregate to form a densely filled glycocalyx beneath the mucin cover. The trans-sialidase family of glycoproteins is another molecule found in the cell surface of *T. cruzi*, playing a pivotal role in escaping from host immune surveillance [84,92–95].

T. brucei membrane surface coats are composed mainly of the variant surface glycoproteins (VSG) and are anchored to the outer membrane by a GPI-anchor [84]. *T. brucei* is an extracellular parasite in all developmental forms; consequently, these surface molecules are not used in cell attachment [96], but the VSG layer acts as a molecular sieve for particles over 20 kDa [97], besides protecting it from host complement via the alternative pathway. The parasite avoids the immune system thanks to its ability to express different VSGs and replaces them periodically, a phenomenon known as antigenic variation, allowing that *T. brucei* trypomastigotes persist for long periods in the human bloodstream [98,99].

During the intracellular life stage, *P. falciparum*–infected red blood cells (PfRBC) diverge from healthy red blood cells (RBC), mainly by an increase in phosphatidylinositol and phosphatidic acid and a decrease in sphingomyelin in the outer membrane [100]. These changes in RBC glycocalyx seem to be related to an electrostatic change in the outer membrane of PfRBC, explaining in part why cationic AMPs preferentially interact with cationic PfRBC glycocalyx and barely affect healthy RBC [101,102].

Tachyzoites is the motile, fast-growing, and intracellular stage of *T. gondii*. During this developmental form, it expresses a huge amount of GPI and free GPI in its glycocalyx. The free GPI has a glucose α1-4GalNAcβ1-4 disaccharide side chain, and when released from the parasite, generates a high immune response, activating macrophages and inducing the production of IgM antibody by the human host [103,104].

4. Mode of Action of Antiprotozoal AMPs

Since protozoan membranes are composed basically of negatively charged lipids and AMPs are cationic and amphipathic, electrostatic interactions between membrane and peptide must be related in the disruption mechanism of the surface-membranes. Conventional AMPs most likely target the cytoplasmic membrane, acting through permeabilization of the plasma membrane, disorganizing the electrochemical gradient, and consequently disrupting the cellular homeostasis of parasite cells [83]. Researchers believed that membrane targeting was AMPs' only mode of action, but the mechanisms of action of these biotoxins have been considerably studied since their discovery [63]. Although investigations focus mainly on bacteria and fungi, targets and effects of AMPs against protozoa were elucidated, especially in *Leishmania* and trypanosomatidae parasites [61,70,105].

The mode of action of AMPs can be divided into two major groups—direct microbial action in protozoan parasites (direct killing) and immune modulation of the host. In turn, direct action can be subdivided into AMPs targeting membrane and internal targets (Figure 1) [61,63,70,83,106,107].

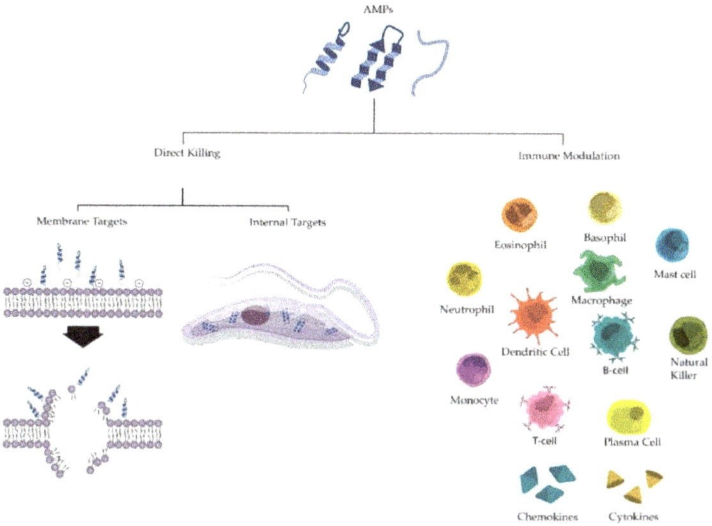

Figure 1. Mode of action of antiprotozoal AMPs. (**left**): Direct microbial action and possible membrane/internal targets of AMPs. (**right**): Modulation caused by AMPs in different types of cells, molecules and processes in mammals' immune system.

4.1. Direct Killing

In the classical models of targeting membrane, the AMPs lying on the membrane must reach a critical concentration, capable of triggering the mechanism of membrane disarrangement. The interaction between the AMP and the parasite membrane does not involve receptor-specific interaction in most cases [108]. AMPs can have one or multiple microbial targets simultaneously, presenting a broad range of action against bacteria, viruses, parasites, and also anticancer activity [109]. Moreover, AMPs can show toxicity against different life cycles of the protozoa and sometimes even divergent mode of action for distinct developmental forms of the same organism [61].

Several models were suggested to explain the process induced by AMPs targeting membrane. The classical models of membrane disruption include the carpet model (detergent-like), the barrel-stave and the toroidal pore [70,83,110]. The carpet model proposes that electrostatic interactions cause peptide coating on the surface of the membrane and formation of a carpet structure, changing the fluidity and properties of the membrane, which will destabilize the bilayer through solubilization into micellar structures [108,111]. In the barrel-stave model, peptides self-aggregate and spontaneously insert themselves into the membrane, forming different sized pores, which grow in diameters according to the addition of new peptides [108,112]. The toroidal pore pattern shares common features with the barrel-stave, forming a membrane pore, but in this mechanism, peptides interact with the membrane, and transient pores are formed with peptides and lipids alternated in the arrangement. AMPs have been shown to translocate through the open pores, suggesting that this mechanism may be associated with potential intracellular targets [108,113]. Other modes of action models that try to describe targeting membrane were suggested, like molecular electroporation [110], sinking-raft model [114], Shai-Huang-Matsazuki model [115], the interfacial activity model [115], targeting of oxidized phospholipids [116], and anion carrier [117].

Several internal targets were described for different parasiticidal AMPs, aiming at key cellular molecules and processes including DNA, RNA, and protein synthesis [118–122], protein degradation by proteasome [123], lysosomal bilayer [78], disrupting key enzymatic activities [124], organelles related with calcium storage (acidocalcisomes, glycosomes and/or endoplasmic reticulum) [125–127], and mitochondria (Figure 2) [79,128].

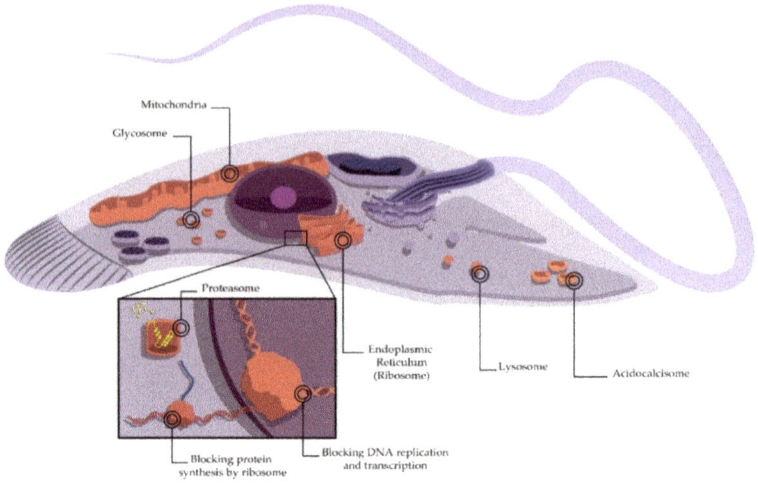

Figure 2. Schematic overview of a protozoan cell with various internal targets (highlighted in red) of AMPs.

4.2. Immune Modulatory Effects

Several AMPs also are able to modulate the host immune system, displaying specificity toward a variety of immune responses: activation, chemotaxis, and differentiation of leukocytes, macrophage activation, degranulation of mast cells, changes in dendritic cell and adaptive immune responses, angiogenesis, cell proliferation, suppressing lactic acid formation, wound healing, controlling reactive oxygen, and nitrogen compounds and repressing inflammation through down-regulation of proinflammatory chemokines and pathogen antigens [107,129–139]. Generally, studies involving immune modulation of mammals by AMPs are done with bacteria. However, in view of some similarities in immune system responses against microorganisms, mammals' immune modulation against protozoan parasites may present great similarities or in some cases even be identical to the bacterial model [140].

Most AMPs act through upregulation and activation of human immune system; however some AMPs work in a totally opposite way, inhibiting the inflammatory response through suppression of pro-inflammatory cytokines [132,140,141]. Innate defense regulators (IDR) are synthetic versions of natural AMPs, like IDR-1018. These peptides could be potential new drugs for treatment of severe malaria, since they decrease the harmful neural inflammation caused by *Plasmodium* infection, which is related to malaria patients' mortality [132,141]. Phospholipase A2 from *Bothrops marajoensis* and *Apis mellifera* venom has shown antiparasiticial and immunomodulatory activities on *L. infantum*, *T. cruzi*, *T. brucei*, and *P. falciparum*. Besides that, temporins, magainin 2, and indolicidin can improve the efficiency of these venom enzymes through modulation of hydrolytic activity [137,142–145]. Because of that, some AMPs such as temporin and IDR-1018 may act as adjuvants, improving the effects and acting synergistically with other molecules, including AMPs [146].

5. Protozoonosis

5.1. Chagas Disease

T. cruzi is a parasitic protozoan and the causative agent of American trypanosomiasis, also known as Chagas disease (CD). CD is a vector-borne illness transmitted to animals and people predominantly by blood-sucking bugs (kissing bugs), mediated via infected insect's feces, released during blood meals (Figure 3) [147–149]. The most important insects responsible for transmission of *T. cruzi* are members of *Rhodnius*, *Triatoma*, and *Panstrongylus* genera, which belong to the Triatominae subfamily [150]. Only two drugs are currently used in the clinical treatment of CD—benznidazole and nifurtimox. In spite of the fact that they are highly toxic, and their efficacy profile is far from ideal, both medicaments have been the frontline treatment for *T. cruzi* for nearly 50 years. Although both drugs are classified as essential by the WHO, they are not yet registered in Europe [148,150,151]. The use of benznidazole is approved by the FDA, but the need of high administered doses, the long period of treatment, the high incidence of side effects and the marked adverse reactions are some problems reported in its use. On the other hand, Nifurtimox is not currently FDA-approved [148,152,153]. Alongside this, *T. cruzi* strains resistant to these drugs were reported [154]. Therefore, there is a great need for new and safe parasitic drugs, especially due to the lack of efficiency of the main drugs on the market.

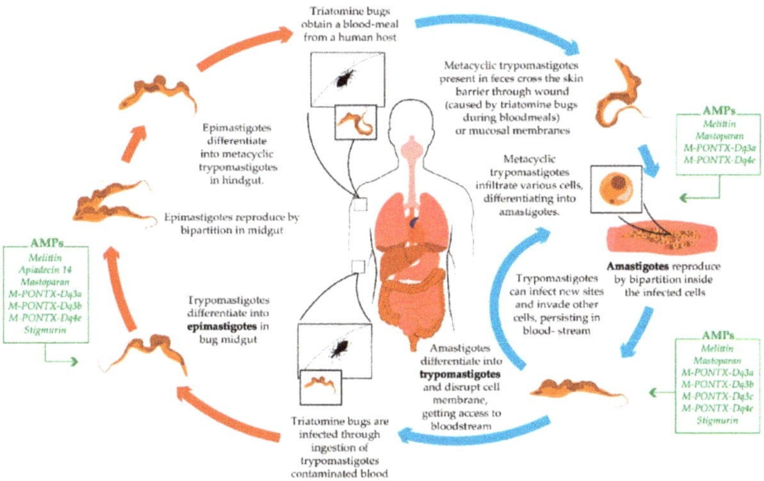

Figure 3. Schematic life cycle of *T. cruzi*. The blue arrows indicate life stages in the definitive host (human). The red arrows indicate life stages in the vector of CD. The green boxes illustrate the AMPs described with activity against each specific developmental form of the parasite.

Anti-Chagas diseaseAMPs

The AMPs that exhibited toxicity and anti-*Trypanosoma cruzi* activity are summarized in Table 1, and the activity of the listed AMPs on specific stages of the life cycles is highlighted in Figure 3.

Melittin is an AMP from the western honeybee, *A. mellifera*, and the most abundant compound found in this insect venom. It is a 26-residue highly hydrophobic peptide, with 2.85 kDa molecular weight, presenting a small hydrophilic C-terminus, due to the presence of lysine and arginine amino acids. These features suggest that the peptide exerts its initial action at the parasitic membrane, and thanks to its amphipathic nature, the α-helical peptide binds to the membrane, causing destabilization. Melittin-treated epimastigote and amastigote cells presented changes in growth, viability and morphology, suggesting a predominantly autophagic death pathway. In addition, melittin exerts a calcium influx and does not disrupt the membrane permeability of *T. cruzi* bloodstream form, possibly involving apoptosis-like cell death, through an electrogenic process in a receptor-independent way. These results show that the same compound can induce different cell death mechanisms. The hemolytic effect of melittin does not make it so attractive to the pharmaceutical industry, but the use of hybrid AMPs, such as the hybrid of cecropin/melittin, substantially lessens this unwanted effect [155–159].

Apidaecin 14 is another AMP isolated from western honeybee venom. This insect toxin is heat-stable, 18 residues long, with 2.1 kDa, belonging to the proline-rich family of apidaecins, and differently from melittin, it is not an α-helical peptide, but a linear peptide with C-terminal amidation. It was bioassayed against *T. cruzi* epimastigotes with an innovative approach. In 2010, Fieck and co-workers used paratransgenesis to control *T. cruzi* in the vector *Rhodnius prolixus*. For this, they heterologously expressed different AMPs, using the symbiont microorganism *Rhodococcus rhodnii*, present in the same niche as the *T. cruzi* parasite: the insect's gut. Apidaecin 14 showed lethality to *T. cruzi* with low toxicity to *R. rhodnii*. Surprisingly, the synergistic treatment of apidaecin with other AMPs (cecropin, magainin 2, or melittin) demonstrated high efficiency with half maximal inhibitory concentration values on the nanomolar scale [160]. The mode of action of apidaecin 14 seems to be related to the interaction and inactivation of the heat shock protein DnaK, an essential chaperone in several cytoplasmic cellular processes, including folding of nascent polypeptide chains, avoiding aggregation of partially folded proteins, remodeling folding pathways, and regulating activity [161,162].

Table 1. AMPs isolated from different venomous arthropods with activity against *T. cruzi*.

Source	AMP	Parasite Stage	Inhibition Activity [a]	Reference
		Insect		
Apis mellifera	Melittin	Epimastigote Trypomastigote Amastigote	IC_{50} = 2.44 μg/mL IC_{50} = 0.14 μg/mL IC_{50} = 0.22 μg/mL	[155]
A. mellifera	Apiadecin 14	Epimastigote	LD_{100} = 199 μM	[160]
Polybia paulista	Mastoparan	Epimastigote Trypomastigote Amastigote	IC_{50} = 61.4 μM IC_{50} = 5.31 μM [b]	[124]
Dinoponera quadriceps	M-PONTX-Dq3a	Epimastigote Trypomastigote Amastigote	IC_{50} = 4.7 μM IC_{50} = 0.32 μM [b]	[163]
D. quadriceps	M-PONTX-Dq3b	Epimastigote Trypomastigote	IC_{50} = 48.8 μM IC_{50} = 7.4 μM	[163]
D. quadriceps	M-PONTX-Dq3c	Trypomastigote	IC_{50} = 34.8 μM	[163]
D. quadriceps	M-PONTX-Dq4e	Epimastigote Trypomastigote Amastigote	IC_{50} = 23.5 μM IC_{50} = 4.7 μM [b]	[163]
		Scorpion		
Tityus stigmurus	Stigmurin	Epimastigote Trypomastigote	GI = 90% (25μM) GI = 100% (25μM)	[164]
		Spider		
Cupiennius salei	Cupiennin 1a	Amastigote	IC_{50} = 0.92 μM	[165]

IC_{50}: Half maximal inhibitory concentration. LD_{100}: Absolute lethal dose. GI: growth inhibition. [a] 24 h of treatment. [b] Exhibited inhibition, but IC_{50} was not calculated.

Mastoparan is 14 amino acids in length and amidated in the C-terminus, isolated from *Polybia paulista* wasp venom with a molecular weight of 1.66k Da. The peptide is rich in hydrophobic and basic residues, which enable the formation of the secondary α-helical structure of the peptide. Unlike other AMPs, mastoparan exerts its toxicity by a unique mechanism. It inhibits glyceraldehyde-3-phosphate dehydrogenase from *T. cruzi* (TcGAPDH), a key enzyme in the glycolytic pathway. In addition, this peptide is related to ROS induction and mitochondrial disruption in all *T. cruzi* morphological forms, leading the cells to energy collapse [124].

Four different biotoxins active against *T. cruzi* were isolated from the venom of the New World giant ant *D. quadriceps*: M-PONTX-Dq3a, M-PONTX-Dq3b, M-PONTX-Dq3c, and M-PONTX-Dq4e. M-PONTX-Dq3b (13-residue peptide) and M-PONTX-Dq3c (11-residue peptide) are fragments of

M-PONTX-Dq3a (23-residue peptide), with molecular weights of 1.5 kDa, 1.32 kDa, and 2.56 kDa, respectively. M-PONTX-Dq4e is the longest dinoponeratoxin, with 30 amino acids in length and 3.35 kDa. The four toxins present amidation at their C-terminus by post-translation modifications and the α-helical secondary structure. Among these, M-PONTX-Dq3a represents the most promising peptide from *D. quadriceps*, since it inhibits all *T. cruzi* developmental forms, including intracellular amastigotes. M-PONTX-Dq3a toxin has a high molecular weight and net charge, when compared to other dinoponeratoxins. This could be correlated with the high susceptibility of trypomastigote against this peptide, since this developmental form shows overexpression of sialic acid and mucin glycoproteins, negatively charged components of the parasitic plasmatic membrane. Against epimastigotes, M-PONTX-Dq3a showed inhibition rates 45 times lower than benznidazole, the first-line treatment for CD. Biochemical and morphological evidences suggest necrosis as the major death pathway of this AMP. These results against the developmental forms of *T. cruzi* are in agreement with the WHO guidelines for prospection of new drugs [163,166].

The α-helical peptide stigmurin, isolated from venom of the scorpion *T. stigmurus*, showed high antiparasitic activity on trypomastigote and epimastigote forms. This cationic peptide is formed by 17 amino acid residues and has 1.79 kDa molecular weight, with low hemolytic activity. Total growth inhibition of trypomastigote was achieved with a concentration of 25 μM of the toxin. Bioassays against epimastigotes with the same peptide concentration were able to inhibit 90% of parasite growth. Interestingly, rational designed peptides (StigA6, StigA16, StigA25, and StigA31) with higher net charge, increase in α-helix percentage and hydrophobic moment were able to inhibit the parasites with lower concentrations, when compared to native stigmurin. The analog peptides StigA6 and StigA16 presented 100% growth inhibition with a tenfold smaller dose, showing that rational design could be a promising tool to obtain effective new drugs. Stigmurin and the analogue peptides probably cause parasite death through interaction and destabilization of the cell membrane [164,167].

5.2. Human African Trypanosomiasis

T. brucei is a microscopic parasite and the disease-causing agent of Human African trypanosomiasis (HAT), also known as sleeping sickness, an illness spread via the bite of infected blood-feeding tsetse fly (genus *Glossina*) (Figure 4). Two different forms of the disease are known, depending of the subspecies of the parasite involved—West African trypanosomiasis (Gambian sleeping sickness) caused by *T. brucei gambiense* is responsible for the slow-progressing form. *T. brucei rhodesiense* is, in turn, behind the faster-progressing form, East African trypanosomiasis (Rhodesian sleeping sickness). Each subspecies of *T. brucei* is transmitted by different species or subspecies of *Glossina* [105,148,168]. Gambian sleeping sickness is doubtless the most common and widespread form of HAT, representing 98% of reported cases. In contrast, Rhodesian sleeping sickness is a zoonotic pathogen, affecting humans sporadically and responsible for only 2% of reported cases [168–170].

Sleeping sickness is curable with the right diagnostic approach and treatment but is lethal if untreated. The treatment in most cases needs much effort, mainly because of the logistic difficulties of drug delivery and access by professionals in rural areas for diagnosis and therapy administration.

The selection of therapy depends on both disease stage and the subspecies of the parasite. Currently, there are five first-line drugs routinely used against HAT. Pentamidine and suramin are used to treat first stage of Gambian and Rhodesian sleeping sickness, respectively. The second stage of *T. brucei gambiense* is treated with a combination of nifurtimox-eflornithine, which presents high trypanocidal efficiency, but the need for daily intravenous infusion and multiple administrations make this therapy regime difficult. For more than 70 years, the only treatment against East HAT has been Merlarsoprol, an arsenic-derived drug that presents many adverse reactions and highly toxicity, including encephalopathic reaction with mortality rate of approximately 10% of treated individuals. A new and revolutionary oral treatment, fexinidazole, was developed in 2018, and is able to cure both late and first stages of Gambian sleeping sickness. This pill-based therapy has received a positive scientific opinion from the European Medicines Agency and is already registered in the country with the highest incidence of cases, Congo [105,168,171].

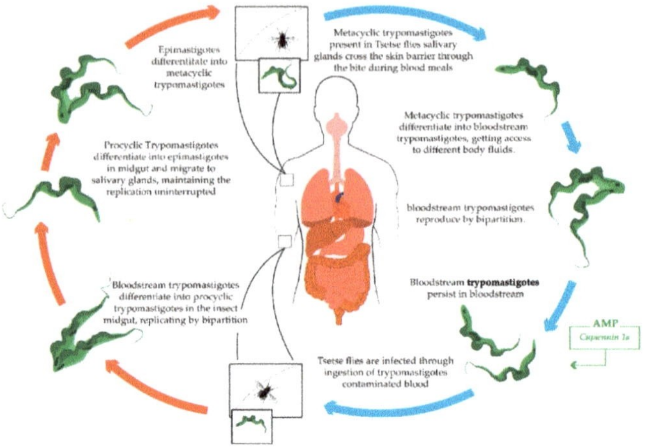

Figure 4. Schematic life cycle of *T. brucei*. The blue arrows indicate life stages in the definitive host (human). The red arrows indicate life stages in the vector of human African trypanosomiasis. The green box illustrates the AMP described with activity against the specific developmental form of the parasite.

Anti-Human African Trypanosomiasis AMPs

The only described AMP isolated from a venomous arthropod and active against *T. brucei* is the α-helical spider toxin Cupiennin 1a, a 35-residue cytolytic peptide isolated from the venom of the tiger wandering spider *Cupiennius salei* (Figure 4). This 3.5 kDa peptide exhibits broad activity against the parasites *T. brucei rhodesiense*, *T. cruzi*, and *P. falciparum*, with growth inhibition values at the nanomolar scale against *T. brucei rhodesiense* bloodstream forms. On the other hand, it also shows high cytolytic activity against negatively charged mammalian cells, mediated especially by sialic acid present in cell membranes, contributing to toxin-membrane interaction [165].

5.3. *Leishmaniasis*

Leishmaniasis is a vector-borne disease that is caused by obligate intracellular protozoan of the *Leishmania* genus [172,173]. Dipterans from the *Phlebotomus* genus are responsible for parasite transmission in the new world, while *Lutzomyia* genus causes transmission in the old world [173,174]. *Leishmania* are a complex group of unicellular parasites that alternately infect insects (intermediate host) and mammals (definitive host). About 70 different animal species are considered natural reservoir hosts of *Leishmania* parasites and more than 20 *Leishmania* species related to human infection [175,176]. There are several clinical presentation forms of leishmaniasis in humans. The three most common forms are cutaneous leishmaniasis (CL), visceral leishmaniasis (VL), and mucocutaneous leishmaniasis (MC). The *Leishmania* parasite, differently from other protozoan parasites, has a simple life cycle with only two digenic forms during the whole life cycle (Figure 5) [177,178].

Leishmanial treatment is conditioned by several factors, comprising type of disease, concomitant pathologies, parasite species and geographic location [173]. A huge number of drugs for the treatment of each leishmaniasis form are available, but pentavalent antimonials (stibogluconate and meglumine antimoniate) have been the first line and most used compounds in the treatment of all leishmaniasis forms for decades [179,180]. Pentavalent antimony administration is done parenterally for 28 days, making monitoring by health professionals necessary. In addition, these medicaments present high toxicity, adverse effects and an increase in parasite drug resistance [181–183]. For CL, other drugs like pentamidine and miltefosine are used, despite the excessive price, high toxicity and possible teratogenic side effects [181,184]. In India, miltefosine was used also to treat VL through oral administration [185], but a long treatment period increases the possibility of developing drug resistance [186]. The use of Amphotericin B has increased worldwide for VL treatment, but it causes significant nephrotoxicity [175,187,188].

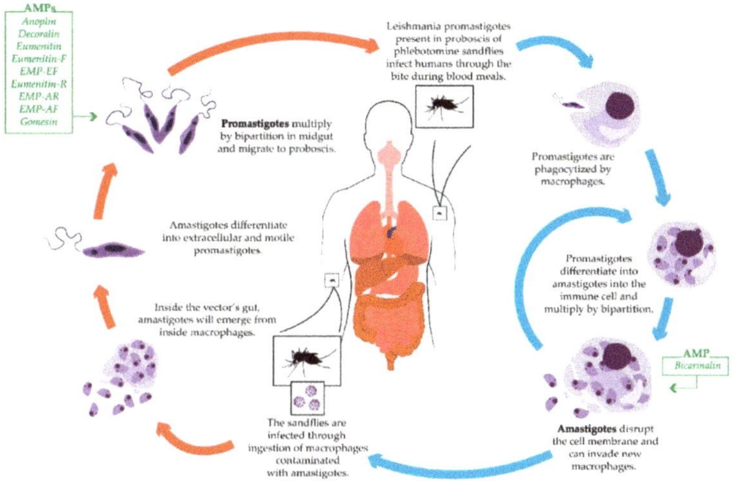

Figure 5. Schematic life cycle of *Leishmania*. The blue arrows indicate life stages in the definitive host (human). The red arrows indicate life stages in the vector of leishmaniasis. The green boxes illustrate the AMPs described with activity against each specific developmental form of the parasite.

Antileishmanial AMPs

The AMPs that exhibited toxicity and anti-*Leishmania* activity are summarized in Table 2, and the activity of the listed AMPs on specific stages of the life cycles is highlighted in Figure 5.

Gomesin was the first AMP isolated from a spider with toxicity against protozoan parasites. This defensin-type peptide was isolated from *Acanthoscurria gomesiana* hemocytes, possessing 18 amino acid residues and 2.27 kDa with four cysteine residues that form two internal disulfide bridges, contributing to stability and also responsible for the β-sheet structure of the peptide. Gomesin causes in vitro inhibition growth of *L. amazonensis* and *L. major* promastigotes at micromolar concentrations, which could be related to the high presence of anionic phospholipids and ergosterol in the plasma membrane of these parasites, causing a more negative net charge when compared with mammalian cells. This will allow the peptide to interact with the membrane, causing rupture and loss of cellular homeostasis [189,190].

Solitary wasp venoms can be a rich source of linear cationic α-helical peptides, killing parasites through membrane targeting. Decoralin (1.25 kDa), isolated from the venom of the solitary eumenine wasp *Oreumene decorates*, together with anoplin (1.15 kDa) from *Anoplius samariensis*, were bioassayed against *L. major* promastigotes. These peptides present some structural similarity, although decoralin has a linear chain length of 11 amino acid residues, one more residue than anoplin. Both peptides exhibited inhibition of promastigotes, despite a slightly high peptide concentration, but their hemolytic effect was quite low. The native peptide decoralin was synthesized with a C-terminal amidation (decoralin-NH_2), and the analogous peptide demonstrated a sixfold reduction in the peptide concentration to exert the same growth inhibition as native decoralin, with no changes in hemolysis, possibly because C-terminal amidation stabilizes the α-helical conformation. All these features make the use of these toxins advantageous for chemical structure modifications and the improvement of biological properties [191]. A similar study carried out by Rangel and co-workers isolated four new linear cationic α-helical insect toxins from another two species of solitary wasps: two mastoparan peptides were isolated from *Eumenes rubrofemoratus*, the toxins eumenitin-R and eumenine mastoparan-ER (EMP-ER), and other two from *E. fraterculus*, eumenitin-F and eumenine mastoparan-EF (EMP-EF). Additionally, other two previously reported peptides were tested against *L. major* promastigotes, eumenitin from *E. rubronotatus* [192], and eumenine mastoparan-AF (EMP-AF) from *Anterhynchium flavomarginatum micado* [193]. All these six peptides showed some physicochemical and biological similarities: antileishmanial activity, short linear length (14 to 15 amino acids long), small molecular weight (1.48 to 1.65 kDa), polycationic features, and α-helical configuration after electrostatic interaction with anionic membrane. Among these peptides, EMP-ER, EMP-EF, EMP-AF present a C-terminal amidation, which may explain why EMP-ER demonstrates greater inhibitory effect against the promastigote form of the parasite [194]. Melittin showed robust inhibitory activity against *L. major* promastigotes, despite also exhibiting toxic effects on human dendritic cells [195]. A hybrid synthetic peptide using part of the melittin sequence and Cecropin A exhibited an enhancement in leishmanicidal activity and a decrease in host immune cell toxicity [196].

Table 2. AMPs isolated from different venomous arthropods with activity against *Leishmania*.

Source	AMP	Activity against	Parasite Stage	Inhibition Activity [a]	Reference
		Insect			
Apis mellifera	Melittin	*L. major* *L. panamensis*	Promastigote	EC_{50} = 74.01 µg/mL EC_{50} ≥ 100 µg /mL	[195]
Anoplius samariensis	Anoplin	*L. major*	Promastigote	IC_{50} ≥ 87 µM	[191]
Oreumenes decoratus	Decoralin	*L. major*	Promastigote	IC_{50} = 72 µM	[191]
Eumenes rubronotatus	Eumenitin	*L. major*	Promastigote	IC_{50} = 35 µM	[191]
Eumenes fraterculus	Eumenitin-F	*L. major*	Promastigote	IC_{50} = 52 µM	[194]
E. fraterculus	Eumenine mastoparan-EF (EMP-EF)	*L. major*	Promastigote	IC_{50} = 40 µM	[194]
E. rubrofemoratus	eumenitin-R	*L. major*	Promastigote	IC_{50} ≥ 62 µM	[194]
E. rubrofemoratus	Eumenine mastoparan-ER (EMP-AR)	*L. major*	Promastigote	IC_{50} = 20 µM	[194]
Anterhynchium flavomarginatum micado	Eumenine mastoparan-AF (EMP-AF)	*L. major*	Promastigote	IC_{50} = 35 µM	[194]
Tetramorium bicarinatum	Bicarinalin	*L. infantum*	Amastigote	IC_{50} = 1.5 µM	[197]
		Spider			
Acanthoscurria gomesiana	Gomesin *	*L. amazonensis* *L. major*	Promastigote	IC_{50} = ~5.0 µM IC_{50} = ~2.5 µM	[189,190]

* Peptides isolated from venomous animals, but not from venom glands. EC_{50}: Half maximal effective concentration. IC_{50}: Half maximal inhibitory concentration. [a] 24 h of treatment.

Bicarinalin is a recently characterized α-helical peptide and the first isolated from ants' venom (*Tetramorium bicarinatum*) with trypanocidal activity. This biotoxin is a cystein-free polycationic peptide, with amidated C-terminal, 20 residues in length and 2.21 kDa, presenting very low hemolytic activity against human erythrocytes. Bicarinalin showed a broad spectrum of antimicrobial activities, a relatively long half-life stability for blood proteases (about 15 h) and slight cytotoxicity on human lymphocytes; in vitro bioassays against *L. infantum* intracellular amastigotes indicated parasiticidal activity at low concentrations. Thus, the membrane targeting bicarinalin shows signs of being a possible candidate for the development of a new leishmanicidal drug [197].

Promising studies showed the crude venom of *Tityus discrepans*, a medically important Venezuelan scorpion, inhibited the growth of *L. mexicana*, *L. braziliensis*, and *L. chagasi* promastigote forms, leading to drastic morphological alterations and consequently parasite death [198]. A preliminary study with crude venom of *D. quadriceps* giant ant displayed inhibition of promastigote forms of *L. amazonensis*. Flow cytometry and confocal microscopy analyses suggested involvement of necrotic and apoptotic pathways [199]. Interestingly, hybrid AMPs present notable in vitro antileishmanial activity with enhanced activity on the parental peptides and less hemolytic effects, in both life forms of *Leishmania*, intracellular amastigotes and extracellular promastigotes, besides a broad spectrum against different varieties of *Leishmania* [159,196,200].

5.4. Malaria

There are five possible protozoa that may be related to malaria, all belonging to the *Plasmodium* genus: *P. vivax*, *P. falciparum*, *P. malariae*, *P. ovale*, and *P. knowlesi* [201]. Transmission occurs through the bite of female mosquitoes of the genus *Anopheles* carrying the protozoan (Figure 6) [202]. The chosen treatment depends on the type of *Plasmodium*, the severity of the disease and the locality in which the disease was acquired [148]. This identification is important to determine the resistance probability of the organism to a particular drug. Among the antimalarial drugs used, the first-line drugs are chloroquine, atovaquone-lumefantrine (Malarone), artemether-lumefantrine (Coartem), doxycycline, primaquine, and tafenoquine [203–205].

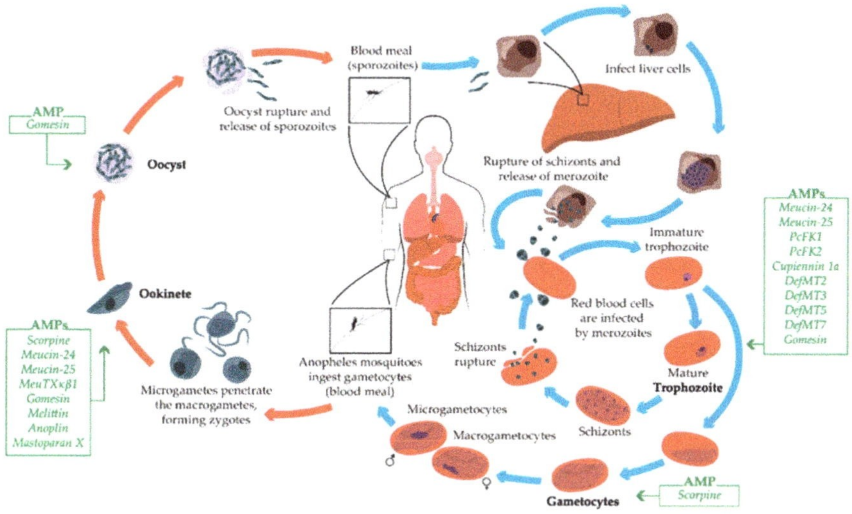

Figure 6. Schematic life cycle of *Plasmodium*. The blue arrows indicate life stages in the definitive host (human). The red arrows indicate life stages in the vector of malaria. The green boxes illustrate the AMPs described with activity against each specific developmental form of the parasite.

Antimalarial AMPs

The AMPs that exhibited toxicity and anti-malaria activity are summarized in Table 3, and the activity of the listed AMPs on specific stages of the life cycles is highlighted in Figure 6.

Scorpine, an AMP from *Pandinus imperator* scorpion venom, has 75 amino acids in length, a molecular mass of 8.3 kDa and three disulfide bridges, and it presents anti-bacterial and anti-malarial activities. The results showed that the peptide was active in the sexual stages of the parasite. Scorpine inhibited ookinete and gamete development. When compared with shiva-3, a synthetic analog of cecropin peptide with antiparasitic activity, scorpine exhibited more potent toxicity in gametes and ookinetes than shiva-3 [206].

Meucin-24 and Meucin-25 are *Mesobuthus eupeus* scorpion venom AMPs, discovered through investigation of the cDNA venom gland library. Meucin-24 has 24 amino acids, 2.75 kDa and a high sequence identity with antimicrobial and K^+-channel blocker toxins, also possessing N-terminus homology with melittin. Meucin-25 has 25 amino acids, 3.1 kDa, but no sequence identity with antimicrobial toxins described. They exhibited activity against *P. berghei*, *P. falciparum*, and also dipteran cells, making them potentially attractive for use with double action as a disease vector control tool and also as an antimalarial molecule. In water, meucin-24 showed a random coil conformation and meucin-25 a β-sheet structure. In TFE, both showed an α-helical formation [207].

MeuTXKβ1, a *Mesobuthus eupeus* venom toxin, did not show an effect on Na_V and K_V channels tested at concentration of 1 μM, and presented low antibacterial action, with a lethal concentration of 21 μM. However, activity against *P. berghei* development was stronger than the activity presented by other synthetic peptides, like shiva-3 [208]. In water, meuTXKβ1 showed 17% of α-Helix and 21% of β-sheet conformation and, in 50% of TFE, it showed 55% of α-Helix and 17% of β-sheets [209].

Psalmopeotoxin I and psalmopeotoxin II are AMPs isolated from *Psalmopoeus cambridgei*, the Trinidad chevron tarantula, also known as *Psalmopoeus cambridgei Falciparum* killer (PcFK). Both psalmopeotoxin I (PcFK1) and psalmopeotoxin II (PcFK2) peptides present three disulfide bridges, differing in the number and composition of amino acids in their structure. PcFK1 is a 33-residue peptide with 3.63 kDA, while PcFK2 is shorter, with a length of 28 amino acids and 2.96 kDa [210].

Gomesin showed activity against some bacteria and fungi and recently was compared to another five peptides with the same structure, in order to comprise the interconnection between the structural properties and the antimicrobial activity, deducing that high amphipathicity and low hydrophobicity of AMPs are related to more toxicity activity [211]. Moreira and co-workers tested gomesin against *P. berghei* and *P. falciparum*, besides analyzing the effect on the mosquito, aiming for antimalarial activity on the vector. The results showed an inhibition of gamete development and also of ookinete formation in *P. berghei*. In addition, the spider peptide displayed inhibition against the intraerythrocytic stage of *P. falciparum*. Gomesin manifested activity against oocysts in vivo for both parasite species, in the vector *A. stephensi*, and did not affect the mosquito's development [212].

Table 3. AMPs isolated from different venomous arthropods with activity against *Plasmodium*.

Source	AMP	Activity against	Parasite Stage	Inhibition Activity	Reference
		Insect			
Apis mellifera	Melittin	*P. berghei* *P. falciparum*	Ookinete	GI = 100% (50 μM) GI = 60% (50 μM)	[213]
Anoplius samariensis	Anoplin	*P. berghei*	Ookinete	GI = 100% (100 μM)	[213]
Vespula lewisii	Mastoparan X	*P. berghei* *P. falciparum*	Ookinete	GI = 100% (100 μM)	[213]
		Scorpion			
Pandinus imperator	Scorpine	*P. berghei*	Gametocyte Ookinete	ED_{50} = 10 μM ED_{50} = 0.7 μM	[206]
Mesobuthus eupeus	Meucin-24	*P. berghei* *P. falciparum*	Ookinete Trophozoite	GI = 40% (20 μM) GI = 100% (10 μM)	[207]
M. eupeus	Meucin-25	*P. berghei* *P. falciparum*	Ookinete Trophozoite	GI = 50% (20 μM) GI = 100% (10 μM)	[207]
M. eupeus	MeuTXKβ1	*P. berghei*	Ookinete	GI = 89–98.8% (10-20 μM)	[209]
		Spider			
Psalmopoeus cambridgei	Psalmopeotoxin I (PcFK1)	*P. falciparum*	Trophozoite	$IC_{50}{}^{c}$ = 1.59 μM	[210]
P. cambridgei	Psalmopeotoxin II (PcFK2)	*P. falciparum*	Trophozoite	IC_{50} = 1.15 μM	[210]
Acanthoscurria gomesiana	Gomesin *	*P. berghei* *P. falciparum*	Trophozoite Ookinete Oocysts	IC_{50} = 46.8 μM GI = 100% (50 μM) GI = 86% (100 μM)	[212]
A. gomesiana	Gomesin *	*P. falciparum*	Oocysts	GI = 100% (100 μM)	[212]
Cupiennius salei	Cupiennin 1a	*P. falciparum*	Trophozoite	IC_{50} = 0.032 μM	[165]
		Tick			
Ixodes ricinus	DefMT2 *	*P. falciparum*	Trophozoite	GI = 70% (50 μM)	[214]
I. ricinus	DefMT3 *	*P. falciparum*	Trophozoite	GI = 50% (50 μM)	[214]
I. ricinus	DefMT5 *	*P. falciparum*	Trophozoite	GI = 100% (50 μM)	[214]
I. ricinus	DefMT7 *	*P. falciparum*	Trophozoite	GI = 30% (50 μM)	[214]

* Peptides isolated from venomous animals, but not from venom glands. GI: growth inhibition. ED_{50}: Median effective dose. IC_{50}: Half maximal inhibitory concentration.

Cupiennin 1a displayed a non-stereospecific cytolytic activity against cancer cells, human blood, bacteria, trypanosomes and *Plasmodium*. This toxin was bioassayed against *P. falciparum* showing very low IC_{50} values, but a high hemolytic activity [165].

I. ricinus is a European tick that encodes antimicrobial peptides with action on pathogens such as bacteria and fungi. Cabezas-Cruz and co-workers studied the defensin peptides DefMT2, DefMT3, DefMT5, DefMT6 and DefMT7 against the malaria parasite. The results showed that the most effective peptide against *P. falciparum* was DefMT5. In contrast, DefMT6 did not show activity against *P. falciparum*, despite the similarity of these peptides. Regarding antibacterial and antifungal actions, DefMT3, DefMT5, and DefMT6 showed activity against both microorganisms, but DefMT2 and DefMT7 were not able to inhibit these pathogens [214]. All peptides have α-helix (N-terminus) and antiparallel β strand (C-terminus). Only DefMT7 does not present a β strand at the C-terminus [215].

Carter and co-workers tested several Hymenopteran AMPs that could show toxic effects on *Plasmodium* development (*P. berghei* and *P. falciparium*), namely melittin, anoplin, and mastoparan X isolated from *A. mellifera* [216], *A. samariensis* [217], and *V. lewisii* [218], respectively. Synergistic effects were also observed in treatments with two different peptides. Higher inhibition effect on the development of *Plasmodium* was observed when instead of using a single peptide (50 μM), two different peptides were administered together (25 μM each). For example, anoplin (25 μM) and mastoparan X (25 μM) showed a better inhibition effect than only mastoparan X (50 μM) [213].

5.5. Toxoplasmosis

T. gondii is a protozoan that causes toxoplasmosis [219]. More than 40 million people worldwide have the parasite, although few have symptoms. Therefore, this disease is considered one of the neglected parasite infections (Figure 7) [148]. A few drugs for the treatment of toxoplasmosis are available, such as pyrimethamine and sulfadiazine [220], but studies using AMPs in this area are promising. So far, anti-*Toxoplasma* peptides were isolated from spider and tick, namely Lycosin-I [221] and Longicin [222], respectively.

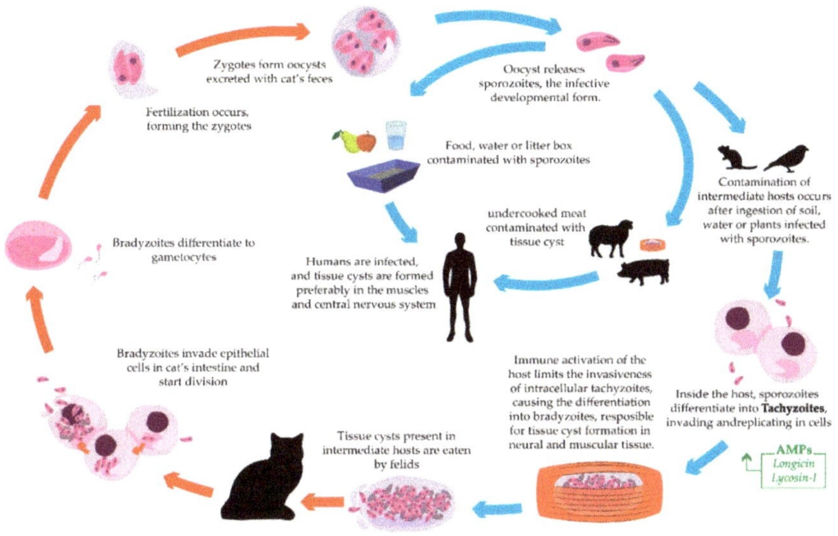

Figure 7. Schematic life cycle of *T. gondii*. The blue arrows indicate life stages in the intermediate hosts (exo-enteric cycle). The red arrows indicate life stages in the definitive host of toxoplasmosis (enteric cycle). The green box illustrates the AMPs described with activity against the specific developmental form of the parasite.

Anti-*Toxoplasma* AMPs

The AMPs that exhibited toxicity and anti-toxoplasmosis activity are summarized in Table 4, and the activity of the listed AMPs on specific stages of the life cycles are highlighted in Figure 7.

Table 4. AMPs isolated from different venomous arthropods with activity against *T. gondii.*

Source	AMP	Activity Against	Parasite Stage	Inhibition Activity [a]	Reference
		Spider			
Lycosa singoriensis	Lycosin-I	*T. gondii*	Tachyzoite	IC_{50} [b] = 28 μM IC_{50} [c] = 10.08 μM	[221]
		Tick			
Haemaphysalis longicornis	Longicin *	*T. gondii*	Tachyzoite	- [d]	[222]

* Peptides isolated from venomous animals, but not from venom glands. [a] 24 h of treatment. [b] Inhibitory effects on proliferation of intracellular tachyzoites. [c] Inhibitory effects on invasion of parasite into host cells. [d] Exhibited inhibition, but IC_{50} was not calculated.

Lycosin-I, from *L. singoriensis*, is a linear α-helical peptide with 24 amino acids and molecular weight of 2.89 kDa that inhibited *T. gondii* proliferation and invasion. The peptide was able to cause morphological changes in the parasite, causing damage to organelles, and vacuolization, signs of apoptosis-like death, but further studies are necessary to elucidate the death pathway caused by this spider toxin [221]. Longicin is a *H. longicornis* defensin peptide with β-sheet at the C terminus [223] that showed antibacterial and antiparasitic activities. The peptide precursor is formed by a 74-amino acids signal peptide, and the mature toxin is 52 residues in length, with 5.82 kDa. Tanaka and co-workers studied the peptide's effect against *T. gondii* during the tachyzoite stage. The results showed morphological cell changes in cytoplasm and nuclei, consequently growth inhibition and parasite death, but the death pathway related to this peptide is still unclear [222].

6. Future Prospects

Several studies have been developed over the years, involving a wide variety of venomous animal AMPs tested against pathogenic protozoa, resulting in a bank with over 100 active molecules and potential agents for the development of novel peptide-based antiprotozoal chemotherapies [54]. Nevertheless, the need for new antiparasitic drugs is still urgent, making the prospection of new sources of bioactive molecules very attractive. Among the venomous arthropods, the centipedes (Chilopoda) comprise over 3000 species and are amongst the most remarkable sources of venom peptides. Several studies showed a significant antibacterial activity with over 30 AMPs isolated from these venomous animals; they are therefore a possible source of new compounds against protozoonosis [224,225].

Bioengineering tools to circumvent cytotoxicity and hemolysis problems, as well to enhance parasiticidal activity, were explored to overcome the drawbacks of therapeutic natural peptides. Structural analogs of natural AMPs and hybrid peptide formulations performed well in improving biological activity, including the analogs of stigmurin, stigA6, and stigA16, or CM11 and Oct-CA(1–7)M(2–9), melittin/cecropin A hybrids [164,167,196]. Moreover, C-terminal amidation of decoralin significantly decreased the values of IC_{50} when compared with the native peptide [191]. In order to make the net charge of the peptide more negative, amino acid substitutions could be another strategy to improve the biological activity. AMPs also demonstrated the potential for technological innovation due to synergistic interactions exhibited when used in combination with conventional antibiotics and other AMPs, drastically decreasing antimicrobial resistance [160,226].

The use of synthetic AMPs is still limited by the high production price when compared to conventional organic molecule drugs, and isolation from natural sources is not a viable solution. Studies have been carried out in the development of recombinant DNA methods to successfully synthesize and purify AMPs for cost-effective therapeutic application, but the commercial viability of these methods has yet to be evaluated [227–229]. In addition, since ribosome-synthesized AMPs are expressed by unique genes, they can be considered for use in gene therapy for introduction directly into infected tissue [61], possibly promoting a reduction in the cost associated with large-scale production and purification of AMPs. Application of new computational and experimental strategies aimed at downsizing, stabilization and other druggability issues are likely to reduce prices in the near future.

Nevertheless, it is known that a long test period is required before AMPs are available on the pharmaceutical market, as some adverse effects have yet to be overcome, such as hemolytic activity and cytotoxicity. Until now, no AMPs from venomous arthropods have become available for the treatment of parasitic diseases, but despite all the challenges involved in making AMPs a real treatment for protozoan diseases, at least six AMPs are currently undergoing clinical development in various therapeutic areas [63]. Pexiganan, the synthetic magainin analog, has reached phase III clinical trials. This arginine-rich variant peptide is capable of inducing apoptosis in *Leishmania* [230–232]. Clinical assays of the synthetic cecropin/melittin hybrid Oct-CA(1–7)M(2–9) were performed against naturally acquired leishmaniasis in dogs. The effectiveness of the peptide was confirmed with the cure of canine leishmaniasis after intravenous injection therapy, without observing side effects, even after six months of treatment [200].

7. Conclusions

Due to poor sanitation, difficult access to safe water, and scarcity of basic care policies, protozoan parasites still cause debilitating human diseases across the globe. In addition, there is a lack of interest from the pharmaceutical market in chemotherapy treatments, lack of research for more effective vaccines, and adverse effects of long-term parenteral treatments that cause toxicity in patients. Recently, the WHO brought to the public a new prevention weapon and hope in the fight against malaria, the first vaccine against *P. falciparum*. RTS, S/AS01 is the name of the vaccine that will provide partial protection against malaria in young children, especially in Africa, through routine immunization programs [233]. However, there is still a need for innovative treatments and tools to treat those who cannot benefit from this immunization. Compared to other drugs developed for chronic and noninfectious diseases, the use of protozoan-directed AMPs is still in its initial phase, although it indicates attractive pharmaceutical action to combat parasitic diseases [234]. Although their application is taking place very gradually, the new discoveries and research into medicinal peptides are proving to be a reality for the treatment of protozoonosis. It is hoped that this compilation will develop prospects for new strategies and paradigms in the application of AMPs, and AMP-based drugs should become a reality in upcoming years.

Author Contributions: All authors listed have made a substantial, direct and intellectual contribution to the work, and approved it for publication.

Funding: This study was supported by CNPq (407625/2013-5).

Acknowledgments: This work was supported by Conselho Nacional de Desenvolvimento Científico e Tecnológico—CNPq (407625/2013-5). The authors thank the Programa de Pós-graduação em Biologia Animal from the University of Brasilia, and Coordenação de Aperfeiçoamento de Pessoal de Nível Superior (CAPES-PROAP) for supporting this publication. LFSM and EFS received scholarships from CNPq.

Conflicts of Interest: The authors declare that there is no conflict of interest.

References

1. Junior, V.H.; De Amorim, P.C.H.; Junior, W.T.H.; Cardoso, J.L.C. Venomous and poisonous arthropods: Identification, clinical manifestations of envenomation, and treatments used in human injuries. *Rev. Soc. Bras. Med. Trop.* **2015**, *48*, 650–657. [CrossRef] [PubMed]
2. Giribet, G.; Edgecombe, G.D. Reevaluating the arthropod tree of life. *Annu. Rev. Èntomol.* **2012**, *57*, 167–186. [CrossRef] [PubMed]
3. Schwartz, E.F.; Mourão, C.B.F.; Moreira, K.G.; Camargos, T.S.; Mortari, M.R. Arthropod venoms: A vast arsenal of insecticidal neuropeptides. *Biopolymers* **2012**, *98*, 385–405. [CrossRef] [PubMed]
4. Daly, N.L.; Wilson, D. Structural diversity of arthropod venom toxins. *Toxicon* **2018**, *152*, 46–56. [CrossRef] [PubMed]

5. Zhang, Z.-Q. Animal biodiversity: An outline of higher-level classification and survey of taxonomic richness (COVER). *Zootaxa* **2011**, *3148*, 1–2. [CrossRef]
6. Stork, N.E.; Mc Broom, J.; Gely, C.; Hamilton, A.J. New approaches narrow global species estimates for beetles, insects, and terrestrial arthropods. *Proc. Natl. Acad. Sci. USA* **2015**, *112*, 7519–7523. [CrossRef] [PubMed]
7. Eyun, S.-I.; Soh, H.Y.; Posavi, M.; Munro, J.B.; Hughes, D.S.; Murali, S.C.; Qu, J.; Dugan, S.; Lee, S.L.; Chao, H.; et al. Evolutionary History of Chemosensory-Related Gene Families across the Arthropoda. *Mol. Boil. Evol.* **2017**, *34*, 1838–1862. [CrossRef]
8. Cloudsley-Thompson, J.L. Adaptations of Arthropoda to arid environments. *Annu. Rev. Èntomol.* **1975**, *20*, 261–283. [CrossRef]
9. Sømme, L. Adaptations Of Terrestrial Arthropods To The Alpine Environment. *Boil. Rev.* **1989**, *64*, 367–407. [CrossRef]
10. Glenner, H.; Thomsen, P.F.; Hebsgaard, M.B.; Sørensen, M.V.; Willerslev, E. The origin of insects. *Science* **2006**, *314*, 1883–1884. [CrossRef]
11. Kelley, J.L.; Peyton, J.T.; Fiston-Lavier, A.-S.; Teets, N.M.; Yee, M.-C.; Johnston, J.S.; Bustamante, C.D.; Lee, R.E.; Denlinger, D.L. Compact genome of the Antarctic midge is likely an adaptation to an extreme environment. *Nat. Commun.* **2014**, *5*, 4611. [CrossRef] [PubMed]
12. Marcussi, S.; Arantes, E.C.; Soares, A.M. *Escorpiões: Biologia, Envenenamento e Mecanismos de Ação de Suas Toxinas*, 1ª edição; FUNPEC Editora: Ribeirão Preto, SP, Brasil, 2011.
13. Senji Laxme, R.R.; Suranse, V.; Sunagar, K. Arthropod venoms: Biochemistry, ecology and evolution. *Toxicon* **2019**, *158*, 84–103. [CrossRef] [PubMed]
14. Walker, A.A.; Robinson, S.D.; Yeates, D.K.; Jin, J.; Baumann, K.; Dobson, J.; Fry, B.G.; King, G.F. Entomo-venomics: The evolution, biology and biochemistry of insect venoms. *Toxicon* **2018**, *154*, 15–27. [CrossRef] [PubMed]
15. Casewell, N.R.; Wüster, W.; Vonk, F.J.; Harrison, R.A.; Fry, B.G. Complex cocktails: The evolutionary novelty of venoms. *Trends Ecol. Evol.* **2013**, *28*, 219–229. [CrossRef] [PubMed]
16. Suranse, V.; Srikanthan, A.; Sunagar, K. Animal Venoms: Origin, diversity and evolution. In *eLS*; John Wiley & Sons, Ltd.: Chichester, UK, 2018; pp. 1–20.
17. Schmidt, J.O. Biochemistry of Insect Venoms. *Annu. Rev. Entomol.* **1982**, *27*, 339–368. [CrossRef] [PubMed]
18. Beard, R.L. Insect Toxins and Venoms. *Annu. Rev. Entomol.* **1963**, *8*, 1–18. [CrossRef] [PubMed]
19. Herzig, V. Arthropod assassins: Crawling biochemists with diverse toxin pharmacopeias. *Toxicon* **2019**, *158*, 33–37. [CrossRef]
20. Walker, A.A.; Hernández-Vargas, M.J.; Corzo, G.; Fry, B.G.; King, G.F. Giant fish-killing water bug reveals ancient and dynamic venom evolution in Heteroptera. *Cell. Mol. Life Sci.* **2018**, *75*, 3215–3229. [CrossRef]
21. Rong, M.; Yang, S.; Wen, B.; Mo, G.; Kang, D.; Liu, J.; Lin, Z.; Jiang, W.; Li, B.; Du, C.; et al. Peptidomics combined with cDNA library unravel the diversity of centipede venom. *J. Proteom.* **2015**, *114*, 28–37. [CrossRef]
22. Hakim, M.A.; Yang, S.; Lai, R. Centipede Venoms and Their Components: Resources for Potential Therapeutic Applications. *Toxins* **2015**, *7*, 4832–4851. [CrossRef]
23. Amorim, F.G.; Longhim, H.T.; Cologna, C.T.; Degueldre, M.; De Pauw, E.; Quinton, L.; Arantes, E.C. Proteome of fraction from *Tityus serrulatus* venom reveals new enzymes and toxins. *J. Venom. Anim. Toxins Incl. Trop. Dis.* **2019**, *25*, 25. [CrossRef]
24. Escoubas, P. Structure and pharmacology of spider venom neurotoxins. *Biochimie* **2000**, *82*, 893–907. [CrossRef]
25. García-Arredondo, A.; Rodríguez-Rios, L.; Díaz-Peña, L.F.; Vega-Ángeles, R. Pharmacological characterization of venoms from three theraphosid spiders: *Poecilotheria regalis*, *Ceratogyrus darlingi* and *Brachypelma epicureanum*. *J. Venom. Anim. Toxins Incl. Trop. Dis.* **2015**, *21*, 555. [CrossRef]
26. Von Reumont, B.M.; Blanke, A.; Richter, S.; Alvarez, F.; Bleidorn, C.; Jenner, R.A. The first venomous crustacean revealed by transcriptomics and functional morphology: Remipede venom glands express a unique toxin cocktail dominated by enzymes and a neurotoxin. *Mol. Biol. Evol.* **2014**, *31*, 48–58. [CrossRef]
27. Stork, N.E. How many species of insects and other terrestrial arthropods are there on Earth? *Annu. Rev. Entomol.* **2018**, *63*, 31–45. [CrossRef]

28. Bonato, L.; Chagas, A., Jr.; Edgecombe, G.D.; Lewis, J.G.E.; Minelli, A.; Pereira, L.A.; Shelley, R.M.; Stoev, P.; Zapparoli, M. ChiloBase 2.0—A World Catalogue of Centipedes (Chilopoda). Available online: http://chilobase.biologia.unipd.it/ (accessed on 12 July 2019).
29. Rein, J.O. The Scorpion Files. Available online: https://www.ntnu.no/ub/scorpion-files/ (accessed on 12 July 2019).
30. Natural History Museum Bern World Spider Catalog. Version 20.0. Available online: https://wsc.nmbe.ch/ (accessed on 12 July 2019).
31. Cabezas-Cruz, A.; Valdés, J.J. Are ticks venomous animals? *Front. Zool.* **2014**, *11*, 47. [CrossRef]
32. Wermeling, D.; Drass, M.; Ellis, D.; Mayo, M.; McGuire, D.; O'Connell, D.; Hale, V.; Chao, S. Pharmacokinetics and Pharmacodynamics of Intrathecal Ziconotide in Chronic Pain Patients. *J. Clin. Pharmacol.* **2003**, *43*, 624–636. [CrossRef]
33. Ferreira, S.H.; Greene, L.J.; Alabaster, V.A.; Bakhle, Y.S.; Vane, J.R. Activity of various fractions of bradykinin potentiating factor against angiotensin I converting enzyme. *Nature* **1970**, *225*, 33. [CrossRef]
34. Furman, B.L. The development of Byetta (exenatide) from the venom of the Gila monster as an anti-diabetic agent. *Toxicon* **2012**, *59*, 464–471. [CrossRef]
35. Hultmark, D. *Drosophila* immunity: Paths and patterns. *Curr. Opin. Immunol.* **2003**, *15*, 12–19. [CrossRef]
36. Barra, D.; Simmaco, M. Amphibian skin: A promising resource for antimicrobial peptides. *Trends Biotechnol.* **1995**, *13*, 205–209. [CrossRef]
37. Reddy, K.; Yedery, R.; Aranha, C. Antimicrobial peptides: Premises and promises. *Int. J. Antimicrob. Agents* **2004**, *24*, 536–547. [CrossRef]
38. Brogden, K.A.; Ackermann, M.; McCray, P.B., Jr.; Tack, B.F. Antimicrobial peptides in animals and their role in host defences. *Int. J. Antimicrob. Agents* **2003**, *22*, 465–478. [CrossRef]
39. Brown, K.L.; Hancock, R.E. Cationic host defense (antimicrobial) peptides. *Curr. Opin. Immunol.* **2006**, *18*, 24–30. [CrossRef]
40. Gentilucci, L.; Tolomelli, A.; Squassabia, F. Peptides and peptidomimetics in medicine, surgery and biotechnology. *Curr. Med. Chem.* **2006**, *13*, 2449–2466. [CrossRef]
41. Bessalle, R.; Haas, H.; Goria, A.; Shalit, I.; Fridkin, M. Augmentation of the antibacterial activity of magainin by positive-charge chain extension. *Antimicrob. Agents Chemother.* **1992**, *36*, 313–317. [CrossRef]
42. Finger, S.; Kerth, A.; Dathe, M.; Blume, A. The efficacy of trivalent cyclic hexapeptides to induce lipid clustering in PG/PE membranes correlates with their antimicrobial activity. *Biochim. Biophys. Acta-Biomembr.* **2015**, *1848*, 2998–3006. [CrossRef]
43. Patterson-Delafield, J.; Szklarek, D.; Martinez, R.J.; Lehrer, R.I. Microbicidal cationic proteins of rabbit alveolar macrophages: Amino acid composition and functional attributes. *Infect. Immun.* **1981**, *31*, 723–731.
44. Mygind, P.H.; Fischer, R.L.; Schnorr, K.M.; Hansen, M.T.; Sönksen, C.P.; Ludvigsen, S.; Raventós, D.; Buskov, S.; Christensen, B.; De Maria, L.; et al. Plectasin is a peptide antibiotic with therapeutic potential from a saprophytic fungus. *Nature* **2005**, *437*, 975–980. [CrossRef]
45. Dai, C.; Ma, Y.; Zhao, Z.; Zhao, R.; Wang, Q.; Wu, Y.; Cao, Z.; Li, W. Mucroporin, the first cationic host defense peptide from the venom of *Lychas mucronatus*. *Antimicrob. Agents Chemother.* **2008**, *52*, 3967–3972. [CrossRef]
46. Zhao, Z.; Ma, Y.; Dai, C.; Zhao, R.; Li, S.; Wu, Y.; Cao, Z.; Li, W. Imcroporin, a new cationic antimicrobial peptide from the venom of the scorpion *Isometrus maculates*. *Antimicrob. Agents Chemother.* **2009**, *53*, 3472–3477. [CrossRef]
47. Zanjani, N.T.; Miranda-Saksena, M.; Cunningham, A.L.; Dehghani, F. Antimicrobial peptides of marine crustaceans: The potential and challenges of developing therapeutic agents. *Curr. Med. Chem.* **2018**, *25*, 2245–2259. [CrossRef]
48. Nie, Y.; Zeng, X.-C.; Yang, Y.; Luo, F.; Luo, X.; Wu, S.; Zhang, L.; Zhou, J. A novel class of antimicrobial peptides from the scorpion *Heterometrus spinifer*. *Peptides* **2012**, *38*, 389–394. [CrossRef]
49. Harrison, P.L.; Abdel-Rahman, M.A.; Miller, K.; Strong, P.N. Antimicrobial peptides from scorpion venoms. *Toxicon* **2014**, *88*, 115–137. [CrossRef]
50. Hernández-Aponte, C.A.; Silva-Sánchez, J.; Quintero-Hernández, V.; Rodríguez-Romero, A.; Balderas, C.; Possani, L.D.; Gurrola, G.B. Vejovine, a new antibiotic from the scorpion venom of *Vaejovis mexicanus*. *Toxicon* **2011**, *57*, 84–92. [CrossRef]
51. Zhao, X.; Wu, H.; Lü, H.; Li, G.; Huang, Q. LAMP: A Database Linking Antimicrobial Peptides. *PLoS ONE* **2013**, *8*, e66557. [CrossRef]

52. Di Luca, M.; Maccari, G.; Maisetta, G.; Batoni, G. BaAMPs: The database of biofilm-active antimicrobial peptides. *Biofouling* **2015**, *31*, 193–199. [CrossRef]
53. Fan, L.; Sun, J.; Zhou, M.; Zhou, J.; Lao, X.; Zheng, H.; Xu, H. DRAMP: A comprehensive data repository of antimicrobial peptides. *Sci. Rep.* **2016**, *6*, 24482. [CrossRef]
54. Wang, G.; Li, X.; Wang, Z. APD3: The antimicrobial peptide database as a tool for research and education. *Nucleic Acids Res.* **2016**, *44*, D1087–D1093. [CrossRef]
55. Yucesoy, D.T.; Hnilova, M.; Boone, K.; Arnold, P.M.; Snead, M.L.; Tamerler, C. Chimeric peptides as implant functionalization agents for titanium alloy implants with antimicrobial properties. *JOM* **2015**, *67*, 754–766. [CrossRef]
56. Wisdom, C.; Van Oosten, S.K.; Boone, K.W.; Khvostenko, D.; Arnold, P.M.; Snead, M.L.; Tamerler, C. Controlling the Biomimetic Implant Interface: Modulating Antimicrobial Activity by Spacer Design. *J. Mol. Eng. Mater.* **2016**, *4*, 1640005. [CrossRef]
57. Tajbakhsh, M.; Karimi, A.; Tohidpour, A.; Abbasi, N.; Fallah, F.; Akhavan, M.M. The antimicrobial potential of a new derivative of cathelicidin from *Bungarus fasciatus* against methicillin-resistant *Staphylococcus aureus*. *J. Microbiol.* **2018**, *56*, 128–137. [CrossRef]
58. Takahashi, D.; Shukla, S.K.; Prakash, O.; Zhang, G. Structural determinants of host defense peptides for antimicrobial activity and target cell selectivity. *Biochimie* **2010**, *92*, 1236–1241. [CrossRef]
59. Huang, Y.; Huang, J.; Chen, Y. Alpha-helical cationic antimicrobial peptides: Relationships of structure and function. *Protein Cell* **2010**, *1*, 143–152. [CrossRef]
60. Scocchi, M.; Wang, S.; Zanetti, M. Structural organization of the bovine cathelicidin gene family and identification of a novel member 1. *FEBS Lett.* **1997**, *417*, 311–315. [CrossRef]
61. Lewies, A.; Wentzel, J.F.; Jacobs, G.; Du Plessis, L.H. The Potential Use of natural and structural analogues of antimicrobial peptides in the fight against neglected tropical diseases. *Molecules* **2015**, *20*, 15392–15433. [CrossRef]
62. Ciumac, D.; Gong, H.; Hu, X.; Lu, J.R. Membrane targeting cationic antimicrobial peptides. *J. Colloid Interface Sci.* **2019**, *537*, 163–185. [CrossRef]
63. Kumar, P.; Kizhakkedathu, J.N.; Straus, S.K. Antimicrobial peptides: diversity, mechanism of action and strategies to improve the activity and biocompatibility in vivo. *Biomolecules* **2018**, *8*, 4. [CrossRef]
64. Doherty, T.; Waring, A.J.; Hong, M. Peptide–lipid interactions of the β-hairpin antimicrobial peptide tachyplesin and its linear derivatives from solid-state NMR. *Biochim. Biophys. Acta-Biomembr.* **2006**, *1758*, 1285–1291. [CrossRef]
65. Sitaram, N.; Subbalakshmi, C.; Nagaraj, R. Indolicidin, a 13-residue basic antimicrobial peptide rich in tryptophan and proline, interacts with Ca^{2+}-calmodulin. *Biochem. Biophys. Res. Commun.* **2003**, *309*, 879–884. [CrossRef]
66. Shi, J.; Ross, C.R.; Leto, T.L.; Blecha, F. PR-39, a proline-rich antibacterial peptide that inhibits phagocyte NADPH oxidase activity by binding to Src homology 3 domains of p47 phox. *Proc. Natl. Acad. Sci. USA* **1996**, *93*, 6014–6018. [CrossRef]
67. Van Dijk, I.A.; Nazmi, K.; Bolscher, J.G.M.; Veerman, E.C.I.; Stap, J. Histatin-1, a histidine-rich peptide in human saliva, promotes cell-substrate and cell-cell adhesion. *FASEB J.* **2015**, *29*, 3124–3132. [CrossRef]
68. Stepensky, D. Pharmacokinetics of Toxin-Derived Peptide Drugs. *Toxins* **2018**, *10*, 483. [CrossRef]
69. Fjell, C.D.; Hiss, J.A.; Hancock, R.E.W.; Schneider, G. Designing antimicrobial peptides: Form follows function. *Nat. Rev. Drug Discov.* **2012**, *11*, 37–51. [CrossRef]
70. Marr, A.K.; McGwire, B.S.; McMaster, W.R. Modes of action of Leishmanicidal antimicrobial peptides. *Future Microbiol.* **2012**, *7*, 1047–1059. [CrossRef]
71. Robbel, L.; Marahiel, M.A. Daptomycin, a bacterial lipopeptide synthesized by a nonribosomal machinery. *J. Boil. Chem.* **2010**, *285*, 27501–27508. [CrossRef]
72. Pogliano, J.; Pogliano, N.; Silverman, J.A. Daptomycin-mediated reorganization of membrane architecture causes mislocalization of essential cell division proteins. *J. Bacteriol.* **2012**, *194*, 4494–4504. [CrossRef]
73. Mosaheb, M.U.W.F.Z.; Khan, N.A.; Siddiqui, R. Cockroaches, locusts, and envenomating arthropods: A promising source of antimicrobials. *Iran. J. Basic Med. Sci.* **2018**, *21*, 873–877.
74. Huang, J.; Feigenson, G.W. A microscopic interaction model of maximum solubility of cholesterol in lipid bilayers. *Biophys. J.* **1999**, *76*, 2142–2157. [CrossRef]

75. Ali, M.R.; Cheng, K.H.; Huang, J. Ceramide drives cholesterol out of the ordered lipid bilayer phase into the crystal phase in 1-Palmitoyl-2-oleoyl-sn-glycero-3-phosphocholine/cholesterol/ceramide ternary mixtures. *Biochemistry* **2006**, *45*, 12629–12638. [CrossRef]
76. Matsuzaki, K. Why and how are peptide–lipid interactions utilized for self-defense? Magainins and tachyplesins as archetypes. *Biochim. Biophys. Acta-Biomembr.* **1999**, *1462*, 1–10. [CrossRef]
77. Powers, J.-P.S.; Hancock, R.E. The relationship between peptide structure and antibacterial activity. *Peptides* **2003**, *24*, 1681–1691. [CrossRef] [PubMed]
78. Delgado, M.; Anderson, P.; Garcia-Salcedo, J.A.; Caro, M.; Gonzalez-Rey, E. Neuropeptides kill African trypanosomes by targeting intracellular compartments and inducing autophagic-like cell death. *Cell Death Differ.* **2009**, *16*, 406–416. [CrossRef] [PubMed]
79. Luque-Ortega, J.R.; Hof, W.V.; Veerman, E.C.I.; Saugar, J.M.; Rivas, L. Human antimicrobial peptide histatin 5 is a cell-penetrating peptide targeting mitochondrial ATP synthesis in *Leishmania*. *FASEB J.* **2008**, *22*, 1817–1828. [CrossRef] [PubMed]
80. Ferguson, M.A.J.; Hart, G.W.; Kinoshita, T. *Essentials of Glycobiology*, 3rd ed.; Cold Spring Harbor Laboratory Press: Cold Spring Harbor, NY, USA, 2015.
81. Barreto-Bergter, E. Structures of glycolipids found in trypanosomatids: contribution to parasite functions. *Open Parasitol. J.* **2010**, *4*, 84–97. [CrossRef]
82. Souto-Padrón, T. The surface charge of trypanosomatids. *An. Acad. Bras. Cienc.* **2002**, *74*, 649–675. [CrossRef]
83. Torrent, M.; Pulido, D.; Rivas, L.; Andreu, D. Antimicrobial peptide action on parasites. *Curr. Drug Targets* **2012**, *13*, 1138–1147. [CrossRef]
84. McConville, M.J.; Mullin, K.A.; Ilgoutz, S.C.; Teasdale, R.D. Secretory pathway of trypanosomatid parasites. *Microbiol. Mol. Boil. Rev.* **2002**, *66*, 122–154. [CrossRef]
85. Kulkarni, M.M.; McMaster, W.R.; Kamysz, E.; Kamysz, W.; Engman, D.M.; McGwire, B.S. The major surface-metalloprotease of the parasitic protozoan, *Leishmania*, protects against antimicrobial peptide-induced apoptotic killing. *Mol. Microbiol.* **2006**, *62*, 1484–1497. [CrossRef]
86. Homans, S.W.; Mehlert, A.; Turco, S.J. Solution structure of the lipophosphoglycan of *Leishmania donovani*. *Biochemistry* **1992**, *31*, 654–661. [CrossRef]
87. Razzazan, A.; Saberi, M.R.; Jaafari, M.R. Hypothesis Insights from the analysis of a predicted model of gp63 in *Leishmania donovani*. *Bioinformation* **2008**, *3*, 114. [CrossRef]
88. Mangoni, M.L.; Maisetta, G.; Di Luca, M.; Gaddi, L.M.H.; Esin, S.; Florio, W.; Brancatisano, F.L.; Barra, D.; Campa, M.; Batoni, G. Comparative analysis of the bactericidal activities of amphibian peptide analogues against multidrug-resistant nosocomial bacterial strains. *Antimicrob. Agents Chemother.* **2008**, *52*, 85. [CrossRef]
89. Mangoni, M.L.; Marcellini HG, L.; Simmaco, M. Biological characterization and modes of action of temporins and bombinins H, multiple forms of short and mildly cationic anti-microbial peptides from amphibian skin. *J. Pept. Sci.* **2007**, *13*, 603–613. [CrossRef]
90. Späth, G.F.; Epstein, L.; Leader, B.; Singer, S.M.; Avila, H.A.; Turco, S.J.; Beverley, S.M. Lipophosphoglycan is a virulence factor distinct from related glycoconjugates in the protozoan parasite *Leishmania major*. *Proc. Natl. Acad. Sci. USA* **2000**, *97*, 9258–9263. [CrossRef]
91. Pimenta, P.F.; De Souza, W. *Leishmania mexicana amazonensis*: Surface charge of amastigote and promastigote forms. *Exp. Parasitol.* **1983**, *56*, 194–206. [CrossRef]
92. Burleigh, B.A.; Andrews, N.W. The Mechanisms of *Trypanosoma cruzi* invasion of mammalian cells. *Annu. Rev. Microbiol.* **1995**, *49*, 175–200. [CrossRef]
93. De Lederkremer, R.M.; Colli, W. Galactofuranose-containing glycoconjugates in trypanosomatids. *Glycobiology* **1995**, *5*, 547–552. [CrossRef]
94. Nardy, A.F.F.R.; Freire-De-Lima, C.G.; Pérez, A.R.; Morrot, A. Role of *Trypanosoma cruzi* trans-sialidase on the escape from host immune surveillance. *Front. Microbiol.* **2016**, *7*, 784. [CrossRef]
95. Acosta-Serrano, A. The mucin-like glycoprotein super-family of *Trypanosoma cruzi*: Structure and biological roles. *Mol. Biochem. Parasitol.* **2001**, *114*, 143–150. [CrossRef]
96. Yao, C. Major surface protease of trypanosomatids: One size fits all? *Infect. Immun.* **2010**, *78*, 22–31. [CrossRef]
97. Mehlert, A.; Bond, C.S.; Ferguson, M.A. The glycoforms of a *Trypanosoma brucei* variant surface glycoprotein and molecular modeling of a glycosylated surface coat. *Glycobiology* **2002**, *12*, 607–612. [CrossRef]

98. Pays, E.; Vanhamme, L.; Perez-Morga, D. Antigenic variation in *Trypanosoma brucei*: Facts, challenges and mysteries. *Curr. Opin. Microbiol.* **2004**, *7*, 369–374. [CrossRef]
99. Pays, E. Expression and function of surface proteins in *Trypanosoma brucei*. *Mol. Biochem. Parasitol.* **1998**, *91*, 3–36. [CrossRef]
100. Hsiao, L.L.; Howard, R.J.; Aikawa, M.; Taraschi, T.F. Modification of host cell membrane lipid composition by the intra-erythrocytic human malaria parasite *Plasmodium falciparum*. *Biochem. J.* **1991**, *274*, 121–132. [CrossRef]
101. Gelhaus, C.; Jacobs, T.; Andrä, J.; Leippe, M. The Antimicrobial Peptide NK-2, the Core Region of Mammalian NK-Lysin, Kills Intraerythrocytic *Plasmodium falciparum*. *Antimicrob. Agents Chemother.* **2008**, *52*, 1713–1720. [CrossRef]
102. Vale, N.; Aguiar, L.; Gomes, P.; Aguiar, L. Antimicrobial peptides: A new class of antimalarial drugs? *Front. Pharmacol.* **2014**, *5*, 275. [CrossRef]
103. Weiss, L.M.; Kim, K. *Toxoplasma Gondii: The Model Apicomplexan. Perspectives and Methods*, 2nd ed.; Elsevier: Amsterdam, The Netherlands; Academic Press: Cambridge, MA, USA, 2013; ISBN 9780123964816.
104. Tsai, Y.-H.; Liu, X.; Seeberger, P.H. Chemical Biology of Glycosylphosphatidylinositol Anchors. *Angew. Chem. Int. Ed.* **2012**, *51*, 11438–11456. [CrossRef]
105. Harrington, J.M. Antimicrobial peptide killing of African trypanosomes. *Parasite Immunol.* **2011**, *33*, 461–469. [CrossRef]
106. McGwire, B.S.; Kulkarni, M.M. Interactions of antimicrobial peptides with *Leishmania* and trypanosomes and their functional role in host parasitism. *Exp. Parasitol.* **2010**, *126*, 397–405. [CrossRef]
107. Lacerda, A.F.; Pelegrini, P.B.; De Oliveira, D.M.; Vasconcelos, É.A.; Grossi-De-Sa, M.F. Anti-parasitic Peptides from Arthropods and their Application in Drug Therapy. *Front. Microbiol.* **2016**, *7*, 232. [CrossRef]
108. Yeaman, M.R.; Yount, N.Y.; Hauger, R.L.; Grigoriadis, D.E.; Dallman, M.F.; Plotsky, P.M.; Vale, W.W.; Dautzenberg, F.M. Mechanisms of Antimicrobial Peptide Action and Resistance. *Pharmacol. Rev.* **2003**, *55*, 27–55. [CrossRef]
109. Wang, G.; Li, X.; Wang, Z. APD2: The updated antimicrobial peptide database and its application in peptide design. *Nucleic Acids Res.* **2008**, *37*, D933–D937. [CrossRef]
110. Nguyen, L.T.; Haney, E.F.; Vogel, H.J. The expanding scope of antimicrobial peptide structures and their modes of action. *Trends Biotechnol.* **2011**, *29*, 464–472. [CrossRef]
111. Brogden, K.A. Antimicrobial peptides: Pore formers or metabolic inhibitors in bacteria? *Nat. Rev. Genet.* **2005**, *3*, 238–250. [CrossRef]
112. Lee, M.-T.; Sun, T.-L.; Hung, W.-C.; Huang, H.W. Process of inducing pores in membranes by melittin. *Proc. Natl. Acad. Sci. USA* **2013**, *110*, 14243–14248. [CrossRef]
113. He, Y.; Prieto, L.; Lazaridis, T. Modeling peptide binding to anionic membrane pores. *J. Comput. Chem.* **2013**, *34*, 1463–1475. [CrossRef]
114. Pokorny, A.; Almeida, P.F.F. Kinetics of Dye Efflux and Lipid Flip-Flop Induced by δ-lysin in phosphatidylcholine vesicles and the mechanism of graded release by amphipathic, α-helical peptides. *Biochemistry* **2004**, *43*, 8846–8857. [CrossRef]
115. Lee, T.-H.; N Hall, K.; Aguilar, M.-I. Antimicrobial peptide structure and mechanism of action: A focus on the role of membrane structure. *Curr. Top. Med. Chem.* **2015**, *16*, 25–39. [CrossRef]
116. Mattila, J.-P.; Sabatini, K.; Kinnunen, P.K. Oxidized phospholipids as potential molecular targets for antimicrobial peptides. *Biochim. Biophys. Acta-Biomembr.* **2008**, *1778*, 2041–2050. [CrossRef]
117. Rokitskaya, T.I.; Kolodkin, N.I.; Kotova, E.A.; Antonenko, Y.N. Indolicidin action on membrane permeability: Carrier mechanism versus pore formation. *Biochim. Biophys. Acta-Biomembr.* **2011**, *1808*, 91–97. [CrossRef]
118. Rogers, M.J. Inhibition of *Plasmodium falciparum* protein synthesis. Targeting the plastid-like organelle with thiostrepton. *J. Boil. Chem.* **1997**, *272*, 2046–2049.
119. Clough, B.; Strath, M.; Preiser, P.; Denny, P.; Wilson, I.R.; Wilson, I. Thiostrepton binds to malarial plastid rRNA. *FEBS Lett.* **1997**, *406*, 123–125. [CrossRef]
120. Chen, R.; Mao, Y.; Wang, J.; Liu, M.; Qiao, Y.; Zheng, L.; Su, Y.; Ke, Q.; Zheng, W. Molecular mechanisms of an antimicrobial peptide piscidin (Lc-pis) in a parasitic protozoan, *Cryptocaryon irritans*. *BMC Genom.* **2018**, *19*, 192. [CrossRef]
121. Lin, Q.; Katakura, K.; Suzuki, M. Inhibition of mitochondrial and plastid activity of *Plasmodium falciparum* by minocycline. *FEBS Lett.* **2002**, *515*, 71–74. [CrossRef]

122. Goodman, C.D.; Su, V.; McFadden, G.I. The effects of anti-bacterials on the malaria parasite *Plasmodium falciparum*. *Mol. Biochem. Parasitol.* **2007**, *152*, 181–191. [CrossRef]
123. Aminake, M.N.; Schoof, S.; Sologub, L.; Leubner, M.; Kirschner, M.; Arndt, H.-D.; Pradel, G. Thiostrepton and Derivatives Exhibit Antimalarial and gametocytocidal activity by dually targeting parasite proteasome and apicoplast. *Antimicrob. Agents Chemother.* **2011**, *55*, 1338–1348. [CrossRef]
124. Vinhote, J.F.C.; Lima, D.B.; Mello, C.P.; de Souza, B.M.; Havt, A.; Palma, M.S.; dos Santos, R.P.; de Albuquerque, E.L.; Freire, V.N.; Martins, A.M.C. Trypanocidal activity of mastoparan from *Polybia paulista* wasp venom by interaction with TcGAPDH. *Toxicon* **2017**, *137*, 168–172. [CrossRef]
125. Kulkarni, M.M.; McMaster, W.R.; Kamysz, W.; McGwire, B.S. Antimicrobial peptide-induced apoptotic death of *Leishmania* results from calcium-de pendent, caspase-independent mitochondrial toxicity. *J. Biol. Chem.* **2009**, *284*, 15496–15504. [CrossRef]
126. Moreno, S.N.J.; Docampo, R. Calcium regulation in protozoan parasites. *Curr. Opin. Microbiol.* **2003**, *6*, 359–364. [CrossRef]
127. Gupta, S.; Raychaudhury, B.; Banerjee, S.; Das, B.; Datta, S.C. An intracellular calcium store is present in *Leishmania donovani* glycosomes. *Exp. Parasitol.* **2006**, *113*, 161–167. [CrossRef]
128. Da Costa, J.P.; Cova, M.; Ferreira, R.; Vitorino, R. Antimicrobial peptides: An alternative for innovative medicines? *Appl. Microbiol. Biotechnol.* **2015**, *99*, 2023–2040. [CrossRef]
129. Fura, J.; Sarkar, S.; Pidgeon, S.; Pires, M. Combatting bacterial pathogens with immunomodulation and infection tolerance strategies. *Curr. Top. Med. Chem.* **2016**, *16*, 1. [CrossRef]
130. Niyonsaba, F.; Hirata, M.; Ogawa, H.; Nagaoka, I. Epithelial cell-derived antibacterial peptides human beta-defensins and cathelicidin: Multifunctional activities on mast cells. *Curr. Drug Targets. Inflamm. Allergy* **2003**, *2*, 224–231. [CrossRef]
131. Oppenheim, J.J.; Biragyn, A.; Kwak, L.W.; Yang, D. Roles of antimicrobial peptides such as defensins in innate and adaptive immunity. *Ann. Rheum. Dis.* **2003**, *62*, ii17–ii21. [CrossRef]
132. Yang, R.; Zhang, Z.; Pei, X.; Han, X.; Wang, J.; Wang, L.; Long, Z.; Shen, X.; Li, Y. Immunomodulatory effects of marine oligopeptide preparation from Chum Salmon (*Oncorhynchus keta*) in mice. *Food Chem.* **2009**, *113*, 464–470. [CrossRef]
133. Lahov, E.; Regelson, W. Antibacterial and immunostimulating casein-derived substances from milk: Casecidin, isracidin peptides. *Food Chem. Toxicol.* **1996**, *34*, 131–145. [CrossRef]
134. Hilchie, A.L.; Wuerth, K.; Hancock, R.E.W. Immune modulation by multifaceted cationic host defense (antimicrobial) peptides. *Nat. Methods* **2013**, *9*, 761–768. [CrossRef]
135. Nijnik, A.; Hancock, R. Host defence peptides: Antimicrobial and immunomodulatory activity and potential applications for tackling antibiotic-resistant infections. *Emerg. Heal. Threat. J.* **2009**, *2*, 7078. [CrossRef]
136. Afacan, N.J.; Yeung, A.T.; Pena, O.M.; Hancock, R.E. Therapeutic potential of host defense peptides in antibiotic-resistant infections. *Curr. Pharm. Des.* **2012**, *18*, 807–819. [CrossRef]
137. Lai, Y.; Gallo, R.L. AMPed Up immunity: How antimicrobial peptides have multiple roles in immune defense. *Trends Immunol.* **2009**, *30*, 131–141. [CrossRef]
138. Hancock, R.E.W.; Nijnik, A.; Philpott, D.J. Modulating immunity as a therapy for bacterial infections. *Nat. Rev. Genet.* **2012**, *10*, 243–254. [CrossRef]
139. Bowdish, D.; Davidson, D.; Hancock, R. A Re-evaluation of the role of host defence peptides in mammalian immunity. *Curr. Protein Pept. Sci.* **2005**, *6*, 35–51. [CrossRef]
140. Karaś, M.A.; Turska-Szewczuk, A.; Janczarek, M.; Szuster-Ciesielska, A. Glycoconjugates of Gram-negative bacteria and parasitic protozoa—Are they similar in orchestrating the innate immune response? *Innate Immun.* **2019**, *25*, 73–96. [CrossRef]
141. Achtman, A.H.; Pilat, S.; Law, C.W.; Lynn, D.J.; Janot, L.; Mayer, M.L.; Ma, S.; Kindrachuk, J.; Finlay, B.B.; Brinkman, F.S.L. Effective adjunctive therapy by an innate defense regulatory peptide in a preclinical model of severe malaria. *Sci. Transl. Med.* **2012**, *4*, 135ra64. [CrossRef]
142. Zhao, H.; Kinnunen, P.K.J. Modulation of the activity of secretory phospholipase A2 by antimicrobial peptides. *Antimicrob. Agents Chemother.* **2003**, *47*, 965–971. [CrossRef]
143. Boutrin, M.-C.; Foster, H.; Pentreath, V.; Foster, H. The effects of bee (*Apis mellifera*) venom phospholipase A2 on *Trypanosoma brucei brucei* and enterobacteria. *Exp. Parasitol.* **2008**, *119*, 246–251. [CrossRef]

144. Grabner, A.N.; Alfonso, J.; Kayano, A.M.; Moreira-Dill, L.S.; Santos, A.P.D.A.D.; Caldeira, C.A.; Sobrinho, J.C.; Gómez, A.; Grabner, F.P.; Cardoso, F.F.; et al. BmajPLA 2-II, a basic Lys49-phospholipase A2 homologue from *Bothrops marajoensis* snake venom with parasiticidal potential. *Int. J. Boil. Macromol.* **2017**, *102*, 571–581. [CrossRef]
145. Barros, G.A.C.; Pereira, A.V.; Barros, L.C.; Lourenco, A.L., Jr.; Calvi, S.A.; Santos, L.D.; Barraviera, B.; Ferreira, R.S. In vitro activity of phospholipase A2 and of peptides from *Crotalus durissus terrificus* venom against amastigote and promastigote forms *of Leishmania* (L.) *infantum chagasi*. *J. Venom. Anim. Toxins Incl. Trop. Dis.* **2015**, *21*, 537. [CrossRef]
146. Nicholls, E.F.; Madera, L.; Hancock, R.E.W. Immunomodulators as adjuvants for vaccines and antimicrobial therapy. *Ann. N. Y. Acad. Sci.* **2010**, *1213*, 46–61. [CrossRef]
147. Steverding, D. The history of Chagas disease. *Parasit. Vectors* **2014**, *7*, 317. [CrossRef]
148. Centers for Disease Control and Prevention; Global Health, D. of P.D. and M. CDC—American trypanosomiasis. Available online: https://www.cdc.gov/parasites (accessed on 25 June 2019).
149. World Health Organization. WHO Chagas disease (American trypanosomiasis). Available online: https://www.who.int/chagas/en/ (accessed on 25 June 2019).
150. Antinori, S.; Galimberti, L.; Bianco, R.; Grande, R.; Galli, M.; Corbellino, M. Chagas disease in Europe: A review for the internist in the globalized world. *Eur. J. Intern. Med.* **2017**, *43*, 6–15. [CrossRef]
151. Pérez-Molina, J.A.; Molina, I. Chagas disease. *Lancet* **2018**, *391*, 82–94. [CrossRef]
152. Bermudez, J.; Davies, C.; Simonazzi, A.; Real, J.P.; Palma, S. Current drug therapy and pharmaceutical challenges for Chagas disease. *Acta Trop.* **2016**, *156*, 1–16. [CrossRef]
153. Palmeiro-Roldán, R.; Fonseca-Berzal, C.; Gómez-Barrio, A.; Arán, V.J.; Escario, J.A.; Torrado-Duran, S.; Torrado-Santiago, S. Development of novel benznidazole formulations: Physicochemical characterization and in vivo evaluation on parasitemia reduction in Chagas disease. *Int. J. Pharm.* **2014**, *472*, 110–117. [CrossRef]
154. Mejia, A.M.; Hall, B.S.; Taylor, M.C.; Gómez-Palacio, A.; Wilkinson, S.R.; Triana-Chávez, O.; Kelly, J.M. Benznidazole-Resistance in *Trypanosoma cruzi* is a readily acquired trait that can arise independently in a single population. *J. Infect. Dis.* **2012**, *206*, 220–228. [CrossRef]
155. Adade, C.M.; Oliveira, I.R.; Pais, J.A.; Souto-Padrón, T. Melittin peptide kills *Trypanosoma cruzi* parasites by inducing different cell death pathways. *Toxicon* **2013**, *69*, 227–239. [CrossRef]
156. Adade, C.M.; Chagas, G.S.F.; Souto-Padrón, T. *Apis mellifera* venom induces different cell death pathways in *Trypanosoma cruzi*. *Parasitology* **2012**, *139*, 1444–1461. [CrossRef]
157. Ruben, L.; Akins, C.D.; Haghighat, N.G.; Xue, L. Calcium influx in *Trypanosoma brucei* can be induced by amphiphilic peptides and amines. *Mol. Biochem. Parasitol.* **1996**, *81*, 191–200. [CrossRef]
158. Chicharro, C.; Granata, C.; Lozano, R.; Andreu, D.; Rivas, L. N-terminal fatty acid substitution increases the leishmanicidal activity of CA(1-7)M(2-9), a cecropin-melittin hybrid peptide. *Antimicrob. Agents Chemother.* **2001**, *45*, 2441–2449. [CrossRef]
159. Khalili, S.; Mohebali, M.; Ebrahimzadeh, E.; Shayan, E.; Mohammadi-Yeganeh, S.; Moghaddam, M.M.; Elikaee, S.; Akhoundi, B.; Sharifi-Yazdi, M.K. Antimicrobial activity of an antimicrobial peptide against amastigote forms of *Leishmania major*. *Veter-Res. Forum Int. Q. J.* **2018**, *9*, 323–328.
160. Fieck, A.; Hurwitz, I.; Kang, A.S.; Durvasula, R. *Trypanosoma cruzi*: Synergistic cytotoxicity of multiple amphipathic anti-microbial peptides to *T. cruzi* and potential bacterial hosts. *Exp. Parasitol.* **2010**, *125*, 342–347. [CrossRef]
161. Lima, D.B.; Mello, C.P.; Bandeira, I.C.J.; De Menezes, R.R.P.P.B.; Sampaio, T.L.; Falcão, C.B.; Morlighem, J.-R.L.; Rádis-Baptista, G.; Martins, A.M.C. The dinoponeratoxin peptides from the giant ant *Dinoponera quadriceps* display in vitro antitrypanosomal activity. *Boil. Chem.* **2018**, *399*, 187–196. [CrossRef]
162. Parente, A.M.S.; Daniele-Silva, A.; Furtado, A.A.; Melo, M.A.; Lacerda, A.F.; Queiroz, M.; Moreno, C.; Santos, E.; Rocha, H.A.O.; Barbosa, E.G.; et al. Analogs of the scorpion venom peptide Stigmurin: Structural assessment, toxicity, and increased antimicrobial activity. *Toxins* **2018**, *10*, 161. [CrossRef]
163. Kuhn-Nentwig, L.; Willems, J.; Seebeck, T.; Shalaby, T.; Kaiser, M.; Nentwig, W. Cupiennin 1a exhibits a remarkably broad, non-stereospecific cytolytic activity on bacteria, protozoan parasites, insects, and human cancer cells. *Amino Acids* **2011**, *40*, 69–76. [CrossRef]

164. Mashaghi, A.; Bezrukavnikov, S.; Minde, D.P.; Wentink, A.S.; Kityk, R.; Zachmann-Brand, B.; Mayer, M.P.; Kramer, G.; Bukau, B.; Tans, S.J. Alternative modes of client binding enable functional plasticity of Hsp70. *Nature* **2016**, *539*, 448–451. [CrossRef]
165. Kragol, G.; Lovas, S.; Váradi, G.; Condie, B.A.; Hoffmann, R.; Otvos, L. The antibacterial peptide pyrrhocoricin inhibits the atpase actions of DnaK and prevents chaperone-assisted protein folding. *Biochemistry* **2001**, *40*, 3016–3026. [CrossRef]
166. Nwaka, S.; Hudson, A. Innovative lead discovery strategies for tropical diseases. *Nat. Rev. Drug Discov.* **2006**, *5*, 941–955. [CrossRef]
167. Amorim-Carmo, B.; Daniele-Silva, A.; Parente, A.M.S.; Furtado, A.A.; Carvalho, E.; Oliveira, J.W.F.; Santos, E.C.G.; Silva, M.S.; Silva, S.R.B.; Silva-Júnior, A.A.; et al. Potent and broad-spectrum antimicrobial activity of analogs from the scorpion peptide stigmurin. *Int. J. Mol. Sci.* **2019**, *20*, 623. [CrossRef]
168. World Health Organization. WHO Trypanosomiasis, Human African (Sleeping Sickness). Available online: https://www.who.int/news-room/fact-sheets/detail/trypanosomiasis-human-african-(sleeping-sickness) (accessed on 8 July 2019).
169. Pays, E.; Vanhollebeke, B.; Uzureau, P.; Lecordier, L.; Perez-Morga, D. The molecular arms race between African trypanosomes and humans. *Nat. Rev. Genet.* **2014**, *12*, 575–584. [CrossRef]
170. Tiberti, N.; Sanchez, J.C. Sleeping Sickness in the 'Omics Era. *Proteom.-Clin. Appl.* **2018**, *12*, 1–10. [CrossRef]
171. Maxmen, A. Pill treats sleeping sickness Scientists seek approval from regulators for this relatively quick and easy therapy. *Nature* **2017**, *550*, 441. [CrossRef]
172. Pink, R.; Hudson, A.; Mouriès, M.-A.; Bendig, M. Opportunities and Challenges in Antiparasitic Drug Discovery. *Nat. Rev. Drug Discov.* **2005**, *4*, 727–740. [CrossRef]
173. World Health Organization. WHO Leishmaniasis. Available online: https://www.who.int/en/news-room/fact-sheets/detail/leishmaniasis (accessed on 23 July 2019).
174. Myler, P.J.; Fasel, N. *Leishmania: After the Genome*; Caister Academic: Poole, UK, 2008; ISBN 9781904455288.
175. McGwire, B.S.; Satoskar, A.R. Leishmaniasis: Clinical syndromes and treatment. *QJM* **2014**, *107*, 7–14. [CrossRef]
176. Alvar, J.; Velez, I.D.; Bern, C.; Herrero, M.; Desjeux, P.; Cano, J.; Jannin, J.; Boer, M.D. Leishmaniasis worldwide and global estimates of its incidence. *PLoS ONE* **2012**, *7*, e35671. [CrossRef]
177. Kaye, P.; Scott, P. Leishmaniasis: Complexity at the host–pathogen interface. *Nat. Rev. Genet.* **2011**, *9*, 604–615. [CrossRef]
178. Zahedifard, F.; Rafati, S. Prospects for antimicrobial peptide-based immunotherapy approaches in *Leishmania* control. *Expert Rev. Anti-Infect. Ther.* **2018**, *16*, 461–469. [CrossRef]
179. Ali, M.; Hofland, H.; Zijlstra, E.; El-Hassan, A.; El-Toum, I.; Satti, M.; Ghalib, H. The treatment of kala-azar in the Sudan with sodium stibogluconate: A randomized trial of three dosage regimens. *Trans. R. Soc. Trop. Med. Hyg.* **1993**, *87*, 307–309.
180. Baiocco, P.; Colotti, G.; Franceschini, S.; Ilari, A. Molecular basis of antimony treatment in leishmaniasis. *J. Med. Chem.* **2009**, *52*, 2603–2612. [CrossRef]
181. Ameen, M. Cutaneous and mucocutaneous leishmaniasis: Emerging therapies and progress in disease management. *Expert Opin. Pharmacother.* **2010**, *11*, 557–569. [CrossRef]
182. Rojas, R.; Valderrama, L.; Valderrama, M.; Varona, M.X.; Ouellette, M.; Saravia, N.G. Resistance to Antimony and Treatment Failure in Human *Leishmania* (*Viannia*) Infection. *J. Infect. Dis.* **2006**, *193*, 1375–1383. [CrossRef]
183. Croft, S.L.; Sundar, S.; Fairlamb, A.H. Drug resistance in leishmaniasis. *Clin. Microbiol. Rev.* **2006**, *19*, 111–126. [CrossRef]
184. De Menezes, J.P.B.; Guedes, C.E.S.; Petersen, A.L.D.O.A.; Fraga, D.B.M.; Veras, P.S.T. Advances in development of new treatment for leishmaniasis. *Biomed Res. Int.* **2015**, *2015*, 815023. [CrossRef]
185. Berman, J. Clinical status of agents being developed for leishmaniasis. *Expert Opin. Investig. Drugs* **2005**, *14*, 1337–1346. [CrossRef]
186. Sundar, S.; Olliaro, P.L. Miltefosine in the treatment of leishmaniasis: Clinical evidence for informed clinical risk management. *Ther. Clin. Risk Manag.* **2007**, *3*, 733–740.
187. Chattopadhyay, A.; Jafurulla, M. A novel mechanism for an old drug: Amphotericin B in the treatment of visceral leishmaniasis. *Biochem. Biophys. Res. Commun.* **2011**, *416*, 7–12. [CrossRef]

188. Sundar, S.; Rai, M.; Chakravarty, J.; Agarwal, D.; Agrawal, N.; Vaillant, M.; Olliaro, P.; Murray, H.W. New treatment approach in indian visceral leishmaniasis: Single-dose liposomal amphotericin b followed by short-course oral miltefosine. *Clin. Infect. Dis.* **2008**, *47*, 1000–1006. [CrossRef]
189. Silva, P.I.; Daffre, S.; Bulet, P. Isolation and characterization of gomesin, an 18-residue cysteine-rich defense peptide from the spider *Acanthoscurria gomesiana* hemocytes with sequence similarities to horseshoe crab antimicrobial peptides of the tachyplesin family. *J. Biol. Chem.* **2000**, *275*, 33464–33470. [CrossRef]
190. Schaeffer, M.; De Miranda, A.; Mottram, J.C.; Coombs, G.H. Differentiation of *Leishmania major* is impaired by over-expression of pyroglutamyl peptidase I. *Mol. Biochem. Parasitol.* **2006**, *150*, 318–329. [CrossRef]
191. Konno, K.; Rangel, M.; Oliveira, J.S.; dos Santos Cabrera, M.P.; Fontana, R.; Hirata, I.Y.; Hide, I.; Nakata, Y.; Mori, K.; Kawano, M.; et al. Decoralin, a novel linear cationic α-helical peptide from the venom of the solitary eumenine wasp *Oreumenes decoratus*. *Peptides* **2007**, *28*, 2320–2327. [CrossRef]
192. Konno, K.; Hisada, M.; Naoki, H.; Itagaki, Y.; Fontana, R.; Rangel, M.; Oliveira, J.S.; Cabrera, M.P.D.S.; Neto, J.R.; Hide, I.; et al. Eumenitin, a novel antimicrobial peptide from the venom of the solitary eumenine wasp *Eumenes rubronotatus*. *Peptides* **2006**, *27*, 2624–2631. [CrossRef]
193. Konno, K.; Hisada, M.; Naoki, H.; Itagaki, Y.; Kawai, N.; Miwa, A.; Yasuhara, T.; Morimoto, Y.; Nakata, Y. Structure and biological activities of eumenine mastoparan-AF (EMP-AF), a new mast cell degranulating peptide in the venom of the solitary wasp (*Anterhynchium flavomarginatum micado*). *Toxicon* **2000**, *38*, 1505–1515. [CrossRef]
194. Rangel, M.; Cabrera, M.P.D.S.; Kazuma, K.; Ando, K.; Wang, X.; Kato, M.; Nihei, K.-I.; Hirata, I.Y.; Cross, T.J.; Garcia, A.N.; et al. Chemical and biological characterization of four new linear cationic α-helical peptides from the venoms of two solitary eumenine wasps. *Toxicon* **2011**, *57*, 1081–1092. [CrossRef]
195. Pérez-Cordero, J.J.; Lozano, J.M.; Cortés, J.; Delgado, G. Leishmanicidal activity of synthetic antimicrobial peptides in an infection model with human dendritic cells. *Peptides* **2011**, *32*, 683–690. [CrossRef]
196. Diaz-Achirica, P.; Ubach, J.; Guinea, A.; Andreu, D.; Rivas, L. The plasma membrane of *Leishmania donovani* promastigotes is the main target for CA(1–8)M(1–18), a synthetic cecropin A–melittin hybrid peptide. *Biochem. J.* **1998**, *330*, 453–460. [CrossRef]
197. Téné, N.; Bonnafé, E.; Berger, F.; Rifflet, A.; Guilhaudis, L.; Ségalas-Milazzo, I.; Pipy, B.; Coste, A.; Leprince, J.; Treilhou, M. Biochemical and biophysical combined study of bicarinalin, an ant venom antimicrobial peptide. *Peptides* **2016**, *79*, 103–113. [CrossRef]
198. Borges, A.; Silva, S.; Camp, H.J.O.D.; Velasco, E.; Alvarez, M.; Alfonzo, M.J.; Jorquera, A.; De Sousa, L.; Delgado, O.; De Sousa, J.L. In vitro leishmanicidal activity of *Tityus discrepans* scorpion venom. *Parasitol. Res.* **2006**, *99*, 167–173. [CrossRef]
199. Lima, D.B.; Sousa, P.L.; Torres, A.F.C.; Rodrigues, K.A.D.F.; Mello, C.P.; De Menezes, R.R.P.P.B.; Tessarolo, L.D.; Quinet, Y.P.; De Oliveira, M.R.; Martins, A.M.C. Antiparasitic effect of *Dinoponera quadriceps* giant ant venom. *Toxicon* **2016**, *120*, 128–132. [CrossRef]
200. Alberola, J.; Rodriguez, A.; Francino, O.; Roura, X.; Rivas, L.; Andreu, D. Safety and efficacy of antimicrobial peptides against naturally acquired leishmaniasis. *Antimicrob. Agents Chemother.* **2004**, *48*, 641–643. [CrossRef]
201. White, N.J.; Pukrittayakamee, S.; Hien, T.T.; Faiz, M.A.; Mokuolu, O.A.; Dondorp, A.M. Malaria. *Lancet* **2014**, *383*, 723–735. [CrossRef]
202. Wang, X.; Zhao, X.-Q. A Malaria transmission model with temperature-dependent incubation period. *Bull. Math. Boil.* **2017**, *72*, 1155–1182. [CrossRef]
203. Watson, J.; Taylor, W.R.J.; Bancone, G.; Chu, C.S.; Jittamala, P.; White, N.J. Implications of current therapeutic restrictions for primaquine and tafenoquine in the radical cure of *vivax* malaria. *PLoS Negl. Trop. Dis.* **2018**, *12*, e0006440. [CrossRef]
204. Sawa, P.; Shekalaghe, S.A.; Drakeley, C.J.; Sutherland, C.J.; Mweresa, C.K.; Baidjoe, A.Y.; Manjurano, A.; Kavishe, R.A.; Beshir, K.B.; Yussuf, R.U.; et al. Malaria transmission after artemether-lumefantrine and dihydroartemisinin-piperaquine: A randomized trial. *J. Infect. Dis.* **2013**, *207*, 1637–1645. [CrossRef]
205. Jones, J.G. Malaria chemoprophylaxis and travel immunizations. *Am. Fam. Physician* **2010**, *82*, 583–584.
206. Conde, R.; Zamudio, F.Z.; Rodr, M.H. Scorpine, an anti-malaria and anti-bacterial agent purified from scorpion venom. *FEBS Lett.* **2000**, *471*, 165–168. [CrossRef]
207. Gao, B.; Xu, J.; Rodriguez, M.D.C.; Lanz-Mendoza, H.; Hernández-Rivas, R.; Du, W.; Zhu, S. Characterization of two linear cationic antimalarial peptides in the scorpion *Mesobuthus eupeus*. *Biochimie* **2010**, *92*, 350–359. [CrossRef]

208. Vizioli, J.; Bulet, P.; Hoffmann, J.A.; Kafatos, F.C.; Müller, H.-M.; Dimopoulos, G. Gambicin: A novel immune responsive antimicrobial peptide from the malaria vector *Anopheles gambiae*. *Proc. Natl. Acad. Sci. USA* **2001**, *98*, 12630–12635. [CrossRef]
209. Zhu, S.; Gao, B.; Aumelas, A.; Rodriguez, M.D.C.; Lanz-Mendoza, H.; Peigneur, S.; Diego-Garcia, E.; Martin-Eauclaire, M.-F.; Tytgat, J.; Possani, L.D. MeuTXKβ1, a scorpion venom-derived two-domain potassium channel toxin-like peptide with cytolytic activity. *Biochim. Biophys. Acta-Proteins Proteom.* **2010**, *1804*, 872–883. [CrossRef]
210. Choi, S.-J.; Parent, R.; Guillaume, C.; Deregnaucourt, C.; Delarbre, C.; Ojcius, D.M.; Montagne, J.-J.; Célérier, M.-L.; Phelipot, A.; Amiche, M.; et al. Isolation and characterization of Psalmopeotoxin I and II: Two novel antimalarial peptides from the venom of the tarantula *Psalmopoeus cambridgei*. *FEBS Lett.* **2004**, *572*, 109–117. [CrossRef]
211. Edwards, I.A.; Elliott, A.G.; Kavanagh, A.M.; Zuegg, J.; Blaskovich, M.A.T.; Cooper, M.A. Contribution of amphipathicity and hydrophobicity to the antimicrobial activity and cytotoxicity of β-hairpin peptides. *ACS Infect. Dis.* **2016**, *2*, 442–450. [CrossRef]
212. Moreira, C.K.; Rodrigues, F.G.; Ghosh, A.; Varotti, F.D.P.; Miranda, A.; Daffre, S.; Jacobs-Lorena, M.; Moreira, L.A. Effect of the antimicrobial peptide Gomesin against different life stages of *Plasmodium* spp. *Exp. Parasitol.* **2007**, *116*, 346–353. [CrossRef]
213. Carter, V.; Underhill, A.; Baber, I.; Sylla, L.; Baby, M.; Larget-Thiery, I.; Zettor, A.; Bourgouin, C.; Langel, Ü.; Faye, I.; et al. Killer bee molecules: antimicrobial peptides as effector molecules to target sporogonic stages of *Plasmodium*. *PLoS Pathog.* **2013**, *9*, e1003790. [CrossRef] [PubMed]
214. Cabezas-Cruz, A.; Tonk, M.; Bouchut, A.; Pierrot, C.; Pierce, R.J.; Kotsyfakis, M.; Rahnamaeian, M.; Vilcinskas, A.; Khalife, J.; Valdés, J.J. Antiplasmodial activity is an ancient and conserved feature of tick defensins. *Front. Microbiol.* **2016**, *7*, 2954. [CrossRef] [PubMed]
215. Tonk, M.; Cabezas-Cruz, A.; Valdés, J.J.; Rego, R.O.; Rudenko, N.; Golovchenko, M.; Bell-Sakyi, L.; De La Fuente, J.; Grubhoffer, L. Identification and partial characterisation of new members of the *Ixodes ricinus* defensin family. *Gene* **2014**, *540*, 146–152. [CrossRef] [PubMed]
216. Asthana, N.; Yadav, S.P.; Ghosh, J.K. Dissection of antibacterial and toxic activity of melittin. *J. Biol. Chem.* **2004**, *279*, 55042–55050. [CrossRef] [PubMed]
217. Konno, K.; Hisada, M.; Fontana, R.; Lorenzi, C.C.; Naoki, H.; Itagaki, Y.; Miwa, A.; Kawai, N.; Nakata, Y.; Yasuhara, T.; et al. Anoplin, a novel antimicrobial peptide from the venom of the solitary wasp *Anoplius samariensis*. *Biochim. Biophys. Acta-Protein Struct. Mol. Enzym.* **2001**, *1550*, 70–80. [CrossRef]
218. Hirai, Y.; Yasuhara, T.; Yoshida, H.; Nakajima, T.; Fujino, M.; Kitada, C. A new mast cell degranulating peptide "mastoparan" in the venom of *Vespula lewisii*. *Chem. Pharm. Bull.* **1979**, *27*, 1942–1944. [CrossRef]
219. Khan, K.; Khan, W. Congenital toxoplasmosis: An overview of the neurological and ocular manifestations. *Parasitol. Int.* **2018**, *67*, 715–721. [CrossRef]
220. Martins-Duarte, E.S.; De Souza, W.; Vommaro, R.C. *Toxoplasma gondii*: The effect of fluconazole combined with sulfadiazine and pyrimethamine against acute toxoplasmosis in murine model. *Exp. Parasitol.* **2013**, *133*, 294–299. [CrossRef]
221. Tang, Y.; Hou, S.; Li, X.; Wu, M.; Ma, B.; Wang, Z.; Jiang, J.; Deng, M.; Duan, Z.; Tang, X.; et al. Anti-parasitic effect on *Toxoplasma gondii* induced by a spider peptide lycosin-I. *Exp. Parasitol.* **2019**, *198*, 17–25. [CrossRef]
222. Tanaka, T.; Maeda, H.; Galay, R.L.; Boldbattar, D.; Umemiya-Shirafuji, R.; Suzuki, H.; Xuan, X.; Tsuji, N.; Fujisaki, K. tick longicin implicated in the arthropod transmission of *Toxoplasma Gondii*. *J. Vet. Sci. Technol.* **2012**, *3*, 3633–3640.
223. Tsuji, N.; Battsetseg, B.; Boldbaatar, D.; Miyoshi, T.; Xuan, X.; Oliver, J.H.; Fujisaki, K. Babesial vector tick defensin against *Babesia* sp. Parasites. *Infect. Immun.* **2007**, *75*, 3633–3640. [CrossRef] [PubMed]
224. Fratini, F.; Cilia, G.; Turchi, B.; Felicioli, A. Insects, arachnids and centipedes venom: A powerful weapon against bacteria. A literature review. *Toxicon* **2017**, *130*, 91–103. [CrossRef] [PubMed]
225. Primon-Barros, M.; Macedo, A.J. Animal venom peptides: potential for new antimicrobial agents. *Curr. Top. Med. Chem.* **2017**, *17*, 1119–1156. [CrossRef]
226. Rajamuthiah, R.; Jayamani, E.; Conery, A.L.; Fuchs, B.B.; Kim, W.; Johnston, T.; Vilcinskas, A.; Ausubel, F.M.; Mylonakis, E. A defensin from the model beetle *Tribolium castaneum* acts synergistically with telavancin and daptomycin against multidrug resistant *Staphylococcus aureus*. *PLoS ONE* **2015**, *10*, e0128576. [CrossRef] [PubMed]

227. Ali, M.P.; Yoshimatsu, K.; Suzuki, T.; Kato, T.; Park, E.Y. Expression and purification of cyto-insectotoxin (Cit1a) using silkworm larvae targeting for an antimicrobial therapeutic agent. *Appl. Microbiol. Biotechnol.* **2014**, *98*, 6973–6982. [CrossRef] [PubMed]
228. Bommarius, B.; Jenssen, H.; Elliott, M.; Kindrachuk, J.; Pasupuleti, M.; Gieren, H.; Jaeger, K.-E.; Hancock, R.W.; Kalman, D. Cost-effective expression and purification of antimicrobial and host defense peptides in *Escherichia coli*. *Peptides* **2010**, *31*, 1957–1965. [CrossRef] [PubMed]
229. Li, Y. Recombinant production of antimicrobial peptides in *Escherichia coli*: A review. *Protein Expr. Purif.* **2011**, *80*, 260–267. [CrossRef]
230. Kulkarni, M.M.; Karafova, A.; Kamysz, W.; McGwire, B.S. Design of protease-resistant pexiganan enhances antileishmanial activity. *Parasitol. Res.* **2014**, *113*, 1971–1976. [CrossRef]
231. Lipsky, B.A.; Holroyd, K.J.; Zasloff, M. Topical versus systemic antimicrobial therapy for treating mildly infected diabetic foot ulcers: A randomized, controlled, double-blinded, multicenter trial of pexiganan cream. *Clin. Infect. Dis.* **2008**, *47*, 1537–1545. [CrossRef]
232. Fox, J.L. Antimicrobial peptides stage a comeback. *Nat. Biotechnol.* **2013**, *31*, 379–382. [CrossRef]
233. World Health Organization. WHO Malaria. Available online: https://www.who.int/malaria/en/ (accessed on 28 July 2019).
234. Wanted: A reward for antibiotic development. *Nat. Biotechnol.* **2018**, *36*, 555. [CrossRef] [PubMed]

toxins

MDPI

Article

Fire Ant Venom Alkaloids Inhibit Biofilm Formation

Danielle Bruno de Carvalho [1,†], Eduardo Gonçalves Paterson Fox [2,*,†], Diogo Gama dos Santos [1], Joab Sampaio de Sousa [3], Denise Maria Guimarães Freire [3], Fabio C. S. Nogueira [3], Gilberto B. Domont [3], Livia Vieira Araujo de Castilho [3] and Ednildo de Alcântara Machado [1,*]

[1] Departamento de Parasitologia, Instituto de Biofísica Carlos, Chagas Filho (IBCCF), Universidade Federal do Rio de Janeiro, Rio de Janeiro 21044-020, Brazil

[2] Red Imported Fire Ant Research Centre, South China Agricultural University (SCAU), Guangzhou 510642, China

[3] Departamento de Bioquímica (DBq), Instituto de Química, Universidade Federal do Rio de Janeiro, Rio de Janeiro 21044-020, Brazil

* Correspondence: ofoxofox@gmail.com (E.G.P.F.); ednildo.machado@gmail.com (E.d.A.M.)

† These authors contributed equally to this work.

Received: 18 May 2019; Accepted: 12 July 2019; Published: 18 July 2019

Abstract: Biofilm formation on exposed surfaces is a serious issue for the food industry and medical health facilities. There are many proposed strategies to delay, reduce, or even eliminate biofilm formation on surfaces. The present study focuses on the applicability of fire ant venom alkaloids (aka 'solenopsins', from *Solenopsis invicta*) tested on polystyrene and stainless steel surfaces relative to the adhesion and biofilm-formation by the bacterium *Pseudomonas fluorescens*. Conditioning with solenopsins demonstrates significant reduction of bacterial adhesion. Inhibition rates were 62.7% on polystyrene and 59.0% on stainless steel surfaces. In addition, solenopsins drastically reduced cell populations already growing on conditioned surfaces. Contrary to assumptions by previous authors, solenopsins tested negative for amphipathic properties, thus understanding the mechanisms behind the observed effects still relies on further investigation.

Keywords: natural antibiotics; piperidine heterocyclic amines; industrial biotechnology; LTQ Orbitrap Hybrid Mass Spectrometer; myrmecology

Key Contribution: The formation of biofilm on two commonly-employed surface materials is strongly inhibited by conditioning with fire ant venom alkaloids, biofilm inhibition is associated with marked antimicrobial activity, venom solenopsins do not show chemical evidence of detergent-like activity.

1. Introduction

Any exposed surface, ranging from biological tissues to stainless steel, is vulnerable to the adhesion of microorganisms, whose accumulated secreted factors may lead to the formation of a biofilm matrix [1,2]. Biofilm formation is a primary cause of urinary tract inflammations, rejection of surgically implanted parts and prostheses, and of dental plaque formation [3,4]. Furthermore, major economic losses associated to biofilm formation can result from biological corrosion of duct pipes and connections, disruption of heat modulators, accelerated material degradation, and food contamination [4–6]. As a result, the formation of biofilm is a major health and industrial concern.

When immersed within their secreted biofilm, microorganisms may become thousands of times more resistant to methods of control (e.g., antibiotics, disinfectants) as compared to their free-living state [6,7]. The acquired resistance makes the removal of microorganisms more difficult, which poses a problem in industrial and medical spheres [7–9]. The most commonly employed chemicals against biofilm formation are organic halogen compounds, peroxides, inorganic acids, anionic detergents, and surfactants [6]. Because of their high toxicity, low biodegradability, and high surface abrasion [10,11], these chemicals become additional hazards to humans and the environment.

A range of microorganisms can form biofilms, of which the gram-negative bacterium *Pseudomonas fluorescens* (Flügge 1886) is one of the most intensively studied. This aerobic bacterium will rapidly form biofilms on surfaces with different physicochemical properties, including polystyrene, stainless steel, and polyamides [12,13]. Though regarded as non-pathogenic, *P. fluorescens* is often involved in rapid food contamination, leading to gastroenteritis [14,15]. Moreover, *Pseudomonas* spp. are among the most abundant microbes detected in industrial water circuits, and are associated with augmented corrosion and clogging of pipelines, ultimately leading to loss of speed, load capacity, and unnecessary energy expenditure [16,17].

The development of alternative strategies for reducing the negative effects of the harsh chemicals used in suppressing industrial microbial growth and biofilms formation is a necessity. One prophylactic approach is the pretreatment of surfaces with organic molecules that can later inhibit microbial adhesion [18,19]. Examples of low-toxicity biomolecules currently under investigation for their anti-biofilm activity include natural biosurfactants, such as surfactins and rhamnolipids [17–19]. The heterogeneous class of bioactive amines known as 'alkaloids' has, however, been largely overlooked in this context. A group of alkaloids derived from the venom of fire ants (Insecta: Hymenoptera: Formicidae: *Solenopsis*) trivially known as 'solenopsins' (reviewed in [20]) has been recently proposed as a potential candidate for biofilm inhibition [21] but remains mostly untested. In this context, the present report adds further information on the anti-biofilm effects from conditioning surfaces with solenopsin alkaloids obtained from solvent extraction of red imported fire ants.

2. Results

2.1. Solenopsins Extraction and Purification

The relative composition of solenopsin analogues obtained by hexane extraction of fire ants is given in Table 1 (and a chromatogram in Figure S1).

Table 1. Composition of solenopsins from a whole-nest extraction of the fire ant *Solenopsis invicta.*

Compound Name	Short Trivial Name	Chemical Formula	Diagnostic Ions-*m/z*	RT (Initial)	Relative Abundance (Area %)
cis-2-Me-6-Tridecyl-Piperidine	C13	$C_{19}H_{39}N$	280 (M^+), 266, 98	19.942	2.594
trans-2-Me-6-Tridecenyl-Piperidine	C13:1	$C_{19}H_{38}N$	279 (M^+), 264, 180, 124, 111, 98	20.167	76.528
trans-2-Me-6-Tridecyl-Piperidine	C13	$C_{19}H_{39}N$	280 (M^+), 266, 98	20.375	6.349
cis-2-Me-6-Pentadecyl-Piperidine	C15	$C_{21}H_{43}N$	309 (M^+), 308, 294, 98	21.550	0.394
trans-2-Me-6-Pentadecenyl-Piperidine	C15:1	$C_{21}H_{42}N$	307 (M^+), 292, 228, 154, 124, 111, 98	21.833	11.554
trans-2-Me-6-Pentadecyl-Piperidine	C15	$C_{21}H_{43}N$	309 (M^+), 308, 294, 98	22.025	2.580

2.2. Antimicrobial Activity

Obtained inhibition haloes against Petri dish-grown *P. fluorescens* were largest for the highest tested concentrations of solenopsins, providing evidence for antimicrobial activity (Figure 1). The solenopsin alkaloids presented antimicrobial activity at concentrations ranging from 750 to 5000 μg/mL, yielding mean diameters of inhibition halos between 8 and 14 mm (Figure 1). The minimum inhibitory concentration (MIC), estimated by log linear regression, was 370.4 μg/mL (Figure S2).

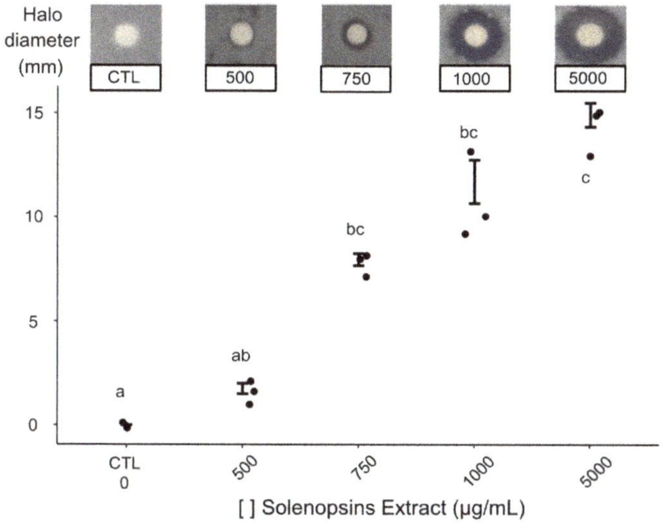

Figure 1. Diameters of inhibition zones resulting from the antimicrobial activity of solenopsins by the paper disk diffusion method. Points are raw data and vertical whiskers represent SD around the mean. Disks impregnated with different concentrations (µg/mL) of solenopsins were added to a confluent *Pseudomonas fluorescens* growth plate and incubated at 25 °C for 24 h. Treatments topped by same letters were statistically similar based on Dunn's test at alpha = 0.05.

2.3. *Effect of Preconditioning on Cell Adhesion and Biofilm Formation*

Figure 2 illustrates anti-biofilm activity from polystyrene and stainless steel surfaces preconditioned with solenopsins. Conditioning yielded maximal inhibitions of cell adhesion of 80.7% on polystyrene and 63.9% on stainless steel under the concentration of 5000 µg/mL, although no significant difference is observed from 1000 µg/mL (*p*-values: 0.3318, 0.5000).

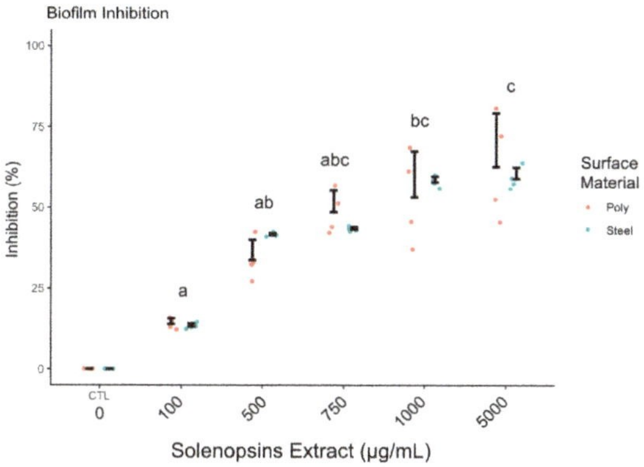

Figure 2. Inhibition of biofilm formation (as discounted % relative to control) by *Pseudomonas fluorescens* ATCC 13525 on surfaces of polystyrene and stainless steel 304 conditioned with solenopsin alkaloids at different concentrations. Points are raw data and vertical whiskers represent SD around the mean; 'CTL' stands for negative control and 'poly' for polystyrene. Treatments accompanied by same letters were statistically similar based on Dunn's test at alpha = 0.05: no difference was observed between results with different surface materials.

In addition to an antiadhesive effect, solenopsins had some capacity of reducing mature biofilms (i.e., preformed biofilm) growing on non-conditioned polystyrene (Figure 3, in red), though complete eradication was not observed. No effect was observed on mature biofilm grown on non-conditioned steel (Figure 3, in blue).

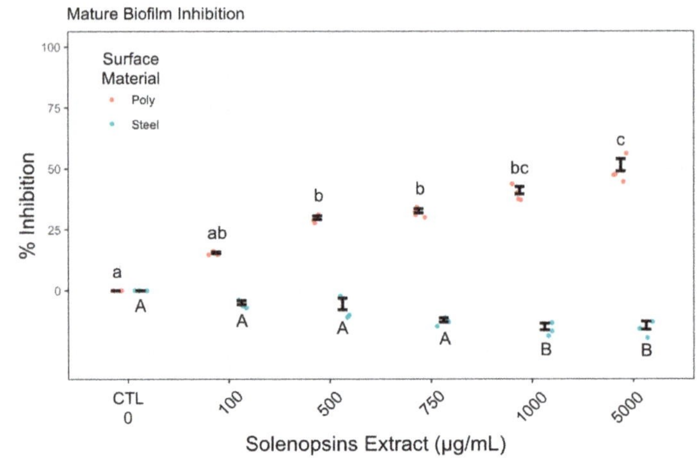

Figure 3. Reduction of mature biofilm (as % discounted of controls) by *Pseudomonas fluorescens* ATCC 13525 on non-conditioned surfaces of polystyrene (red) and stainless steel 304 (blue) by solenopsin alkaloids at different concentrations. Points are raw data and vertical whiskers represent SD around the mean; 'CTL' stands for negative control and 'poly' for polystyrene. Concentration groups within the same surface treatment accompanied by the same letter did not differ significantly by Dunn's test at alpha = 0.05 (polystyrene: lowercase on top; stainless steel: uppercase below).

2.4. *Quantification of Viable Cells*

Colony-forming unit counts indicated a decrease of viable cells recovered from biofilm grown on surfaces conditioned with solenopsins (Supplementary Table; Kruskal–Wallis chi-squared = 12.3579, df = 4, p-value = 0.01) relative to non-conditioned controls (Figure 4). The number of viable cells recovered from biofilms grown on polystyrene conditioned with solenopsins was remarkably lower than in non-conditioned controls (Figure 4), and cells recovered from the conditioned steel surface were not viable (Table S1). The pattern observed was congruent with observations by epifluorescence microscopy (Figure 5). Controls had many layers of adhered cells (Figure 5A,B).

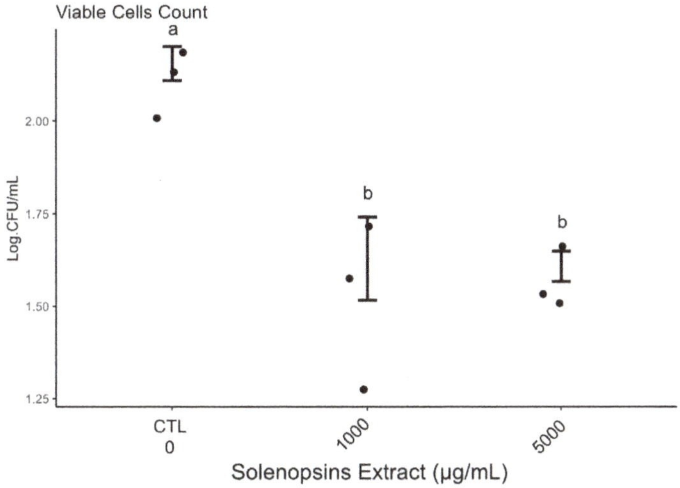

Figure 4. Viability of cells (in log/mL) recovered from biofilm of *Pseudomonas fluorescens* ATCC 13525 formed on surfaces of polystyrene conditioned with extracted solenopsins. No viable cells were recovered from a conditioned stainless steel coupon. Points are raw data and vertical whiskers represent SD around the mean; 'CTL' is negative control, and concentration groups topped by the same letter did not differ significantly by Dunn's test at alpha = 0.05.

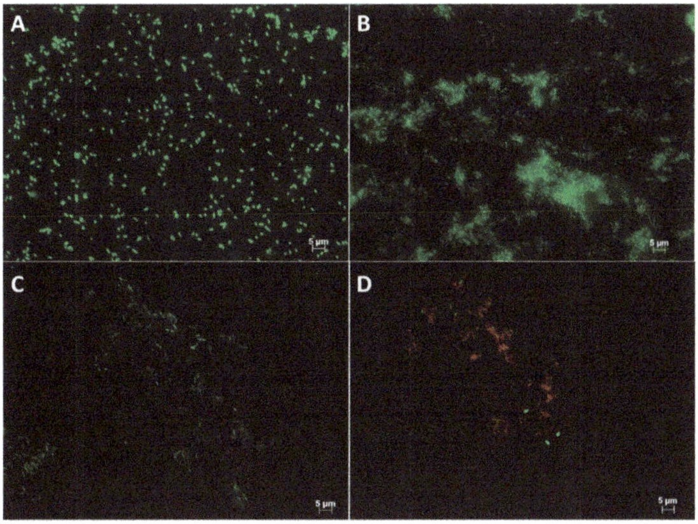

Figure 5. Surface adhesion by *Pseudomonas fluorescens* ATCC 13525 on polystyrene (left-hand panels) and stainless steel (right-hand panels) coupons after 24 h of incubation, as shown by epifluorescence of viable cells: Top panels (**A**,**B**) are negative non-conditioned controls; panels (**C**,**D**) are surfaces conditioned with 1000 µg/mL solenopsin alkaloids.

2.5. Physicochemical Properties: Surface Characteristics

Surface conditioning works by inhibiting microbial adhesion. This may be due to physicochemical surface alterations by amphiphilic (surface-active) compounds [19]. Therefore we tested the obtained solenopsins for a potential amphiphilic character, using the biosurfactant rhamnolipids as positive controls. Obtained contact angle measurements (Θ_W) and energetic characteristics of polystyrene and stainless steel coupons conditioned with solenopsins and rhamnolipids are shown in Table S1. Non-conditioned polystyrene and stainless steel surfaces were shown as hydrophobic, and become more hydrophilic only from conditioning with rhamnolipids. Accordingly, as illustrated by results in Table S2, conditioning with solenopsins does not change the hydrophobic character of these surfaces.

3. Discussion

Surfaces made of polystyrene and stainless steel AISI 304 are widely employed in industrial and healthcare facilities, where they frequently come into contact with organic material. The formation of surface biofilms offers a permanent source of food and instrumental contamination. Currently, disinfectants and harsh chemicals are used in preventing industrial biofilms, with limited efficiency. For instance, the most commonly-employed sanitisers in Brazilian food facilities are industrial chemicals based on the following active principles: quaternary ammonium amines, active chlorine released from bleaches and NaDCC, organic peroxide from peracetic acid, inorganic peroxide from oxygenated water, and iodine solutions [22]. Milk processing lines worldwide employ a cleaning protocol called Cleaning-in-Place (CIP) that is based on a series of surface washing steps using water and disinfectants at high temperatures. However, a systematic assessment of CIP demonstrates it is inefficient in controlling biofilm formation (e.g., [23]) and will not completely remove attached bacteria [24].

New strategies to improve the efficiency of surface cleaning are continuously proposed. For example, biodegradable low-toxicity biosurfactant extracts from microbes have gathered considerable attention for their antimicrobial and anti-adhesive activities [17–19]. Also, a number of plant-derived alkaloids have been demonstrated to inhibit the formation of and disperse bacterial biofilms [25–28] that are often attributed to either intrinsic direct antimicrobial activity [29] or unknown effects [26,28]. Solenopsins are animal-derived alkaloids active against a number of microbes [20,30,31] that have been demonstrated to affect biofilm formation via a molecular disruption of quorum sensing in *Pseudomonas aeruginosa* (Schroeter 1872) [21].

No previous investigation on the potential of solenopsin alkaloids for surface conditioning has been published to date, although the possibility was raised by Fox [20]. Herein we demonstrate conditioning of polystyrene and stainless steel surfaces with solenopsins from *S. invicta* results in inhibited posterior microbial adhesion.

3.1. Compounds Production/Extraction

It should be noted that the venom alkaloids extraction method [32] resulted (Table 1) in considerable variation in the relative proportions of solenopsin B (aka 'C13') and solenopsins C (aka 'C15') in comparison to a typical venom profile of *S. invicta* workers (e.g., compare with patterns presented in [33]). Whether the obtained pattern was a natural alteration associated with uncontrolled variables such as environmental conditions and relative proportions of collected castes, or representative of a local cryptic species (e.g., as in [33,34]) is the subject of ongoing investigation.

The properties of natural extracts are defined by their relative chemical composition, which ultimately depends on extraction methods. This leaves a number of open questions such as: What are the effects of the isolated isomers and their relative contributions to the observed effects? Would different combinations (or relative proportions) of isomers differently affect biofilm formation? These questions are currently under investigation in parallel studies using synthetic solenopsin analogues.

There are a number of published methods for the extraction and purification of venom alkaloids [32,35,36] that enable obtaining gram-amounts of solenopsins in different degrees of purity. Minding that fire ants are a top-concern world invasive species [37], harvesting solenopsins from highly infested areas may be feasible for small-scale applications. Concerning artificial synthesis, despite several published methods, purchasing artificial solenopsins is restricted to few companies (e.g., WuXi AppTec of Shanghai, China) and can be prohibitively expensive for large-scale applications. Nonetheless, remaining obstacles for obtaining the compounds are likely circumventable by a sudden increase in market demand, particularly considering the number of other biotech applications proposed for solenopsin alkaloids (reviewed in [20]).

3.2. Antimicrobial Activity

Figure 1 clearly illustrates dose-dependent antimicrobial activity of solenopsins against biofilm-secreting *P. fluorescens*. Following a similar test, Jouvenaz et al. [31] found limited antimicrobial activity of synthetic solenopsins diluted 1:1000 against four out of 12 tested Gram-negative bacteria, namely *Shigella flexneri*, *Sh. boydii*, *Salmonella typhimurium*, and *Sa. paratyphi* (Table 1 of p. 292 in [31]). All the active solenopsin analogues tested by Jouvenaz et al. [31] exhibited inhibition haloes of 8 mm diameter or less, which are suggestive of a weaker effect than the observed in our study for the extract doses of 750 µg/mL and above (Figure 1). As discussed in the previous section, some augmented effect may have resulted from a natural combination of different solenopsin analogues, which awaits further evaluation using synthetic mixtures simulating natural venoms. Another study testing the antimicrobial activities of solenopsins extracted from *S. invicta* reported a growth inhibition halo of about 15 mm using 3800 µg/mL of solenopsins against the Gram-positive bacterium *Clavibacter michiganensis*; this was roughly the same inhibition halo diameter observed in our study against *P. fluorescens*, but with the higher concentration of 5000 µg/mL. It should be minded that Gram-positive bacteria such as *C. michiganensis* are reported to be more susceptible to the effects of solenopsins than Gram-negative bacteria like *P. fluorescens*, as observed by Sullivan et al. [38] and Jouvenaz et al. [31]. Further dedicated studies screening natural and synthetic solenopsins against a range of microorganisms are needed in order to elucidate their relative antibiotic potential and microbial resistance.

The mechanism of antimicrobial action of solenopsins has remained unclear, but according to Lind [39], they may induce a permeability change in the plasmatic membrane, promoting leakage of cellular components. The same authors have proposed an amphipathic nature of the molecules as the origin of this property. We have, however, found no evidence of chemical surface-activity for solenopsins based on pilot tests compared with detergent controls (Table S3).

Other alkaloids of plant origin are known to present a broad spectrum of activity against bacteria and fungi [2,40], including active inhibition of biofilm formation. For example, Robbers et al. [41] observed that benzophenantridine from the roots of the bloodroot *Sanguinaria canadensis* suppresses bacteria from causing dental plaques. Also, Pereira et al. [42] demonstrated that alkaloids from the pomegranate *Punica granatum* reduced the adhesion of five strains of *Streptococcus* to glass surfaces.

3.3. Biofilm Formation and Suppression

Microbial biofilms are secreted by surface-adhered microorganisms. Therefore, inhibition of biofilm formation can be achieved by preventing microbial adhesion. A long-term strategy for protecting exposed surfaces against microbial adhesion is known as surface conditioning, which is based on the adsorption of antimicrobial or anti-adhesive molecules [19]. Preconditioning with solenopsin alkaloids inhibited the formation of biofilm regardless of the treated surfaces material (Figure 2). Lind et al. [39] suggested that solenopsins would have an amphipathic character, which might account for a change in surface physicochemical characteristics resulting in biofilm growth inhibition, as seen with natural detergents such as rhamnolipids and surfactins [17–19]. However, as discussed further in Section 3.5, the surface conditioning effects are not related to some detergent-like amphipathic chemical character of solenopsins, contrary to the proposed by Lind [39].

The effects of solenopsins on biofilms preformed on non-conditioned exposed surfaces (i.e., 'mature' biofilms) were also evaluated. Exposure of mature biofilms to solenopsins somehow resulted in the elimination of up to 56% of the biofilm from a polystyrene surface in a dose-dependent manner (Figure 3). However, on stainless steel surfaces, exposure to solenopsins yielded no reduction, and may have been accompanied by a small increase in secreted biofilm, which could be indicative of a counter-synergistic effect. This possibility deserves deeper investigation. A previous study by Park et al. [21] demonstrated that exposure to synthetic solenopsin A (aka 'C11', Table 1) dissolved in growth medium will inhibit biofilm formation by *P. aeruginosa* on non-conditioned surfaces via quorum sensing signaling interference.

3.4. Quantification of Viable Cells

Cell counts demonstrate a sharp reduction in the density of viable cells on polystyrene surfaces conditioned with solenopsins (Figure 4, Table S1). The same general pattern is confirmed by epifluorescence microscopy (Figure 5). No viable or cultivable cells were recovered from the matrix grown on conditioned steel (Table S1), which is suggestive of a stronger activity of the compounds when applied to the metal. This phenomenon warrants deeper investigation.

3.5. Physico-Chemical Tests for Surfactant Chemistry

The solenopsin alkaloids were tested to investigate their potential chemical characteristics as surfactants (surface-active compounds), since detergent-like (amphipathic properties) were suggested by some authors (e.g., Lind [39], pers. comm. of Dhammika Nanayakkara) as the likely mode of action for the antimicrobial activity of solenopsins. Amphipathic compounds physically interact by decreasing interfacial tension, thus leading to the formation of micelles, microemulsions, and adsorption to available surfaces. In theory, this chain of physicochemical processes could interfere with the microbial adhesion and biofilm formation [43,44].

According to Vogler [42], the degree of hydrophobicity is measured by the contact angle to water, where contact angles below 65° are indicative of hydrophilic surfaces. A surface is considered hydrophilic when the value of ΔGiwi (total free energy) is positive and Θ_W is less than 65°, and hydrophobic when the value of ΔGiwi is negative and Θ_W is greater than 65° [45–47]).

Conditioning with rhamnolipids has been described as affecting surface hydrophobicity [48,49] and the formation of bacterial biofilms [17]. Accordingly, the obtained rhamnolipids extract displayed remarkable tensioactive effects, illustrated by observed reduction in water surface tension. On the other hand, the solenopsins extract did not display any effect on water surface tension, possibly because of their apolar character, as these alkaloids are described to be largely insoluble in water [20]. Therefore, the mechanisms of biofilm inhibition by these alkaloids must be markedly different from that of biosurfactants, and not related to amphipathic chemistry.

4. Conclusions

The solenopsins extract exhibited potential application as a surface conditioning agent while acting as an antibiotic against biofilm formation. This class of compounds provides novel tools for the development of sustainable strategies to prevent or reduce biofilms on surfaces with potential application in different structural systems. Ongoing and future tests will provide further information into their modes of action, particularly for the solenopsin alkaloids of which so little is known.

5. Materials and Methods

5.1. Solenopsins Extraction and Purification

Nests of the fire ant *S. invicta* were collected from the university campus of the Federal University of Rio de Janeiro, Brazil, from which ants and their venom alkaloids were sequentially extracted following procedures detailed in [29]. Species identification was confirmed based on the presence of a clear frontal streak and a well-developed medial clypeal tooth [50]; voucher specimens were deposited at Museu Nacional do Rio de Janeiro (MNRJ). For venom purification, the obtained ants were immersed in a biphasic hexane/water (1:5) mixture, from which the organic phase was collected and passed through a glass column containing ca. 10 g of silica MESH 200–400 (Sigma, Mendota Heights, MN, USA). The column was washed three times with hexane (Merck, Kenilworth, NJ, USA, purity 98%), and finally the alkaloids were eluted with pure acetone (Merck, Kenilworth, NJ, USA, purity 99.8%). Obtained alkaloids were concentrated under a N_2 flux, and weighed with analytical scales.

The isomeric proportions of solenopsins were determined by a Gas Chromatography system coupled with Mass Spectrometry (GCMS, QP2010A Shimadzu, Rio de Janeiro, Brazil) according to procedures detailed in Fox et al. [51] (also see Supplementary Files). Obtained chromatogram peaks were identified as also described in [51] and tentatively quantified by relative area to an external standard (nicotine from Sigma-Aldrich, Mendota Heights, MN, USA) at 0.5 μg/μL using OpenChrom v. 1.1.0 (University of Hamburg, Hamburg, Germany).

5.2. *Microbial Tests*

Antimicrobial tests were performed with *Pseudomonas fluorescens,* which is a safer alternative to testing with the more ubiquitous pathogen *Pseudomonas aeruginosa* [6]. Stocked *P. fluorescens* cultures were inoculated in Petri dishes containing nutrient agar and incubated at 25 °C for 24 h. After this period, standard bacterial suspensions were adjusted to a concentration of 10^9 colony forming units (CFU)/mL, according to [18].

5.2.1. Antimicrobial Activity

Antimicrobial activity was assessed by the method of disc diffusion as described in [52], and the minimum inhibitory concentration (MIC) was estimated by logarithm linear regression [53]. Suspensions of 10^6 CFU/mL of *P. fluorescens* were obtained by serial dilutions, estimated by a spectrophotometer at 600 nm wavelength to a final volume of 100 μL, and spread on a Petri dish containing nutrient agar. Sterile filter paper discs (Whatman 3) of 6 mm diameter were immersed in the different concentrations of solenopsins (500, 750, 1000, and 5000 μg/mL) in ethanol. Negative controls had pure ethanol. Following solvent evaporation, paper discs were placed at the centre of the inoculated Petri dishes, which were incubated at 25 °C for 24 h. The diameter of the inhibition halo was measured from the rim of the paper disc using a caliper. Four independent replications were carried out.

5.2.2. Quantification of Biofilm Formation

Biofilm formation was induced by inoculating 20 μL aliquots of standardised suspensions from Section 5.2.1. into 96-well microplates made of either polystyrene (OLen from Kasvi, São José do Pinhais, Brazil) or stainless steel (AISI 304) containing a nutrient broth. These microplates were kept at 25 °C for different time periods to perform biofilm formation kinetics. At the end of each time period, the growth medium was removed, wells were carefully washed with distilled water, fixed for 15 min with methanol (Merck, São Paulo, Brazil; 99.9% purity), and stained for 20 min with 1% (*w/v*) crystal violet after [54]. Finally, the optical density at 570 nm of the stained solution was measured as an estimation for overall cell adhesion following Stepanovic et al. [55]. Mean values are presented from four independent experiments.

5.2.3. Effect of Surface Conditioning on Cell Adhesion

Microplates, as described in Section 5.2.2, were surface-conditioned according to Nitschke et al. [19]. Surface conditioning solutions of solenopsins were prepared in ethanol (Merck, São Paulo, Brazil; 99.5% purity) at the concentrations of 0, 100, 500, 750, 1000, or 5000 μg/mL. After 24 h of conditioning by immersion, the plate surfaces were washed with sterile distilled water and left to dry at room temperature. Cell adhesion was estimated with crystal violet, as described in Section 5.2.2.

5.2.4. Effect of Surface Conditioning on Cell Viability

Polystyrene and stainless steel surfaces were conditioned as described in Section 5.2.3 and inoculated with a suspension of 10^9 CFU/mL of *P. fluorescens*. Following biofilm formation, surfaces were washed to remove any non-adhered cells, and biofilms were scraped off for analysis. The proportion of viable cells recovered from biofilms growing on conditioned surfaces were estimated by the plate spreading technique. A 100-μL aliquot per sample was spread using a sterile Drigalski loop onto a Petri dish containing nutrient agar. Dishes were incubated at 25 °C for 24 h, and the resulting CFU were visually counted.

5.2.5. Epifluorescence Microscopy Observations

Plate coupons (2 cm^2) of polystyrene and stainless steel were conditioned as described in Section 5.2.3 with 1 mg/mL solenopsins for 24 h at 25 °C, and immersed in a nutrient broth containing 10^9 CFU/mL *P. fluorescens*. These surfaces were incubated at 25 °C for 20 h and 16 h, respectively, washed with distilled water to remove non-adhered cells, and stained with the bacterial cell viability fluorescent marker L7012 LIVE/DEAD® Baclight^{TM} (Molecular Probes Inc., Eugene, OR, USA) according to the manufacturer's manual. Finally, the treated surfaces were observed under a Zeiss Axioplan 2 microscope (Oberkochen, Germany) equipped with an epifluorescence system under excitation/emission wavelengths of 480/500 nm for SYTO 9 and 490/635 nm for propidium iodite. Pictures were taken with a digital camera Color View XS (AnalySIS GmBH, Karlsruhe, Germany).

5.3. *Physico-Chemical Tests for Surfactant Chemistry*

The obtained solenopsins extract was subjected to physicochemical assays to test for a potential amphiphilic character. The natural biosurfactants known as rhamnolipids—well-known amphiphilic compounds with anti-biofilm activity [17,49,56]—were used as positive controls.

5.3.1. Extraction of Biosurfactants (Positive Controls)

Rhamnolipid production from *P. aeruginosa* was induced by procedures described elsewhere [57]. Cells were removed by centrifugation, and the supernatant containing the compounds was sterilised, filtered (pore size 0.45 μm), and stored at 4 °C until use. The supernatant was acidified with 1.0 N HCl to pH 3.5 and directly extracted with ethyl acetate 1:3, from which the organic phase was recovered, and incubated with anhydrous sodium sulfate to remove water residues. The extract was recovered from the solvent using a rotary evaporator, redissolved in methanol, and finally lyophilised. The obtained extract was partitioned with methanol: chloroform: 2-propanol in the ratio of 1:2:4 with 7.5 mM ammonia acetate, and finally centrifuged at 12,000× *g* for 5 min to remove impurities.

5.3.2. Physicochemical Properties

The obtained crude extracts of solenopsins and rhamnolipids were subjected to analyses of surface tension (ST) and critical micellar concentration (CMC). These physicochemical properties were estimated based on the pendant drop technique on a drop shape analyser (DSA 100S Model OF3210) following [58,59]. Measurements for ST and CMC were taken from n = 10 drops at 23 °C and 55% relative humidity.

5.3.3. Surface Characteristics

Small coupons (2 cm^2) of either polystyrene or stainless steel grade 304 were cleaned as in [19], and conditioned with either rhamnolipids or solenopsins. The conditioned surfaces were washed with distilled water and left to dry at room temperature. Finally, the sessile drop method described in Section 5.3.2. was used to measure the contact angle between the surface and 7 μL droplets of distilled water, formamide, and ethylene glycol using a goniometer. The angles were measured as described in [46] at 23 °C and 55% relative humidity.

The surface free energy obtained from the contact angle was calculated from the surface tension components of each tested liquid according to the equation below (as in Van Oss et al. [60]):

$$(1 + cos\theta)\gamma_i^{TOT} = 2\left[\left(\sqrt{\gamma_s^{LW}\gamma_i^{LW}}\right) + \left(\sqrt{\gamma_s^{+}\gamma_i^{-}}\right) + \left(\sqrt{\gamma_s^{-}\gamma_i^{+}}\right)\right]$$

where θ is the contact angle between the liquid and the surface, γ^{TOT} is the total surface free energy, γ^{LW} is the Lifshitz-van der Waals component, γ^{AB} is the Lewis acid-base property, and γ^{+} e γ^{-} are the electron acceptor and donor components, respectively; $\gamma^{TOT} = \gamma^{LW} + \gamma^{AB}$ and $\gamma^{AB} = 2\sqrt{\gamma^{+}\gamma^{-}}$.

Surface hydrophobicity was determined by contact angle measurements using the approach of Van Oss et al. [60] and Van Oss [46]. The results were calculated according to the equation below:

$$\Delta Giwi = -2\left(\sqrt{\gamma_l^{LW} - \gamma_w^{LW}}\right) - 4\left(\sqrt{\gamma_l^{+}\gamma_w^{-}} + \sqrt{\gamma_w^{-}\gamma_l^{+}} - \sqrt{\gamma_l^{+}\gamma_l^{-}} - \sqrt{\gamma_w^{+}\gamma_w^{-}}\right)$$

5.3.4. Hydrophilic-Lipophilic Balance (HLB)

The HLB value indicates whether a surfactant will promote water-in-oil or oil-in-water emulsions. According to Griffin [61], the HLB can be calculated as:

$$\text{HLB} = 20 \times (\text{MWHP}/\text{MWSA})$$

where MWHP is the molecular weight of the hydrophilic part and MWSA is the molecular weight of the whole surface-active agent, giving a result on a scale of 0 to 20. An HLB value of 0 corresponds to a completely lipophilic/hydrophobic molecule, and a value of 20 corresponds to a completely hydrophilic/lipophobic molecule. The HLB value can be used to predict the surfactant properties of a molecule (see Table S2).

5.4. Statistics

All analyses and plots were generated with R v. 3.0.0 using 'ggplot2' and packages 'ddply' and 'reshape2.' Raw data, as well as plotting and analytical scripts, are provided as Supplementary Materials. Results were analysed non-parametrically using Wilcoxon–Mann–Whitney (2-factorial analyses) or Kruskal–Wallis (3-factorial analyses) tests. Equivalent results are obtained by parametric counterparts (not shown).

Supplementary Materials: The following are available online at http://www.mdpi.com/2072-6651/11/7/420/s1, Figure S1: Representative chromatogram of venom alkaloids extracted with hexane, Figure S2: Linear regression from mean obtained inhibition halos from disk-diffusion using different concentrations (µg/mL) of solenopsins added to a confluent Pseudomonas fluorescens growth plate, incubated at 25 °C for 24 h, Table S1: Viability of cells recovered from 1 mL of biofilm of *Pseudomonas fluorescens* formed on surfaces of polystyrene or stainless steel conditioned with venom solenopsins extracted from the fire ant *Solenopsis invicta*, Table S2: Values of surfactants and their respective applications (Adapted from [54]), Table S3: Physicochemical properties of surfaces conditioned with rhamnolipids extracted from *Pseudomonas aeruginosa* and venom solenopsins extracted from red imported fire ants *Solenopsis invicta;* R scripts used for statistical analyses and generating figures, including raw data; Raw chromatogram GM-MS data file of obtained solenopsins, Raw GC-MS method settings file.

Author Contributions: Conceptualization, E.G.P.F. and E.d.A.M.; methodology, E.d.A.M., L.V.A.d.C.; software, E.G.P.F.; formal analysis, D.B.d.C., L.V.A.d.C., E.G.P.F., J.S.d.S.; investigation, D.B.d.C., D.G.d.S., L.V.A.d.C.; resources, E.d.A.M., G.B.D., F.C.S.N.; data curation, D.B.d.C., L.V.A.d.C., E.G.P.F.; writing—original draft preparation, D.B.d.C., L.V.A.d.C.; writing—review and editing, E.G.P.F.; supervision, E.d.A.M., G.B.D., L.V.A.d.C.; project administration, E.d.A.M., D.M.G.F.; funding acquisition, E.d.A.M., D.M.G.F.

Funding: This research was funded by Conselho Nacional de Desenvolvimento Científico e Tecnológico (CNPq) grant no. 150895/2010-0.

Acknowledgments: Authors wish to thank Eric Lucas for grammar revision, and Yijuan Xu for hosting E.G.P.F. during manuscript preparation. Mileane de Souza Busch and Georgia Correa Atella provided access and assistance with GC-MS equipment. Five reviewers contributed with comments and insightful discussions.

Conflicts of Interest: The authors declare no conflict of interest. The funders had no role in the design of the study; in the collection, analyses, or interpretation of data; in the writing of the manuscript, or in the decision to publish the results.

References

1. Dunne, W.M., Jr. Bacterial adhesion: Seen any good biofilms lately? *Clin. Microbiol.* **2002**, *15*, 155–166. [CrossRef] [PubMed]
2. Xu, D.; Jia, R.; Li, Y.; Gu, T. Advances in the treatment of problematic industrial biofilms. *World J. Microbiol. Biotechnol.* **2017**, *33*, 2–10. [CrossRef] [PubMed]
3. Donlan, R.M. Biofilms and device-associated infections. *Emerg. Infect. Dis.* **2001**, *7*, 277–281. [CrossRef] [PubMed]
4. Kumar, C.G.; Anand, S.K. Significance of microbial biofilms in food industry: A review. *Int. J. Food Microbiol.* **1998**, *42*, 9–27. [CrossRef]
5. Costernon, J.W.; Irving, R.T.; Chen, K.J. The bacterial glycocalix in nature and disease. *Annu. Rev. Microbiol.* **1981**, *35*, 299–304. [CrossRef] [PubMed]
6. Costerton, J.W.; Korber, D.R.; Lappin-Scott, H.M. Microbial biofilms. *Annu. Rev. Microbiol.* **1995**, *49*, 711–745. [CrossRef] [PubMed]
7. Drenkard, E. Antimicrobial resistance of *Pseudomonas aeruginosa* biofilms. *Microbes Infect. Inst. Pasteur* **2003**, *5*, 1213–1219. [CrossRef]
8. Hood, S.K.; Zottola, E. Biofilms in food processing. *Food Control. Oxf.* **1995**, *6*, 9–18. [CrossRef]
9. Jenkinson, H.F.; Lappin-Scott, H.M. Biofilms adhere to stay. *Trends Microbiol.* **2001**, *9*, 9–10. [CrossRef]
10. Djordjevic, D.; Wiedmann, M.; McLandsborough, L.A. Microtiter plate assay for assessment of *Listeria monocytogenes* biofilm formation. *Appl. Environ. Microbiol.* **2002**, *68*, 2950–2958. [CrossRef]
11. Klosowska-Chomiczewska, I.; Medrzycka, K.; Karpenko, E. Biosurfactants—Biodegradability, toxicity, efficiency in comparison with synthetic surfactants. *Adv. Chem. Mech. Eng.* **2011**, *2*, 1–9.
12. O'Toole, G.A.; Kolter, R. Initiation of biofilm formation in *Pseudomonas fluorescens* WCS365 proceeds via multiple, convergent signalling pathways: A genetic analysis. *Mol. Microbiol.* **1998**, *28*, 449–461. [CrossRef] [PubMed]
13. Hinsa, S.M.; Espinosa-Urgel, M.; Ramos, J.L.; O'Toole, G.A. Transition from reversible to irreversible attachment during biofilm formation by *Pseudomonas fluorescens* requires an ABC transporter and a large secreted protein. *Mol. Microbiol.* **2003**, *49*, 905–918. [CrossRef] [PubMed]
14. Wiedmann, M.; Weilmeier, D.; Dineen, S.S.; Ralyea, R.; Boor, K.J. Molecular and Phenotypic characterization of *Pseudomonas* spisolated from milk. *Appl. Environ. Microbiol.* **2000**, *66*, 2085–2095. [CrossRef] [PubMed]
15. Rawat, S. Food Spoilage: Microorganisms and their prevention. *Asian J. Plant. Sci. Res.* **2015**, *5*, 47–56.
16. Mattila-Sandholm, T.; Wirtanen, G. Biofilm formation in the industry: A review. *Food Rev. Int.* **1992**, *8*, 573–603. [CrossRef]
17. Araujo, L.V.; Freire, D.M.G.; Nitschke, M. Biossurfactantes: Propriedades anticorrosivas, antibiofilmes e antimicrobianas. *Quim. Nova* **2013**, *36*, 848–858. [CrossRef]
18. Araujo, L.V.; Abreu, F.; Lins, U.; Anna, L.M.M.; Nitschke, M.; Freire, D.M.G. Rhamnolipid and surfactin inhibit *Listeria monocytogenes* adhesion. *Food Res. Int.* **2011**, *44*, 481–488. [CrossRef]
19. Nitschke, M.; Araújo, V.; Costa, S.G.V.A.O.; Pires, R.C.; Zeraik, A.E.; Fernandes, A.C.L.B.; Freire, D.M.G.; Contiero, J. Surfactin reduces the adhesion of food-borne pathogenic bacteria to solid surface. *Lett. Appl. Microbiol.* **2009**, *49*, 241–247. [CrossRef]
20. Fox, E.G. Venom toxins of fire ants. In *Venom Genomics and Proteomics*; Gopalakrishnakone, P., Calvete, J.J., Eds.; Springer: Dordrecht, The Netherlands, 2014; pp. 1–16.
21. Park, J.; Kaufmann, G.F.; Bowen, J.P.; Arbiser, J.L.; Janda, K.D. Solenopsin A, a venom alkaloid from the fire ant *Solenopsis invicta*, inhibits quorum sensing signalling in *Pseudomonas aeruginosa*. *J. Infect. Dis.* **2008**, *198*, 1198–1201. [CrossRef]
22. Andrade, N.J. Higienização na indústria de alimentos: Avaliação e controle da adesão e formação de biofilmes bacterianos. In *Higienização na Indústria de Alimentos: Avaliação e Controle da Adesão e Formação de Biofilmes Bacterianos*; Livraria Varela: São Paulo, Brazil, 2008.
23. Dufour, M.; Simmonds, R.S.; Bremer, J. Development of a laboratory scale clean-in-place system to test the effectiveness of "natural" antimicrobials against dairy biofilms. *J. Food Prot.* **2004**, *67*, 1438–1443. [CrossRef] [PubMed]

24. Bremer, J.; Fillery, S.; McQuillan, A.J. Laboratory scale clean-in-place (CIP) studies on the effectiveness of different caustic and acid wash steps on the removal of dairy biofilms. *Int. J. Food Microbiol.* **2006**, *106*, 254–262. [CrossRef] [PubMed]
25. Huigens, R.W.; Rogers, S.A.; Steinhauer, A.T.; Melander, C. Inhibition of *Acinetobacter baumannii*, *Staphylococcus aureus* and *Pseudomonas aeruginosa* biofilm formation with a class of TAGE-triazole conjugates. *Org. Biomol. Chem.* **2009**, *7*, 794–802. [CrossRef] [PubMed]
26. Wang, X.; Yao, X.; Zhu, Z.; Tang, T.; Dai, K.; Sadovskaya, I.; Jabbouri, S. Effect of berberine on *Staphylococcus epidermidis* biofilm formation. *Int. J. Antimicrob. Agents* **2009**, *34*, 60–66. [CrossRef] [PubMed]
27. Majik, M.S.; Naik, D.; Bhat, C.; Tilve, S.; Tilvi, S.; D'Souza, L. Synthesis of (R)-norbgugaine and its potential as quorum sensing inhibitor against *Pseudomonas aeruginosa*. *Bioorganic Med. Chem. Lett.* **2013**, *23*, 2353–2356. [CrossRef] [PubMed]
28. Furlani, R.E.; Yeagley, A.A.; Melander, C. A flexible approach to 1,4-di-substituted 2-aminoimidazoles that inhibit and disperse biofilms and potentiate the effects of ß-lactams against multi-drug resistant bacteria. *Eur. J. Med. Chem.* **2013**, *62*, 59–70. [CrossRef] [PubMed]
29. Skogman, M.E.; Kujala, J.; Busygin, I.; Leino, R.; Vuorela, P.M.; Fallarero, A. Evaluation of antibacterial and antibiofilm activities of cinchona alkaloid derivatives against *Staphylococcus aureus*. *Nat. Prod. Commun.* **2012**, *7*, 1173–1176.
30. Li, S.; Jin, X.; Chen, J.; Lu, S. Inhibitory activities of venom alkaloids of Red Imported Fire Ant against *Clavibacter michiganensis* subs*michiganensis* in vitro and the application of piperidine alkaloids to manage symptom development of bacterial canker on tomato in the greenhouse. *Int. J. Pest. Manag.* **2013**, *59*, 150–156. [CrossRef]
31. Jouvenaz, D.P.; Blum, M.S.; MacConnell, J.G. Antibacterial activity of venom alkaloids from the imported fire ant, *Solenopsin invicta* Buren. *Antimicrob. Agents Chemother.* **1972**, *2*, 291–293. [CrossRef]
32. Fox, E.G.P.; Solis, D.R.; Santos, L.D.; Pinto, J.R.A.S.; Menegasso, A.R.S.; Silva, R.C.M.C.; Palma, M.S.; Bueno, O.C.; Machado, E.A. A simple, rapid method for the extraction of whole fire ant venom (Insecta: Formicidae: *Solenopsis*). *Toxicon* **2013**, *65*, 5–8.
33. Fox, E.G.P. Chemical blueprints to identifying fire ants: Overview on venom alkaloids. *BioRxiv* **2018**, *2018*, 407775. [CrossRef]
34. Fox, E.G.P.; Pianaro, A.; Solis, D.R.; Delabie, J.H.C.; Vairo, B.C.; MacHado, E.D.A.; Bueno, O.C. Intraspecific and intracolonial variation in the profile of venom alkaloids and cuticular hydrocarbons of the fire ant *Solenopsis saevissima* Smith (Hymenoptera: Formicidae). *Psyche J. Entomol.* **2012**, *2012*, 398061. [CrossRef]
35. Fox, E.G.P.; Xu, M.; Wang, L.; Chen, L.; Lu, Y.Y. Speedy milking of fresh venom from aculeate hymenopterans. *Toxicon* **2019**, *146*, 120–123. [CrossRef] [PubMed]
36. Shi, Q.-H.; Hu, L.; Wang, W.-K.; Vander Meer, R.K.; Porter, S.D.; Chen, L. Workers and alate queens of *Solenopsis geminata* share qualitatively similar but quantitatively different venom alkaloid chemistry. *Front. Ecol. Evol.* **2015**, *3*. [CrossRef]
37. IUCN. View 100 of the World's Worst Invasive Alien Species [EB/OL]. Available online: http://www.issg.org/worst100_species.html (accessed on 6 May 2019).
38. Sullivan, D.C.; Flowers, H.; Rockhold, R.; Herath, H.M.T.B.; Nanayakkara, N.P.D. Antibacterial activity of synthetic fire ant venom: The solenopsins and isosolenopsins. *Am. J. Med. Sci.* **2009**, *338*, 287–291. [CrossRef] [PubMed]
39. Lind, N.K. Mechanisms of action of fire ant (*Solenopsis*) venom I. Lytic release histamine from mast cells. *Toxicon* **1982**, *20*, 831–840. [CrossRef]
40. Hullin, V.; Mathat, A.G.; Mafart, P.; Dufosé, L. Les proprietés anti-microbiennes des huiles essentielles et composés d'arômes. *Sci. Des. Aliment.* **1998**, *18*, 563–582.
41. Robbers, J.E.; Speedie, M.K.; Tyler, V.E. *Farmacognosia & Farmacobiotecnologia*; Editora Premier: São Paulo, Brazil, 1997.
42. Pereira, J.V.; Pereira, M.S.V.; Sampaio, F.C.; Sampaio, M.C.C.; Alves, P.M.; Araujo, C.R.F.; Higino, J.S. Efeito antibacteriano e antiaderente in vitro do extrato da *Punica granatum* Linn. sobre microrganismos do biofilme dental. *Braz. J. Pharmacogn.* **2006**, *16*, 88–93. [CrossRef]
43. Mclandsborough, L.; Rodriguez, A.; Perez-Conesa, D.; Weiss, J. Biofilms: At the interface between biophysics and microbiology. *Food Biophys.* **2006**, *1*, 94–114. [CrossRef]

44. Nitschke, M.; Costa, S.G.V.A. Biosurfactants in food industry. *Trends Food Sci. Technol.* **2007**, *18*, 252–259. [CrossRef]
45. Vogler, E.A. Structure and reactivity of water at biomaterial surface. *Adv. Colloid Interface Sci.* **1998**, *74*, 69–117. [CrossRef]
46. Van Oss, C.J. Hydrophobicity of biosurfaces origin, quantitative determination and interaction energies. *Colloids Surf. B Biointerfaces* **1995**, *5*, 91–110. [CrossRef]
47. Araujo, E.A.; Andrade, N.J.; Carvalho, A.F.; Ramos, A.M.; Silva, C.A.S.; Silva, L.H.M. Aspectos coloidais da adesão de microrganismos. *Quim. Nova* **2009**, *33*, 1940–1948. [CrossRef]
48. Gomes, M.Z.V.; Nitschke, M. Evaluation of rhamnolipid and surfactin to reduce the adhesion and remove biofilms of individual and mixed cultures of food pathogenic bacteria. *Food Control.* **2012**, *25*, 441–447. [CrossRef]
49. Araujo, L.V.; Guimarães, C.R.; Marquita, R.L.S.; Santiago, V.M.J.; Souza, M.P.; Nitschke, M.; Freire, D.M.G. Rhamnolipid and surfactin: Anti-adhesion/antibiofilm and antimicrobial effects. *Food Control.* **2016**, *63*, 171–178. [CrossRef]
50. Pitts, J.P.; McHugh, J.V.; Ross, K.G. Cladistic analysis of the fire ants of the *Solenopsis saevissima* species-group (Hymenoptera: Formicidae). *Zool. Scr.* **2005**, *34*, 493–505. [CrossRef]
51. Fox, E.G.P.; Solis, D.R.; Lazoski, C.; Mackay, W. Weaving through a cryptic species: Comparing the Neotropical ants *Camponotus senex* and *Camponotus textor* (Hymenoptera: Formicidae). *Micron* **2017**, *99*, 56–66. [CrossRef] [PubMed]
52. Li, L. Screening and partial characterization of *Bacillus* with potential applications in biocontrol of cucumber *Fusarium* wilt. *Crop. Prot. Amst.* **2012**, *35*, 29–35. [CrossRef]
53. Bonev, B.; Hooper, J.; Parisot, J. Principles of assessing bacterial susceptibility to antibiotics using the agar diffusion method. *J. Antimicrob. Chemother.* **2008**, *61*, 1295–1301. [CrossRef]
54. Stepanovic, S.; Cirkovic, I.; Ranin, L.; Svabic-Vlahovic, M. Biofilm formation by *Salmonella* spand *Listeria* monocytogenes on plastic surface. *Lett. Appl. Microbiol.* **2004**, *38*, 428–432. [CrossRef]
55. Stepanovic, S.; Vukovic, D.; Dakic, I.; Savic, B.; Svabic-Vlahovic, M. A modified microtiter-plate test for quantification of staphylococcal biofilm formation. *J. Microbiol. Methods Columbia* **2000**, *40*, 175–179. [CrossRef]
56. Sotirova, A.V.; Spasova, D.I.; Galabova, D.N.; Karpenko, E.; Shulga, A. Rhamnolipid-biosurfactant permeabilizing effects on gram-positive and gram-negative bacterial strains. *Curr. Microbiol.* **2008**, *56*, 639–644. [CrossRef] [PubMed]
57. Santos, S.A.; Sampaio, A.P.; Vasquez, G.S.; Santa Anna, L.M.; Freire, D.M.G. Evaluation of different carbon in nitrogen sources in production of rhamnolipids by a strain of *Pseudomonas aeruginosa*. *Appl. Biochem. Biotechnol.* **2002**, *98*, 1025–1035. [CrossRef]
58. Song, B.; Springer, J. Determination of interfacial tension from the profile of a pendant drop using computer-aided image processing. *J. Colloid Interface Sci.* **1996**, *184*, 64–76. [PubMed]
59. Sheppard, J.D.; Mulligan, C.N. The production of surfactin by *Bacillus subtilis* grown on peat hydrolysate. *Appl. Microbiol. Biotechnol.* **1987**, *27*, 110–116. [CrossRef]
60. Van Oss, C.J.M.; Chaudhury, I.C.; Good, R.J. Interfacial Lifshitz-van der Waals and polar interactions in macroscopic systems. *Chem. Rev.* **1988**, *88*, 927–941. [CrossRef]
61. Griffin, W.C. Classification of surface-active agents by "HLB". *J. Soc. Cosmet. Chem.* **1949**, *1*, 311–326.

toxins

MDPI

Article

Antiparasitic Properties of Cantharidin and the Blister Beetle *Berberomeloe majalis* (Coleoptera: Meloidae)

Douglas W. Whitman [1], Maria Fe Andrés [2], Rafael A. Martínez-Díaz [3], Alexandra Ibáñez-Escribano [4], A. Sonia Olmeda [5] and Azucena González-Coloma [2,*]

1. School of Biological Sciences, Illinois State University, Normal, IL 61790, USA; dwwhitm@ilstu.edu
2. Instituto de Ciencias Agrarias, CSIC, Serrano 115-dpdo, 28006 Madrid, Spain; mafay@ica.csic.es
3. Facultad de Medicina, Universidad Autónoma de Madrid (UAM), Arzobispo Morcillo S/N, 28029 Madrid, Spain; rafael.martinez@uam.es
4. Facultad de Farmacia, Universidad Complutense de Madrid (UCM), CEI Campus Moncloa, 28040 Madrid, Spain; alexandraibanez@ucm.es
5. Facultad de Veterinaria, Universidad Complutense (UCM), 28040 Madrid, Spain; angeles@ucm.es

* Correspondence: azu@ica.csic.es; Tel.: +34-917-452-500

Received: 4 April 2019; Accepted: 18 April 2019; Published: 22 April 2019

check for updates

Abstract: Cantharidin (CTD) is a toxic monoterpene produced by blister beetles (Fam. Meloidae) as a chemical defense against predators. Although CTD is highly poisonous to many predator species, some have evolved the ability to feed on poisonous Meloidae, or otherwise beneficially use blister beetles. Great Bustards, *Otis tarda*, eat CTD-containing *Berberomeloe majalis* blister beetles, and it has been hypothesized that beetle consumption by these birds reduces parasite load (a case of self-medication). We examined this hypothesis by testing diverse organisms against CTD and extracts of *B. majalis* hemolymph and bodies. Our results show that all three preparations (CTD and extracts of *B. majalis*) were toxic to a protozoan (*Trichomonas vaginalis*), a nematode (*Meloidogyne javanica*), two insects (*Myzus persicae* and *Rhopalosiphum padi*) and a tick (*Hyalomma lusitanicum*). This not only supports the anti-parasitic hypothesis for beetle consumption, but suggests potential new roles for CTD, under certain conditions.

Keywords: cantharidin; blister beetle; *Berberomeloe majalis*; nematicide; ixodicide; antifeedant

Key Contribution: Cantharidin is active against a diverse range of organisms including protozoa; nematodes; ticks; and insects; supporting the hypothesis that Great Bustards might reduce parasite loads via ingestion of blister beetles.

1. Introduction

Cantharidin (CTD) is a toxic trycyclic monoterpene with the chemical formula: 3,6-epoxy-1,2-dimethylcyclohexane-1,2-dicarboxylic anhydride (Figure 1). Found in blister beetles, CTD was one of the first pharmacoactive natural products used by humans [1–3], and was long considered a sexual stimulant [4–8]. In the late Middle Ages, *Lytta vesicatoria* blister beetles were collected and sold throughout Europe as an aphrodisiac, known as "Spanish Fly" (Figure 2) [9–13]. Today, CTD is used on humans to treat both common and molluscum warts, to remove tattoos, and as a counterirritant, and, until recently, was used as a sexual stimulant in livestock breeding [4,14]. Against vertebrates, CTD is a powerful vesicant and highly toxic. However, in low doses it "stimulates" or irritates vertebrate mucus membranes [10,15,16]. Human ingestion can result in vomiting, diarrhea, bleeding from the gastrointestinal tract, nephritis, hematuria, proteinuria, liver, kidney and other organ edema and failure, and death [4,16–21]. The consumption of beetles in fresh forage or hay, or drinking beetle- contaminated water, can seriously harm pets, poultry, or livestock [16,18,22,23].

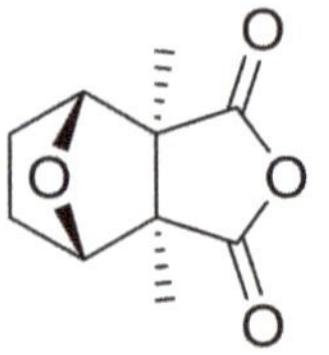

Figure 1. Cantharidin.

Biochemically, CTD acts at multiple levels [16]. It is a potent and specific inhibitor of protein phosphatases 1 (PP1) and 2A (PP2A) [24,25]. It causes the release of serine proteases, which break the peptide bonds in proteins, destroying the adhesion between cells, releasing fluids and causing blistering and bleeding [4]. It disrupts mitosis [16].

CTD was first discovered in blister beetles (Order: Coleoptera; Family: Meloidae), a group of ~3000 species found in temperate and tropical regions world-wide [16,26]. Most meloids are chemically protected from predators by the presence of CTD, which also plays a role in mating [27]. CTD is transferred from males to females during mating in CTD producing insects [28]. Furthermore, CTD synthesis takes place in the male body and is finally deposited in the testes—hemolymph transport is not involved. In females, CTD enters the genitalia from the male as a nuptial gift [28].

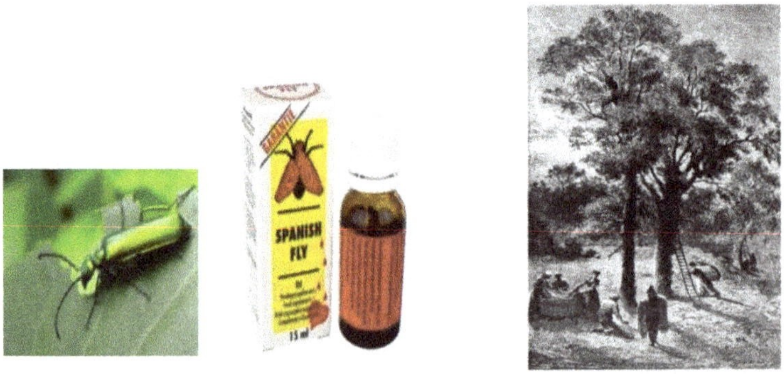

Figure 2. Spanish fly (*Lytta vesicatoria*) (from Stefanie Hamm), an example of commercial cantharadin preparation, and collecting blister beetles in Spain in the 17th Century.

A few insect predators have evolved partial immunity to CTD and, in some cases, actually use this poisonous substance for their own benefit. Some insects [27], frogs, toads [29], birds [30], and mammals [31] consume them in the wild. Other uses described include the protection of white breasted nuthatches nestholes by sweeping the bark with a meloid insect [32] or traditional pharmacological use by humans [33].

For example, great bustards, *Otis tarda*, a vulnerable and protected bird species in Europe, consume red-striped oil beetles, *Berberomeloe majalis*, a common CTD-containing blister beetle in the Mediterranean area, even though the beetle is highly toxic [17,34,35]. Bravo et al. (2014) [36] suggest that beetle consumption by bustards (particularly males) represents CTD self-medication to reduce parasites and diarrhea that impair the appearance of the cloaca of the birds (a central element of courtship), thus increasing their chances of reproduction.

Bravo et al.'s hypothesis is reasonable, considering that CTD is bactericidal [36], and that birds are greatly harmed by a diverse range of pathogens and parasites, including numerous bacteria, protozoa, helminths and arthropods. The protozoans *Eimeria spp.*, *Cryptosporidium spp.*, *Giardia spp.*, *Trichomonas spp.*, *Histomonas spp.* and *Hexamita spp.* commonly infect bird digestive tracts [37]. Two protozoa cause oropharyngeal diseases in bustards: *Trichomonas gallinae* and *Entamoeba anatis* [38]. Cestodes (*Hispaniolepis sp., Raillietina cesticillus, Schistometra (Otiditaenia) conoides*, and *Idiogenes otidis*), nematodes (*Capillaria sp., Syngamus trachea, Cyathostoma sp., Heterakis gallinae, H. isolench, Aprocta orbitalis, Oxyspirura hispanica*, and *Trichostrongylus sp*), insects (including mallophaga such as *Otilipeurus turmalis*, and fly maggots such as *Lucilia sericata*) and ticks (*Rhipicephalus sanguineus*, and *Hyalomma sp.*) also infest bustards [37,39,40].

In this paper, we examine Bravo et al.'s (2014) hypothesis [36], by testing the antiparasitic efficacy of both pure CTD and extracts of *B. majalis* beetles against protozoa (*Trichomonas vaginalis*), a nematode (*Meloidogyne javanica*), and a tick (*Hyalomma lusitanicum*). Additionally, several phytophagous insects (*Myzus persicae, Rhopalosiphum padi, Spodoptera littoralis*) have been tested to include target species other than meloid predators or bird parasites. Our results show strong anti-parasite activity, supporting Bravo et al.'s hypothesis, and suggesting new roles for CTD.

2. Results and Discussion

Cantharidin (CTD) concentrations vary greatly between and within Meloid species. Various studies have found from <0.04 to 30.3 mg CTD/individual beetles [16,41–43]. Variation in arthropod defense titers is well known [44]. In *Berberomeloe majalis* the reported CTD content in adults varied between 0.035–1.89 mg/beetle (0.015–0.845 mg/g) [34] and 1.05–109.2 mg / beetle (1.5–156.7 mg/g) [36]. Our analysis (Table 1) indicated CTD concentrations of 295 and 41.2 μg/mg in our hemolymph extract and body extract, respectively, indicating that the hemolymph extract was ~7 times more concentrated in CTD than the body extract. The total CTD contained in 200 insects was 1819 mg (hemolymph + body), giving an estimated value of 9.1 mg of CTD per beetle. These concentrations are within the ranges reported by Bravo et al. (2014) [36]. We detected relatively low amounts of CTD in *B. majalis* hemolymph as opposed to the beetle bodies (Table 1). This is not surprising, considering that CTD is typically concentrated in meloid reproductive organs [28].

Table 1. Cantharidin (CTD) concentration in *Berberomeloe majalis* blister beetles and their extracts.

Extract	CTD (μg/mg)	Total CTD (mg) [a]	Distribution of Total CTD (%)	CTD Per Beetle (mg) [b]
Body	41.2	1813	99.3	9.06
Hemolymph	295.0	5.9	0.7	0.03
Total	-	1819	100	9.1

[a] Total CTD (for 20 mg and 44 g of hemolymph and body extract respectively). [b] Estimated CTD per beetle, N = 200 beetles.

Our bioassays demonstrated strong effects from *B. majalis* extracts and CTD against nearly all species tested. Population growth of the parasitic protozoan *Trichomonas vaginalis* was strongly suppressed, with 50% growth inhibition (GI_{50}) at 75.7 (body extract), 15.5 (hemolymph), and 5.6 μg/mL (CTD), with consistent dose-responses (Table 2). CTD had a remarkable activity level in comparison with other natural products and extracts screened against this parasite [45].

Table 2. Activity of cantharidin (CTD) and extracts of *Berberomeloe majalis* blister beetles against the parasitic flagellated protozoan, *Trichomonas vaginalis*. Data are expressed as percentages of growth inhibition.

Concentration (μg/mL)	Body Extract	Hemolymph Extract	CTD	Metronidazole
500	92.7 ± 0.8	99.8 ± 0.3	-	-
100	52.7 ± 4.6	77.5 ± 4.1	98.1 ± 0.3	-
GI_{50} (μg/mL) (95% CL)	75.7 (24.6–220.2)	15.5 (1.4–36.2)	5.6 (4.2–7.0)	0.6 (0.3–1.4)

Previously, CTD showed promising effects against *Leishmania major*, both in vitro, with 80% growth inhibition at a concentration of 50 μg/mL, and in vivo in experimentally infected BALB/c mice [46,47]. In addition, norcantharidin and analogs displayed good antiplasmodial activity on sensitive (D6) and chloroquine resistant (W2) strains of *Plasmodium falciparum*, with IC_{50} values close to 3.0 μM [48]. However, ours is the first report on the effects of *B. majalis* extracts and cantharidin on *Trichomonas* sp.

The plant endoparasitic nematode *Meloidogyne javanica* was also very sensitive to the hemolymph extract, with CTD being extremely potent against this parasite (CTD showed 26 and >1000 times more potent LD_{50} and LD_{90} values, respectively, than hemolymph) (Table 3). The activity of the hemolymph did not correlate with its content in CTD, may be due to the lipophilic nature of the extract. This is the first report on the effects of *B. majalis* hemolymph and CTD on nematodes, and specifically on *M. javanica*. Preliminary results on the larvicidal effect of CTD analogs on the parasitic nematode *Haemonchus contortus* lead to the proposal of serine/threonine phosphatase inhibitors as potential nematicidal targets [49,50].

Table 3. The effects of cantharidin (CTD) and *B. majalis* extracts on juvenile mortality in the parasitic nematode *Meloidogyne javanica*.

Treatment	**Dose (μg/μL)**	**Mortality [a] %**	**Lethal Concentrations [b]**	
			LC_{50} (μg/mg)	**LC_{90} (μg/mg)**
Body	**1**	74.9 ± 2.92	nc	
Hemolymph	1	84.05 ± 2.64	0.656 (0.626–0.687)	1.108 (1.054–1.172)
CTD	0.5	100 ± 0	0.0252(0.023–0.027)	0.065 (0.061–0.070)

[a] Data corrected according to Scheider–Orelli's formula. Values are means of four replicates. [b] Lethal doses to give 50% and 90% mortality (95% Confidence Limits).

B. majalis extracts and cantharidin were strong antifeedants against aphids, with *Rhopalosiphum padi* more sensitive than *Myzus persicae*. The antifeedant effects correlated with the CTD content of the extracts (hemolymph > body extract), with pure CTD the strongest aphid antifeedant (Table 4). The feeding behavior of the polyphagous chewing lepidopteran *Spodoptera littoralis* was not affected (data not shown). Previously, cantharidin showed toxicity and growth-regulation effects against *Plutella xylostella* moth caterpillars [51], inhibited glutathione S-transferase from Codling moth caterpillars, *Cydia pomonella* [52] and lepidopteran protein phosphatases [53,54]. Furthermore, CTD and several acylthiourea derivatives showed contact toxicity against the aphid *Brevicoryne brassicae* [55]. However, this is the first report on the antifeedant effects of CTD and CTD-rich extracts against aphids.

Table 4. Insect antifeedant effects of *B. majalis* extracts and cantharidin (CTD).

Treatment	**Concentration (μg/cm^2)**	***Rhopalosiphum Padi***	***Myzus Persicae***
		%SI [b]	
Body	**50**	94.35 ± 2.42	82.75 ± 8.28
	EC_{50} [b]	6.7 (4.63–9.63)	14.3 (8.1–25.3)
Hemolymph	50	96.84 ± 1.94	93.23 ± 5.0
	EC_{50} [b]	0.8 (0.5–1.5)	3.38 (1.98–5.77)
CTD	50	94.7 ± 3.5	91.50 ± 2.31
	EC_{50} [b]	0.098 (0.031–0.3)	0.211 (0.05–0.91)

[a] %SI = (1 − (T/C)) × 100, where T and C are settling on treated and control leaf disks. [b] EC_{50}, effective dose to give a 50% inhibition (95% Confidence Limits).

The extracts and CTD were effective ixodicidal agents with similar effective doses (Table 5). CTD and CTD-rich extracts had LD_{50} concentrations seven times more potent than the positive control, nootkatone [56] but had similar LD_{90} values.

Table 5. Effects of *B. majalis* extracts and cantharidin (CTD) on *Hyalomma lusitanicum* tick larval mortality.

Treatment	Mortality [a]	Lethal Concentrations [b]	
		LC_{50} (µg/mg)	LC_{90} (µg/mg)
Body	81.7 ± 0.9	12.79 (10.84–14.93)	23.93 (20.79–28.94)
Hemolymph	70.2 ± 1.8	12.25 (10.65–13.94)	21.05 (18.74–24.47)
CTD	90 ± 0.1	12.84 (11.55–14.30)	20.31 (18.32–23.11)
Nootkatone [c]	-	4.02 (1.92–7.42)	18.02 (13.60–29.16)

[a] At 20 µg/mg cellulose. Data corrected according to Scheider–Orelli's formula. Values are means of three replicates.
[b] Lethal doses to give 50% and 90% mortality (95% Confidence Limits). [c] From Ruiz–Vázquez et al. [56].

The fact that the hemolymph and the body extracts showed similar effects suggests the presence of additional ixodicidal components in the body extract, which had the lowest CTD concentration. Chemically defended insects often contain multiple classes of toxic compounds [44]. Wang et al. (2014) [55] previously reported the acaricidal effects of CTD on *Tetranychus cinnabarinus*. This is the first report on the ixodicidal effects of cantharidin.

3. Conclusions

Our study documents that CTD is active against a diverse range of organisms including protozoa, nematodes, ticks, and insects. As such, our findings support Bravo et al.'s (2014) [36] hypothesis that Great Bustards might reduce parasite loads via the ingestion of blister beetles, a possible example of self-medication.

On a broader scale, our results (and those of other authors) showing CTD activity against a diverse range of taxa, suggest that this natural product might be developed to combat specific pests or pathogens under certain conditions. Of course, CTD is highly toxic to humans and many vertebrates [57,58], and appropriate safety precautions must be followed. That CTD is currently used in humans to treat common and molluscum warts, to remove tattoos, and as a counterirritant, and that it has commonly been used to encourage livestock breeding, implies that additional (safe) uses might be found.

4. Materials and Methods

4.1. Insect Extracts

Two hundred adult *Berberomeloe majalis* of mixed sex (males averaged 22.3 ± 0.3 mm and 490 ± 34.1 mg; females 30.3 ± 1.4 mm and 1234 ± 138.3 mg) were collected in Central Spain (Finca La Garganta, Ciudad Real) in March 2015. Insects were frozen at −20 °C until use. To obtain hemolymph, we cut the terminal abdomens and allowed hemolymph to drip into a vial. The resulting hemolymph (4.8 mL) was extracted with dichloromethane (DCM) (10 mL, 3 times) and the solvent evaporated to give an extract of beetle hemolymph (20 mg). The remaining insect bodies (~172 g of combined males and females) were macerated with DCM (400 mL, 3 times) at room temperature, filtered, and the solvent evaporated to give 44 g of body extract.

4.2. Cantharidin Quantification

We analyzed the above extracts via GC–MS (Thermo Finnigan Trace GC 2000 coupled with a Trace MS mass selective detector). The chromatographic conditions were controlled using Xcalibur software version 1.2 (Thermo Finnigan, San Jose, CA, USA). The GC column was a SLB-5 ms (30 m, 60.32 mm, 0.25 µm, Supelco Analytical, Bellefonte, PA, USA). The flow rate of helium was 0.8 mL/min. The injection volume was 1 mL in splitless mode for 2 min. Injector conditions were 250 °C in constant flow mode. The column oven had an initial temperature of 50 °C for two minutes. The subsequent temperature was programmed at a heating rate of 10 °C/min to 310 °C. The final temperature was held isothermally for 5 min. Total run time was 30 min. Cantharidin (CTD) detection was performed by selected ion monitoring (SIM), registering m/z = 128 (= the majority ion of CTD´s mass spectra).

CTD identification was performed by comparison with mass spectra available in the NIST MS search 2.0 library. The extracts were dissolved in DCM and the concentrations injected were 0.1 and 0.5 mg of extract/mL DCM for the hemolymph and body extracts, with an injection volume of 1 mL. Confirmation and quantification were achieved with the retention time and calibration curves (range: 0.015–48 mg/mL, slope: 476.401, r^2 = 0.999) obtained from the injection of CTD standard purchased from Sigma–Aldrich (St. Louis, MO, USA).

4.3. Bioassays

In all bioassays we tested various doses of three primary preparations: (1) Extract of beetle hemolymph. (2) Extract of beetle bodies. (3) 99% pure CTD (Sigma–Aldrich, St. Louis, MO, USA).

4.4. Antiprotozoal Activity

Antiprotozoal activity was evaluated on the metronidazole-sensitive *Trichomonas vaginalis* JH31A no.4 isolate (American Type Culture Collection, (ATCC)). The flagellates were cultured in a trypticase-yeast extract-maltose modified medium supplemented with 10% heat-inactivated fetal bovine serum (FBS) and antibiotic solutions at 37 °C and 5% CO_2. Assays were carried out in glass tubes containing 10^5 trophozoites/mL. After 5–6 h of seeding, extracts (1), (2) or CTD were added to log-phase growth cultures at several concentrations (500, 250, 100, 50, 25 and 10 μg/mL for extracts (1) and (2); 100, 50, 25, 10, 5 and 1 μg/mL for CTD). The tubes were incubated for 24 h at 37 °C and 5% CO_2. The trichomonacidal activity was obtained by a fluorimetric method using resazurin (Sigma-Aldrich) as previously described [59,60]. The experiments were performed at least two times in triplicate. GI_{50} values, as well as the 95% CI were calculated by Probit analysis (SPSS v.20, IBM, Armonk, NY, USA).

4.5. Nematicidal Activity

We tested the toxicity of our three preparations against 2nd stage juveniles (J2) of *Meloidogyne javanica* previously maintained on *Lycopersicon esculentum* plants (var. "Marmande") in pot cultures at 25 ± 1 °C and >70% RH. The experiments were carried out in 96-well microplates (Becton, Dickinson), as described per Andrés et al., (2012) [61]. The three preparations were tested at initial concentrations of 1.0 and 0.5 mg/mL (final concentration in the well) and diluted serially if necessary. The number of dead juveniles was recorded after 72 h. All treatments were replicated four times. The data were determined as mortality percentage corrected according to Scheider–Orelli's formula. Effective lethal doses (LC_{50} and LC_{90}) were calculated for the active pure compounds by Probit analysis (five serial dilutions, 0.5–0.01 mg/mL).

4.6. Insect Bioassays

Spodoptera littoralis, *Myzus persicae* and *Rhopalosiphum padi* colonies were reared on an artificial diet, bell pepper (*Capsicum annuum*) and barley (*Hordeum vulgare*) respectively, and maintained at 22 ± 1 °C, >70% relative humidity with a photoperiod of 16:8 h (L:D) in a growth chamber. Choice antifeedant bioassays were conducted in Petri dishes with newly emerged *S. littoralis* sixth instar larvae (at least 10 replicates with 2 insects each to give a SE < 10) or 2 × 2 cm plastic boxes with adults (24–48 h old) of the aphids *M. persicae* and *R. padi* (20 replicates with 10 insects each). Feeding or settling inhibition on treated (10 μL of extract or CTD solution) and untreated (10 μL of solvent) leaf disks of the host plant (%FI or %SI) were calculated as %FI= (1−(T/C)) × 100, where T and C are the consumption of treated and control leaf disks, respectively, or as %SI= (1−10 (%T/%C)) × 100 where %C and %T are percent aphids settled on control and treated leaf disks, respectively, as described [62]. The antifeedant effects (%FI/%SI) were analyzed for significance by the non-parametric Wilcoxon signed-rank test. EC_{50} (effective dose to obtain 50% feeding inhibition) were determined for extracts and CTD (four serial dilutions, 10–1 or 5–0.5 mg/mL) with %FI/%SI values > 75% from a linear regression analysis (%FI/%SI values on log (Dose)) (statistical package: www.statgraphics.com).

4.7. Ixodicidal Activity

Hyalomma lusitanicum engorged female ticks were collected in central Spain (Finca La Garganta, Ciudad Real) from their host (deer) and maintained at 22–24 °C and 70% RH in a growth chamber until oviposition and egg hatch. Resulting larvae (4–6 weeks old) were used for the bioassays. Briefly, 50 µL test solution were added to 25 mg of powdered cellulose at different concentrations and the solvent evaporated. For each test, three replicates with 20 larvae each were used. Larval mortality was checked after 24 h of contact with the treated cellulose in the environmental conditions described [56], using a binocular magnifying glass. The mortality data shown have been corrected with respect to the control according to Schneider–Orelli's formula. Effective lethal doses (LC_{50} and LC_{90}) were calculated by Probit Analysis (5 serial dilutions, STATGRAPHICS Centurion XVI, version 16.1.02).

Author Contributions: Conceptualization, D.W.W. and A.G.-C.; methodology, M.F.A., R.A.M.-D., A.I.-E., A.S.O. and A.G.-C.; investigation, M.F.A., R.A.M.-D., A.I.-E., A.S.O. and A.G.-C.; resources, A.G.-C.; writing—original draft preparation, D.W.W. and A.G.-C..; writing—review and editing, D.W.W. and A.G.-C.; R.A.M.-D., M.F.A., A.S.O. and A.I.-E.; supervision, A.G.-C.; funding acquisition, A.G.-C.

Funding: This research was funded by MINECO/FEDER, Spain, Grant no. CTQ2015-64049-C3-1-R; Ministerio de Economia y Competitividad, Spain (MINECO/FEDER), Grant no. CGL2017-87206-P.

Acknowledgments: The authors are especially grateful to J.M. Tercero (Villamagna SA) and his Grace the Duke of Westminster for providing *B. majalis* and *H. lusitanicum*.

Conflicts of Interest: The authors declare no conflict of interest.

References

1. Gathercoal, E.N.; Wirth, E.H. *Pharmacognosy*; Lea and Febiger: Philadelphia, PA, USA, 1936; pp. 1–852.
2. Wang, G.S. Medical uses of mylabris in ancient China and recent studies. *J. Ethnopharmacol.* **1989**, *26*, 147–162. [CrossRef]
3. Wilson, C.R. Methods for Analysis of Gastrointestinal Toxicants. In *Comprehensive Toxicology*, 2nd ed.; Hooser, S., Mc-Queen, C., Eds.; Elsevier Academic Press: London, UK, 2010; pp. 145–152.
4. Moed, L.; Shwayder, T.A.; Chang, M.W. Cantharidin revisited: A blistering defense of an ancient medicine. *Arch. Dermatol.* **2001**, *137*, 1357–1360. [CrossRef] [PubMed]
5. Pajovic, B.; Radosavljevic, M.; Radunovic, M.; Radojevic, N.; Bjelogrlic, B. Arthropods and their products as aphrodisiacs—Review of literature. *Eur. Rev. Med. Pharmaco.* **2012**, *16*, 539–547.
6. James, P.; Thorpe, N. *Ancient Inventions*; Ballantine Books; The Random House Publishing Group: New York, NY, USA, 1995; pp. 1–672.
7. Ford, P.; Howell, M. *The Beetle of Aphrodite and other Medical Mysteries*; Random House: New York, NY, USA, 1985; pp. 1–358.
8. Schaeffer, N. *The Marquis de Sade: A Life*; Harvard University Press: Cambridge, MA, USA, 2000; pp. 1–557.
9. Robiquet, M. Expériences sur les cantharides. *Annales de Chimie* **1810**, *76*, 302–322.
10. Aggrawal, A. Spanish Fly (Cantharides). In *Textbook of Forensic Medicine and Toxicology*; Avichal Publishing Company: New Delhi, India, 2014; p. 652.
11. Blood, D.C.; Studdert, V.P.; Gay, C.C. *Saunders Comprehensive Veterinary Dictionary*, 3rd ed.; Elsevier: Philadelphia, PA, USA, 2007; pp. 1–2172.
12. Anon. Cantharide. In *Farlex Partner Medical Dictionary*; Farlex: Huntingdon Valley, PA, USA, 2012. Available online: http://medical-dictionary.thefreedictionary.com/ (accessed on 31 January 2017).
13. Taberner, P.V. *Aphrodisiacs: The Science and the Myth*; Springer Science & Business Media: Bristol, UK, 2012; pp. 1–278.
14. Puerto-Galvis, C.E.; Vargas-Méndez, L.Y.; Kouznetsov, V.V. Cantharidin-Based Small Molecules as Potential Therapeutic Agents. *Chem. Biol. Drug Des.* **2013**, *82*, 477–499. [CrossRef] [PubMed]
15. Karras, D.J.; Farrell, S.E.; Harrigan, R.A.; Henretig, F.M.; Gealt, L. Poisoning from "Spanish Fly" (cantharidin). *Am. J. Emerg. Med.* **1996**, *14*, 478–483. [CrossRef]
16. Ghoneim, K. Cantharidin toxicosis to animal and human in the world: A review. *Stand. Res. J. Toxicol. Environ. Health Sci.* **2013**, *1*, 1–16.

17. Cotovio, P.; Silva, C.; Marques, M.G.; Ferrer, F.; Costa, F.; Carreira, A.; Campos, M. Acute kidney injury by cantharidin poisoning following a silly bet on an ugly beetle. *Clin. Kidney J.* **2013**, *6*, 201–203. [CrossRef]
18. Schmitz, D.G. Overview of Cantharidin Poisoning (Blister Beetle Poisoning). In *The Merck Veterinary Manual*; Aiello, S.E., Moses, M.A., Eds.; Merck Sharp & Dohme: Kenilworth, NJ, USA, 2013. Available online: http://www.merckvetmanual.com/ (accessed on 31 January 2017).
19. Nickolls, L.C.; Teare, D. Poisoning by cantharidin. *Br. Med. J.* **1954**, *2*, 384–1386. [CrossRef]
20. Froberg, B.A. Animals. In *Criminal Poisoning: Clinical and Forensic Perspectives*; Jones & Bartlett: Burlington, MA, USA, 2010; pp. 39–48.
21. Al-Rumikan, A.; Al-Hamdan, N.A. Indirect cantharidin food poisoning caused by eating wild birds. *Saudi Epidemiol. Bulll.* **1999**, *6*, 25–26.
22. Penrith, M.L.; Naudé, T.W. Mortality in chickens associated with blíster beetle consumption. *J. S. Afr. Vet. Assoc.* **1996**, *67*, 97–99.
23. Rockett, J.; Bosted, S. *Veterinary Clinical Procedures in Large Animal Practices*; Cengage Learning: Boston, MA, USA, 2015; pp. 1–672.
24. Honkanen, R.E. Cantharidin, another natural toxin that inhibits the activity of serine/threonine protein phosphatases types 1 and 2ª. *FEBS Lett.* **1993**, *330*, 283–286. [CrossRef]
25. Baba, Y.; Hirukawa, N.; Sodeoka, M. Optically active cantharidin analogues possessing selective inhibitory activity on Ser/Thr protein phosphatase 2B (calcineurin): Implications for the binding mode. *Bioorgan. Med. Chem.* **2005**, *13*, 5164–5170. [CrossRef]
26. Bologna, M.A.; Oliverio, M.; Pitzalis, M.; Mariottini, P. Phylogeny and evolutionary history of the blister beetles (Coleoptera, Meloidae). *Mol. Phylogenet. Evol.* **2008**, *48*, 679–693. [CrossRef]
27. Carrel, J.E.; Eisner, T. Cantharidin: Potent feeding deterrent to insects. *Science* **1974**, *183*, 755–757. [CrossRef] [PubMed]
28. Nikbakhtzadeh, N.R.; Dettner, K.; Boland, W.; Gäde, G.; Dötterle, S. Intraspecific transfer of cantharidin within selected members of the family Meloidae (Insecta: Coleoptera). *J. Insect. Physiol.* **2007**, *53*, 890–899. [CrossRef]
29. Eisner, T.; Conner, J.; Carrel, J.E.; McCormick, J.P.; Slagle, A.J.; Gans, C.; O'Reilly, J.C. Systemic retention of ingested cantharidin by frogs. *Chemoecology* **1990**, *1*, 57–62. [CrossRef]
30. Bartram, S.; Boland, W. Chemistry and ecology of toxic birds. *ChemBioChem* **2001**, *2*, 809–811. [CrossRef]
31. Wirtz, W.O.; Austin, D.H.; Dekle, G.W. Food habits of the common long-nosed armadillo *Dasypus movemcinctus* in Florida, 1960–1961. In *Evolution and Ecology of Armadillos, Sloths, and Vermilinguas*; Montgomery, G.G., Ed.; Smithsonian Institution Press: Washington, DC, USA, 1985; pp. 439–451.
32. Larson, N.P. The common toad as an enemy of blíster beetles. *J. Econ. Entomol.* **1943**, *36*, 480. [CrossRef]
33. Kilham, L. Use of blíster beetle in bill-sweeping by White-brested Nuthatch. *Auk Ornithol. Adv.* **1971**, *88*, 175–176.
34. Percino-Daniel, N.; Buckley, D.; García-París, M. Pharmacological properties of blister beetles (Coleoptera: Meloidae) promoted their integration into the cultural heritage of native rural Spain as inferred by vernacular names diversity, traditions, and mitochondrial DNA. *J. Ethnopharmacol.* **2013**, *147*, 570–583. [CrossRef]
35. Sánchez-Barbudo, I.S.; Camarero, P.R.; García-Montijano, M.; Mateo, R. Possible cantharidin poisoning of a great bustard (*Otis tarda*). *Toxicon* **2012**, *59*, 100–103. [CrossRef] [PubMed]
36. Bravo, C.; Bautista, L.M.; García-París, M.; Blanco, G.; Alonso, J.C. Males of a Strongly Polygynous Species Consume More Poisonous Food than Females. *PLoS ONE* **2014**, *9*, e111057. [CrossRef] [PubMed]
37. Bailey, T.A. *Diseases and Medical Management of Houbara Bustards and other Otididae*; Emirates Printing Press LLC: Dubai, UAE, 2008; pp. 1–494.
38. Silvanose, C.; Samour, J.; Naldo, J.; Bailey, T.A. Oro-pharyngeal protozoa in captive bustards: Clinical and pathological considerations. *Avian. Pathol.* **1998**, *27*, 526–530. [CrossRef]
39. Alonso, J.C.; Palacín, C. Avutarda—*Otis tarda*. In *Enciclopedia Virtual de los Vertebrados Españoles*; Salvador, A., Morales, M.B., Eds.; Museo Nacional de Ciencias Naturales: Madrid, Spain, 2015. Available online: http://www.vertebradosibericos.org/ (accessed on 31 January 2017).
40. Cordero del Campillo, M.; Castañón-Ordóñez, L.; Reguera-Feo, A. *Índice Catálogo de Zooparásitos Ibéricos*, 2nd ed.; Universidad de León, Secretariado de Publicaciones: León, Spain, 1994; pp. 1–650.

41. McCormick, J.P.; Carrel, J.E. Cantharidin biosynthesis and function in meloid beetles. In *Pheromone Biochemistry*; Prestwich, G.D., Bloomquist, H.F., Eds.; Harcourt, Brace, & Jovanovich: Orlando, FL, USA, 1987; pp. 307–350.
42. Carrel, J.E.; McCairel, M.H.; Slagle, A.J.; Doom, J.P.; Brill, J.; McCormick, J.P. Cantharidin production in a blister beetle. *Experientia* **1993**, *49*, 171–174. [CrossRef]
43. Mebs, D.; Pogoda, W.; Schneider, M.; Kauert, G. Cantharidin and demethylcantharidin (palasonin) content of blister beetles (Coleoptera: Meloidae) from southern Africa. *Toxicon* **2009**, *53*, 466–468. [CrossRef] [PubMed]
44. Whitman, D.W. Allelochemical interactions among plants, herbivores, and their predators. In *Novel Aspects of Insect-Plant Interactions*; Barbosa, P., Letrourneau, D., Eds.; John Wiley: New York, NY, USA, 1988; pp. 11–64.
45. De Brum Vieira, P.; Brandt Giordani, R.; Macedo, A.J.; Tasca, T. Natural and synthetic compound anti-*Trichomonas vaginalis*: An update review. *Parasitol. Res.* **2015**, *114*, 1249–1261. [CrossRef]
46. Yahya, M.; Fatemeh, G.; Abdolhosein, D.; Zohreh, S.; Zuhair, H. Effect of cantharidin on apoptosis of *the Leishmania major* and on parasite load in BALB/c mice. *Res. J. Parasitol.* **2013**, *8*, 14–25.
47. Ghaffarifar, F. *Leishmania major*: *In vitro* and *in vivo* anti-leishmanial effect of cantharidin. *Exp. Parasitol.* **2010**, *126*, 126–129. [CrossRef]
48. Bajsa, J.; McCluskey, A.; Gordon, C.P.; Stewart, S.G.; Sahu, R.; Duke, S.O.; Tekwan, B.L. The antiplasmodial activity of norcantharidin analogs. *Bioorg. Med. Chem. Lett.* **2010**, *20*, 6688–6695. [CrossRef] [PubMed]
49. Campbell, B.E.; Tarleton, M.; Gordon, C.P.; Sakoff, J.A.; Gilbert, J.; McCluskey, A.; Gasser, R.B. Norcantharidin analogues with nematocidal activity in *Haemonchus contortus*. *Bioorg. Med. Chem. Lett.* **2011**, *21*, 3277–3281. [CrossRef]
50. Campbell, B.E.; Hofmann, A.; McCluskey, A.; Gasser, R.B. Serine/threonine phosphatases in socioeconomically important parasitic nematodes-prospects as novel drug targets? *Biotechnol. Adv.* **2011**, *29*, 28–39. [CrossRef]
51. Huang, Z.; Zhang, Y. Chronic sublethal effects of cantharidin on the diamondback moth *Plutella xylostella* (lepidoptera: Plutellidae). *Toxins* **2015**, *7*, 1962–1978. [CrossRef]
52. Yang, X.; Zhang, Y. Characterization of glutathione S-transferases from *Sus scrofa, Cydia pomonella* and *Triticum aestivum*: Their responses to cantharidin. *Enzyme Microb. Technol.* **2015**, *69*, 1–9. [CrossRef] [PubMed]
53. Chen, X.; Lü, S.; Zhang, Y. Characterization of protein phosphatase 5 from three lepidopteran insects: *Helicoverpa armigera, Mythimna separata* and *Plutella xylostella*. *PLoS ONE* **2014**, *9*, e97437. [CrossRef] [PubMed]
54. Chen, X.; Liu, J.; Zhang, Y. Cantharidin impedes the activity of protein serine/threonine phosphatase in *Plutella xylostella*. *Mol. BioSyst.* **2014**, *10*, 240–250. [CrossRef]
55. Wang, M.; Nan, X.; Feng, G.; Yu, H.; Hu, G.; Liu, Y. Design, synthesis and bioactivity evaluation of novel acylthiourea derivatives of cantharidin. *Ind. Crop. Prod.* **2014**, *55*, 11–18. [CrossRef]
56. Ruiz-Vásquez, L.; Olmeda, A.S.; Zúñiga, G.; Villarroel, L.; Echeverri, L.F.; González-Coloma, A.; Reina, M. Insect antifeedant and ixodicidal compounds from *Senecio adenotrichius*. *Chem. Biodivers.* **2017**, *14*, 1612–1880. [CrossRef] [PubMed]
57. Till, J.S.; Majmudar, B.N. Cantharidin poisoning. *South. Med. J.* **1981**, *74*, 444–447. [CrossRef]
58. Polettini, A.; Crippa, O.; Ravagli, A.; Saragoni, A. A fatal case of poisoning with cantharidin. *Forensic. Sci. Int.* **1992**, *56*, 37–43. [CrossRef]
59. Martínez-Díaz, R.A.; Ibáñez-Escribano, A.; Burillo, J.; de las Heras, L.; del Prado, G.; Agulló-Ortuño, M.T.; Julio, L.F.; González-Coloma, A. Trypanocidal, trichomonacidal and cytotoxic components of cultivated *Artemisia absinthium* Linnaeus (Asteraceae) essential oil. *Mem. Inst. Oswaldo Cruz.* **2015**, *110*, 639–699. [CrossRef] [PubMed]
60. Ibáñez-Escribano, A.; Meneses Marcel, A.; Machado Tugores, Y.; Nogal Ruiz, J.J.; Arán Redó, V.J.; Escario García-Trevijano, J.A.; Gómez Barrio, A. Validation of a modified fluorimetric assay for the screening of trichomonacidal drugs. *Mem. Inst. Oswaldo Cruz.* **2012**, *107*, 637–643. [CrossRef]
61. Andrés, M.F.; González-Coloma, A.; Sanz, J.; Burillo, J.; Sainz, P. Nematocidal activity of essential oils: A review. *Phytochem. Rev.* **2012**, *11*, 371–390. [CrossRef]
62. Burgueño-Tapia, E.; Castillo, L.; González-Coloma, A.; Joseph-Nathan, P. Antifeedant and phytotoxic activity of the sesquiterpene p-benzoquinone perezone and some of its derivatives. *J. Chem. Ecol.* **2008**, *34*, 766–771. [CrossRef] [PubMed]

toxins

MDPI

Review

Potential Therapeutic Applications of Bee Venom on Skin Disease and Its Mechanisms: A Literature Review

Haejoong Kim [1], Soo-Yeon Park [2,*] and Gihyun Lee [1,*]

[1] College of Korean Medicine, Dongshin University, Naju-si, Jeollanam-do 58245, Korea
[2] Department of Ophthalmology, Otolaryngology & Dermatology, College of Korean Medicine, Dongshin University, Naju-si, Jeollanam-do 58245, Korea
* Correspondence: swallow92@dsu.ac.kr (S.-Y.P.); glee@khu.ac.kr (G.L.)

Received: 3 June 2019; Accepted: 25 June 2019; Published: 27 June 2019

Abstract: Skin is larger than any other organ in humans. Like other organs, various bacterial, viral, and inflammatory diseases, as well as cancer, affect the skin. Skin diseases like acne, atopic dermatitis, and psoriasis often reduce the quality of life seriously. Therefore, effective treatment of skin disorders is important despite them not being life-threatening. Conventional medicines for skin diseases include corticosteroids and antimicrobial drugs, which are effective in treating many inflammatory and infectious skin diseases; however, there are growing concerns about the side effects of these therapies, especially during long-term use in relapsing or intractable diseases. Hence, many researchers are trying to develop alternative treatments, especially from natural sources, to resolve these limitations. Bee venom (BV) is an attractive candidate because many experimental and clinical reports show that BV exhibits anti-inflammatory, anti-apoptotic, anti-fibrotic, antibacterial, antiviral, antifungal, and anticancer effects. Here, we review the therapeutic applications of BV in skin diseases, including acne, alopecia, atopic dermatitis, melanoma, morphea, photoaging, psoriasis, wounds, wrinkles, and vitiligo. Moreover, we explore the therapeutic mechanisms of BV in the treatment of skin diseases and killing effects of BV on skin disease-causing pathogens, including bacteria, fungi and viruses.

Keywords: bee venom; alternative treatment; skin; cutaneous disease; mechanism

Key Contribution: This review summarizes the therapeutic applications of BV in skin diseases, including acne, alopecia, atopic dermatitis, melanoma, morphea, photoaging, psoriasis, wounds, wrinkles, and vitiligo. It also deals with the therapeutic mechanisms of BV in the treatment of skin diseases and killing effects of BV on skin disease-causing pathogens, including bacteria, fungi and viruses.

1. Introduction

Bee venom (BV), produced by honeybees (*Apis mellifera*), is one of the most well-known natural toxins. BV is a very diverse set of chemicals. It includes peptides such as melittin, apamine, adolapin, and MCD peptide, enzymes like phospholipase A2 (PLA2), hyaluronidase, acid phosphomonoesterase, and lysophosphofolipase, and it also contains various amines such as histamine, dopamine, and norepinephrine [1].

BV has long been used as a therapeutic substance. It generally has been administrated in the form of piercing directly with bee sting, or injecting extracted and purified BV with a syringe. In oriental medicine, BV is also injected into specific acupoints related with a disorder [2,3]. BV has been broadly used for reducing pain and suppressing inflammation in musculoskeletal disorders, such as osteoarthritis, rheumatoid arthritis, and lumbar pain [2,4–6], and in recent years, its therapeutic effects in treating neurological diseases like chronic neuralgia, Parkinson's disease, and amyotrophic lateral sclerosis have been reported [7,8]. Another recent study also showed that BV has a therapeutic effect on periodontal disease [9]. Accumulated evidence shows that BV has anti-inflammatory, anti-apoptotic, antifibrotic, and anti-atherosclerotic properties which support these therapeutic applications [10]. In addition, a number of recent studies have demonstrated antibacterial, antiviral, antifungal, and anticancer effects of BV [1,11–17].

Many reviews have highlighted the therapeutic value of BV, but none have focused on the effect of BV on skin diseases. To the best of our knowledge, this is the first review that summarizes the potential therapeutic mechanisms and applications of BV in skin diseases. They are shown at ahead of discussion in order of clinical study, in vivo study, and in vitro study (Tables 1–3). To date, skin diseases where therapeutic application of BV has been studied include acne, alopecia, atopic dermatitis, melanoma, morphea, photoaging, psoriasis, wound, wrinkle, and vitiligo (Figure 1). The purpose of this review is to provide the present knowledge from a various experimental and clinical reports and to help researchers design a follow-up study from previous studies and diseases that are yet to be studied.

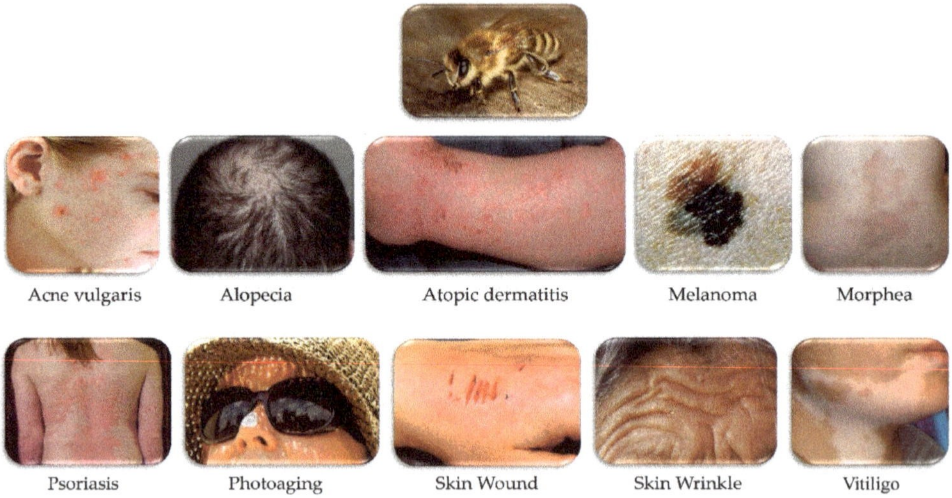

Figure 1. Skin diseases where the therapeutic application of bee venom (BV) has been studied.

2. Therapeutic Effects of BV in Skin Diseases

2.1. Acne

Acne, marked by the development of papules, pustules, and nodules, is an inflammatory disorder which occurred on the sebaceous unit. Acne is generally observed on the skin of the face, breast, and back. Pathological features of acne include increased sebum secretion, inflammation, keratinization of sebaceous ducts, and bacterial colonization of sebaceous ducts [18,19]. Antibiotics, one of the various treatment options for acne, have been utilized to suppress inflammation by killing the causative bacteria [20]. However, frequent use of antibiotics poses the risk of side effects, like the appearance of resistant bacterial strains [21,22]. Therefore, there is a growing interest in acne treatments which have a higher therapeutic effect and fewer side effects [22,23]. There are currently many studies demonstrating that BV might be effective for acne vulgaris.

2.1.1. Clinical Studies

In a randomized double-blind control trial of Han et al., to examine the therapeutic effects of BV on acne, a total of 12 subjects received either skincare products containing BV or products without

BV for 2 weeks. The BV group showed a notable advancement in the grading levels based upon the count of inflammatory and non-inflammatory lesions compared to the control. In the study, patients applying cosmetics containing BV showed a reduction by 57.5% in ATP levels, measured to assess a decrease in the count of skin microbes. These results show that cosmetics containing BV may be good candidates for therapeutic agents for acne [24].

In a prospective, non-comparative study of Han et al., 30 subjects with mild to moderate acne were recruited and managed with cosmetics containing BV twice daily for 6 weeks. All the volunteers showed significant improvement in the average visual acne grade compared to the start. The mean extent of improvement in acne grade after 6-weeks was 52.3%, and 77% of the subjects showed advancement in terms of whiteheads and blackheads, papules, pustules, and nodules 6 weeks later compared with the start of the treatment. There was no skin trouble noticed during the progress of the study. These results demonstrated that cosmetics containing BV showed a marked therapeutic effect on acne [25].

2.1.2. In Vivo Studies

Propionibacterium acnes (*P. acnes*) is the main factor that induces inflammation in acne [26]. As a member of normal bacterial flora, *P. acnes* coexists in our skin, but its excessive proliferation plays a key role in the development of inflammatory acne. It contributes to the inflammatory response of acne by stimulating the production of inflammatory cytokines like IL-8, IL-1β and TNF-α from keratinocytes, sebocytes, and inflammatory cells [27].

An et al. intradermally injected *P.acnes* into the ears of mice, and then BV was applied to the right ear only to examine the therapeutic effects of BV on inflammatory skin disease induced by *P. acnes*. BV treatment significantly decreased the inflammatory cells infiltration, and the expression of TNF-α and IL-1β decreased significantly in the BV-treated ear as compared to the untreated ear. The expression of CD14 and TLR2 was also significantly inhibited by BV treatment in *P. acnes*-treated tissue. In addition, the transcriptional activity of NF-κB and AP-1 was noticeably inhibited after BV injection. These results indicate that BV may be beneficial in treating acne [28].

Melitin, the main component of BV, is cationic and is also a toxic peptide that causes hemolysis [29]. Interestingly, recent in vitro and in vivo studies have shown that these cytotoxic melittins can be used to treat inflammatory diseases by reducing excessive immune responses [30]. Lee et al. investigated the therapeutic efficacy of melitin as an alternative treatment for inflammatory skin diseases caused by *P. acnes*. In this study, melittin significantly decreased the swelling and granulomatous inflammation response, which were induced by intradermal injection of *P. acnes*, in the ear when compared to the ear that only *P. acnes* was injected into. The thickness of the ear injected with melittin showed a 1.3-fold decrease in comparison to the ears that only *P. acnes* was injected into. Moreover, melittin evidently downregulated the expression of TNF-α and IL-1β, which further led to remarkable suppression of CD14 and TLR2 expression. These outcomes indicate that the application of melittin has potential for the treatment of *P. acnes*-induced inflammatory skin disorder [31].

2.1.3. In Vitro Studies

In vitro studies of Hari et al. using human keratinocytes and monocyte cells stimulated by heat-killed *P. acne* showed that BV reduced the production of IL-8, TNF-α, and IFN-γ in HaCaT and THP-1 cells. BV also suppressed TLR2 expression, which was induced by heat-killed *P. acnes*-induced, in HaCaT and THP-1 cells in a dose-dependent manner. The activation of TLR encourages the secretion of chemokines, pro-inflammatory cytokines, leukotrienes, and prostaglandins [32].

In the study of Han et al., BV decreased the production of IL-8 and TNF-α, which was caused by *P. acnes*, in THP-1 cell in a similar manner. In this study, BV showed low cytotoxicity against human keratinocytes and monocyte below 10 μg/mL [33]. These results indicate that BV might alternate antibiotic treatment for acne.

Lee et al. tested melittin as a therapeutic agent in heat-killed *P. acnes*–treated keratinocytes. In this study, the injection of melittin considerably reduced the expression of diverse inflammatory cytokines, such as TNF-α, IL-8, IL-1β, and IFN-γ. Melittin treatment suppressed the expression of TNF-α and IL-1β via regulating NF-κB and MAPK pathways in keratinocytes. In this study, melittin did not influence the cell viability of HaCaT cells during 8 hours of treatment. [31]

2.2. *Alopecia*

Hair is regarded as one of the most crucial parts of a person's look. Therefore, loss of hair could negatively affect self-worth and impair life quality. Genetic predisposition is the most common reason of hair loss, but stress is also believed to play a crucial role, specifically in the younger generation. Inflammation of the scalp is also associated with hair loss. According to a recent study, 74.1% of patients diagnosed with alopecia have inflammatory disorders, such as atopic and contact dermatitis. Mental illnesses account for 25.5% of the cases [34].

2.2.1. In Vivo Studies

Park et al. investigated the preventive effect of BV on alopecia by application of BV or minoxidil (2%) to the dorsal surface of mice for 19 days. Dexamethasone (DEX) was used to induce catagen in mice. In this study, BV promoted hair growth in mice by decreasing the levels of 5α-reductase and increasing keratinocyte growth factor (KGF), which stimulates follicular proliferation [35]. 5α-reductase enzymatically catalyzed the conversion of testosterone into DHT that has a higher affinity against androgen receptors than testosterone, which led to stimulating hair loss by the expression of genes associated with hair follicle minimization [36]. Finasteride and dutasteride, which are currently used as hair loss treatment agents based on inhibiting 5α-reductase, can cause severe side effects, including sexual dysfunction, depression, and gynecomastia, which generally lead to treatment discontinuation [37,38]. In this study, no edema, erythema, irritation, and cytotoxicity were observed after BV treatment. These results suggest that BV may be used as a hair growth-promoting agent [35].

2.2.2. In Vitro Studies

The length of hair relies on the duration of the anagen phase [39]. At any given time, hair, which is in anagen, catagen, and telogen phase, accounts for 90%, 1%, and 9% respectively [40]. In vitro studies using DEX-stimulated human dermal papilla cells (hDPCs) showed that BV elevates the proliferation of hDPCs and upregulates growth factors, including FGF7, FGF2, VEGF, and IGF-1 that keep hair in the anagen stage, and hence encourage hair growth in hDPCs [35]. BV presents the potential to be used as a treatment for hair loss, since it can stimulate hair growth by increasing hair growth factors and suppressing the progression to catagen phase.

2.3. *Atopic Dermatitis (AD)*

Atopic dermatitis (AD) is a chronic and relapsing inflammatory skin disorder that is marked by a defective skin barrier, eczema, pruritus, dry skin, and an abnormal IgE-mediated allergic response to diverse external antigens [41].

The incidence of AD has increased considerably in recent years. About 1 to 3% of adults and a maximum of 20% of children have at some point suffered from AD [42]. Antihistamines, steroids, NSAIDs and immunosuppressants have been utilized to treat AD [43–45]. Regrettably, these medications have serious adverse effects, like nephrotoxicity and neurotoxicity [43,46]. Thus, natural substances have emerged as alternative therapeutic agents for immune disorders, such as AD because they are considered to have strong immunomodulatory effects and fewer side effects [47]. Emerging evidence indicates that BV alleviates AD via its anti-inflammatory mechanisms in clinical trials in vivo and in vitro studies.

2.3.1. Clinical Studies

The disease management for AD is on the basis of hydrating the skin and restoring the collapsed epidermal barrier. Regular use of suitable moisturizer is an important part of therapy for AD because xerosis and barrier malfunction are the major symptoms of AD [48]. In the study of You et al., 136 subjects with diagnosed AD were randomly distributed in different groups and were made to apply either a moisturizer containing BV and silk protein or a moisturizer just without BV for 4 weeks. Subjects who applied emollient with BV showed significantly lower Eczema Area and Severity Index (EASI) and visual analogue scale (VAS) value compared to patients who applied emollient without BV. There were no outstanding differences in the incidence of side effects induced by BV on patients' skin [49].

2.3.2. In Vivo Studies

Gu et al. investigated the advancement of AD-like lesions caused by ovalbumin (OVA), which are major egg white proteins, and the mechanism of therapeutic action of BV simultaneously. Histological analysis of dorsal skin thickness indicated that intraperitoneal administration of BV reduced the symptoms of AD. BV inhibited inflammatory cytokines by decreasing IgE secretion, TNF-α, and thymic stromal lymphopoetin (TSLP). It also suppressed the infiltration of eosinophils and mast cells into the lesion. These outcomes indicate BV has a possibility to be developed as an alternative for AD treatment due to the effective inhibition of allergic skin inflammation in AD [50].

Kim et al. noted the relationship between hyperactivity of the complement system and the inflammatory response of AD. In a mouse model in which atopic lesions were induced by 1-chloro-2,4-dinitrobenzene (DNCB), subcutaneous injection of BV almost completely resolved the symptoms of AD. In this study, BV significantly increased the secretion of CD55, a complement formation inhibitor, from THP-1 cells, resulting in a significant reduction in serum C3C and MAC levels, which were evaluated as an indicator of complement system activation. These results suggest that BV may be able to manage AD by inducing CD55 production that inhibits activity of complement system [51].

Itching, a sensation that causes the desire to scratch, is the most outstanding symptom of AD, and continuous scratching further worsens AD symptoms [52]. In the compound 48/80-induced mouse skin scratching model used in study of Kim et al, intraperitoneal administration of BV mitigated scratching behavior in mice. This anti-scratching effect correlated with vascular permeability effects of BV. In this study, BV also significantly suppressed mast cell degranulation and the production of pro-inflammatory cytokines including TNF-α and IL-1β by downregulating the activation of the NF-κB pathway in compound 48/80-treated epidermal tissues. These outcome indicate that BV might be used to ameliorate compound 48/80-induced AD symptoms [47]. In traditional Oriental medicine, BV acupuncture (BVA), which involves injecting BV into acupoints, has been utilized to treat various chronic inflammatory disorder of humans. In a mouse model of thrombotic micro-angiopathy (TMA)-induced AD used in study of Sur et al., BVA treatment at BL40 acupoint in the ear significantly inhibited the expression of both Th1 and Th2 cytokines in lymph nodes and ear skin. The severity of ear skin infection symptoms as AD-like symptoms, including thickness, inflammation, and increased lymph node weight, were considerably soothed by BVA treatment. The proliferation and infiltration of T cells and the synthesis of IL-4 and IgE, which are typical Th2 allergic responses, were also suppressed by BVA treatment. Interestingly, BVA at BL40 acupoint showed a more pronounced inhibitory effect compared to the non-acupoint placed on the base of the tail. These outcomes suggest that injecting BV at specific acupoints successfully relieves AD-like lesions by suppressing allergic and inflammatory responses in a mouse with TMA-induced AD. [53]

Several studies have investigated the pharmacological effects of melittin, the main component of BV. In the study of An et al. using mouse with DNCB-induced AD, topical application of melittin significantly alleviated AD-like symptoms, such as dorsal skin thickness by decreasing the number of mast cell infiltration, CD4+ T cells and the serum level of IgE, IL-4, IFN-γ, and TSLP. In addition, whole BV and melittin restored the abnormal differentiation of epidermis by recovering the expression of filaggrin. These results indicate that melittin could be a suitable agent for the therapy of AD [54].

In the study of Kim et al., intraperitoneally-injected BV also improved OVA-induced AD-like symptoms, such as an increase in skin thickness, edema, erythema, and excoriation in mice by inhibiting mast cell infiltration, by decreasing filaggrin levels, and secretion of AD-related inflammatory chemokines and cytokines, including CD14, CD11b, IL-1β, TNF-α, TSLP, and an excessive IgE response. Taken together, these results confirm that melittin has therapeutic effects on AD-like symptoms. [55]

PLA2, another major component of BV, plays a central role in various cellular responses, such as signal transduction, and the regulation of inflammatory and immune responses and phospholipid metabolism [56,57]. In *Dermatophagoides farinae* extract (DFE)-induced AD mouse model used in the study of Jung et al., topical application of PLA2 significantly decreased the serum IgE, Th1, and Th2 cytokines. AD-induced histological changes and mast cells infiltration were alleviated by PLA2 application. Meanwhile, the depletion of regulatory T cells eliminated the anti-atopic effects of PLA2, which suggests that anti-atopic effects of PLA2 rely on the functions of regulatory T cells. Overall, the results demonstrated that topical application of PLA2 might ameliorate atopic skin inflammation [58].

2.3.3. In Vitro Studies

The in-vitro study of An et al. using TNF-α/IFN-γ-treated human keratinocytes, melittin suppressed the production of chemokines, including CCL22 and CCL17, and pro-inflammatory cytokines such as IL-6, IL-1β, and IFN-γ by inhibiting the activation of NF-κB, STAT1, and STAT3 pathways. Modulating AD-associated cytokines and chemokines may therefore, offer therapeutic efficacy in patients with AD [54].

Filaggrin plays an important role in epidermal barrier function. The activation of STAT3 downregulates filaggrin and Th2-induced cytokines, including IL-4 and IL-13, which are known as activators of STAT3 signaling [59].

Kim et al. investigated anti-atopic effect of melittin using IL-4 and IL-13-stimulated human keratinocytes. In the study, melittin prevented filaggrin deficiency caused by IL-4/IL-13 and activation of STAT3 in keratinocytes. The report proposes that melittin may have a beneficial effect on the skin barrier function via inhibiting filaggrin deficiency by a reduction of IL-4, IL-13, pSTAT3, and TSLP expression [55].

2.4. Melanoma

Melanoma is a skin cancer which begins in melanocytes, which are cell types generally found in skin, eye and the bowel. The treatment for melanoma involves surgical removal, and adjuvant immuno-, chemo- and radiation therapy, which mainly destroy cancer cells by triggering apoptotic pathways [60].

2.4.1. In Vivo Studies

Soman et al. investigated the anticancer effect of melittin on B16F10 mouse melanoma [61]. Melittin is a cytolytic peptide that inserts itself into lipid bilayer membranes followed by oligomerization to make pores on membrane [62]. Although this action can be used to destroy harmful cells, the nonspecific cytotoxicity, genotoxicity and hemolytic action of melittin have restricted its therapeutic usage [30]. To overcome this limitation, investigators used perfluorocarbon nanoparticles, synthetic nanoscale vehicles, which can deliver melittin to both, targeted tumors and premalignant lesions. After intravenous injection of melittin-loaded nanoparticles, tumor weight decreased significantly (~87% reduction). Melittin loaded on targeted nanoparticles induced cancer cell apoptosis via liberation of cytochrome c from mitochondria. In addition, histological analysis revealed a reduction in the number of proliferating cells, blood vessels and significant areas of necrosis. There were no apparent toxic effects in terms of changes in organ weight or serum chemical profile, and the levels of liver enzyme aspartate aminotransferase were significantly lower in the melittin group than the normal control [61].

2.4.2. In Vitro Studies

BV caused the shift of intracellular Ca^{2+} concentrations in human melanoma A2058 cells. Changes in intracellular Ca^{2+} concentration generated reactive oxygen species (ROS) and collapsed mitochondrial membrane potential. As a result, apoptosis-inducing factor (AIF) and endonuclease G (EndoG) were noted to be translocated from mitochondria into the nucleus to carry out apoptosis. The inactivation of AKT and the activation of JNK were also observed in this process. Taken together, these experimental results supply a probable description for the potential mechanisms of BV in melanoma [60].

2.5. Morphea

Morphea is known as a local scleroderma and is a unique inflammatory disease that affects the skin and subcutaneous tissue, resulting in excessive accumulation of collagen, which eventually leads to fibrosis. Morphea is sometimes itchy but painless. It typically begins in red or purple skin areas and becomes thick and white [63].

The exact pathogenesis of morphea is unknown and the causes of morphea are generally considered as immune activation and inflammatory reaction, vascular endocardial damage, fibrosis, and nodularization. At the present time, there is no recommended medicinal treatment for morphea. Hwang et al, showed the successful outcome of BVA treatment in circumscribed morphea in a patient with systemic sclerosis [64].

Clinical Studies (Case Report)

A 64-year-old female presented with circular white areas (1 and 3 cm in diameter) and a heavy itch in the right lateral iliac crest. Subcutaneously, BVA was administered two times for the 1st week and once a week for the following 3 weeks along the edge of the superficial circumscribed lesions. After the first treatment, scores of sleep disturbance and itchiness dropped from 6 to 2 and from 8 to 4, respectively, on an 11 points numeric scale. At the 3rd visit, the patient reported that her itchiness had almost gone after two treatments, but it appeared intermittently. On the 5th visit, she reported that she did not feel the itchiness any more, and that she could sleep well. Her skin also improved. With a follow-up evaluation for 3 months, it was confirmed that her skin condition had improved drastically to resemble normal skin. Though there was a light itch at the site of BVA for around half a day following treatment, there were no other significant side effects during treatments. The result demonstrates the potential of BVA to be used as a local treatment for morphea [64].

2.6. Photoaging

Human skin is usually damaged by the exposure to ultraviolet (UV) ray of sunlight. Atmospheric ozone layer absorbs UVC, but both UVA and UVB arrive at the ground and have physiological effects [65]. In particular, UVB is regarded as one of the most hazardous environmental carcinogen because UVB irradiation can lead to the production of MMP-1 and MMP-3 in fibroblasts, inducing photoaging of the skin and progression of skin tumor [66].

In Vitro Studies

The in-vitro study of Han et al. using human dermal fibroblasts (HDF) irradiated by UVB, BV significantly decreased UV-induced MMP-1 and MMP-3 by 50–80% and 50–85%, respectively, compared to controls. It also reduced the expression of MMP-1 and MMP-3 mRNA. Moreover, BV promoted the recovery of the damage caused by UVB irradiation in HDF. One microgram/milliliter of BV exerted no remarkable effect on both cell viability and morphology. However, at the higher concentration of 10 μg/mL, BV treatment declined cell viability up to 90% [67]. These results hint that

BV might be utilized as a potential protective agent for inhibiting photoaging. It is considered that BV allergy is mainly due to its allergic components, such as PLA2. Hyunkyoung et al. investigated the efficacy of PLA2-free bee venom (PBV) in preventing photoaging by comparing it with original BV. In this study, both BV and PBV decreased the levels of MMP-1and MMP-13 in HaCaT cells and MMP-1, -2 and -3 in HDF cells, which are induced by UVB, and restored the cell damage and production of collagen. In addition, both BV and PBV downregulated UVB-induced activation of ERK1/2 and p38 in HaCaT and HDF cells. However, the difference between the two is that BV shows a cytotoxic effect, whereas PBV showed some advantages in preventing skin wrinkle formation without significant cytotoxicity [68].

Activities of MMPs induced by UVB caused the degradation of collagen, which led to the loss of elasticity of skin ultimately forming wrinkles [69]. These results suggest that the application of PBV appears to be an effective method in preventing skin wrinkles and protecting the skin from exposure to UVB.

2.7. Psoriasis

Psoriasis is a chronic inflammatory skin disorder marked by well-circumscribed erythematous plaques covered with silvery white scales. The exact pathology is unknown and is believed to be related to the production of inflammatory cytokines and kemokinesis following the activation of T-cells and several types of white blood cells that rule cellular immunity [70]. Unfortunately, current therapies can only suppress psoriasis but not cure it. Studies are being planned to evaluate the efficacy of BV as a new therapy in patients with psoriasis.

Clinical Studies

In the study of Hegazi et al., patients received an intradermal injection of BV. Before treatment and after 3 months of therapy, Psoriasis Area and Severity Index (PASI) score and serum IL-1β were measured to evaluate the outcome of treatment. Both PASI score and serum levels of IL-1β showed a significant decrease upon BV treatment [71]. These results were in accordance with a study which reported a decrease in levels of IL-1β from 289.5 to 29.2 in patients with guttate psoriasis followed by improvement in psoriasis after tonsillectomy [72].

In this study, intradermal injection of BV showed a superior outcome to oral or topical propolis, which were used as positive controls. Interestingly, unlike most treatments used in psoriasis, no systemic adverse effects were observed in all subjects. This indicates that BV might be a safe new treatment option and could be utilized in patients who have renal or liver dysfunctions [71].

Recalcitrant localized plaque psoriasis (RLPP) is characterized by lesions counting under 10% of body surface area which does not respond to any topical and systemic treatment [73]. Eltaher et al. used BV as alternative curative agent for RLPP, and their results exhibited full recovery in 23 out of 25 (92%) of patients, whereas only one patient out of 25 (4%) showed a recovery in symptoms in the placebo group. PGA score and TNF-α levels were remarkably decreased in patients treated with BV compared to the group with placebo. The activity of inflammatory cytokines, including TNF-α, IL-6 and IL-1β, is considered to take responsibility for the development of psoriasis [74]; hence, decreasing their levels might contribute to improvement of the disease. In this study, no adverse effects were observed excluding erythema, mild swelling and slight pain at the spot of BV injection and these troubles eventually got better. Psoriatic lesions did not relapse following 6 months of observation. These results suggested that BV could be safe and effective management for RLPP [75].

2.8. Skin Wounds

Wound healing is the result of a complex and dynamic course of tissue repair that includes various cellular and molecular events [76]. Wound healing is achieved through five interrelated phases; hemostasis and formation of clot, fibroplasias and neovascularization, granulation tissue formation, re-epithelialization, and creation of new ECM and tissue remodeling [77,78]

In Vivo Studies

Han et al. examined the efficacy of BV on healing wound in mice. For research, full-thickness wounds were induced on the dorsal surface of mice, and mice were divided into BV control and Vaseline groups. All the treatments were applied on the gauze covering the wound. The expression of type 1 collagen showed an increase upon BV treatment compared to the other two groups. The speed of wound closure in the BV group was notably faster than in the other two groups. Histology also showed that BV induced remarkable progression of wound healing. In this study, BV reduced the level of fibronectin, TGF-β1, and VEGF but elevated type 1 collagen. The results demonstrated that BV promoted wound healing by inhibiting cytokines related with fibrosis, which led to a reduction of wound size and an increase in propagation of epithelium in mice with full-thickness excision. These results suggest that the topical application of BV could be highly useful in decreasing the sizes of wounds [79].

In diabetic patients, skin wound healing disorders are often the cause of morbidity and mortality. Insufficient recruitment of macrophages and neutrophils at the wound and damage to neovascularization are responsible for impaired diabetic wound healing [80,81].

Hozzein et al. examined the therapeutic effect and mechanism of BV on impaired wound healing caused by diabetes in a mouse model with type I diabetes mellitus. In this study, the rate of wound closure and recovery were increased in the BV-treated group in comparison to the control. Type I collagen showed significant restoration in diabetic mice treated with BV. In addition, the percentage of apoptotic macrophages decreased markedly in BV-treated groups compared to controls, which led to a significant increase of the phagocytic index. Furthermore, BV promoted angiogenesis via recovering Ang-1/Tie-2 signaling and increasing the expression of Nrf2, ERK, Akt/eNOS, and β-defensin-2, which shows a reduction in wound tissues in diabetic mice. These results indicate that BV could be applied as a new potential treatment for encouraging angiogenesis and repairing the impaired wound healing in diabetes [82].

2.9. *Skin Wrinkling*

Wrinkles are a change in appearance induced by ultraviolet rays, and the intrinsic aging process over a prolonged time. Both these factors induce collagen alteration, leading to skin aging. The desire to improve aging skin has led to the development of numerous cosmetics that slow down wrinkle formation. Currently, various ingredients have been added to theses cosmetics and BV is one of the added ingredients.

Clinical Studies

Han et al. assessed the beneficial effects of serum containing BV on facial wrinkles. The results of the application of BV-containing serum decreased average wrinkle depth, the total wrinkle area and count. Topical application of BV is considered to be safe for human skin since it showed no dermal irritation in animal researches [83]. Therefore, BV serum might be effective in improvement of skin wrinkles [84].

2.10. *Vitiligo*

Vitiligo is characterized by depigmentation of skin and hair. It is related to abnormal pigmentation resulting from melanocyte proliferation, melanogenesis, and migration or increases in dendricity [85,86]. Recently, phospholipase A2 of BV has been reported to stimulate melanocyte dendricity and pigmentation [86–88]. According to the authors, pigmentation which occurred around the injection sites and lasted a few months, had been observed after treatment with BV. One study investigated the effect of BV on the proliferation, melanogenesis, migration, dendricity, and signal transduction of human melanocytes.

In Vitro Studies

In the study of Jeon et al., BV treatment elevated the melanocyte proliferation around twice compared to the control in 1 week. By BV treatment, the expression of MITF-M protein increased to the maximum levels on day 3 and slowly decreased till day 5. BV also activated PKA, ERK, and PI3K/Akt signaling. Moreover, BV treatment increased the ratio of cells with more than two dendrites by 23% in a time-dependent manner. The results also showed that BV treatment led to a two-fold increase in the number of migrated cells as compared to the controls. BV-induced melanocyte dendricity and melanocyte migration showed complete inhibition upon pre-treatment with PLA2 inhibitor and aristolochic acid, and this suggests that BV-induced melanocyte dendricity and melanocyte migration occur via the activation of PLA2.

The results of the in-vitro study indicated that BV has a positive effect on melanocyte proliferation, melanogenesis, dendricity, and migration. The result suggest that BV has a potential for treatment of vitiligo by repigmentation in skin [89].

3. Inhibitory Effects of BV against Pathogenic Agent which is Related to Skin Disease

3.1. *Bacteria*

3.1.1. *Propionibacterium Acnes*, Clindamycin-Resistant *P. acnes*, *Staphylococcus epidermidis*, and *Streptococcus pyogenes*

Propionibacterium acnes, *Staphylococcus epidermidis*, *Streptococcus pyrogenes*, and *Staphylococcus aureus* are microorganisms that originally exist on normal skin. During puberty, they proliferate rapidly and often contribute to the development of acne [90,91]. *P. acnes* infections mainly occur in the pilosebaceous unit. In contrast, aerobic organisms like *S. epidermidis*, *S. pyrogenes*, and *S. aureus* generally infect the sebaceous unit [92,93]. In the study of Han et al., BV shows bacteriostatic as well as bactericidal effects against *P. acnes*, clindamycin-resistant *P. acnes*, *S. epidermidis*, and *S. pyrogenes*. In this study, minimum inhibitory concentrations (MIC) of BV against *P. acnes*, clindamycin-resistant *P. acnes*, *S. epidermidis*, and *S. pyrogenes* were 0.086 µg/mL, 0.067 µg/mL, 0.104 µg/mL, and 0.121 µg/mL, respectively [33].

3.1.2. *Staphylococcus aureus* and Methicillin-Resistant *Staphylococcus aureus (MRSA)*

Staphylococcus aureus is the main causative pathogen of Impetigo [94], Paronychia [95], and Staphylococcal-scalded skin syndrome [96]. BV exhibited a significant antibacterial effect against *S. aureus* in an in-vitro study using the disc diffusion method [11]. Although antibiotics effectively deal with *S. aureus* infections these days, the appearance of methicillin-resistant *S. aureus* (MRSA) is posing a challenge to global health systems at present [97].

In the study of Han et al. that investigated the antimicrobial effect of BV on MRSA strain in terms of minimum inhibitory concentrations (MIC) and minimum bactericidal concentrations (MBC), the MIC values of BV against MRSA CCARM 3366 and MRSA CCARM 3708 were 0.085 µg/mL and 0.11 µg/mL separately. Its MBC against MRSA 3366 and MRSA 3708 were 0.106 µg/mL and 0.14 µg/mL respectively. Interestingly, MRSA strains were more sensitive to the mix of BV and vancomycin or gentamicin than either ampicillin or penicillin alone. These outcomes showed that BV exhibits antimicrobial and enhancing antibacterial effects versus MRSA strains [13].

Choi et al. examined whether BV and melittin could suppress MRSA infections in vitro and in vivo. Surprisingly, BV showed outstanding antimicrobial effect in vitro, but strengthened the proliferation and infection of MRSA in vivo. All the mice, injected with MRSA USA300 and BV, died 18 h after infection, while only five died in the control 24 hours after infection. In addition, no outstanding difference was noticed in terms of the diameter of abscesses formed by MRSA USA300 even after BV treatment.

Unlike BV, melittin showed remarkably better protection in the mice models of bacteremia and skin infection. Half of the mice survived over 24 h when 5mg/kg of melittin was injected 1 hour after bacterial infection and the abscess diameters were notably lower than the control [98].

3.2. Fungi

3.2.1. Dermatophytes, *Trichophyton mentagrophytes*, and *Trichophyton rubrum*

Trichophyton mentagrophytes and *Trichophyton rubrum*, common dermatophytes, are known to cause various skin infections in humans and animals. Dermatophytes infect keratinized epithelium, the hair and nails. Tinea pedis is described as a dermatophyte infection on the soles of the feet and interdigital spaces; tinea cruris as an infection of the groin; tinea faciei as the facial infection; and tinea corporis as a fungal infection of the rest of the skin [99].

Yu et al. reported that BV showed significant antifungal effects against the two dermatophytes. In this study, 0.63 ppm of BV inhibited the growing of *T. menatgrophytes* by roughly 92% and *T. rubrum* by 26% after 1 h of incubation. Furthermore, BV exhibited much stronger antifungal activities than that of fluconazole, a standard antifungal agent utilized for the prevention and management of fungal infections. The results of this study suggest that BV could be developed as a natural antifungal drug [100].

Onychomycosis or tinea unguium which accounts for about half of all nail abnormalities is also caused due to dermatophytes, with the most common agent being *Trichophyton rubrum*. In the study of Park et al. that investigated the antifungal effects of BV, mellitin, apamin, and BV-based mists on *T. rubrum* indicated that BV and BV-based mist exhibited strong antifungal effect on *T. rubrum*. However, the isolated BV components, such as mellitin and apamin, showed no significant effect in hindering the growth of the fungal colonies [101].

3.2.2. *Candida Albicans*

Cutaneous candidiasis is typically caused by *Candida albicans*, which exists as normal flora of human skin as well as in the gastrointestinal and genitourinary systems [102]. In the study of Lee et al., Sweet BV (SBV), which is made by removing enzymes and histamine known as allergens from BV, and BV exhibited an antifungal effect against 10 clinical isolates of *C. albicans* that were incubated from blood and the vagina.

In this study, SBV was noted to have much stronger antifungal activity than that of BV. The MIC values measured by the broth microdilution method diverge from 62.5 μg/mL to 125 μg/mL for BV, and in the case of SBV, from 15.63 μg/mL to 62.5 μg/mL. on the kill-curve assay, SBV acted similar to amphotericin B that was utilized as a positive control [103].

Park et al. demonstrated that melittin exerts its antifungal effect by inducing apoptosis. *C. albicans* treated with melittin exhibited an increase of ROS. In addition, markers that are indicators of apoptosis in yeast, involving externalization of phosphatidylserine, and fragmentation of DNA and nucleus fragmentation were observed. This study suggests that melittin exerts an antifungal effect by promoting apoptosis [104].

3.2.3. *Malassezia furfur*

Malassezia furfur, a lipophilic yeast-like fungus exists as an opportunistic pathogen in human skin and causes disorders such as dandruff and pityriasis versicolor.

In the study of Prakash et al., wherein 5 mg/mL BV was loaded onto the disc spread with *M. furfur*, a large zone of inhibition with an area of 86.9 mm^2 was observed. Ketoconazole (200 mg/mL) was used as a standard reference and it showed an area of inhibition of 156.1 mm^2. Since the doses of BV were in the range of 1–5 mg/mL, ketoconazole was applied at 5 mg/mL and it exhibited a suppression zone of 38.8 mm^2.

In this study, BV showed good inhibition against *M. furfur*. Shampoos that can be bought in the commercial market are mostly made of chemicals and have many side effects. Therefore, supplements with natural compounds such as BV can be a better treatment for skin diseases caused by *M. furfur*. [105].

3.3. Viruses

Herpes Simplex Virus

Herpes simplex virus (HSV) invades skin and mucous membranes, harming keratinocytes and causing severe inflammation which is accompanied by small blister on the Erythema. Genital infections are mainly caused by HSV-2, while infections of other areas and the mouth are mostly caused by HSV-1 [106].

In the study of Uddin et al., a non-cytotoxic quantity of BV significantly suppressed the replication of HSV. These antiviral properties are mainly based on the virucidal activity of BV. Apart from antiviral activity, BV stimulated IFN-1, which could subsequently initiate antiviral signaling in the host cell and additionally suppress the replication of the virus.

Uddin et al. also examined the antiviral effect of several components of BV to know which compounds in BV played a critical role in the virucidal effect of BV. Among those, only melittin in non-cytotoxic amounts exhibited similar effects to BV. Melittin directly destabilized the structure of virus particle, thereby suppressing viral infectivity. However, melittin was unable to interrupt the cell attachment and entry of the virus into the cells, and hence, once the cells were infected, it could not suppress viral infection and replication [12]. These results indicate that BV or melittin has the possibility to be a prophylactic or therapeutic agent in viral skin diseases.

4. Therapeutic Mechanisms of BV on Skin Diseases

Collective evidence from in-vitro experiments, in-vivo studies and clinical trials showed that BV has a potential therapeutic effect on skin diseases. The therapeutic mechanisms of BV mentioned above are as follows:

(1) In acne, TNF-α, IL-1β, TLR2, and CD14 expressions were remarkably decreased by BV treatment in *P. acnes*-injected tissues. In addition, the DNA-binding activity of NF-κB and AP-1 was noticeably inhibited by BV treatment [28]. BV reduced the expression of IL-8, TNF-α, and IFN-γ in HaCaT (keratinocyte) and THP-1 (monocytes) cells. It also suppressed TLR2 expression induced by heat-killed *P. acnes* in HaCaT and THP-1 cells [107]. Melittin significantly decreased TNF-α and IL-1β expression, leading to a noticeable suppression of TLR2 and CD14 expression in keratinocytes [31].

(2) In alopecia, BV promotes hair growth by reducing 5α-reductase expression and increasing KGF which stimulates follicular proliferation. BV increases the proliferation of hDPCs and upregulates growth factors, such as FGF7, FGF2, IGF-1, and VEGF, which maintain hair follicles in the anagen phase [35].

(3) In AD, BV suppressed the inflammatory cytokines by decreasing IgE, TNF-α, and TSLP levels. It also suppressed the infiltration of mast cells and eosinophils [50]. BV significantly increased the secretion of CD55, a complement formation inhibitor, from THP-1 cells, resulting in a significant reduction in serum C3C and MAC levels, which were evaluated as an indicator of complement system activation [51]. BV significantly inhibited mast cell degranulation and synthesis of pro-inflammatory cytokines, like TNF-α and IL-1β, by downregulating NF-κB activation [47]. The propagation and infiltration of T lymphocyte and the production of IL-4 and IgE, which are induced by Th2 type allergic responses, were suppressed by BV treatment [53].

Melittin decreased CD4+ T lymphocytes, mast cell infiltration and serum levels of IgE, IFN-γ, IL-4, and TSLP. Melittin also suppressed the production of chemokines, like CCL17 and CCL22, and pro-inflammatory cytokines involving IL-6, IL-1β, and IFN-γ by inhibiting the activation of NF-κB, STAT1, and STAT3 signaling pathways in keratinocytes [54]. Moreover, melittin inhibited filaggrin deficiency induced by IL-4 and IL-13 in keratinocytes. In addition, it suppressed mast cell infiltration and AD-related inflammatory molecules, such as CD14, CD11b, IL-1β, TNF-α, and TSLP and exaggerated IgE response [55]. The application of PLA2 significantly suppressed the increase in serum IgE and Th1 and Th2 cytokines. It also attenuated the infiltration of mast cells and histological changes [58].

(4) In melanoma, BV induced fluctuation in intracellular Ca^{2+} concentrations which increased the levels of ROS and collapse of membrane potential of mitochondria. As a result, AIF and EndoG are translocated from mitochondria into the nucleus to initiate apoptosis [60]. Melittin, loaded on targeted nanoparticles, induced apoptosis of cancer cell via release of cytochrome c from mitochondria [61].

(5) In morphea, the therapeutic mechanism of BV has not been studied yet.

(6) In photoaging, BV significantly decreased UVB-induced MMP-1 and MMP-3 expression in HDFs [67]. BV also decreased the levels of MMP-1 and MMP-13 in HaCaT cells, and MMP-1, -2, and -3 in HDF cells, which are induced by UVB. Moreover, cell damage and production of collagen were restored by BV treatment. Furthermore, BV treatment downregulated UVB0-induced activation of p38 and ERK1/2 in HaCaT and HDF cells [68].

(7) In psoriasis, a notable reduction in the serum level of IL-1β was observed upon BV treatment [71].

(8) In skin wound healing, BV treatment elevated type 1 collagen expression and decreased the levels of TGF-β1, VEGF, and fibronectin, which are cytokines associated with fibrosis [79]. In diabetic wound healing, BV treatment markedly restored type 1 collagen expression. BV significantly decreased the percentage of apoptotic macrophages. In addition, BV promotes angiogenesis via recovering Ang-1/Tie-2 signaling and increasing the expression of Nrf2, ERK, Akt/eNOS and β-defensin-2, which are normally downregulated in wounded tissues [82].

(9) In wrinkled skin, the therapeutic mechanism of BV action is yet to be explored.

(10) In vitiligo, BV significantly increased melanocyte proliferation, melanogenesis, dendricity, and migration. Hence, BV activated PKA, ERK, and PI3K/Akt signaling and increased MITF-M protein expression [89].

Table 1. Clinical study on therapeutic application of bee venom for skin disease.

Disease	Model	Venom/Compound/(Bee Species)	Dose (Administration Method)	Results	Mechanism/Molecular Response	Reference
Acne	Human DB, RCT (n = 12)	Cosmetic containing BV (*Apis melifera*)	0.06 mg/mL, Cosmetic 4 mL twice daily for 2 weeks (Applied to whole face)	Significant improvement of KAGS score ($p < 0.01$), 57.5% decrease of ATP level which indicate MO level ($p < 0.01$)	Not reported	[24]
Acne	Human (n = 30)	Serum containing BV (*Apis melifera*)	Not reported, Serum 0.7–0.9 g twice daily for 6 weeks (Applied to whole face)	Significant improvement (52.3%) of MCAGS score after 6 weeks ($p < 0.001$) Open and closed comedones were significantly decreased ($p < 0.001$). Significant decrease in papules ($p < 0.05$)	Not reported	[25]
Atopic dermatitis	Human DB, RCT (n = 114)	Emollient containing BV (*Apis melifera*)	Not reported, twice daily for 4 weeks (Applied to entire body)	Remarkable reduction of EASI score in comparison to control ($p < 0.05$). VAS score for pruritus was notably declined compared with control ($p < 0.05$). TEWL value were not notably different between two groups.	Not reported	[49]
Psoriasis	Human RLPP patients DB, RCT (n = 50)	BV (*Apis melifera*)	0.05 mL/cm^2 (intradermal injection around psoriatic lesion)	BV treatment group showed significant lower PGA scores against placebo group ($p < 0.001$). During the follow-up period of 6 months, psoriasis did not recur.	TNF-α was notably decreased compared to control ($p < 0.05$).	[75]
Psoriasis	Human patients with localized plaque psoriasis (n = 48)	BV (*Apis melifera*)	Starting with 0.01 μL, increasing 0.01 μL every injection untill arriving 1 μL (Intradermal, twice weekly) TP: topical propolis twice daily OP: oral propolis 1 g/day by capsule	PASI score was significantly decreased decreased after treatment ($p < 0.01$). Much more reduction than TP and OP. The highest reduction in (TP + OP + BV) group.	Serum IL-1β was significantly decreased after treatment ($p < 0.05$). Much more decrease than TP and OP.The highest decrease in (TP + OP + BV) group.	[71]

Table 1. *Cont.*

Disease	Model	Venom/Compound/(Bee Species)	Dose (Administration Method)	Results	Mechanism/Molecular Response	Reference
Scleroderma	A case report: 64-year-old Korean woman, White circular lesion on the right lateral iliac crest	BV (*Apis melifera*)	Dried BV 1 g dissolved in 10000cc water. Total volume under 0.2 mL. twice weekly (subcutaneous, along the margins of the lesion)	On a 11-point numeric scale (NRS 11), average score of itch declined from 8 to 4 and sleep disturbance from 6 to 2, respectively. On the fifth visit, patient stated that she no longer felt an itch and had no sleep disturbance due to itching. Three months later, the follow-up evaluation showed that the condition of the skin was close to normal skin.	Not reported	[64]
Wrinkle	Human, Double blind (n = 22)	Serum containing BV (*Apis melifera*)	BV 0.006% serum 4 mL twice daily for 12 weeks (Applied to whole face)	The average visual grade (SKWGS) of all patients with BV serum significantly improved (11.83% decrement) ($p < 0.001$). Total area, count and average depth of wrinkle were significantly decreased ($p < 0.05$).	Not reported	[84]

Abbreviations: ATP: Adenosine triphosphate, DB: double-blind, EASI: eczema area and severity index, KAGS: Korean Acne Grading System, MCAGS: Modified Cook's Acne Grading Scale, MO: micro-organism, PASI: psoriasis area and severity index, PASI: psoriasis area and severity index, PGA: physician global Assessment, RCT: randomized controlled trial, RLPP: recalcitrant localized plaque psoriasis, SKWGS: south Korean wrinkle-grading system, TEWL: transepidermal water loss, TNF-α: tumor necrosis factor-α, VAS: visual analog scale.

Table 2. In vivo studies on therapeutic application of bee venom for skin disease.

Disease	Model	Venom/Compound/(Bee Species)/	Dose (Administration Method)/Control	Results	Mechanism/Molecular Response	Reference
Acne	8-week ICR mice, P. acnes intradermally injected into both ears. (n = 30)	BV (*Apis melifera*)	1 μg blended with 0.05 g Vaseline (topical, on the right ear) NC: P.acnes only PC: vaseline applied to left ear	Ear thickness was reduced three-fold after 24 h compared to NC ($p < 0.05$). Swelling, erythema and inflammatory reactions were reduced.	TLR2 and CD14 expression is significantly inhibited. DNA-binding activity of NF-κB and AP-1 is remarkably inhibited compared to NC and PC ($p < 0.05$). Inhibiting the NF- κB signaling pathways.	[28]

Table 2. *Cont.*

Disease	Model	Venom/Compound/(Bee Species)/	Dose (Administration Method)/Control	Results	Mechanism/Molecular Response	Reference
Acne	8-week ICR mice, P. acnes intradermally injected into both ear. (n = 30)	Melittin (*Apis melifera*)	100 µg blended with 0.05 g Vaseline (topical, on the right ear) NC: P.acnes only PC: vaseline applied to left ear	Ear thickness was reduced 1.3-fold after 24 h compared with NC ($p <$ 0.05). Swelling and granulomatous response were markedly reduced.	Significant reduction of TNF-α, IL-1β, IL-8, IFN-γ compared with NC and PC ($p < 0.05$). DNA-binding activity of NF-κB and AP-1 is remarkably inhibited compared to NC and PC ($p < 0.05$). Melittin significantly reduced the phosphorylation of IKK, IκB and NF- κB. Inhibiting the NF- κB and MAPK signaling pathways.	[31]
Alopecia	6-week female C57BL/6 mice, catagen phase induced on dorsal skin by dexamethasone.	BV (*Apis melifera*)	Three CONC: 0.001% 0.005% 0.01% 100 µL each Once daily for 19 day (Applied to dorsal skin) NC:dexamethasone only PC: minoxidil 2% 100 µL	Hair growth promoted notably in a dose-dependent manner at all doses. 0.01% BV resulted in the greatest increase in hair growth compared to PC ($p < 0.05$).	KGF expression is significantly increased compared with NC ($p < 0.05$). 5α-reductase significantly decreased compared with NC ($p < 0.05$).	[35]
Atopic dermatitis	DNCB induced atopic dermatitis in 7-week male Balb/c mice (n = 8)	BV (*Apis melifera*)	0.3 mg/kg (subcutaneous) PBS	Dryness, hemorrhage, excoriation, edema and redness were almost completely restored.	Serum C3C and MAC were significantly decreased after BV injection compared to PBS injection ($p < 0.001$). Serum-secreted CD55 were significantly elevated compared with PBS injection ($p < 0.001$). BV increased CD55 production in THP-1 cells	[51]
Atopic dermatitis	OVA-induced atopic dermatitis in 6-week female Balb/c mice (n = 25)	BV (*Apis melifera*)	Three doses: 1 µg/Kg, 10 µg/Kg, 100 µg/Kg twice a week for 2 weeks (intraperitoneal) NC: untreated PC: OVA only	Bleeding, erythema, eczema, and dryness were significantly reduced. Dorsal skin thickness was remarkably reduced in a dose-dependent manner compared to PC ($p < 0.05$), the greatest decrease in BV 100 group.	Significant reduction of mast cell infiltration in BV 10 and 100 group compared with PC ($p < 0.05$). Serum IgE levels were reduced, the greatest decrease in BV 100 group. Significant reduction of TNF-α in BV 10 and 100 and TSLP in BV 100 group compared with PC ($p < 0.05$).	[50]

Table 2. *Cont.*

Disease	Model	Venom/Compound/ (Bee Species)/	Dose (Administration Method)/Control	Results	Mechanism/Molecular Response	Reference
Atopic dermatitis	DNCB induced atopic dermatitis in 6-week female Balb/c mice (n = 45)	Melittin (*Apis melifera*)	Three doses: 100 µg, 200 µg, 500 µg blended with placebo (topical, to dorsal skin) Placebo only	Dorsal skin thickness was notably decreased in comparison to placebo group ($p < 0.05$)	Mast cell infiltration was significantly decreased compared with control ($p < 0.05$). Serum IFN-γ, IL-4, IgE and TSLP were markedly decreased in melittin 200 and 500 group compared to placebo group ($p < 0.05$). $CD4^+$ and $CD3^+$ were significantly decreased in melittin 500 ($p < 0.05$).	[54]
Atopic dermatitis	Chicken OVA-induced atopic dermatitis in 6-week female Balb/c mice (n = 25)	Melittin (*Apis melifera*)	Three CONC: 1 µg/Kg, 10 µg/Kg, 100 µg/Kg (intraperitoneal) NC: untreated PC: OVA only	Dorsal skin thickness was significantly reduced in comparison to PC ($p < 0.05$), the greatest decrease in BV 100 group. Edema, erythema and excoriation were improved in melittin group.	Melittin significantly improved OVA-induced filaggrin deficiency ($p < 0.05$). CD14 and CD11b were significantly decreased in melittin 100 group compared to PC ($p < 0.05$). Mast cell infiltration was remarkably decreased in melittin 10 and 100 group compared to PC ($p < 0.05$). Serum IL-1β, TNF-α was notably decreased in all dose compared to PC ($p < 0.05$). Serum TSLP was remarkably decreased in melittin 100 compared to PC ($p < 0.05$). Skin IL-13 mRNA was significantly declined in melittin 100 compared with PC ($p < 0.05$).	[55]
Atopic dermatitis	DFE/DNCB-induced atopic dermatitis in 7–8-week female Balb/c mice (n = 25)	PLA2 (*Apis melifera*)	Two doses: 16 ng/ear, 80 ng/ear (Applied to ear skin) NC: DFE/DNCB only PC :dexamethasone 50 µg /ear	Ear thickness was notably decreased in all doses compared to NC ($p < 0.001$), not more than PC. AD-like skin lesions were significantly suppressed by PLA2.	Th1 cytokines (TNF- α, IL-6 and IFN-) and Th2 cytokines (IL-4 and IL-13) were remarkably decreased in comparison to NC ($p < 0.05$), no more effective than PC. Epidermal hyperplasia and lymphocyte infiltration were significantly attenuated by PLA2 in a dose-dependent manner compared with control ($p < 0.01$–$p < 0.05$), no more effective than PC. PLA2 has the potential to counteract AD-like skin lesion-associated inflammation responses via the induction of Tregs.	[58]

Table 2. *Cont.*

Disease	Model	Venom/Compound/ (Bee Species)/	Dose (Administration Method)/Control	Results	Mechanism/Molecular Response	Reference
Atopic dermatitis	Compound 48/80-induced atopic dermatitis in 6-week Balb/c mice (n = 32).	BV (*Apis melifera*)	Two doses: 0.01 mg/Kg 0.1 mg/Kg (intraperitoneal) PC: Compound 48/80 only	Scratching behavior caused by compound 48/80 was decreased by 75% and 87% compared with PC in BV 0.01 and 0.1 respectively. ($p < 0.05$) Vascular permeability of the skin was decreased by 33.3% and 70.7% compared with PC in BV 0.01 and 0.1 respectively. ($p < 0.05$)	Mast cell degranulation was remarkably decreased in a dose-dependent manner compared to PC ($p < 0.05$). TNF-α and IL-1β were significantly suppressed in skin tissue by BV treatment. BV inhibited activation of NF- κB, which was induced by compound 48/80.	[47]
Atopic dermatitis	Trimellitic anhydride -induced atopic dermatitis on ear skin in 10-week male Balb/c mice (n = 50).	BV (*Apis melifera*)	0.3 mg/Kg, Once daily for 14 day (subcutaneous, acupuncture bilateral point BL40) NC: TMA treated PC: prednisone BVNA: BV at non acupoint; base of tail	BV at BL40 acupoint significantly relieved the AD symptoms. Thickness of ear and weight of lymph node were remarkably decreased compared to NC ($p < 0.001$). All results not better than PC but similar to BVNA indicated no healing effect on AD-like symptoms.	Serum IL-4 and IgE was notably declined compared to NC ($p < 0.001$). Number of CD4 and CD8 positive cells was notably declined in comparison to NC ($p < 0.01$). TNF-α, IFN-γ, IL-2, IL-4, IL-10 and IL-12 concentration in auricular lymph node were remarkably decreased compared to NC ($p < 0.001$–$p < 0.05$).	[53]
Melanoma	B16F10 murine melanoma was implanted subcutaneously in C57BL/6 mice (n = 15)	Melittin (*Apis melifera*)	8.5 mg/Kg, 4 injections every other day starting at day 5 (intravenous, Melittin is loaded on molecularly targeted nanoparticles.) S: saline only N: nanoparticle only	Tumor weight was significantly decreased on day 14 compared with S (~88% reduction) and N (~87% reduction) ($p < 0.01$). Decrease in the number of blood vessels in proliferating cells, and significant areas of necrosis in melittin-treated-tumor.	Melittin-loaded nanoparticles cause apoptosis of cancer cell via release of cytochrome c from mitochondria.	[61]
Wound (Diabetic wound)	Diabetic 12-week male Balb/c mice wounded on back (n = 45)	BV (*Apis melifera*)	200 μg/kg for 15 day (subcutaneous, on wound area) NC: wound on non-diabetic mice PC: diabetic mice without BV treatment	Degree of wound closure was similar to NC, markedly higher than PC ($p < 0.05$).	Type I collagen expression was significantly recovered in BV-treated diabetic mice compared with PC ($p < 0.05$), lower than NC. Ang-1, Nrf2, p-Tyr, p-eNOS, p-AKT, p-ERK, CD31, CCL2, CCL3, CXCL2 and β-Defensin-2 expression were significantly recovered in BV-treated diabetic mice compared with PC ($p < 0.05$).	[82]

Table 2. *Cont.*

Disease	Model	Venom/Compound/ (Bee Species)/	Dose (Administration Method)/Control	Results	Mechanism/Molecular Response	Reference
Wound	7-week male HR-1 mice wounded on back (n = 30)	BV (*Apis melifera*)	1 μg/gauze (Wound was covered with an equal size of gauze treated with BV for 7 day) NC: untreatedPC: treated with Vaseline	Dramatic decrease of wound size was observed in BV group compared to NC and PC ($p < 0.05$).	Type 1 collagen was remarkably elevated in BV group in comparison to NC and Vaseline. TGF-b1 and fibronectin were significantly decreased in BV group in comparison to control and Vaseline. VEGF was remarkably declined in BV and PC compared to NC ($p < 0.05$).	[79]

Abbreviations: AP-1: activator protein-1, CONC: concentration, DEX: dexamethasone, DFE: *Dermatophagoides farinae* extract, DNCB: 1-chloro-2,4-dinitrobenzene, i.p.: intraperitoneally, i.v.: intravenous, KGF: keratinocyte growth factor, MAPKs: mitogen-activated protein kinases, NC: normal control, OVA: ovalbumin, P. acnes: Propionibacterium acnes, PC: positive control, PLA2: phospholipase A2, s.c:. subcutaneous, TGF-b1: transforming growth factor-b1, TNF-α: tumor necrosis factor- α, Tregs: regulatory T cell, TSLP: thymic stromal lymphopoietin, VEGF: vascular endothelial growth factor.

Table 3. In vitro studies on the therapeutic application of bee venom for skin disease.

Disease	Model	Venom/Compound/ (Bee Species)	Dose	Results	Mechanism/Molecular Response	Reference
Acne	THP-1 cell dealt with heat-killed P. acnes	BV (*Apis melifera*)	Three CONC: 0.1 μg/mL, 1 μg/mL, 5 μg/mL for 48 h	Significant reduction of TNF-α, IL-8 in a concentration-dependent manner ($p < 0.05$). Lowest TNF-α at 5 μg/mL Lowest IL-8 at 1 μg/mL	Not reported	[32]
Acne	THP-1 cell dealt with heat-killed P. acnes	BV (*Apis melifera*)	Three CONC: 1 ng/mL, 10 ng/mL, 100 ng/mL for 8 h	Significant reduction of TNF-α, IL-8, IFN-γ at all doses compared to control ($p < 0.05$). Reduced in dose dependent manner.	TLR2 expression significantly suppressed	[107]
Acne	THP-1 cell treated with heat-killed P. acnes	Melittin (*Apis melifera*)	Three CONC: 0.1 ng/mL, 0.5 ng/mL, 1 ng/mL. for 8 h	Significant reduction of TNF-α, IL-8 at all doses compared to control ($p < 0.05$). Reduced in dose-dependent manner.	Melittin significantly reduced the phosphorylation of IKK, IκB and NF- κB. Inhibiting the NF- κB signaling pathways.	[107]
Acne	HaCat cell treated with heat-killed P. acnes	BV (*Apis melifera*)	Three CONC: 1 ng/mL, 10 ng/mL, 100 ng/mL for 8 h	Significant reduction of TNF-α, IL-8, IFN-γ at 10, 100 ng/mL in comparison to control ($p < 0.05$). Reduced in dose-dependent manner.	TLR2 expression significantly suppressed	[107]

Table 3. *Cont.*

Disease	Model	Venom/Compound/ (Bee Species)	Dose	Results	Mechanism/Molecular Response	Reference
Acne	HaCat cell dealt with heat-killed P. acnes	Melittin (*Apis melifera*)	1 μg/mL	Significant reduction of TNF-α, IL-1β, IL-8, IFN-γ compared with control ($p < 0.05$).	TLR2 and 4 expression significantly decreased. Melittin significantly reduced the phosphorylation of IKK, IκB, NF- κB and p-38. Inhibiting the NF-κB and MAPK signaling pathways.	[31]
Alopecia	hDPC treated with 0.1% dexamethasone	BV (*Apis melifera*)	Three CONC: 100 ng/mL, 200 ng/mL, 500 ng/mL for 24 h	Significant increase of FGF-2, FGF-7, IGF-1R and VEGF compared with DEX only. ($p < 0.001$–$p < 0.05$). Protein-level of VEGF is increased 1.95-, 2.95-, 2.08 and 1.47-fold with 100, 200, 500 ng/mL BV and 2% minoxidil respectively.	Not reported	[35]
Atopic dermatitis	Hacat cell treated with TNF-α and IFN-γ	Melittin (*Apis melifera*)	Three CONC: 0.1 μg/mL, 0.5 μg/mL, 1 μg/mL.	IL-1β, IL-6 and IFN-γ were decreased in a dose-dependent manner. mRNA of CCL17 and CCL22 were significantly decreased in a dose-dependent manner in melitin 0.5 and 1 in comparison to control ($p < 0.05$). pJAK2, pSTAT1 and pSTAT3 expression was decreased in melittin 1 μg/mL	NF- κB DNA-binding activity was markedly reduced.	[54]
Atopic dermatitis	Hacat cell treated by 50 ng/mL of IL-4 and IL-13	Melittin (*Apis melifera*)	Three CONC: 0.1 μg/mL, 0.5 μg/mL, 1 μg/mL. for 24 h	Filaggrin expression was remarkably elevated in a dose-dependent manner in all doses compared to control ($p < 0.05$) pSTAT3 expression was significantly decreased in melittin 1 μg/mL	Not reported	[55]

Table 3. *Cont.*

Disease	Model	Venom/Compound/ (Bee Species)	Dose	Results	Mechanism/Molecular Response	Reference
Melanoma	Human melanoma A2058 cells	BV (*Apis melifera*)	4 μg/mL	Application of 4 mg/mL BV for 2 h resulted in the death of approximately 80% of A2058 cells.	BV generated reactive oxygen species (ROS) and altered mitochondrial membrane potential transition. BV causes apoptosis in AIF/EndoG-dependent but caspase-independent manner. BV interfered with AKT and MAPK family kinase activation. BV treatment significantly reduced phosphorylated AKT and p38 BV made ER and extracellular Ca^{2+} drift to the cytosol.	[60]
Photoaging	HDF cell irradiated by UVB (312 nm)	PLA2-free BV(PBV) and BV (*Apis melifera*)	PBV: 1.5 μg/mL, 3.0 μg/mL, BV 1.5 μg/mL, 3.0 μg/mL	Both PBV and BV significantly restored Type 1 procollagen synthesis in UVB-irradiated HDF cells except for BV 3 μg/mL ($p < 0.05$). Type 1 collagen significantly increased in both BV, PBV compared with control ($p < 0.05$). (Degree: 3.0 BV > 1.5 BV > 3.0 PBV > 1.5 PBV)	PBV and BV treatments significantly attenuated the MMP-1, 2 and 3 expressions ($p < 0.05$). Both PBV and BV significantly inhibited the UVB-stimulated phosphorylations of ERK1/2 and p38 ($p < 0.05$).	[68]
Photoaging	Hacat cell irradiated by UVB (312 nm)	PLA2-free BV(PBV) and BV (*Apis melifera*)	PBV: 1.5 μg/mL, 3.0 μg/mL, BV: 1.5 μg/mL, 3.0 μg/mL.	PBV and BV treatments significantly attenuated the MMP-1, 13 expressions ($p < 0.05$). Both PBV and BV significantly inhibited the UVB-stimulated phosphorylations of ERK1/2 and p38 ($p < 0.05$).		[68]
Photoaging	HDF cell irradiated by UVB (280–350 nm)	BV (*Apis melifera*)	Three CONC: 0.01 μg/mL, 0.1 μg/mL, 1 μg/mL for 24 h	BV significantly decreased MMP-1 expressions by 50–80% while MMP-3 expression by 50–85% compared to controls ($p < 0.05$). The biggest MMP-1 and MMP-3 inhibitions were observed at a 0.1 μg/mL.	Not reported	[67]
Vitiligo	Human epidermal melanocyte	BV (*Apis melifera*)	10 μg/mL	Melanocyte proliferation and melanin content were remarkably increased compared to control ($p < 0.05$), similar to melanocyte treated with 10 μM forskolin but no more than.	Forskolin increased the cAMP level 40-fold, but BV only tripled. Based on this, the cAMP level does not appear to be the deciding factor	[89]

Abbreviations: AIF: apoptosis-inducing factor, AKT: protein kinase B, cAMP: cyclic adenosine monophosphate, CONC: concentration, DEX: dexamethasone, EndoG: endonuclease G, ER: endoplasmic reticulum, ERK1/2: extracellular signal-regulated kinase 1 and 2, FGF: fibroblast growth factor, HaCat: human keratocyte, HDF: human dermal fibroblasts, hDPC: human dermal papilla cell, HEK: human epidermal keratinocyte, IGF-1R: insulin-like growth factor 1 receptor, MAPK: mitogen-activated protein kinase, *P. acnes*: *Propionibacterium acnes*, pJAK: phosphorylated janus kinases, pSTAT3: phosphorylated signal transducer and activator of transcription, TLR2: Toll-like receptor 2, UVB: ultraviolet, VEGF: vascular endothelial growth factor.

5. Discussion

Although no severe adverse effects were accounted from the studies reviewed here (Table 4), it cannot be ruled out that BV might cause fatal adverse reactions such as anaphylaxis [108]. Thus, physicians who use BV should be careful when administering BV to patients. In clinics, a skin test is used to determine whether BV treatment is suitable for individual patients, however, negative results of a skin test do not always guarantee safety [109]. Furthermore, one case report showed that anaphylaxis may occur in patients who have had no adverse reaction after former BV therapy [110]. Since anaphylaxis can occur under any circumstances, an emergency kit in accordance with the guidelines for management of anaphylaxis should always be kept ready. Meanwhile, one retrospective case study reported that the mean time to onset of anaphylaxis after BV therapy was 21.75 min [111], therefore, it is necessary to monitor the patient for at least 30 min after BV treatment. One recent study reported that high levels of basal serum tryptase increased the risk of severe anaxphylaxis [110]. As per this information, even if an injection of BV did not cause anaphylaxis in the past, if the basal serum tryptase is elevated at a certain time for some reason, anaphylaxis may occur when BV is injected. If this hypothesis is correct, the specific physiological state of the body at the point of BV injection may be a strong risk factor for the development of anaphylaxis. The analysis of safety of BV treatment will be a crucial factor in determining the value of BV as a therapeutic agent. We hope that further studies on prediction factors to prevent anaphylaxis upon BV administration will be conducted.

Table 4. Adverse effects reported in clinical studies and in in vivo studies.

Disease	Type of Study	Venom/Compound/(Bee Species)	Adverse Effect (Severity)	Reference
Atopic dermatitis	Clinical	Emollient containing BV (*Apis melifera*)	Irritation, pruritus, erythema, urticaria and disease exacerbation (mild). No significant differences in the incidence compared with control.	[49]
Psoriasis	Clinical	BV (*Apis melifera*)	Mild pain, redness and swelling at the site of apitheraphy injection	[75]
Psoriasis	Clinical	BV (*Apis melifera*)	4patients experienced itching but not significant. No systemic adverse effect.	[71]
Scleroderma	Clinical	BV (*Apis melifera*)	Slight itchiness at the location of inoculation for 1 half-day.	[64]

In this review, we surveyed the reports that showed the cytocidal effect of BV on pathogenic microorganisms that cause skin diseases as well as have a therapeutic effect on skin diseases. BV showed a significant inhibitory effect against various bacteria, fungi and viruses, and these results show potential applications of BV for diseases wherein the microbial agent is the main therapeutic agent. We expect further studies that examine the effect of BV on the treatment of various skin infections.

Treatment of warts by subcutaneous injection of BV is already being practiced in oriental medicine clinics in Korea. So, we believe that there would be a study that shows the therapeutic effects of BV on warts, but there have been no documented reports were warts were treated by using BV. Warts is known to be caused by skin infection with human papilloma virus (HPV). BV may also have a virucidal effect on the HPV virus that causes warts, as it is reported to have antiviral properties [12]. We look forward to further research about using BV in the management of warts. Furthermore, we hope that clinicians who use BV for the treatment of skin disorder actively report their cases.

Treatment with natural substances is expected to have fewer side effects than with conventional medicine, but this comparison should ensure sufficient therapeutic effects. Many studies reviewed here have shown the ability of BV to reduce inflammatory cytokines and the disease-causing microbes; however, the status of BV among the current treatments is not very clear. Using current commercial drugs as positive controls in the future studies will help assess the precise therapeutic effect of BV. However, it may not be accurate to conclude that BV is meaningless as an alternative treatment because conventional medicine shows a greater magnitude of change in vitro studies. Because life has a very complex and organic structure, reactions to certain substances can be different between at the cell level and at the living level. Therefore, in order to ultimately determine whether BV has a therapeutic effect or not, it is necessary to evaluate how much change is made by BV in the lesion in the animal or human, not just in the cell. In addition, even if the efficacy of BV is lower than conventional therapy, it can be valuable as a therapeutic agent if it can make enough improvement of disease.Of course, in-vitro study can easily help in the analysis of molecular mechanisms and it plays an important role in providing hypotheses for follow-up research at a low cost; however, clinical trial and in-vivo study are necessary to decide the dosage and appropriate use of BV. Meanwhile, such studies are also very important in identifying the side effects of BV. Choi et al. conducted in vitro and in vivo studies to examine whether BV and melittin are able to suppress MRSA infections. Surprisingly, BV showed outstanding antimicrobial activity in vitro, but strengthened the proliferation and infection of MRSA in vivo [98]. Among 25 studies on 10 diseases surveyed this time, 15 studies were on acne and AD. The number of studies on the other eight diseases was not sufficient to conclusively assert the therapeutic role of BV. Especially, for vitiligo and photoaging, only in vitro studies have been carried out. We look forward to additional studies in the form of a clinical trials and more in vivo studies for the remaining eight diseases.

In this review, we have tried to investigate not only the therapeutic effects of BV, but also its acting mechanism. In the case of much studied acne and AD, there is considerable information about the mechanism of BV action. However, despite a limited number of studies, therapeutic mechanisms of BV action in alopecia, melanoma, photoaging, wound healing, and vitiligo were also found. However, no studies have been carried out for morphea, psoriasis and skin wrinkles. Despite many studies, the precise use of BV in treatment has not been accurately identified. We look forward to further studies that examine the molecular mechanism of BV treatment.

This review only dealt with melanoma in relation to skin cancer, but there was also a study that tested the efficacy of melittin in relation to the treatment of squamous cell carcinoma (SCC). SCC has the second highest prevalence of skin cancer after melanoma [112], with 700,000 new cases occurring each year [113]. The major risk factors of SCC are ultraviolet light and ultraviolet light absorbed by skin cells' DNA, including keratinocyte, causing genetic and epigenetic changes in these cells. In particular, studies have shown that p53 and the RAS pathway are responsible for this malignant transformation [114]. Do et al. demonstrated that the combination of melittin and 5-FU, which is used as topical treatment for SCC, increased the cancer-killing effect and reduced the cytotoxicity on normal keratinocyte [115]. Despite delicate data collection, there were studies that were missed. In the data collection process for preparing a review paper, a search method that can scan not only the title of the paper but also the contents of the paper should be considered.

It is not necessary to use only one method to treat diseases nor is it needed to replace the conventional drugs completely with natural substances. We expect that there is potential that a combination of BV and conventional medicine could prove to be a valuable therapeutic asset and could minimize adverse effects. We look forward to various types of follow-up research using BV.

Funding: This research received no external funding.

Conflicts of Interest: The authors declare no conflict of interest.

References

1. Son, D.J.; Lee, J.W.; Lee, Y.H.; Song, H.S.; Lee, C.K.; Hong, J.T. Therapeutic application of anti-arthritis, pain-releasing, and anti-cancer effects of bee venom and its constituent compounds. *Pharmacol. Ther.* **2007**, *115*, 246–270. [CrossRef] [PubMed]
2. Lee, M.S.; Pittler, M.H.; Shin, B.C.; Kong, J.C.; Ernst, E. Bee venom acupuncture for musculoskeletal pain: A review. *J. Pain* **2008**, *9*, 289–297. [CrossRef] [PubMed]
3. Han, C.H.; Lee, Y.S.; Sung, S.H.; Lee, B.H.; Shin, H.Y.; Lee, Y.J. Trend analysis of the research on bee venom acupuncture in south korea, based on published articles. *J. Korean Med.* **2015**, *36*, 80–103. [CrossRef]
4. Lee, J.A.; Son, M.J.; Choi, J.; Jun, J.H.; Kim, J.I.; Lee, M.S. Bee venom acupuncture for rheumatoid arthritis: A systematic review of randomised clinical trials. *BMJ Open* **2014**, *4*, e006140. [CrossRef] [PubMed]
5. Seo, B.K.; Lee, J.H.; Sung, W.S.; Song, E.M.; Jo, D.J. Bee venom acupuncture for the treatment of chronic low back pain: Study protocol for a randomized, double-blinded, sham-controlled trial. *Trials* **2013**, *14*, 16. [CrossRef] [PubMed]
6. Nitecka-Buchta, A.; Buchta, P.; Tabenska-Bosakowska, E.; Walczynska-Dragon, K.; Baron, S. Myorelaxant effect of bee venom topical skin application in patients with rdc/tmd ia and rdc/tmd ib: A randomized, double blinded study. *Biomed. Res. Int.* **2014**, *2014*, 296053. [CrossRef] [PubMed]
7. Hwang, D.S.; Kim, S.K.; Bae, H. Therapeutic effects of bee venom on immunological and neurological diseases. *Toxins* **2015**, *7*, 2413–2421. [CrossRef]
8. Yang, E.J.; Jiang, J.H.; Lee, S.M.; Yang, S.C.; Hwang, H.S.; Lee, M.S.; Choi, S.M. Bee venom attenuates neuroinflammatory events and extends survival in amyotrophic lateral sclerosis models. *J. Neuroinflamm.* **2010**, *7*, 69. [CrossRef]
9. Gu, H.; An, H.J.; Kim, J.Y.; Kim, W.H.; Gwon, M.G.; Kim, H.J.; Han, S.M.; Park, I.; Park, S.C.; Leem, J.; et al. Bee venom attenuates porphyromonas gingivalis and rankl-induced bone resorption with osteoclastogenic differentiation. *Food Chem. Toxicol.* **2019**, *129*, 344–353. [CrossRef]
10. Zhang, S.; Liu, Y.; Ye, Y.; Wang, X.R.; Lin, L.T.; Xiao, L.Y.; Zhou, P.; Shi, G.X.; Liu, C.Z. Bee venom therapy: Potential mechanisms and therapeutic applications. *Toxicon* **2018**, *148*, 64–73. [CrossRef]
11. Zolfagharian, H.; Mohajeri, M.; Babaie, M. Bee venom (apis mellifera) an effective potential alternative to gentamicin for specific bacteria strains: Bee venom an effective potential for bacteria. *J. Pharmacopunct.* **2016**, *19*, 225–230. [CrossRef] [PubMed]
12. Uddin, M.B.; Lee, B.H.; Nikapitiya, C.; Kim, J.H.; Kim, T.H.; Lee, H.C.; Kim, C.G.; Lee, J.S.; Kim, C.J. Inhibitory effects of bee venom and its components against viruses in vitro and in vivo. *J. Microbiol.* **2016**, *54*, 853–866. [CrossRef] [PubMed]
13. Han, S.M.; Kim, J.M.; Hong, I.P.; Woo, S.O.; Kim, S.G.; Jang, H.R.; Pak, S.C. Antibacterial activity and antibiotic-enhancing effects of honeybee venom against methicillin-resistant staphylococcus aureus. *Molecules* **2016**, *21*, 79. [CrossRef] [PubMed]
14. Socarras, K.M.; Theophilus, P.A.S.; Torres, J.P.; Gupta, K.; Sapi, E. Antimicrobial activity of bee venom and melittin against borrelia burgdorferi. *Antibiotics* **2017**, *6*, 31. [CrossRef] [PubMed]
15. Lyu, C.; Fang, F.; Li, B. Anti-tumor effects of melittin and its potential applications in clinic. *Curr. Protein Pept. Sci.* **2019**, *20*, 240–250. [CrossRef] [PubMed]
16. Rady, I.; Siddiqui, I.A.; Rady, M.; Mukhtar, H. Melittin, a major peptide component of bee venom, and its conjugates in cancer therapy. *Cancer Lett.* **2017**, *402*, 16–31. [CrossRef]
17. Memariani, H.; Memariani, M.; Shahidi-Dadras, M.; Nasiri, S.; Akhavan, M.M.; Moravvej, H. Melittin: From honeybees to superbugs. *Appl. Microbiol. Biotechnol.* **2019**, *103*, 3265–3276. [CrossRef] [PubMed]
18. Jappe, U. Pathological mechanisms of acne with special emphasis on propionibacterium acnes and related therapy. *Acta Derm. Venereol.* **2003**, *83*, 241–248. [CrossRef]
19. Toyoda, M.; Morohashi, M. Pathogenesis of acne. *Med. Electron Microsc.* **2001**, *34*, 29–40. [CrossRef]
20. Ochsendorf, F. Systemic antibiotic therapy of acne vulgaris. *J. Dtsch. Dermatol. Ges.* **2006**, *4*, 828–841. [CrossRef]
21. Eady, E.A. Bacterial resistance in acne. *Dermatology* **1998**, *196*, 59–66. [CrossRef] [PubMed]
22. Eady, E.A.; Cove, J.H.; Holland, K.T.; Cunliffe, W.J. Erythromycin resistant propionibacteria in antibiotic treated acne patients: Association with therapeutic failure. *Br. J. Dermatol.* **1989**, *121*, 51–57. [CrossRef]

23. Tan, H.H. Antibacterial therapy for acne: A guide to selection and use of systemic agents. *Am. J. Clin. Dermatol.* **2003**, *4*, 307–314. [CrossRef]
24. Han, S.M.; Lee, K.G.; Pak, S.C. Effects of cosmetics containing purified honeybee (apis mellifera l.) venom on acne vulgaris. *J. Integr. Med.* **2013**, *11*, 320–326. [CrossRef] [PubMed]
25. Han, S.M.; Pak, S.C.; Nicholls, Y.M.; Macfarlane, N. Evaluation of anti-acne property of purified bee venom serum in humans. *J. Cosmet. Dermatol.* **2016**, *15*, 324–329. [CrossRef] [PubMed]
26. Leyden, J.J.; McGinley, K.J.; Mills, O.H.; Kligman, A.M. Propionibacterium levels in patients with and without acne vulgaris. *J. Investig. Dermatol.* **1975**, *65*, 382–384. [CrossRef] [PubMed]
27. Vowels, B.R.; Yang, S.; Leyden, J.J. Induction of proinflammatory cytokines by a soluble factor of propionibacterium acnes: Implications for chronic inflammatory acne. *Infect. Immun.* **1995**, *63*, 3158–3165. [PubMed]
28. An, H.J.; Lee, W.R.; Kim, K.H.; Kim, J.Y.; Lee, S.J.; Han, S.M.; Lee, K.G.; Lee, C.K.; Park, K.K. Inhibitory effects of bee venom on propionibacterium acnes-induced inflammatory skin disease in an animal model. *Int. J. Mol. Med.* **2014**, *34*, 1341–1348. [CrossRef] [PubMed]
29. Raghuraman, H.; Chattopadhyay, A. Melittin: A membrane-active peptide with diverse functions. *Biosci. Rep.* **2007**, *27*, 189–223. [CrossRef]
30. Lee, G.; Bae, H. Anti-inflammatory applications of melittin, a major component of bee venom: Detailed mechanism of action and adverse effects. *Molecules* **2016**, *21*, 616. [CrossRef] [PubMed]
31. Lee, W.R.; Kim, K.H.; An, H.J.; Kim, J.Y.; Chang, Y.C.; Chung, H.; Park, Y.Y.; Lee, M.L.; Park, K.K. The protective effects of melittin on propionibacterium acnes-induced inflammatory responses in vitro and in vivo. *J. Investig. Dermatol.* **2014**, *134*, 1922–1930. [CrossRef] [PubMed]
32. Hari, A.; Flach, T.L.; Shi, Y.; Mydlarski, P.R. Toll-like receptors: Role in dermatological disease. *Mediat. Inflamm.* **2010**, *2010*, 16. [CrossRef] [PubMed]
33. Han, S.; Lee, K.; Yeo, J.; Baek, H.; Park, K. Antibacterial and anti-inflammatory effects of honeybee (apis mellifera) venom against acne-inducing bacteria. *J. Med. Plants Res.* **2010**, *4*, 459–464.
34. Huang, K.P.; Mullangi, S.; Guo, Y.; Qureshi, A.A. Autoimmune, atopic, and mental health comorbid conditions associated with alopecia areata in the united states. *JAMA Dermatol.* **2013**, *149*, 789–794. [CrossRef] [PubMed]
35. Park, S.; Erdogan, S.; Hwang, D.; Hwang, S.; Han, E.H.; Lim, Y.H. Bee venom promotes hair growth in association with inhibiting 5alpha-reductase expression. *Biol. Pharm. Bull.* **2016**, *39*, 1060–1068. [CrossRef] [PubMed]
36. Yim, E.; Nole, K.L.; Tosti, A. 5alpha-reductase inhibitors in androgenetic alopecia. *Curr. Opin. Endocrinol. Diabetes Obes.* **2014**, *21*, 493–498. [CrossRef]
37. Amory, J.K.; Wang, C.; Swerdloff, R.S.; Anawalt, B.D.; Matsumoto, A.M.; Bremner, W.J.; Walker, S.E.; Haberer, L.J.; Clark, R.V. The effect of 5alpha-reductase inhibition with dutasteride and finasteride on semen parameters and serum hormones in healthy men. *J. Clin. Endocrinol. Metab.* **2007**, *92*, 1659–1665. [CrossRef] [PubMed]
38. Traish, A.M.; Hassani, J.; Guay, A.T.; Zitzmann, M.; Hansen, M.L. Adverse side effects of 5alpha-reductase inhibitors therapy: Persistent diminished libido and erectile dysfunction and depression in a subset of patients. *J. Sex. Med.* **2011**, *8*, 872–884. [CrossRef]
39. Cotsarelis, G.; Millar, S.E. Towards a molecular understanding of hair loss and its treatment. *Trends Mol. Med.* **2001**, *7*, 293–301. [CrossRef]
40. Stough, D.; Stenn, K.; Haber, R.; Parsley, W.M.; Vogel, J.E.; Whiting, D.A.; Washenik, K. Psychological effect, pathophysiology, and management of androgenetic alopecia in men. *Mayo Clin. Proc.* **2005**, *80*, 1316–1322. [CrossRef]
41. Lee, H.J.; Lee, S.H. Epidermal permeability barrier defects and barrier repair therapy in atopic dermatitis. *Allergy Asthma Immunol. Res.* **2014**, *6*, 276–287. [CrossRef] [PubMed]
42. Leung, D.Y. Atopic dermatitis: New insights and opportunities for therapeutic intervention. *J. Allergy Clin. Immunol.* **2000**, *105*, 860–876. [CrossRef] [PubMed]
43. Friedman, E.S.; LaNatra, N.; Stiller, M.J. Nsaids in dermatologic therapy: Review and preview. *J. Cutan. Med. Surg.* **2002**, *6*, 449–459. [CrossRef] [PubMed]
44. Belvisi, M.G.; Hele, D.J. Soft steroids: A new approach to the treatment of inflammatory airways diseases. *Pulm. Pharmacol. Ther.* **2003**, *16*, 321–325. [CrossRef]

45. Simons, F.E. The antiallergic effects of antihistamines (h1-receptor antagonists). *J. Allergy Clin. Immunol.* **1992**, *90*, 705–715. [CrossRef]
46. Schafer-Korting, M.; Schmid, M.H.; Korting, H.C. Topical glucocorticoids with improved risk-benefit ratio. Rationale of a new concept. *Drug Saf.* **1996**, *14*, 375–385. [CrossRef] [PubMed]
47. Kim, K.H.; Lee, W.R.; An, H.J.; Kim, J.Y.; Chung, H.; Han, S.M.; Lee, M.L.; Lee, K.G.; Pak, S.C.; Park, K.K. Bee venom ameliorates compound 48/80-induced atopic dermatitis-related symptoms. *Int. J. Clin. Exp. Pathol.* **2013**, *6*, 2896–2903. [PubMed]
48. Wakao, S.; Kuroda, Y.; Ogura, F.; Shigemoto, T.; Dezawa, M. Regenerative effects of mesenchymal stem cells: Contribution of muse cells, a novel pluripotent stem cell type that resides in mesenchymal cells. *Cells* **2012**, *1*, 1045–1060. [CrossRef]
49. You, C.E.; Moon, S.H.; Lee, K.H.; Kim, K.H.; Park, C.W.; Seo, S.J.; Cho, S.H. Effects of emollient containing bee venom on atopic dermatitis: A double-blinded, randomized, base-controlled, multicenter study of 136 patients. *Ann. Dermatol.* **2016**, *28*, 593–599. [CrossRef]
50. Gu, H.; Kim, W.H.; An, H.J.; Kim, J.Y.; Gwon, M.G.; Han, S.M.; Leem, J.; Park, K.K. Therapeutic effects of bee venom on experimental atopic dermatitis. *Mol. Med. Rep.* **2018**, *18*, 3711–3718. [CrossRef]
51. Kim, Y.; Lee, Y.-W.; Kim, H.; Chung, D.K. Bee venom alleviates atopic dermatitis symptoms through the upregulation of decay-accelerating factor (daf/cd55). *Toxins* **2019**, *11*, 239. [CrossRef]
52. Leung, D.Y.; Hanifin, J.M.; Charlesworth, E.N.; Li, J.T.; Bernstein, I.L.; Berger, W.E.; Blessing-Moore, J.; Fineman, S.; Lee, F.E.; Nicklas, R.A.; et al. Disease management of atopic dermatitis: A practice parameter. *Ann. Allergy Asthma Immunol.* **1997**, *79*, 197–211.
53. Sur, B.; Lee, B.; Yeom, M.; Hong, J.H.; Kwon, S.; Kim, S.T.; Lee, H.S.; Park, H.J.; Lee, H.; Hahm, D.H. Bee venom acupuncture alleviates trimellitic anhydride-induced atopic dermatitis-like skin lesions in mice. *BMC Complement. Altern. Med.* **2016**, *16*, 38. [CrossRef]
54. An, H.J.; Kim, J.Y.; Kim, W.H.; Gwon, M.G.; Gu, H.M.; Jeon, M.J.; Han, S.M.; Pak, S.C.; Lee, C.K.; Park, I.S.; et al. Therapeutic effects of bee venom and its major component, melittin, on atopic dermatitis in vivo and in vitro. *Br. J. Pharmacol.* **2018**, *175*, 4310–4324. [CrossRef]
55. Kim, W.H.; An, H.J.; Kim, J.Y.; Gwon, M.G.; Gu, H.; Jeon, M.; Sung, W.J.; Han, S.M.; Pak, S.C.; Kim, M.K.; et al. Beneficial effects of melittin on ovalbumin-induced atopic dermatitis in mouse. *Sci. Rep.* **2017**, *7*, 17679. [CrossRef]
56. Dennis, E.A.; Rhee, S.G.; Billah, M.M.; Hannun, Y.A. Role of phospholipase in generating lipid second messengers in signal transduction. *FASEB J.* **1991**, *5*, 2068–2077. [CrossRef]
57. Mukherjee, A.B.; Miele, L.; Pattabiraman, N. Phospholipase A_2 enzymes: Regulation and physiological role. *Biochem. Pharmacol.* **1994**, *48*, 1–10. [CrossRef]
58. Jung, K.H.; Baek, H.; Kang, M.; Kim, N.; Lee, S.Y.; Bae, H. Bee venom phospholipase a2 ameliorates house dust mite extract induced atopic dermatitis like skin lesions in mice. *Toxins* **2017**, *9*, 68. [CrossRef]
59. Amano, W.; Nakajima, S.; Kunugi, H.; Numata, Y.; Kitoh, A.; Egawa, G.; Dainichi, T.; Honda, T.; Otsuka, A.; Kimoto, Y.; et al. The janus kinase inhibitor jte-052 improves skin barrier function through suppressing signal transducer and activator of transcription 3 signaling. *J. Allergy Clin. Immunol.* **2015**, *136*, 667–677. [CrossRef]
60. Tu, W.C.; Wu, C.C.; Hsieh, H.L.; Chen, C.Y.; Hsu, S.L. Honeybee venom induces calcium-dependent but caspase-independent apoptotic cell death in human melanoma a2058 cells. *Toxicon* **2008**, *52*, 318–329. [CrossRef]
61. Soman, N.R.; Baldwin, S.L.; Hu, G.; Marsh, J.N.; Lanza, G.M.; Heuser, J.E.; Arbeit, J.M.; Wickline, S.A.; Schlesinger, P.H. Molecularly targeted nanocarriers deliver the cytolytic peptide melittin specifically to tumor cells in mice, reducing tumor growth. *J. Clin. Investig.* **2009**, *119*, 2830–2842. [CrossRef]
62. Shai, Y. Mechanism of the binding, insertion and destabilization of phospholipid bilayer membranes by alpha-helical antimicrobial and cell non-selective membrane-lytic peptides. *Biochim. Biophys. Acta* **1999**, *1462*, 55–70. [CrossRef]
63. Fett, N.M. Morphea (localized scleroderma). *JAMA Dermatol.* **2013**, *149*, 1124. [CrossRef]
64. Hwang, J.H.; Kim, K.H. Bee venom acupuncture for circumscribed morphea in a patient with systemic sclerosis: A case report. *Medicine* **2018**, *97*, e13404. [CrossRef]
65. Jones, S.A.; McArdle, F.; Jack, C.I.; Jackson, M.J. Effect of antioxidant supplementation on the adaptive response of human skin fibroblasts to uv-induced oxidative stress. *Redox Rep.* **1999**, *4*, 291–299. [CrossRef]

66. Katiyar, S.K.; Bergamo, B.M.; Vyalil, P.K.; Elmets, C.A. Green tea polyphenols: DNA photodamage and photoimmunology. *J. Photochem. Photobiol. B* **2001**, *65*, 109–114. [CrossRef]
67. Han, S.; Lee, K.; Yeo, J.; Kweon, H.; Woo, S.; Lee, M.; Baek, H.; Park, K. Inhibitory effect of bee venom against ultraviolet b induced mmp-11 and mmp-3 in human dermal fibroblasts. *J. Apic. Res.* **2007**, *46*, 94–98. [CrossRef]
68. Lee, H.; Bae, S.K.; Pyo, M.; Heo, Y.; Kim, C.G.; Kang, C.; Kim, E. Anti-wrinkle effect of pla2-free bee venom against uvb-irradiated human skin cells. *J. Agric. Life Sci.* **2015**, *49*, 125–135.
69. Makrantonaki, E.; Zouboulis, C.C. Molecular mechanisms of skin aging: State of the art. *Ann. N. Y. Acad. Sci.* **2007**, *1119*, 40–50. [CrossRef]
70. Schon, M.P.; Boehncke, W.H. Psoriasis. *N. Engl. J. Med.* **2005**, *352*, 1899–1912. [CrossRef]
71. Hegazi, A.G.; Raboh, F.A.A.; Ramzy, N.E.; Shaaban, D.M.; Khader, D.Y. Bee venom and propolis as new treatment modality in patients with localized plaque psoriases. *Int. Res. J. Med. Med. Sci.* **2013**, *1*, 27–33.
72. Mizutani, H.; Ohmoto, Y.; Mizutani, T.; Murata, M.; Shimizu, M. Role of increased production of monocytes TNF-α, IL-1β and IL-6 in psoriasis: Relation to focal infection, disease activity and responses to treatments. *J. Dermatol. Sci.* **1997**, *14*, 145–153. [CrossRef]
73. Feldman, S. Advances in psoriasis treatment. *Dermatol. Online J.* **2000**, *6*, 4.
74. Williams, I.R.; Kupper, T.S. Immunity at the surface: Homeostatic mechanisms of the skin immune system. *Life Sci.* **1996**, *58*, 1485–1507. [CrossRef]
75. Eltaher, S.; Mohammed, G.F.; Younes, S.; Elakhras, A. Efficacy of the apitherapy in the treatment of recalcitrant localized plaque psoriasis and evaluation of tumor necrosis factor-alpha (tnf-alpha) serum level: A double-blind randomized clinical trial. *J. Dermatol. Treat.* **2015**, *26*, 335–339. [CrossRef]
76. Coenen, J. Late results of a triple-layer artificial skin. In Proceedings of the European Burn Association 5th Congres, Brighton, UK, 20–23 September 1993.
77. Rothe, M.; Falanga, V. Growth factors: Their biology and promise in dermatologic diseases and tissue repair. *JAMA Dermatol.* **1989**, *125*, 1390–1398. [CrossRef]
78. Singer, A.J.; Clark, R.A. Cutaneous wound healing. *N. Engl. J. Med.* **1999**, *341*, 738–746. [CrossRef]
79. Han, S.; Lee, K.; Yeo, J.; Kim, W.; Park, K. Biological effects of treatment of an animal skin wound with honeybee (*apis mellifera*. L) venom. *J. Plast. Reconstr. Aesthet. Surg.* **2011**, *64*, e67–e72. [CrossRef]
80. Galkowska, H.; Wojewodzka, U.; Olszewski, W.L. Chemokines, cytokines, and growth factors in keratinocytes and dermal endothelial cells in the margin of chronic diabetic foot ulcers. *Wound Repair Regen* **2006**, *14*, 558–565. [CrossRef]
81. Goren, I.; Muller, E.; Pfeilschifter, J.; Frank, S. Severely impaired insulin signaling in chronic wounds of diabetic ob/ob mice: A potential role of tumor necrosis factor-alpha. *Am. J. Pathol.* **2006**, *168*, 765–777. [CrossRef]
82. Hozzein, W.N.; Badr, G.; Badr, B.M.; Allam, A.; Ghamdi, A.A.; Al-Wadaan, M.A.; Al-Waili, N.S. Bee venom improves diabetic wound healing by protecting functional macrophages from apoptosis and enhancing nrf2, ang-1 and tie-2 signaling. *Mol. Immunol.* **2018**, *103*, 322–335. [CrossRef]
83. Han, S.M.; Lee, K.G.; Park, K.K.; Pak, S.C. Skin sensitization study of bee venom (*Apis mellifera* L.) in guinea pigs and rats. *Cutan. Ocul. Toxicol.* **2013**, *32*, 27–30. [CrossRef]
84. Han, S.M.; Hong, I.P.; Woo, S.O.; Chun, S.N.; Park, K.K.; Nicholls, Y.M.; Pak, S.C. The beneficial effects of honeybee-venom serum on facial wrinkles in humans. *Clin. Interv. Aging* **2015**, *10*, 1587–1592. [CrossRef]
85. Lan, C.C.; Chen, G.S.; Chiou, M.H.; Wu, C.S.; Chang, C.H.; Yu, H.S. Fk506 promotes melanocyte and melanoblast growth and creates a favourable milieu for cell migration via keratinocytes: Possible mechanisms of how tacrolimus ointment induces repigmentation in patients with vitiligo. *Br. J. Dermatol.* **2005**, *153*, 498–505. [CrossRef]
86. Scott, G.A.; Jacobs, S.E.; Pentland, A.P. Spla2-x stimulates cutaneous melanocyte dendricity and pigmentation through a lysophosphatidylcholine-dependent mechanism. *J. Investig. Dermatol.* **2006**, *126*, 855–861. [CrossRef]
87. Maeda, K.; Tomita, Y.; Naganuma, M.; Tagami, H. Phospholipases induce melanogenesis in organ-cultured skin. *Photochem. Photobiol.* **1996**, *64*, 220–223. [CrossRef]
88. Maeda, K.; Naganuma, M. Melanocyte-stimulating properties of secretory phospholipase A_2. *Photochem. Photobiol.* **1997**, *65*, 145–149. [CrossRef]

89. Jeon, S.; Kim, N.H.; Koo, B.S.; Lee, H.J.; Lee, A.Y. Bee venom stimulates human melanocyte proliferation, melanogenesis, dendricity and migration. *Exp. Mol. Med.* **2007**, *39*, 603–613. [CrossRef]
90. Chomnawang, M.T.; Surassmo, S.; Nukoolkarn, V.S.; Gritsanapan, W. Antimicrobial effects of thai medicinal plants against acne-inducing bacteria. *J. Ethnopharmacol.* **2005**, *101*, 330–333. [CrossRef]
91. Nakatsuji, T.; Kao, M.C.; Fang, J.Y.; Zouboulis, C.C.; Zhang, L.; Gallo, R.L.; Huang, C.M. Antimicrobial property of lauric acid against propionibacterium acnes: Its therapeutic potential for inflammatory acne vulgaris. *J. Investig. Dermatol.* **2009**, *129*, 2480–2488. [CrossRef]
92. Leyden, J.J.; Del Rosso, J.Q.; Webster, G.F. Clinical considerations in the treatment of acne vulgaris and other inflammatory skin disorders: A status report. *Dermatol. Clin.* **2009**, *27*, 1–15. [CrossRef] [PubMed]
93. Bojar, R.A.; Holland, K.T. Acne and propionibacterium acnes. *Clin. Dermatol.* **2004**, *22*, 375–379. [CrossRef] [PubMed]
94. Lebwohl, M.G.; Heymann, W.R.; Berth-Jones, J.; Coulson, I. Impetigo. In *Treatment of Skin Disease E-Book: Comprehensive Therapeutic Strategies*, 4th ed.; Elsevier Health Sciences: Amsterdam, The Netherlands, 2013; p. 332.
95. Lebwohl, M.G.; Heymann, W.R.; Berth-Jones, J.; Coulson, I. Paronychia. In *Treatment of Skin Disease E-Book: Comprehensive Therapeutic Strategies*, 4th ed.; Elsevier Health Sciences: Amsterdam, The Netherlands, 2013; p. 542.
96. Lebwohl, M.G.; Heymann, W.R.; Berth-Jones, J.; Coulson, I. Staphylococcal Scalded Skin Syndrome. In *Treatment of Skin Disease E-Book: Comprehensive Therapeutic Strategies*, 4th ed.; Elsevier Health Sciences: Amsterdam, The Netherlands, 2013; p. 723.
97. Taylor, A.R. Methicillin-resistant staphylococcus aureus infections. *Prim. Care Clin. Off. Pract.* **2013**, *40*, 637–654. [CrossRef] [PubMed]
98. Choi, J.H.; Jang, A.Y.; Lin, S.; Lim, S.; Kim, D.; Park, K.; Han, S.-M.; Yeo, J.-H.; Seo, H.S. Melittin, a honeybee venom-derived antimicrobial peptide, may target methicillin-resistant staphylococcus aureus. *Mol. Med. Rep.* **2015**, *12*, 6483–6490. [CrossRef] [PubMed]
99. Lebwohl, M.G.; Heymann, W.R.; Berth-Jones, J.; Coulson, I. Tinea Pedis and Skin Dermatophytosis. In *Treatment of Skin Disease E-Book: Comprehensive Therapeutic Strategies*, 4th ed.; Elsevier Health Sciences: Amsterdam, The Netherlands, 2013; p. 756.
100. Yu, A.R.; Kim, J.J.; Park, G.S.; Oh, S.M.; Han, C.S.; Lee, M.Y. Biochemistry: The antifungal activity of bee venom against dermatophytes. *J. Appl. Biol. Chem.* **2012**, *55*, 7–11. [CrossRef]
101. Park, J.; Kwon, O.; An, H.J.; Park, K.K. Antifungal effects of bee venom components on trichophyton rubrum: A novel approach of bee venom study for possible emerging antifungal agent. *Ann. Dermatol.* **2018**, *30*, 202–210. [CrossRef] [PubMed]
102. Lebwohl, M.G.; Heymann, W.R.; Berth-Jones, J.; Coulson, I. Cutaneous Candidiasis and Chronic Mucocutaneous Candidasis. In *Treatment of Skin Disease E-Book: Comprehensive Therapeutic Strategies*, 4th ed.; Elsevier Health Sciences: Amsterdam, The Netherlands, 2013; p. 157.
103. Lee, S.B. Antifungal activity of bee venom and sweet bee venom against clinically isolated candida albicans. *J. Pharmacopunct.* **2016**, *19*, 45–50. [CrossRef]
104. Park, C.; Lee, D.G. Melittin induces apoptotic features in candida albicans. *Biochem. Biophys. Res. Commun.* **2010**, *394*, 170–172. [CrossRef]
105. Prakash, S.; Bhargava, H. Apis cerana bee venom: It's antidiabetic and anti-dandruff activity against malassezia furfur. *World Appl. Sci. J.* **2014**, *32*, 343–348.
106. Lebwohl, M.G.; Heymann, W.R.; Berth-Jones, J.; Coulson, I. Herpes Labialis. In *Treatment of Skin Disease E-Book: Comprehensive Therapeutic Strategies*, 4th ed.; Elsevier Health Sciences: Amsterdam, The Netherlands, 2013; p. 308.
107. Kim, J.-Y.; Lee, W.-R.; Kim, K.-H.; An, H.-J.; Chang, Y.-C.; Han, S.-M.; Park, Y.-Y.; Pak, S.C.; Park, K.-K. Effects of bee venom against propionibacterium acnes-induced inflammation in human keratinocytes and monocytes. *Int. J. Mol. Med.* **2015**, *35*, 1651–1656. [CrossRef]
108. Park, J.H.; Yim, B.K.; Lee, J.H.; Lee, S.; Kim, T.H. Risk associated with bee venom therapy: A systematic review and meta-analysis. *PLoS ONE* **2015**, *10*, e0126971. [CrossRef] [PubMed]

109. Cavallucci, E.; Ramondo, S.; Renzetti, A.; Turi, M.C.; Di Claudio, F.; Braga, M.; Incorvaia, C.; Schiavone, C.; Ballone, E.; Di Gioacchino, M. Maintenance venom immunotherapy administered at a 3-month interval preserves safety and efficacy and improves adherence. *J. Investig. Allergol. Clin. Immunol.* **2010**, *20*, 63–68. [PubMed]
110. Kim, J.-H.; Kim, M.-S.; Lee, J.-Y.; Yeom, S.-R.; Kwon, Y.-D.; Kim, D.-W. The case report of anaphylaxis after treated with bee-venom acupuncture. *J. Korean Med. Rehabil.* **2015**, *25*, 175–182. [CrossRef]
111. Lee, S.-K.; Ye, Y.-M.; Park, H.-S.; Jang, G.C.; Jee, Y.-K.; Park, H.-K.; Koh, Y.-I.; Kim, J.-H.; Kim, C.-W.; Hur, G.-Y. Hymenoptera venom anaphylaxis in adult korean: A multicenter retrospective case study. *Allergy Asthma Respir. Dis.* **2014**, *2*, 344–351.
112. Alam, M.; Ratner, D. Cutaneous squamous-cell carcinoma. *N. Engl. J. Med.* **2001**, *344*, 975–983. [CrossRef] [PubMed]
113. Lomas, A.; Leonardi-Bee, J.; Bath-Hextall, F. A systematic review of worldwide incidence of nonmelanoma skin cancer. *Br. J. Dermatol.* **2012**, *166*, 1069–1080. [CrossRef]
114. Grossman, D.; Leffell, D.J. The molecular basis of nonmelanoma skin cancer: New understanding. *Arch. Dermatol.* **1997**, *133*, 1263–1270. [CrossRef]
115. Do, N.; Weindl, G.; Grohmann, L.; Salwiczek, M.; Koksch, B.; Korting, H.C.; Schafer-Korting, M. Cationic membrane-active peptides - anticancer and antifungal activity as well as penetration into human skin. *Exp. Dermatol.* **2014**, *23*, 326–331. [CrossRef]

toxins

MDPI

Communication

The Influence of Bee Venom Melittin on the Functioning of the Immune System and the Contractile Activity of the Insect Heart—A Preliminary Study

Jan Lubawy [1,*,†], Arkadiusz Urbański [1,*,†], Lucyna Mrówczyńska [2], Eliza Matuszewska [3], Agata Światły-Błaszkiewicz [3], Jan Matysiak [3] and Grzegorz Rosiński [1]

1 Department of Animal Physiology and Development, Faculty of Biology, Adam Mickiewicz University in Poznań, 61-614 Poznań, Poland
2 Department of Cell Biology, Faculty of Biology, Adam Mickiewicz University in Poznań, 61-614 Poznań, Poland
3 Department of Inorganic and Analytical Chemistry, Poznan University of Medical Sciences, 60-780 Poznan, Poland
* Correspondence: j.lubawy@amu.edu.pl (J.L.); arur@amu.edu.pl (A.U.)
† Authors have contributed equally.

Received: 23 July 2019; Accepted: 23 August 2019; Published: 27 August 2019

check for updates

Abstract: Melittin (MEL) is a basic polypeptide originally purified from honeybee venom. MEL exhibits a broad spectrum of biological activity. However, almost all studies on MEL activity have been carried out on vertebrate models or cell lines. Recently, due to cheap breeding and the possibility of extrapolating the results of the research to vertebrates, insects have been used for various bioassays and comparative physiological studies. For these reasons, it is valuable to examine the influence of melittin on insect physiology. Here, for the first time, we report the immunotropic and cardiotropic effects of melittin on the beetle *Tenebrio molitor* as a model insect. After melittin injection at 10^{-7} M and 10^{-3} M, the number of apoptotic cells in the haemolymph increased in a dose-dependent manner. The pro-apoptotic action of MEL was likely compensated by increasing the total number of haemocytes. However, the injection of MEL did not cause any changes in the percent of phagocytic haemocytes or in the phenoloxidase activity. In an in vitro bioassay with a semi-isolated *Tenebrio* heart, MEL induced a slight chronotropic-positive effect only at a higher concentration (10^{-4} M). Preliminary results indicated that melittin exerts pleiotropic effects on the functioning of the immune system and the endogenous contractile activity of the heart. Some of the induced responses in *T. molitor* resemble the reactions observed in vertebrate models. Therefore, the *T. molitor* beetle may be a convenient invertebrate model organism for comparative physiological studies and for the identification of new properties and mechanisms of action of melittin and related compounds.

Keywords: melittin; insect immune system; apoptosis; heart contractility; *Tenebrio molitor*

Key Contribution: In this report, for the first time, we describe the immunotropic and cardiotropic activity of melittin in heterologous bioassays with a model insect species—*T. molitor* beetle.

1. Introduction

Venomous animals have been a focus of interest for humans for years due to the danger associated with them and the possibility of taking advantage of venom action and utilizing it in medicine [1,2]. Animal venoms are immensely complex mixtures composed of proteins, peptides, biogenic amines, and other substances of low-molecular weight, which are often enzymatically active [3–5]. Especially, the great interest is related to the biological activity of proteins isolated from bee (melittin, apamina and tertiapin) and wasp (mastoparan and bradykinin) venoms [2].

Melittin (MEL), a 26-amino-acid amphiphilic polypeptide with a hydrophobic *N*-terminal and a hydrophilic *C*-terminal end, is one of the most important bee venom compounds. MEL is the major active component of apitoxin (honeybee venom), constituting from 40% to 60% of whole dry venom [6]. Melittin has various biological, pharmacological, and toxicological actions, including strong surface activity on cell lipid membranes, and haemolytic, antibacterial, antifungal, and potential anti-tumour activities [6–9]. Melittin is also known as a membrane pore-forming agent that in a dose-dependent manner interacts with the phospholipid bilayer, and the molecular mechanism of interactions between biomembranes and peptides and proteins can be studied using MEL-biological activity [10–12]. When MEL binds to cell membranes, it forms toroid-shaped pores that enable the leakage of molecules of tens of kDa in size. This leakage results in a dose-dependent increase in membrane permeability and cell lysis. As a peptide that forms pores, melittin has been extensively studied from diverse aspects, including its structure, binding properties and mechanisms, and disruption of phospholipid bilayer structure processes (reviewed by Chen, et al. [13]). Due to its fascinating interaction with the lipids of the plasma membrane and its capability to form pores, melittin has the potential to be used as an antimicrobial agent, for cell-selective attack, and for the translocation of materials by increasing the membrane permeability [14–16]. Melittin binds to negatively charged membrane surfaces with ease and then disturbs the integrity of phospholipid bilayers either by forming a transmembrane pore or ion channel or by exhibiting surfactant activity, accompanied by the enhancement of permeability and the leakage of ions and molecules as a consequence [17–19]. The mode of MEL action can be influenced by the compositions of lipid membranes (electric charge or packing density) [20]. Due to its well-defined effect against the plasma membrane, MEL has consistently been used as an antimicrobial peptide (AMP). For example, Lee and Lee [21] showed that MEL has a dual antimicrobial mechanism against *Candida albicans*, disrupting target microorganism membranes and triggering apoptosis through the mitochondria/caspase-dependent pathway [21]. MEL and its derivatives and analogues also show anti-leishmanial activity in vitro. It was shown that hybrids of melittin and other AMPs cause a decrease in electrical potential and morphological changes in the membranes of *Leishmania donovani* with a fast loss of ATP (reviewed by McGwire and Kulkarni [22]). These MEL-induced morphological changes in membranes could be attributed to membrane protein aggregation, hormone secretion, and/or membrane potential alterations. Furthermore, MEL can increase the activity of several enzymes, such as G-protein, protein kinase C, adenylate cyclase, and phospholipases [23], including phospholipase A_2 (PLA_2). MEL also exerts potent cardioactive effects. It produces dose- and time-dependent increases in mean arterial pressure (MAP) and heart rate (HR) [24] and inhibits the activity of Na^+K^+-ATPase [25]. Due to the increase of the permeability of the plasma membrane to ions, especially Na^+ and Ca^{2+}, melittin causes significant morphological and functional cell changes, especially in excitable tissues, such as cardiac myocytes ([26] and references therein). Since MEL is a nonspecific cytolytic peptide that attacks all lipid membranes, leading to significant toxicity, it has been proposed that this peptide could also be used in fighting many disorders, with high therapeutic benefits [2,27]. Jeong, et al. [28] showed that melittin significantly suppresses matrix metalloproteinase-9 (MMP-9), which plays a role in atherosclerosis, and TNF-α-induced MMP-9 expression in human aortic smooth muscle cells (HASMCs). Additionally, melittin decreases the expression levels of many cytokines and growth factors in an atherosclerotic mouse model [26], affecting the processes of the immune and haematopoietic systems [29]. Melittin also inhibits transcriptional activators and simultaneously increases the expression of death receptors on the surface of cells, leading to apoptosis [30]. Due to this and many other biological actions of melittin, this polypeptide is considered a potential compound that may be useful in various medical treatments [31,32]. However, almost all studies concerning melittin bioactions have been performed on vertebrate models or cell lines. Recently, due to cheap and easy breeding and the possibility of obtaining a large number of individuals in a short time, every year, the number of examples of replacing vertebrate models in basic biomedical research by insect species has increased, especially by beetles [33]. The most important argument for this is the high level of structural and functional homology between the molecular pathways involved in the regulation of basic life processes in beetles and vertebrates [33]. For this reason, beetles may be promising model organisms and may also be of use in screening studies concerning MEL biological activities to follow the rule of the 3Rs (replacement, reduction, refinement). However, it is very important to first evaluate whether MEL acts in similar manner on beetles and vertebrate tissues.

Thus far, few attempts have been made to study the effects of bee venom and its components on invertebrates, especially insects. Galdiero et al. [34] observed the ecotoxic and genotoxic effects of MEL on *Daphnia magna*, and Söderhäll [35] found that this peptide induces rapid degranulation and the lysis of isolated granular cells and blocks the prophenoloxidase-activating system in the fresh water crayfish *Pacifastacus leniusculus*. In addition, Mitchell et al. [36] showed that MEL noncompetitively inhibits acetylcholinesterase activity in the third-instar larva of *Drosophila melanogaster*.

In this short report, we present the initial data from studies on the impact of melittin on the functioning of the immune system and the contractile activity of the heart in the *T. molitor* beetle. Because of the cheap and easy breeding, as well as the possibility of extrapolating the results of research on vertebrates [33], employing an "easier" insect model can bring benefits, such as research on a wider scale to explore many properties of melittin. For these reasons, it is valuable to examine the influence of melittin on insect physiology. We show that in the case of haemocytes, insect "blood" cells, melittin acts in a similar way as in vertebrates, and the same applies to heart activity, although the effect is marginal, which can be modulated by many different compounds [37]. Our results indicate the possibility of using this model in the early steps of pharmacological studies of new melittin-based compounds.

2. Results

2.1. Pro-Apoptotic Activity of Melittin on Haemocytes

Injection of melittin into 4-day-old males of *T. molitor* beetles resulted in an increased number of apoptotic cells in the haemolymph (Figures 1 and 2A). The increase in the number of apoptotic haemocytes showed a dependence on the dose, increasing by 14.03% at a concentration of 10^{-7} M (Student's t-test, $t = 1.183$; $p = 0.276$) and by 24.02% at a concentration of 10^{-3} M (Student's t-test, $t = 4.545$, $p \leq 0.001$) compared to the control level of 20% of cells.

2.2. Total Haemocyte Count

Measurements of the total haemocyte count (THC) showed statistically significant differences between the groups in the number of cells (Kruskal-Wallis test, $H = 9.402$, $p \leq 0.01$). Interestingly, the changes were reported only after administration of melittin at a concentration of 10^{-3} M. Compared to the control, these differences were statistically significant (Student's t-test, $t = 3.057$, $p \leq 0.01$) (Figure 2B).

2.3. Phagocytic Assay

In the case of the phagocytic bioassay, no statistically significant changes were noted. No changes in the number of haemocytes involved in phagocytosis were observed during the direct effect of melittin on insect haemocytes and 24 h after melittin injection (one-way ANOVA, $F = 0.185$, $p = 0.833$ and $F = 2.967$, $p = 0.079$) (Figure 3A,B).

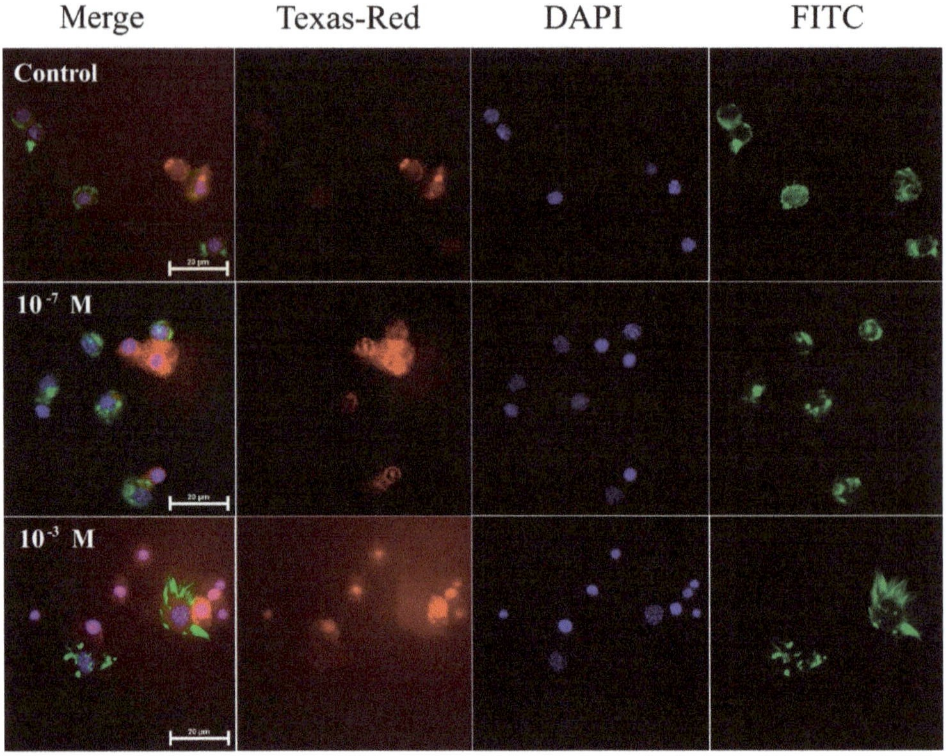

Figure 1. Representative fluorescence microscopic images showing induced apoptosis in haemocytes from 4-day-old male *T. molitor* beetles after an application of physiological saline (control) and melittin at concentrations of 10^{-7} M and 10^{-3} M. Merge—merged photos of the presented fluorescent channels; Texas-Red—haemocytes were stained with SR-VAD-FMK for the detection of caspase activity (red); DAPI—DNA staining (blue); FITC—haemocytes stained with Oregon Green® 488 phalloidin to visualize F-actin cytoskeleton (green). The bar shows a 20 μm scale.

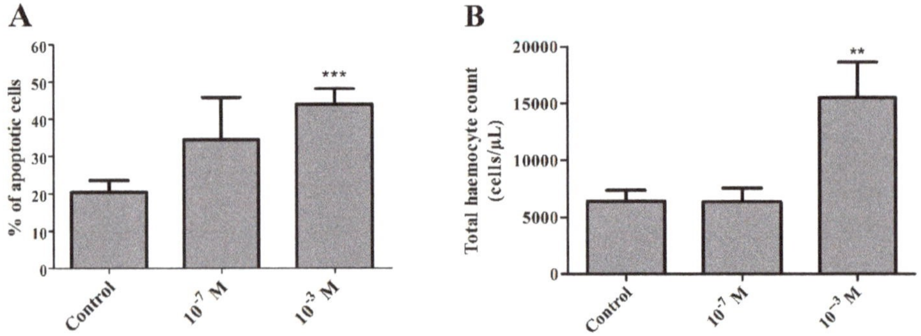

Figure 2. Percentage ratio of apoptotic haemocytes (**A**) and total haemocyte count (THC) in the haemolymph (**B**) of 4-day-old male *T. molitor* beetles after the application of melittin at 10^{-7} M and 10^{-3} M concentrations. Values are presented as the mean ± SEM; **, $p \leq 0.01$, ***, $p \leq 0.01$.

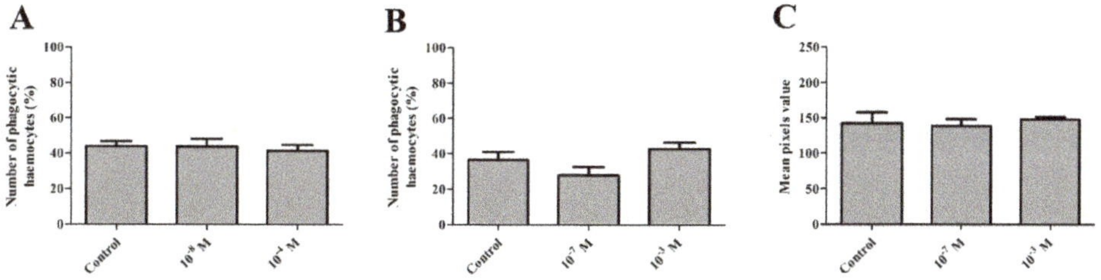

Figure 3. Percentage of phagocytic haemocytes after the direct application of melittin (**A**) and at 24 h after the injection of melittin (**B**), as well as the phenoloxidase (PO) activity (**C**) in the haemolymph of 4-day-old male *T. molitor* beetles at 24 h after the application of peptide. Direct application—haemocytes collected from non-injected individuals; the direct effect was examined by adding melittin to incubation solution at a concentration corresponding to the polypeptide concentration in beetle haemolymph at a 10^{-7} M and 10^{-3} M dilution (final concentration 10^{-8} M and 10^{-4} M). PO activity is based on the mean pixel value of the images. Means ± SEM are given, $n \geq 8$.

2.4. Phenoloxidase Activity

The activity of phenoloxidase in the haemolymph of male *T. molitor* beetles did not change at 24 h after injections of melittin at concentrations of 10^{-7} and 10^{-3} M (Kruskal-Wallis test, $H = 5.146$, $p = 0.76$) (Figure 3C).

2.5. Heart Assay

In the bioassay, we tested the effects of melittin on the contractile activity of the myocardium of the *T. molitor* beetle at a concentration range from 10^{-12} M to 10^{-4} M. Changes in the amplitude (inotropic effect) and frequency of contractions (chronotropic effect) were measured. Under control conditions, during continuous perfusion with physiological saline (PS), the average heart rate was 86.2 beats per minute. The application of an additional 10 µL of PS did not cause any significant changes in the heart rhythm. Additionally, the application of melittin at a concentration range from 10^{-12} M to 10^{-6} M did not cause any significant difference in the contractile activity. However, when MEL was applied at 10^{-4} M, the heart rate increased (positive chronotropic effect) by approximately 9% compared to the control, leaving the amplitude of contractions at the same level (Figure 4). This effect was slight but statistically significant (one-way ANOVA, $F = 2.594$; $p \leq 0.001$) compared to the control. The calculated EC_{50} value for melittin was 5.13×10^{-6} M.

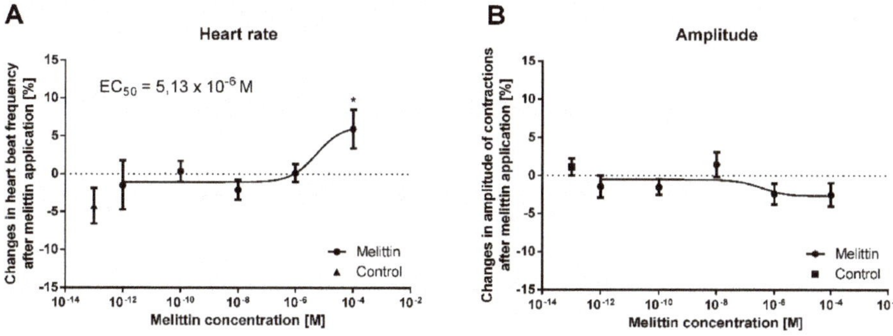

Figure 4. Percentage changes in the mean frequency (**A**) and amplitude (**B**) of heart contractions in *T. molitor* compared to the control after melittin application. Means ± SEM are given for $n = 6$. Significant differences from the control (saline application) are indicated by *, $p \leq 0.05$, (one-way ANOVA test).

3. Discussion

In this report, for the first time, we describe the immunotropic and cardiotropic activity of melittin in heterologous bioassays with the beetle *T. molitor*, a model insect species. The present research is a preliminary study that may indicate the direction of more complex future studies on the impact of melittin on insect physiology.

Many cytotoxic activities of melittin are associated with the pro-apoptotic properties of this polypeptide. Apoptosis, known as programmed cell death, is a key process associated with many cellular events, and melittin-induced apoptosis has been extensively studied. This peptide leads to the apoptosis of various cell types, including erythrocytes and leukocytes, as well as the full spectrum of cancer cells [27,38]. The pro-apoptotic action of melittin was also observed in arthropod cells. Söderhäll [35] showed that melittin induced the degranulation and lysis of granular cells isolated from crayfish *P. leniusculus*. Our study also revealed that melittin induces apoptosis in *Tenebrio* haemocytes. Interestingly, this effect was only observed when MEL was injected at a concentration of 10^{-3} M. Moreover, the apoptotic response was correlated with a simultaneous increase in the number of haemocytes in the haemolymph. This effect is likely related to the mobilization of haemocytes adhered to insect tissues [39]. A possible explanation may be related to compensation for the high ratio of apoptotic cells, which was observed after the application of melittin at a concentration of 10^{-3} M. Simultaneously, in a comparative experiment, we examined the cytotoxic activity of melittin at a concentration range of 10^{-9}–10^{-5} M on human red blood cells, the most numerous cells in the circulatory system, to confirm the literature data [29,39] on the haemolytic activity of this compound. We observed that the threshold of the haemolytic activity of this peptide on erythrocytes began at a concentration of 10^{-8} M (results not shown). The results regarding the effect of melittin on the number of haemocytes and their apoptosis closely correspond with the phagocytic response of haemocytes. The percentage of haemocytes involved in the phagocytosis of latex beads was not changed, regardless of the time of cell contact with melittin. Similar results were obtained by Lee et al. [40], who showed that melittin administration did not affect the phagocytic activity of mouse bone marrow-derived macrophages (BMDMs). The results of the phagocytic assay support our hypothesis about the compensation of the pro-apoptotic action of melittin on insect haemocytes by mobilization of an additional pool of these cells to haemolymph. This mechanism likely ensures the activity of the cellular response at the appropriate level.

One of the most important mechanisms that connect cellular and humoral responses in arthropods is the activity of phenoloxidase (PO) [41]. This enzyme participates not only in cuticle melanisation but also in the pathogen recognition process [42]. The research conducted on the crayfish *P. leniusculus* showed that melittin may reduce the activity of this enzyme in arthropod haemolymph, but only during the co-injection with laminarin, a stimulator of arthropod immune system activity [35]. As in crayfish, a single injection of melittin in the beetle *T. molitor* did not lead to changes in PO activity. Generally, melittin influences the humoral response of vertebrates and acts as an anti-inflammatory compound by suppressing innate immune signalling pathways, including Toll-like receptors 2 and 4 (TLR2, TLR4), CD14, Nuclear factor-kappa B Essential Modulator (NEMO), and Platelet-Derived Growth Factor Receptor β (PDGFRβ) [38,43]. This immunosuppressive action of melittin leads to a reduction in the inflammatory process in various tissues and organs, such as joints, skin, or neuronal tissue [38]. Moreover, melittin can inhibit the innate humoral response during infection. Research by Park et al. [44] showed that melittin suppresses the release of prostaglandin E2 (PGE2) and nitric oxide (NO) from lipopolysaccharide (LPS)-treated RAW264.7 cells. On the other hand, much evidence indicates the pro-inflammatory action of this polypeptide [45]. For example, the expression of genes encoding TNF-α, IL-1, and IL-6 cytokines in PMA-differentiated U937 cells was increased after the co-administration of melittin and LPS compared to LPS stimulation alone [45,46]. For these reasons, the next step will be to evaluate the role of melittin in the modulation of the insect immune system during pathogen infection, including the specificity of the effect of MEL on the molecular pathways associated with the insect immune response. Due to the high level of homology at the molecular level between insect and vertebrate innate immune responses, confirmation of a similar mode of action of melittin on immune-related pathways, such as Toll, IMD, or JAK/STAT, may be useful for searching an alternative model organism in screening research concerning MEL biomedical applications [33].

No less important are the results of melittin influence on insect heart contractile activity. As in the previous section regarding the immune system, our knowledge about the action of melittin on the heart is based only on research conducted on the vertebrate model. Because melittin directly influences Ca^{2+} influx and Na^{+} channels in excitable tissues, this polypeptide affects the action of the vertebrate heart [47]. For example, Brovkovich and Moibenko [48] showed that immediately after application, melittin causes an increase in the contractility of the isolated papillary muscle of the rat heart. After this phase, a dose-dependent decrease in the strength of heart contractions was noted [48]. The bimodal effect of melittin application was also reported in research performed on the isolated guinea pig atria. In this study, at a concentration of 0.1–0.8 µmol/dL, melittin enhanced the contraction of the left atria. However, the use of melittin at higher concentrations (1.6–12.8 µmol/dL) led to the suppression of atrial contractions. Additionally, at a concentration of 0.1–30 µmol/dL, melittin increased the frequency of contractions of isolated right atria [49]. However, there is also evidence of the irreversible paralysis of isolated rat hearts after using 20–40 µg of melittin [50].

In our study, the application of melittin at a concentration of 10^{-4} M to the semi-isolated heart of the *Tenebrio* beetle caused a slight (approximately 9% compared to the control) but significant positive chronotropic effect without simultaneous inotropic changes in the contractile activity of the myocardium. Due to the already known action of MEL on ion channels in vertebrates, a weak *Tenebrio* heart response after the application of this polypeptide may indicate some species-specific activity. Interestingly, whole bee venom caused the strong stimulation of *Tenebrio* heart contractility, which also led to cardiac arrest during the systolic phase (unpublished data). This result suggested that other compounds identified in bee venom may be crucial for exerting a positive chronotropic effect. This effect may be related to the action of tertiapin, which selectively blocks G-protein–gated inwardly rectifying K^{+} channel (IK_{Ach}) [51]. However, we did not exclude the synergistic effect of various components of bee venom. For this reason, in our future research, we will evaluate the cardiotropic properties and potential synergistic actions of other main components of bee venom.

In summary, the presented results clearly showed that melittin affects basic insect immune mechanisms and elicits effects resembling the reactions observed in vertebrate models. These results may be useful for identifying new models for screening biomedical research regarding the influence of melittin and its derivatives on innate immune mechanisms. For this reason, the continuation of the presented work and the determination of how melittin acts on, homological to vertebrates, insect immune-related molecular pathways, such as Toll, IMD, or JAK/STAT, are crucial. Further research on the effect of melittin activity on insect physiology is also necessary due to the different responses of insect hearts compared to vertebrate hearts to melittin application. An explanation of the physiological and biochemical basis of this phenomenon and further research concerning other components of bee venom may be important for identifying new anaphylactic substances.

4. Materials and Methods

4.1. Insects

In all bioassays, adult males of the mealworm beetle *Tenebrio molitor* were used. Individuals were obtained from the culture maintained at the Department of Animal Physiology and Development at Adam Mickiewicz University in Poznań (AMU) according to a method described by Rosinski [52]. To avoid immune-senescence and sex-specific differences in immune system activity, all bioassays concerning this part of the present study were conducted on 4-day-old males. In the heart assay, 30-day-old individuals were used. Although the EU legislation on care and use of experimental animals does not require any permits from the ethics committee, all insects were handled carefully, and the number of animals used was the minimum necessary to achieve the aims of this study.

4.2. *Melittin Injection and Haemolymph Collection*

Before the injection of melittin (Sigma-Aldrich, St. Louis, MO, USA) and haemolymph collection, individuals were anaesthetized with endogenous CO_2. Then, the beetles were disinfected with 70% ethanol (Avantor Performance Materials Poland S.A., Gliwice, Poland) and washed with distilled water.

The beetles were injected with 2 µL of melittin (Sigma-Aldrich, St. Louis, MO, USA) at concentrations of 10^{-7} and 10^{-3} M or 2 µL of physiological saline (PS; 274 mM NaCl, 19 mM KCl, 9 mM $CaCl_2$) as a control. Injections were made with a Hamilton syringe (Hamilton Co., Reno, Nevada, USA) on the ventral side of the body of the beetles under the third pair of legs, inserting the needle towards the head. The melittin concentration used was based on literature data on the concentration of this polypeptide in a single dose of venom applied by bees (10^{-4} M) [53] and the threshold value for melittin-induced haemolysis (10^{-8} M) [30,54]. Due to the average volume of 20 µL of haemolymph in adult *Tenebrio molitor* beetles and the injection of 2 µL of melittin solution, the concentration of this polypeptide in the haemocoel was ten-fold lower [55].

The haemolymph was collected by cutting the tibia of the first pair of legs.

4.3. *Apoptosis*

To detect active caspases in haemocytes, the sulforhodamine derivative of valyl alanyl aspartic acid fluoromethyl ketone, a potent inhibitor of caspase activity (SR-VAD-FMK, Enzo Life Sciences, Inc., New York, NY, USA) was used according to the manufacturer's instructions. Haemocytes were allowed to adhere for 30 min and then washed 3 times with PS, incubated in reaction medium (1/3 × SR-VAD-FMK) for 30 min at room temperature in the dark, washed again 3 times with wash buffer for 5 min at room temperature, and fixed in 4% paraformaldehyde for 10 min. Next, the haemocytes were permeabilized in PS containing 0.1% Triton X-100 (Sigma-Aldrich, St. Louis, MO, USA) for 10 min at room temperature and then washed again with PS. To visualize the F-actin cytoskeleton, the haemocytes were stained with Oregon Green® 488 phalloidin (Invitrogen Carlsbad, CA, USA) for 20 min at room temperature in the dark. After washing with physiological saline, the haemocytes were stained with DAPI solution (Sigma-Aldrich) for 5 min at room temperature in the dark to visualize the nuclei. Finally, the preparations were washed with distilled water and mounted using mounting medium (95% glycerol with 2.5% 1,4-diazabicyclo[2.2.2]octane (DABCO) in PBS; Sigma-Aldrich, St. Louis, MO, USA). The haemocytes prepared in this way were examined using a Nikon Eclipse TE 2000-U fluorescence microscope (Nikon, Tokyo, Japan).

4.4. *Total Haemocyte Count*

The total haemocyte count was determined based on a method previously described by Urbanski et al. [56]. The samples of *Tenebrio* haemolymph (2 µL) were diluted in physiological saline containing anticoagulation buffer (4.5 mM citric acid and 9 mM sodium citrate, Sigma-Aldrich, St. Louis, MO, USA) (5:1 *v*/*v*). Then, the prepared suspension was examined with a Bürker chamber (Waldemar Knittel Glasbearbeitungs- GmbH, Braunschweig, Germany) and a Nikon PrimoStar light microscope (Nikon, Tokyo, Japan).

4.5. *Phagocytic Assay*

A phagocytic assay was performed according to the method described by Urbanski et al. [57]. Phagocytosis was conducted in vitro using fluorescently labelled latex beads (Sigma-Aldrich, St. Louis, MO, USA). The samples of haemolymph (2 µL) were incubated for 30 min with suspension of PS containing anticoagulation buffer and latex beads. The specimens were analysed using Nikon Eclipse fluorescence microscope (Nikon, Tokyo, Japan). The results are expressed as a percentage ratio of haemocytes with fully phagocytosed latex beads to the overall number of haemocytes visible on a single photo. In each biological repetition, the number of haemocytes participating in phagocytosis was estimated based on 5 random photos.

In the case of the phagocytic assay, despite melittin administration by injection, the direct effect of this compound was also tested. For this purpose, melittin was added to the suspension of latex beads with anticoagulant buffer. The melittin concentrations in this suspension corresponded to the final concentration of MEL in the insect after haemolymph injection (10^{-8} and 10^{-4} M, respectively). The haemocytes were incubated in a suspension of latex beads with the tested polypeptide for 30 min.

4.6. Phenoloxidase Activity

Phenoloxidase activity was analysed based on the colorimetric method described by Sorrentino et al. [58]. Haemolymph samples (1 µL) were placed on Whatman No. 52 filter paper soaked with phosphate buffer (10 mM; Sigma-Aldrich, St. Louis, MO, USA) and 3,4-Dihydroxy-DL-phenylalanine (DL-DOPA; 2 mg/ mL, Sigma-Aldrich, St. Louis, MO, USA). After 30 min of incubation, the samples were air dried and scanned using Sharp AR 153EN (600 dpi, 8 bits, grey scale; Sharp Corporation, Osaka, Japan). The PO activity was determined by measuring the intensity of colour in the central part of the obtained spots. The results were expressed as the mean pixel value.

4.7. Heart Bioassay

To measure the activity of melittin on semi-isolated heart preparations, the microdensitometric method, coupled with a computer-based data analysis, was used as previously described [59–61]. After anaesthesia, insects were decapitated, and the abdomen was removed. A cut was then made on the ventral side of the abdomen, and viscera were removed leaving only the dorsal vessel and alary muscles—semi-isolated heart preparation. Next, the preparation in incubation chamber was installed on the microdensitometer MD-100 (Carl Zeiss, Oberkochen, Germany) connected to a computer. The heart was subjected to constant perfusion with fresh PS at a rate of 140 µL/min. Melittin was applied at the injection port using a Hamilton syringe. After 15–20 min of acclimatization, the activity of the isolated heart was recorded for 120 s. The activity of the beetles' myocardium under perfusion with PS was recorded for 30 s. Next, the tested peptide was applied, and the activity of the heart was recorded for an additional 90 s. This procedure was repeated at 5-min intervals for each concentration tested. To test whether the semi-isolated heart preparations functioned properly, the cardiostimulatory peptide proctolin was used as an internal standard. The activity of melittin was presented as a percentage change in the control frequency of heart contractions.

4.8. Statistical Analysis

For statistical analysis of the obtained data, we used GraphPad software ver. 6 (GraphPad Software, San Diego, CA, USA) (Department of Animal Physiology and Development AMU license). Before statistical analysis, the normality of distribution (the Shapiro-Wilk test) and the homogeneity of variance (the Brown-Forsythe test and the Levene test) were checked. For the analysis of groups with normal distribution, one-way ANOVA with Tukey's post hoc or Student's *t*-test were used. The data without normal distribution were analysed with the Kruskal-Wallis test. Values of $p \leq 0.05$ (*), $p \leq 0.01$ (**) or $p \leq 0.001$ (***) were considered statistically significant.

Author Contributions: Conceptualization, J.L. and A.U.; methodology, J.L., A.U., L.M. and G.R.; validation, J.L. and A.U.; investigation, J.L. and A.U.; resources, J.M.; writing—original draft preparation, J.L. and A.U.; writing—review and editing, J.L., A.U., L.M., E.M., A.Ś.-B., J.M. and G.R.; supervision, G.R. and J.M.; funding acquisition, J.M.

Funding: This work was supported by a grant from the National Science Centre, Poland [no. 2016/23/D/NZ7/03949].

Conflicts of Interest: The authors declare no conflicts of interest. The funders had no role in the design of the study; in the collection, analyses, or interpretation of data; in the writing of the manuscript, or in the decision to publish the results.

References

1. Klupczynska, A.; Pawlak, M.; Kokot, Z.J.; Matysiak, J. Application of Metabolomic Tools for Studying Low Molecular-Weight Fraction of Animal Venoms and Poisons. *Toxins* **2018**, *10*, 306. [CrossRef] [PubMed]
2. Moreno, M.; Giralt, E. Three Valuable Peptides from Bee and Wasp Venoms for Therapeutic and Biotechnological Use: Melittin, Apamin and Mastoparan. *Toxins* **2015**, *7*, 1126–1150. [CrossRef] [PubMed]
3. Utkin, Y.N. Animal venom studies: Current benefits and future developments. *World J. Biol. Chem.* **2015**, *6*, 28–33. [CrossRef] [PubMed]
4. Kalogeropoulos, K.; Treschow, A.F.; Escalante, T.; Rucavado, A.; Gutiérrez, J.M.; Laustsen, A.H.; Workman, C.T. Protease activity profiling of snake venoms using high-throughput peptide screening. *Toxins* **2019**, *11*, 170. [CrossRef] [PubMed]
5. Frangieh, J.; Salma, Y.; Haddad, K.; Mattei, C.; Legros, C.; Fajloun, Z.; El Obeid, D. First Characterization of The Venom from Apis mellifera syriaca, A Honeybee from The Middle East Region. *Toxins* **2019**, *11*, 191. [CrossRef] [PubMed]
6. Habermann, E. Bee and wasp venoms. *Science* **1972**, *177*, 314–322. [CrossRef] [PubMed]
7. Chen, J.; Lariviere, W.R. The nociceptive and anti-nociceptive effects of bee venom injection and therapy: A double-edged sword. *Prog. Neurobiol.* **2010**, *92*, 151–183. [CrossRef]
8. Son, D.J.; Lee, J.W.; Lee, Y.H.; Song, H.S.; Lee, C.K.; Hong, J.T. Therapeutic application of anti-arthritis, pain-releasing, and anti-cancer effects of bee venom and its constituent compounds. *Pharmacol. Ther.* **2007**, *115*, 246–270. [CrossRef]
9. Wu, Q.; Patocka, J.; Kuca, K. Insect Antimicrobial Peptides, a Mini Review. *Toxins* **2018**, *10*, 461. [CrossRef]
10. Chen, L.Y.; Cheng, C.W.; Lin, J.J.; Chen, W.Y. Exploring the effect of cholesterol in lipid bilayer membrane on the melittin penetration mechanism. *Anal. Biochem.* **2007**, *367*, 49–55. [CrossRef]
11. Chen, X.; Wang, J.; Kristalyn, C.B.; Chen, Z. Real-time structural investigation of a lipid bilayer during its interaction with melittin using sum frequency generation vibrational spectroscopy. *Biophys. J.* **2007**, *93*, 866–875. [CrossRef]
12. Klocek, G.; Schulthess, T.; Shai, Y.; Seelig, J. Thermodynamics of melittin binding to lipid bilayers. Aggregation and pore formation. *Biochemistry* **2009**, *48*, 2586–2596. [CrossRef]
13. Chen, J.; Guan, S.M.; Sun, W.; Fu, H. Melittin, the Major Pain-Producing Substance of Bee Venom. *Neurosci. Bull.* **2016**, *32*, 265–272. [CrossRef]
14. Boman, H.; Wade, D.; Boman, I.; Wåhlin, B.; Merrifield, R. Antibacterial and antimalarial properties of peptides that are cecropin-melittin hybrids. *FEBS Lett.* **1989**, *259*, 103–106. [CrossRef]
15. Pandey, B.K.; Ahmad, A.; Asthana, N.; Azmi, S.; Srivastava, R.M.; Srivastava, S.; Verma, R.; Vishwakarma, A.L.; Ghosh, J.K. Cell-selective lysis by novel analogues of melittin against human red blood cells and *Escherichia coli*. *Biochemistry* **2010**, *49*, 7920–7929. [CrossRef]
16. Soman, N.R.; Baldwin, S.L.; Hu, G.; Marsh, J.N.; Lanza, G.M.; Heuser, J.E.; Arbeit, J.M.; Wickline, S.A.; Schlesinger, P.H. Molecularly targeted nanocarriers deliver the cytolytic peptide melittin specifically to tumor cells in mice, reducing tumor growth. *J. Clin. Investig.* **2009**, *119*, 2830–2842. [CrossRef]
17. Jamasbi, E.; Ciccotosto, G.D.; Tailhades, J.; Robins-Browne, R.M.; Ugalde, C.L.; Sharples, R.A.; Patil, N.; Wade, J.D.; Hossain, M.A.; Separovic, F. Site of fluorescent label modifies interaction of melittin with live cells and model membranes. *Biochim. Biophys. Acta* **2015**, *1848*, 2031–2039. [CrossRef]
18. Katsu, T.; Kuroko, M.; Morikawa, T.; Sanchika, K.; Fujita, Y.; Yamamura, H.; Uda, M. Mechanism of membrane damage induced by the amphipathic peptides gramicidin S and melittin. *Biochim. Biophys. Acta* **1989**, *983*, 135–141. [CrossRef]
19. Lee, S.Y.; Park, H.S.; Lee, S.J.; Choi, M.U. Melittin exerts multiple effects on the release of free fatty acids from L1210 cells: Lack of selective activation of phospholipase A2 by melittin. *Arch. Biochem. Biophys.* **2001**, *389*, 57–67. [CrossRef]
20. Juhaniewicz, J.; Sek, S. Interaction of melittin with negatively charged lipid bilayers supported on gold electrodes. *Electrochim. Acta* **2016**, *197*, 336–343. [CrossRef]
21. Lee, J.; Lee, D.G. Melittin triggers apoptosis in Candida albicans through the reactive oxygen species-mediated mitochondria/caspase-dependent pathway. *FEMS Microbiol. Lett.* **2014**, *355*, 36–42. [CrossRef] [PubMed]
22. McGwire, B.S.; Kulkarni, M.M. Interactions of antimicrobial peptides with Leishmania and trypanosomes and their functional role in host parasitism. *Exp. Parasitol.* **2010**, *126*, 397–405. [CrossRef] [PubMed]

23. Orsolic, N. Bee venom in cancer therapy. *Cancer Metastasis Rev.* **2012**, *31*, 173–194. [CrossRef] [PubMed]
24. Yalcin, M.; Aydin, C.; Savci, V. Cardiovascular effect of peripheral injected melittin in normotensive conscious rats: Mediation of the central cholinergic system. *Prostaglandins Leukot. Essent. Fat. Acids* **2009**, *81*, 341–347. [CrossRef] [PubMed]
25. Yang, S.; Zhang, X.M.; Jiang, M.H. Inhibitory effect of melittin on Na^+,K^+-ATPase from guinea pig myocardial mitochondria. *Acta Pharm. Sin.* **2001**, *22*, 279–282.
26. Kim, S.J.; Park, J.H.; Kim, K.H.; Lee, W.R.; Kim, K.S.; Park, K.K. Melittin inhibits atherosclerosis in LPS/high-fat treated mice through atheroprotective actions. *J. Atheroscler. Thromb.* **2011**, *18*, 1117–1126. [CrossRef] [PubMed]
27. Gajski, G.; Garaj-Vrhovac, V. Melittin: A lytic peptide with anticancer properties. *Environ. Toxicol. Pharmacol.* **2013**, *36*, 697–705. [CrossRef] [PubMed]
28. Jeong, Y.J.; Cho, H.J.; Whang, K.; Lee, I.S.; Park, K.K.; Choe, J.Y.; Han, S.M.; Kim, C.H.; Chang, H.W.; Moon, S.K.; et al. Melittin has an inhibitory effect on TNF-alpha-induced migration of human aortic smooth muscle cells by blocking the MMP-9 expression. *Food Chem. Toxicol.* **2012**, *50*, 3996–4002. [CrossRef] [PubMed]
29. Gajski, G.; Domijan, A.M.; Zegura, B.; Stern, A.; Geric, M.; Novak Jovanovic, I.; Vrhovac, I.; Madunic, J.; Breljak, D.; Filipic, M.; et al. Melittin induced cytogenetic damage, oxidative stress and changes in gene expression in human peripheral blood lymphocytes. *Toxicon* **2016**, *110*, 56–67. [CrossRef]
30. Zarrinnahad, H.; Mahmoodzadeh, A.; Hamidi, M.P.; Mahdavi, M.; Moradi, A.; Bagheri, K.P.; Shahbazzadeh, D. Apoptotic Effect of Melittin Purified from Iranian Honey Bee Venom on Human Cervical Cancer HeLa Cell Line. *Int. J. Pept. Res. Ther.* **2018**, *24*, 563–570. [CrossRef]
31. Chowanski, S.; Adamski, Z.; Lubawy, J.; Marciniak, P.; Pacholska-Bogalska, J.; Slocinska, M.; Spochacz, M.; Szymczak, M.; Urbanski, A.; Walkowiak-Nowicka, K.; et al. Insect Peptides - Perspectives in Human Diseases Treatment. *Curr. Med. Chem.* **2017**, *24*, 3116–3152. [CrossRef] [PubMed]
32. Silva, J.; Monge-Fuentes, V.; Gomes, F.; Lopes, K.; dos Anjos, L.; Campos, G.; Arenas, C.; Biolchi, A.; Goncalves, J.; Galante, P.; et al. Pharmacological Alternatives for the Treatment of Neurodegenerative Disorders: Wasp and Bee Venoms and Their Components as New Neuroactive Tools. *Toxins* **2015**, *7*, 3179–3209. [CrossRef] [PubMed]
33. Adamski, Z.; Bufo, S.A.; Chowanski, S.; Falabella, P.; Lubawy, J.; Marciniak, P.; Pacholska-Bogalska, J.; Salvia, R.; Scrano, L.; Slocinska, M.; et al. Beetles as Model Organisms in Physiological, Biomedical and Environmental Studies—A Review. *Front. Physiol.* **2019**, *10*, 319. [CrossRef] [PubMed]
34. Galdiero, E.; Maselli, V.; Falanga, A.; Gesuele, R.; Galdiero, S.; Fulgione, D.; Guida, M. Integrated analysis of the ecotoxicological and genotoxic effects of the antimicrobial peptide melittin on Daphnia magna and Pseudokirchneriella subcapitata. *Environ. Pollut.* **2015**, *203*, 145–152. [CrossRef]
35. Söderhäll, K. The bee venom melittin induces lysis of arthropod granular cells and inhibits activation of the prophenoloxidase-activating system. *FEBS Lett.* **1985**, *192*, 109–112. [CrossRef]
36. Mitchell, H.K.; Lowy, P.H.; Sarmiento, L.; Dickson, L. Melittin: Toxicity to Drosophila and inhibition of acetylcholinesterase. *Arch. Biochem. Biophys.* **1971**, *145*, 344–348. [CrossRef]
37. Chowanski, S.; Lubawy, J.; Urbanski, A.; Rosinski, G. Cardioregulatory Functions of Neuropeptides and Peptide Hormones in Insects. *Protein Pept. Lett.* **2016**, *23*, 913–931. [CrossRef]
38. Lee, G.; Bae, H. Anti-Inflammatory Applications of Melittin, a Major Component of Bee Venom: Detailed Mechanism of Action and Adverse Effects. *Molecules* **2016**, *21*, 616. [CrossRef]
39. Rowley, A.F.; Ratcliffe, N.A. A histological study of wound healing and hemocyte function in the wax-moth Galleria mellonella. *J. Morphol.* **1978**, *157*, 181–199. [CrossRef]
40. Lee, C.; Bae, S.S.; Joo, H.; Bae, H. Melittin suppresses tumor progression by regulating tumor-associated macrophages in a Lewis lung carcinoma mouse model. *Oncotarget* **2017**, *8*, 54951–54965. [CrossRef]
41. Strand, M. The insect cellular immune response. *Insect Sci.* **2008**, *15*, 1–14. [CrossRef]
42. Gonzalez-Santoyo, I.; Cordoba-Aguilar, A. Phenoloxidase: A key component of the insect immune system. *Entomol. Exp. Appl.* **2012**, *142*, 1–16. [CrossRef]
43. Choi, J.; Jeon, C.; Lee, J.H.; Jang, J.U.; Quan, F.S.; Lee, K.; Kim, W.; Kim, S.K. Suppressive Effects of Bee Venom Acupuncture on Paclitaxel-Induced Neuropathic Pain in Rats: Mediation by Spinal alpha(2)-Adrenergic Receptor. *Toxins* **2017**, *9*, 351. [CrossRef]

44. Park, H.J.; Lee, S.H.; Son, D.J.; Oh, K.W.; Kim, K.H.; Song, H.S.; Kim, G.J.; Oh, G.T.; Yoon, D.Y.; Hong, J.T. Antiarthritic effect of bee venom–Inhibition of inflammation mediator generation by suppression of NF-kappa B through interaction with the p50 subunit. *Arthritis Rheum.* **2004**, *50*, 3504–3515. [CrossRef]
45. Alqarni, A.M.; Ferro, V.A.; Parkinson, J.A.; Dufton, M.J.; Watson, D.G. Effect of Melittin on Metabolomic Profile and Cytokine Production in PMA-Differentiated THP-1 Cells. *Vaccines* **2018**, *6*, 72. [CrossRef]
46. Tusiimire, J.; Wallace, J.; Woods, N.; Dufton, M.J.; Parkinson, J.A.; Abbott, G.; Clements, C.J.; Young, L.; Park, J.K.; Jeon, J.W.; et al. Effect of Bee Venom and Its Fractions on the Release of Pro-Inflammatory Cytokines in PMA-Differentiated U937 Cells Co-Stimulated with LPS. *Vaccines* **2016**, *4*, 11. [CrossRef]
47. Bkaily, G.; Simaan, M.; Jaalouk, D.; Pothier, P. Effect of apamin and melittin on ion channels and intracellular calcium of heart cells. In *Bee Products*; Mizrahi, A., Lensky, Y., Eds.; Springer: Boston, MA, USA, 1997; pp. 203–211.
48. Brovkovich, V.M.; Moibenko, A.A. Effect of melittin on the contractility of rat papillary muscle. *Bull. Exp. Biol. Med.* **1997**, *124*, 642–644. [CrossRef]
49. Yang, S.; Liu, J.E.; Zhang, A.Z.; Jiang, M.H. Biphasic manner of melittin on isolated guinea pig atria. *Acta Pharm. Sin.* **2000**, *21*, 221–224.
50. Marsh, N.A.; Whaler, B.C. The effects of honey bee (*Apis mellifera* L.) venom and two of its constituents, melittin and phospholipase A2, on the cardiovascular system of the rat. *Toxicon* **1980**, *18*, 427–435. [CrossRef]
51. Drici, M.D.; Diochot, S.; Terrenoire, C.; Romey, G.; Lazdunski, M. The bee venom peptide tertiapin underlines the role of I-KACh in acetylcholine-induced atrioventricular blocks. *Br. J. Pharm.* **2000**, *131*, 569–577. [CrossRef]
52. Rosinski, G. Metabolic and myotropic neuropeptides in insects. *Adam Mickiewicz PressZool. Ser.* **1995**, *22*, 148.
53. Bilo, B.M.; Rueff, F.; Mosbech, H.; Bonifazi, F.; Oude-Elberink, J.N. Diagnosis of Hymenoptera venom allergy. *Allergy* **2005**, *60*, 1339–1349. [CrossRef]
54. Tosteson, M.T.; Holmes, S.J.; Razin, M.; Tosteson, D.C. Melittin lysis of red cells. *J. Membr. Biol.* **1985**, *87*, 35–44. [CrossRef]
55. Marciniak, P.; Urbanski, A.; Kudlewska, M.; Szymczak, M.; Rosinski, G. Peptide hormones regulate the physiological functions of reproductive organs in Tenebrio molitor males. *Peptides* **2017**, *98*, 35–42. [CrossRef]
56. Urbanski, A.; Adamski, Z.; Rosinski, G. Developmental changes in haemocyte morphology in response to *Staphylococcus aureus* and latex beads in the beetle *Tenebrio molitor* L. *Micron* **2018**, *104*, 8–20. [CrossRef]
57. Urbanski, A.; Czarniewska, E.; Baraniak, E.; Rosinski, G. Developmental changes in cellular and humoral responses of the burying beetle Nicrophorus vespilloides (Coleoptera, Silphidae). *J. Insect Physiol.* **2014**, *60*, 98–103. [CrossRef]
58. Sorrentino, R.P.; Small, C.N.; Govind, S. Quantitative analysis of phenol oxidase activity in insect hemolymph. *Biotechniques* **2002**, *32*, 815–823. [CrossRef]
59. Lubawy, J.; Marciniak, P.; Kuczer, M.; Rosiński, G. Myotropic activity of allatostatins in tenebrionid beetles. *Neuropeptides* **2018**, *70*, 26–36. [CrossRef]
60. Urbanski, A.; Lubawy, J.; Marciniak, P.; Rosinski, G. Myotropic activity and immunolocalization of selected neuropeptides of the burying beetle Nicrophorus vespilloides (Coleoptera: Silphidae). *Insect Sci.* **2019**, *26*, 656–670. [CrossRef]
61. Rosinski, G.; Gade, G. Hyperglycemic and myoactive factors in the corpora cardiaca of the mealworm, Tenebrio molitor. *J. Insect Physiol.* **1988**, *34*, 1035–1042. [CrossRef]

toxins

MDPI

Article

Analgesic Effect of Melittin on Oxaliplatin-Induced Peripheral Neuropathy in Rats

Seunghwan Choi [1], Hyeon Kyeong Chae [2], Ho Heo [3], Dae-Hyun Hahm [4], Woojin Kim [1,5,*] and Sun Kwang Kim [1,2,5,*]

1 Department of East-West Medicine, Graduate School, Kyung Hee University, Seoul 02447, Korea
2 Department of Science in Korean Medicine, Graduate School, Kyung Hee University, Seoul 02447, Korea
3 Anapn Korean Traditional Medical Clinic, 11, Seongnae-ro, Gangdong-gu, Seoul 05392, Korea
4 Department of Physiology, School of Medicine, Kyung Hee University, Seoul 02447, Korea
5 Department of Physiology, College of Korean Medicine, Kyung Hee University, Seoul 02447, Korea
* Correspondence: wjkim@khu.ac.kr (W.K.); skkim77@khu.ac.kr (S.K.K.)

Received: 6 June 2019; Accepted: 2 July 2019; Published: 8 July 2019

Abstract: Oxaliplatin is a chemotherapeutic agent used for metastatic colon and other advanced cancers. Most common side effect of oxaliplatin is peripheral neuropathy, manifested in mechanical and cold allodynia. Although the analgesic effect of bee venom has been proven to be effective against oxaliplatin-induced peripheral neuropathy, the effect of its major component; melittin has not been studied yet. Thus, in this study, we investigated whether melittin has an analgesic effect on oxaliplatin-induced allodynia. Intraperitoneal single injection of oxaliplatin (6 mg/kg) induced mechanical and cold allodynia, resulting in increased withdrawal behavior in response to von Frey filaments and acetone drop on hind paw. Subcutaneous melittin injection on acupoint ST36 (0.5 mg/kg) alleviated oxaliplatin-induced mechanical and cold allodynia. In electrophysiological study, using spinal in vivo extracellular recording, it was shown that oxaliplatin-induced hyperexcitation of spinal wide dynamic range neurons in response to peripheral stimuli, and melittin administration inhibited this neuronal activity. In behavioral assessment, analgesic effect of melittin was blocked by intrathecal α1- and α2- adrenergic receptor antagonists administration. Based on these results, we suggest that melittin could be used as an analgesic on oxaliplatin-induced peripheral neuropathy, and that its effect is mediated by activating the spinal α1- and α2-adrenergic receptors.

Keywords: chemotherapy; cold allodynia; mechanical allodynia; melittin; neuropathic pain; oxaliplatin

Key Contribution: Subcutaneous melittin injection on acupoint ST36 (0.5 mg/kg) reduced oxaliplatin-induced cold and mechanical allodynia by activating the spinal α1- and α2-adrenergic receptors.

1. Introduction

Oxaliplatin is the third-generation platinum based chemotherapeutic agent, which is combined with fluorouracil and leucovorin for metastatic colorectal cancer [1]. Also, it has been proven to be effective for advanced esophagogastric [2] and pancreatic cancer [3]. However, oxaliplatin treatment can induce peripheral neuropathy expressed in sensitivity to cold, numbness and tingling in hands and feet [4,5]. These sensory neuropathies have long been recognized as the major dose-limiting adverse events of oxaliplatin treatment [6]. So far, several agents showed potentiality to prevent and treat oxaliplatin-induced peripheral neuropathy [7,8]. However, these agents also have limitations including side effects such as fatigue, insomnia, and nausea [8].

Melittin, which consists of 26 amino acids, is a major component of bee venom [9,10]. Bee venom has been shown to be effective on a variety of pain models, such as cancer pain [11], inflammatory pain [12], and neuropathic pain [13]. In our previous study, we demonstrated that subcutaneous bee venom (1 mg/kg) and melittin (0.5 mg/kg) administration on ipsilateral ST36 alleviated paclitaxel-induced mechanical allodynia [14]. Also, it was reported that melittin injection on ST36 reduced pain caused by complete Freund's adjuvant-induced rheumatoid arthritis [15]. However, the analgesic effect of melittin on oxaliplatin-induced peripheral neuropathy has not been studied yet, and its neuropharmacological mechanism remains undiscovered.

In this study, first, we conducted behavioral tests to assess whether melittin can relieve oxaliplatin-induced mechanical and cold allodynia in rats. Secondly, by using in vivo electrophysiological method, we observed the activities of wide dynamic range (WDR) neurons in the spinal cord after oxaliplatin and melittin injection. Finally, by administrating receptor antagonists intrathecally, we determined whether spinal adrenergic receptors, which are known to be the key mechanisms of bee venom analgesia, are involved in the effect of melittin.

2. Results

2.1. Mechanical and Cold Allodynia Induced by Oxaliplatin Administration in Rats

Single intraperitoneal injection of oxaliplatin at a dose of 6 mg/kg induced mechanical and cold allodynia in rats. As reported in our previous studies, these behavioral changes were shown significantly from three to seven days after the injection [16,17]. Figure 1A shows the results of behavior response to von Frey filament stimuli, exhibiting lowered withdrawal threshold after oxaliplatin administration. Responses to cold stimuli (10 μL of acetone application on ventral side of right hind paw) were also exaggerated in terms of intensity (Figure 1B). We interpreted these deteriorated responses to peripheral stimuli as mechanical and cold allodynia.

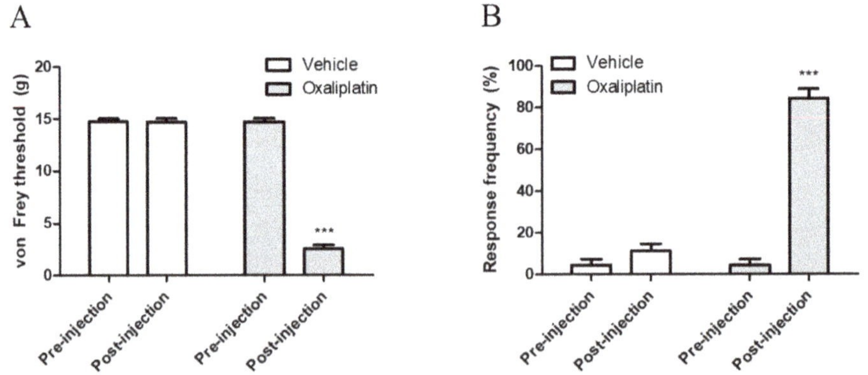

Figure 1. Oxaliplatin administration induces increased behavioral response to mechanical and cold stimulation. Three days after intraperitoneal injection of 6 mg/kg of oxaliplatin, mechanical (**A**) and cold (**B**) allodynia were induced. Behavioral tests were conducted by using von Frey filament and acetone, to assess mechanical and cold allodynia, respectively. Nine rats were allocated in each group. Data is presented as the mean ± standard error of the mean (S.E.M); *** $p < 0.001$, by Bonferroni post-test after two-way analysis of variance (ANOVA).

2.2. Melittin Alleviates Oxaliplatin Induced Mechanical and Cold Allodynia

To verify the analgesic effect of melittin on oxaliplatin-induced peripheral neuropathy, 0.5 mg/kg of melittin was injected subcutaneously on acupoint ST36. Behavioral assessments were done before and after melittin injection. Both the mechanical and cold allodynia were significantly attenuated 30 min after melittin injection (Figure 2A,B, respectively). These results indicate that subcutaneous melittin injection on ipsilateral acupoint can alleviates oxaliplatin-induced peripheral neuropathic pain.

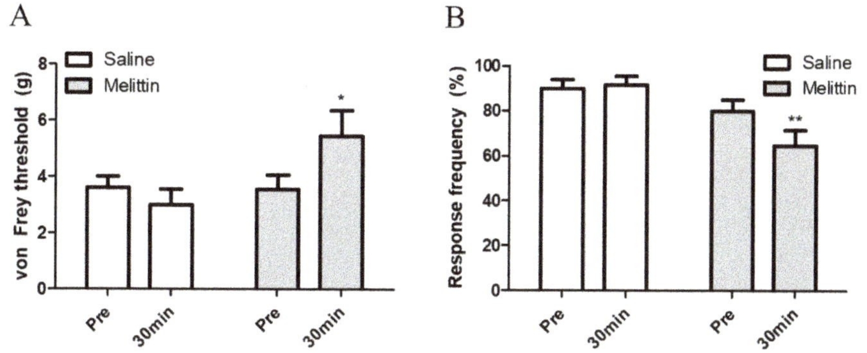

Figure 2. Subcutaneous melittin injection on acupoint ST36 alleviated mechanical and cold allodynia caused by oxaliplatin injection. Rats showing significant mechanical and cold allodynia after oxaliplatin injection were divided into two groups. Saline (n = 13) and melittin (n = 18). Melittin alleviated both the mechanical allodynia (**A**) and cold allodynia (**B**). Data is presented as the mean ± S.E.M.; * $p < 0.05$, ** $p < 0.01$; by Bonferroni post-test after two-way ANOVA.

2.3. Mellitin Inhibits Oxaliplatin-Induced Hyperexcitated Spinal WDR Neuronal Activity

We investigated whether melittin could inhibit the increased spinal WDR neuronal activity to peripheral stimuli after oxaliplatin injection. Figure 3A shows the representative raw trace of the spinal WDR neuronal responding to three seconds of pressure before and after melittin injection. Melittin significantly inhibited mechanical (press and pinch, but not brush) and cold (acetone drop) stimuli, which is quantified by spike number decrement (Figure 3B–E). These electrophysiological results correlate to melittin analgesia shown in behavioral assessment (Figure 2).

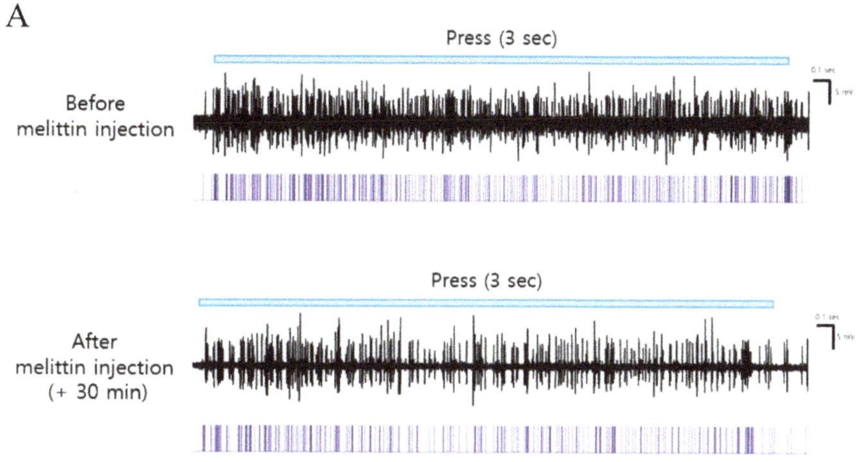

Figure 3. *Cont.*

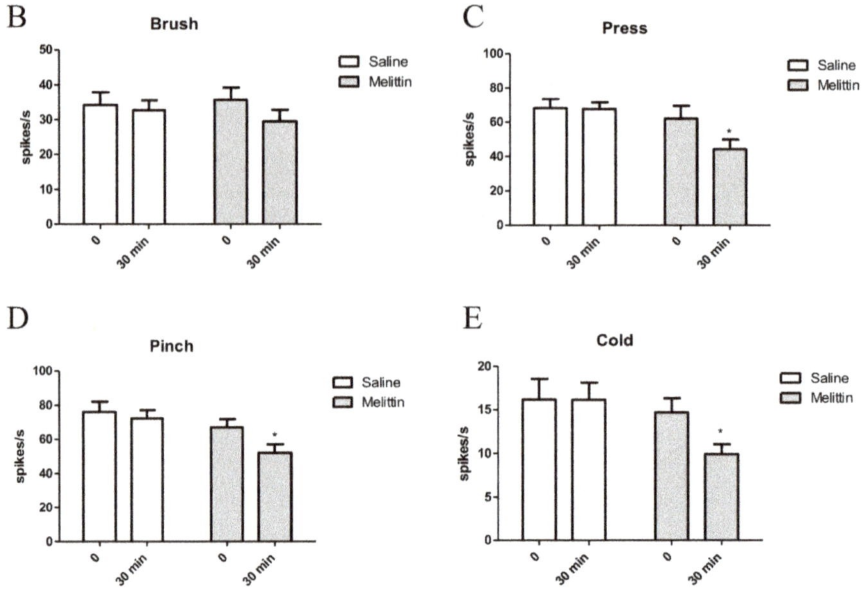

Figure 3. Inhibitory effects of melittin on increased firing of spinal WDR neurons in response to peripheral stimulation in oxaliplatin-injected rats. (**A**) Representative raw trace of spinal WDR neuronal activity altered by melittin injection. (**B–E**) Spike numbers of spinal WDR neuron reacting to peripheral stimuli (brush, press, pinch, and cold) 30 min after 0.5 mg/kg of melittin administration. $N = 11$ for each group. Data is presented as the mean ± SEM.; * $p < 0.05$; by Bonferroni post-test after two-way ANOVA (B–E).

2.4. Both Spinal α1- and 2- Adrenergic Receptors are Involved in the Analgesic Effects of Melittin

To elucidate the spinal mechanism of the analgesic effect of melittin, α-adrenergic receptor antagonists were injected intrathecally before melittin injection. Figure 4A represents the time schedule of the behavioral study. Prazosin (α1-adrenergic receptor antagonist, 30 μg, i.t.) or idazoxan (α2-adrenergic receptor antagonist, 50 μg, i.t.) was administered 20 min before treatments. Both prazosin and idazoxan blocked the melittin analgesia on mechanical and cold allodynia (Figure 4B,C). In contrast, the control of these antagonists (Dimethyl sulfoxide (DMSO) and phosphate-buffered saline (PBS), respectively) did not cause any significant effect on the analgesic effect of melittin. Taken together, both spinal α1- and 2-adrenergic receptors are shown to be involved in the analgesia action of melittin on oxaliplatin-induced peripheral neuropathy.

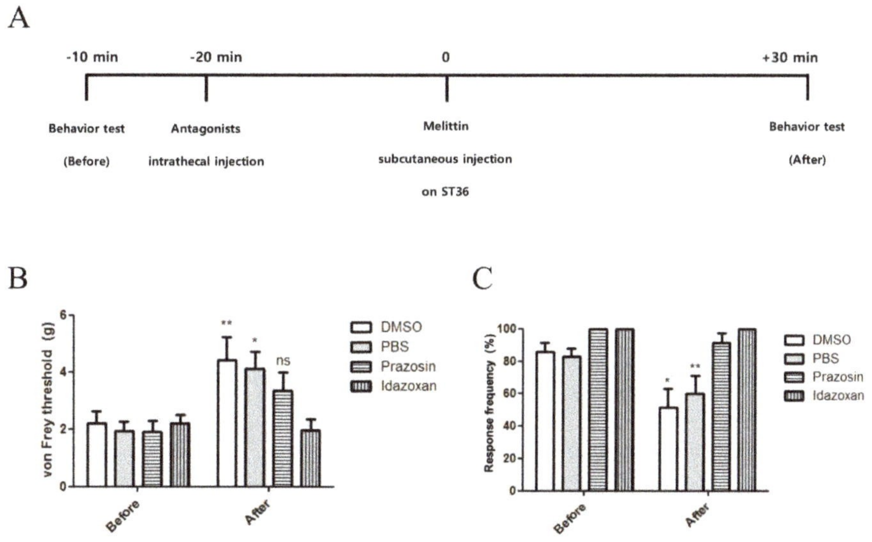

Figure 4. Intrathecal α-adrenergic receptor antagonists reversed the analgesic effect of melittin on mechanical and cold allodynia. (**A**) Timeline of behavioral test conducted with adrenergic antagonists injection. (**B**,**C**) Both α1 and α2-adrenergic receptor antagonists blocked the analgesic effect of melittin. All drugs were injected at ST36. DMSO and PBS were used as control to prazosin and idazoxan, respectively. $N = 7$ for each group. Behavioral tests were conducted 30 min after the melittin administration. Data are presented as mean ± SEM; ns; non-significant, * $p < 0.05$, ** $p < 0.01$; by Bonferroni post-test after two-way ANOVA.

3. Discussion

Oxaliplatin has a broad spectrum of anticancer activity and a better safety profile than cisplatin, which is the first platinum based drug to enter clinical use, but with a significant side toxicity [18]. Nonetheless, oxaliplatin-induced peripheral neuropathy, characterized by mechanical and cold allodynia, could be the main cause of dose reduction and treatment cessation [19]. Although a variety of agents including opioids, antidepressant, antiepileptics, or topical liniments are used to manage this neuropathy; so far, there is no ideal therapeutic agent due to their own side effects or low efficacy [20]. Thus, it would be valuable to discover novel analgesics with satisfactory efficacy and minimal side effects.

For several years, our lab has focused on the analgesic effects of bee venom acupuncture on various chemotherapy-induced peripheral neuropathic pain [14,16,21–23]. In one of our previous studies conducted on paclitaxel-induced peripheral neuropathy animal model, both bee venom acupuncture and melittin were shown to significantly attenuate the pain behavior [14]. It was clear that the mechanism of bee venom acupuncture analgesia involves the spinal α2-adrenergic receptor activation, however, the spinal mechanism of melittin analgesia remained unclear.

In this study, we showed that single oxaliplatin injection (6 mg/kg) produced mechanical and cold allodynia in rats (Figure 1). Subcutaneous melittin injection on ST36 alleviated pain response of ipsilateral hind paw to mechanical and cold stimuli (Figure 2). Like the results of behavioral assessments, on in vivo electrophysiological study, spike numbers of hyperexcitated spinal WDR neuron in response to peripheral mechanical and cold stimuli were inhibited by melittin administration (Figure 3). Furthermore, the analgesic effect of melittin was blocked by intrathecal adrenergic receptor antagonists, both α1 and α2 (Figure 4).

In the spinal dorsal horn, all α1, α2, and β adrenergic receptors are present. Especially, activation of α1 and α2-adrenergic receptor are known to be able to mediate the anti-nociceptive action:

α1-adrenergic receptor has an excitatory effect on inhibitory interneurons, which can increase the release of inhibitory transmitters, while α2-adrenergic receptor has an inhibitory effect by decreasing the activation of both Aδ and C afferent fibers [24]. Based on our previous study [17], it was shown that oxaliplatin-induced allodynic behavior and spinal neuronal hyperexcitation can be modulated by spinal noradrenaline or its receptor agonists. Inhibitory efficacy was shown in α2 and α1-adrenergic receptor agonists, but not in β. Between α2 and α1, α2-adrenergic receptor agonists showed a greater inhibitory effect. This result implies that the activation of spinal noradrenergic inhibitory system can modulate the oxaliplatin-induced peripheral neuropathy. Although the mechanism of bee venom analgesia depends on the pain model employed, spinal α2-adrenergic receptor has been reported to be generally involved [14,25,26]. Phospholipase A2, another major component of bee venom, also induced analgesic effect in oxaliplatin-induced peripheral neuropathy and its action was blocked by intraperitoneal α2-, but not by α1-adrenergic receptor antagonist [27].

In this study, we discovered the potentiality of melittin as an analgesic agent in chemotherapy induced peripheral neuropathy. So far, melittin has been regarded as a pain producing substance, because of its strong surface activity on lipid membranes followed by releasing inflammatory mediators and activating primary nociceptor cells [28]. Actually, subcutaneous injection of melittin on posterior surface of hind paw produced spontaneous paw flinching reflex and an increase in the frequency of the spinal WDR neuron's spontaneous discharges on cutaneous receptive field of hind paw [29]. However, in our behavior study (Figure 2), subcutaneous melittin administration on ST36 did not induce spontaneous painful behavior. Furthermore, it did not generate spontaneous discharge of WDR neuron responding to receptive filed of hind paw. ST36 is the representative acupoint of Korean medicine, which has been reported to be effective on relieving various pain [30,31]. As other papers reported that the analgesic effect of acupuncture or electroacupuncture on ST36 was mediated by activating the descending pain inhibitory system [32–34], melittin injection on ST36 may also have activated the noradrenergic descending inhibitory system.

The advantage of injecting melittin on ipsilateral acupoint than intraperitoneal has two strong points. First, ST36 is anatomically located near the ascending nerve pathways from hind limb, thus the analgesic effect could be more efficient than systemic administration. The other is minimizing adverse effect of melittin. Systemic injection such as intravenous or intraperitoneal might be accompanied by hemolysis. Although the cytotoxicity of melittin is dependent on its concentration, given that it has affinity to erythrocyte membrane, intradermal or subcutaneous injection of low dose of melittin may be a safe method to prevent hemolysis [35].

Although there is no clinical trial that assessed the effect of melittin on humans, Park et al. investigated the effect and safety of sweet bee venom pharmacoacupuncture on five patients with chemotherapy-induced peripheral neuropathy (CIPN) [36]. Patients' visual analogue scale and world health organization (WHO) CIPN grade as primary results were shown to be effective without causing significant adverse effects such as allergic reaction. As the major component of sweet bee venom is melittin, this result shows that melittin may be used safely to patient in the future

Furthermore, another critical value of melittin as an analgesic dealing with chemotherapy-induced peripheral neuropathy is that it has an anticancer activity [9]. Melittin exerted its anticancer effect by modulating tumor-associated macrophage, which inhibited tumor angiogenesis without non selective cytotoxicity when injected at low dose (0.5 mg/kg) [37]. Therefore, as the same dose of melittin significantly suppressed oxaliplatin-induced peripheral neuropathy in our experiments, we suggest that melittin could act as an adjuvant anticancer and an analgesic agent.

4. Conclusion

The results of the present study demonstrate that melittin administration on ST36 can relive the mechanical and cold allodynia induced by a single injection of oxaliplatin in rats. Furthermore, by in vivo electrophysiolgical study, we demonstrated that melittin can inhibit the hyperexcitation of spinal WDR neuron in response to peripheral stimuli. This analgesic effect of melittin was shown to be mediated by spinal α1 and α2-adrenergic receptor activation. Collectively, these results suggest that melittin has analgesic effect on oxaliplatin-induced peripheral neuropathy and the effect is mediated by activating the spinal α1 and α2-adrenergic receptor. Thus, based on these results, melittin could be used as an analgesic on oxaliplatin-induced peripheral neuropathy.

5. Materials and Methods

5.1. Animals

Sprague-Dawley (SD) rats (7–8 weeks old, 180–210 g, n= 99 in total) were purchased from Young Bio (Gyeonggi, Korea) and housed in cages with free water and food. The room was maintained with a 12 h light/dark cycle and kept at 23 ± 2 °C. All procedures involving animals were approved by the Institutional Animal Care and Use Committee of Kyung Hee University (KHUASP(SE)-19-047; approved 12 June 2019, KHUASP(SE)-18-153; approved 29 January 2019) and performed according to the ethical guidelines of the International Association Of the Study of Pain [38]. At the end of the study, the animals were killed by injecting an overdose of urethane.

5.2. Oxaliplatin Administration

Oxaliplatin (Wako Pure Chemical Industries, Osaka, Japan) was dissolved in a 5% glucose solution at a concentration of 2 mg/mL and was intraperitoneally injected at a dose of 6 mg/kg [23]. The same volume of 5% glucose solution was injected to control group.

5.3. Behavioral Tests

Rats were habituated to the circumstances for 30 min before all behavioral tests. All experimenters conducting behavioral tests were blinded to the groups. Rats were placed on a wired mash and enclosed in a clear plastic box (20 × 20 × 14 cm).

To assess mechanical allodynia, paw withdrawal thresholds were measured by applying the von Frey filaments in the center of the right hind paw. Dixon's up-down method and Chaplan's calculation methods were used and withdrawal cut-off values was 15 g [39,40].

Cold allodynia test was conducted as in our previous study [17]. Acetone (10 μL) was applied to the ventral surface of the right hind paw five times by using a pipette with polyethylene tube, and the experimenter monitored the behavioral response for 40 s [41,42].

5.4. Melittin Administration

Melittin (Melittin from honey bee venom; Sigma, St. Louis, MO, USA; 0.5 mg/kg) was dissolved in saline [14], and it was injected once subcutaneously on ipsilateral acupoint, Zusanli (ST 36) of right leg between three and seven days after oxaliplatin administration in rats showing allodynic behavior. ST36 is located in the anterior tibial muscle, 5 mm lateral and distal to the anterior tubercle of the tibia [43].

5.5. In vivo Extracellular Recording

In vivo extracellular recording was done according to our previous studies [17,44,45]. Briefly, rats were anesthetized with urethane (Sigma, St. Louis, MO, USA; 1.2–1.5 g/kg, intraperitoneal (i.p.)) and the procedures were conducted on a warm plate for maintenance of body temperature. Thoracolumbar vertebral laminectomy was performed at the level of T13–L2 to expose the spinal segment L3–L5. Once the laminectomy was done, the rats were placed in a stereotaxic apparatus to fix the vertebrae. On the surface of exposed spinal cord, Krebs solution (in mM: 117 NaCl, 3.6 KCl, 2.5 $CaCl_2$, 1.2 $MgCl_2$, 1.2 NaH_2PO_4, 11 glucose and 25 $NaHCO_3$) with oxygenated of 95% O_2-5% CO_2 gas was continuously irrigated at a flow rate of 10 to 15 mL/min at 38 ± 1 °C. With the solution perfused, dura mater was removed, and pia-arachnoid mater was cut ot make a small opening to insert the tungsten electrode (impedance of 10 MΩ, FHC, ME, USA) smoothly without adjacent tissue suppression.

To identify the receptive filed of WDR neurons, electrode was inserted slowly into the dorsal horn while stimulating the hind paw with light touch (brushing or tapping), pinching (forceps), and acetone drop. After determining the receptive field, brush stimulus was given by applying the camel brush 5 times during 3 s. Press stimulus was given by pressing the center of the receptive field for 3 s, using the blunt tip of the brush with a diameter of 0.5 cm and a magnitude of about 20 g. Pinch stimulus was done by pinching the skin with toothed forceps (11022-14, Fine Science Tools, Heidelberg, Germany) for 3 s. For cold stimulation, 10 μL of acetone drop was applied to the receptive field. Recorded action potentials were amplified with the bioamplifier (DAM80, WPI, Sarasota, FL, USA). The data were digitized (Digidata 1440A, Axon instruments, Foster City, CA, USA) and stored in a personal computer using pClamp 10 software (Axon instruments, Foster City, CA, USA). Recorded data were spiked-sorted with Spike2 (version 6, Cambridge Electronic Design, Cambridge, UK) and produced spike number.

5.6. Antagonist Treatment

To investigate the spinal involvement of noradrenergic receptors, oxaliplatin administered rats were divided randomly into four groups: dimethyl sulfoxide (DMSO; Sigma, St. Louis, MO, USA) + melittin, prazosin + melittin, PBS + melittin, and idazoxan + melittin. α1-adrenoceptor antagonist prazosin (Sigma, St. Louis, MO, USA; 30 μg) was dissolved in 20% DMSO. α2-adrenoceptor antagonist idazoxan (Sigma, St. Louis, MO, USA; 50 μg) was dissolved in PBS. Under isoflurane anesthesia (Hana Pharm. Co., Hwaseong-si, Kyeonggi-Do, Korea), all antagonists were treated intrathecally with a direct lumbar puncture as previously described [14,16,17].

5.7. Statistics

Statistical analysis was conducted with the software of Prism 5.0 (GraphPad software, La Jolla, CA, USA, 2008). All data are presented as the mean ± SEM. $p < 0.05$ was considered significant.

Author Contributions: W.K. and S.K.K. conceived and designed the experiments; S.C. and H.K.C. performed the experiments; S.C., W.K. and S.K.K. analyzed the data; H.H. and D.-H.H. contributed reagents and materials; S.C., W.K. and S.K.K. wrote the paper. All authors read and approved the final manuscript.

Funding: This work was supported by the National Research Foundation of Korea (NRF) grant funded by the Korea government (NRF-2017M3A9E4057926), and by a grant from the Immune and Pain Society.

Acknowledgments: We wish to thank Professor Hyunsu Bae and Chanju Lee for their valuable comments.

Conflicts of Interest: The authors declare no conflict of interest. The funding sponsors had no role in the design of the study; in the collection, analyses, or interpretation of data; in the writing of the manuscript, and in the decision to publish the results

References

1. André, T.; Boni, C.; Mounedji-Boudiaf, L.; Navarro, M.; Tabernero, J.; Hickish, T.; Topham, C.; Zaninelli, M.; Clingan, P.; Bridgewater, J.; et al. Oxaliplatin, Fluorouracil, and Leucovorin as Adjuvant Treatment for Colon Cancer. *N. Engl. J. Med.* **2004**, *350*, 2343–2351. [CrossRef] [PubMed]
2. Cunningham, D.; Starling, N.; Rao, S.; Iveson, T.; Nicolson, M.; Coxon, F.; Middleton, G.; Daniel, F.; Oates, J.; Norman, A.R. Capecitabine and Oxaliplatin for Advanced Esophagogastric Cancer. *N. Engl. J. Med.* **2008**, *358*, 36–46. [CrossRef] [PubMed]
3. Suker, M.; Beumer, B.R.; Sadot, E.; Marthey, L.; Faris, J.E.; Mellon, E.A.; El-Rayes, B.F.; Wang-Gillam, A.; Lacy, J.; Hosein, P.J.; et al. FOLFIRINOX for locally advanced pancreatic cancer: A systematic review and patient-level meta-analysis. *Lancet Oncol.* **2016**, *17*, 801–810. [CrossRef]
4. Pachman, D.R.; Qin, R.; Seisler, D.K.; Smith, E.M.; Beutler, A.S.; Ta, L.E.; Lafky, J.M.; Wagner-Johnston, N.D.; Ruddy, K.J.; Dakhil, S.; et al. Clinical Course of Oxaliplatin-Induced Neuropathy: Results From the Randomized Phase III Trial N08CB (Alliance). *J. Clin. Oncol. Off. J. Am. Soc. Clin. Oncol.* **2015**, *33*, 3416–3422. [CrossRef] [PubMed]

5. Kidwell, K.M.; Yothers, G.; Ganz, P.A.; Land, S.R.; Ko, C.Y.; Cecchini, R.S.; Kopec, J.A.; Wolmark, N. Long-term neurotoxicity effects of oxaliplatin added to fluorouracil and leucovorin as adjuvant therapy for colon cancer: Results from National Surgical Adjuvant Breast and Bowel Project trials C-07 and LTS-01. *Cancer* **2012**, *118*, 5614–5622. [CrossRef] [PubMed]
6. Park, S.B.; Lin, C.S.; Krishnan, A.V.; Goldstein, D.; Friedlander, M.L.; Kiernan, M.C. Long-term neuropathy after oxaliplatin treatment: Challenging the dictum of reversibility. *Oncologist* **2011**, *16*, 708–716. [CrossRef] [PubMed]
7. Argyriou, A.A. Updates on Oxaliplatin-Induced Peripheral Neurotoxicity (OXAIPN). *Toxics* **2015**, *3*, 187–197. [CrossRef] [PubMed]
8. Smith, E.M.; Pang, H.; Cirrincione, C.; Fleishman, S.; Paskett, E.D.; Ahles, T.; Bressler, L.R.; Fadul, C.E.; Knox, C.; Le-Lindqwister, N.; et al. Effect of duloxetine on pain, function, and quality of life among patients with chemotherapy-induced painful peripheral neuropathy: A randomized clinical trial. *JAMA* **2013**, *309*, 1359–1367. [CrossRef] [PubMed]
9. Rady, I.; Siddiqui, I.A.; Rady, M.; Mukhtar, H. Melittin, a major peptide component of bee venom, and its conjugates in cancer therapy. *Cancer Lett.* **2017**, *402*, 16–31. [CrossRef]
10. Lee, G.; Bae, H. Anti-Inflammatory Applications of Melittin, a Major Component of Bee Venom: Detailed Mechanism of Action and Adverse Effects. *Molecules (Basel Switz.)* **2016**, *21*, 616. [CrossRef]
11. Ryu, H.K.; Baek, Y.H.; Park, Y.C.; Seo, B.K. Current studies of acupuncture in cancer-induced bone pain animal models. *Evid.-Based Complement. Altern. Med. eCAM* **2014**, *2014*, 191347. [CrossRef] [PubMed]
12. Chen, H.S.; Qu, F.; He, X.; Liao, D.; Kang, S.M.; Lu, S.J. The anti-nociceptive effect and the possible mechanism of acupoint stimulation caused by chemical irritants in the bee venom pain model. *Brain Res.* **2010**, *1355*, 61–69. [CrossRef] [PubMed]
13. Yoon, S.Y.; Roh, D.H.; Kwon, Y.B.; Kim, H.W.; Seo, H.S.; Han, H.J.; Lee, H.J.; Beitz, A.J.; Lee, J.H. Acupoint stimulation with diluted bee venom (apipuncture) potentiates the analgesic effect of intrathecal clonidine in the rodent formalin test and in a neuropathic pain model. *J. Pain Off. J. Am. Pain Soc.* **2009**, *10*, 253–263. [CrossRef]
14. Choi, J.; Jeon, C.; Lee, J.H.; Jang, J.U.; Quan, F.S.; Lee, K.; Kim, W.; Kim, S.K. Suppressive Effects of Bee Venom Acupuncture on Paclitaxel-Induced Neuropathic Pain in Rats: Mediation by Spinal α_2-Adrenergic Receptor. *Toxins* **2017**, *9*, 351. [CrossRef]
15. Li, J.; Ke, T.; He, C.; Cao, W.; Wei, M.; Zhang, L.; Zhang, J.X.; Wang, W.; Ma, J.; Wang, Z.R.; et al. The anti-arthritic effects of synthetic melittin on the complete Freund's adjuvant-induced rheumatoid arthritis model in rats. *Am. J. Chin. Med.* **2010**, *38*, 1039–1049. [CrossRef]
16. Kim, W.; Kim, M.J.; Go, D.; Min, B.-I.; Na, H.S.; Kim, S.K. Combined Effects of Bee Venom Acupuncture and Morphine on Oxaliplatin-Induced Neuropathic Pain in Mice. *Toxins* **2016**, *8*, 33. [CrossRef] [PubMed]
17. Choi, S.; Yamada, A.; Kim, W.; Kim, S.K.; Furue, H. Noradrenergic inhibition of spinal hyperexcitation elicited by cutaneous cold stimuli in rats with oxaliplatin-induced allodynia: Electrophysiological and behavioral assessments. *J. Physiol. Sci. JPS* **2017**, *67*, 431–438. [CrossRef] [PubMed]
18. Graham, J.; Muhsin, M.; Kirkpatrick, P. Oxaliplatin. *Nat. Rev. Drug Discov.* **2004**, *3*, 11–12. [CrossRef]
19. Dault, R.; Rousseau, M.P.; Beaudoin, A.; Frenette, M.A.; Lemay, F.; Beauchesne, M.F. Impact of oxaliplatin-induced neuropathy in patients with colorectal cancer: A prospective evaluation at a single institution. *Curr. Oncol.* **2016**, *23*, e65–e69. [CrossRef]
20. Fradkin, M.; Batash, R.; Elmaleh, S.; Debi, R.; Schaffer, P.; Schaffer, M.; Asna, N. Management of peripheral neuropathy induced by chemotherapy. *Curr. Med. Chem.* **2019**. [CrossRef]
21. Yoon, H.; Kim, M.J.; Yoon, I.; Li, D.X.; Bae, H.; Kim, S.K. Nicotinic Acetylcholine Receptors Mediate the Suppressive Effect of an Injection of Diluted Bee Venom into the GV3 Acupoint on Oxaliplatin-Induced Neuropathic Cold Allodynia in Rats. *Biol. Pharm. Bull.* **2015**, *38*, 710–714. [CrossRef] [PubMed]
22. Lim, B.-S.; Moon, H.J.; Li, D.X.; Gil, M.; Min, J.K.; Lee, G.; Bae, H.; Kim, S.K.; Min, B.-I. Effect of Bee Venom Acupuncture on Oxaliplatin-Induced Cold Allodynia in Rats. *Evid.-Based Complement. Altern. Med.* **2013**, *2013*, 369324. [CrossRef] [PubMed]
23. Lee, J.H.; Li, D.X.; Yoon, H.; Go, D.; Quan, F.S.; Min, B.I.; Kim, S.K. Serotonergic mechanism of the relieving effect of bee venom acupuncture on oxaliplatin-induced neuropathic cold allodynia in rats. *BMC Complement. Altern. Med.* **2014**, *14*, 471. [CrossRef] [PubMed]

24. Yoshimura, M.; Furue, H. Mechanisms for the anti-nociceptive actions of the descending noradrenergic and serotonergic systems in the spinal cord. *J. Pharmacol. Sci.* **2006**, *101*, 107–117. [CrossRef] [PubMed]
25. Huh, J.E.; Seo, B.K.; Lee, J.W.; Park, Y.C.; Baek, Y.H. Analgesic Effects of Diluted Bee Venom Acupuncture Mediated by delta-Opioid and alpha2-Adrenergic Receptors in Osteoarthritic Rats. *Altern. Ther. Health Med.* **2018**, *24*, 28–35. [PubMed]
26. Yeo, J.H.; Yoon, S.Y.; Kwon, S.K.; Kim, S.J.; Lee, J.H.; Beitz, A.J.; Roh, D.H. Repetitive Acupuncture Point Treatment with Diluted Bee Venom Relieves Mechanical Allodynia and Restores Intraepidermal Nerve Fiber Loss in Oxaliplatin-Induced Neuropathic Mice. *J. Pain Off. J. Am. Pain Soc.* **2016**, *17*, 298–309. [CrossRef] [PubMed]
27. Li, D.; Lee, Y.; Kim, W.; Lee, K.; Bae, H.; Kim, S.K. Analgesic Effects of Bee Venom Derived Phospholipase A(2) in a Mouse Model of Oxaliplatin-Induced Neuropathic Pain. *Toxins* **2015**, *7*, 2422–2434. [CrossRef] [PubMed]
28. Chen, J.; Guan, S.M.; Sun, W.; Fu, H. Melittin, the Major Pain-Producing Substance of Bee Venom. *Neurosci. Bull.* **2016**, *32*, 265–272. [CrossRef] [PubMed]
29. Li, K.C.; Chen, J. Altered pain-related behaviors and spinal neuronal responses produced by s.c. injection of melittin in rats. *Neuroscience* **2004**, *126*, 753–762. [CrossRef]
30. Lu, K.W.; Hsu, C.K.; Hsieh, C.L.; Yang, J.; Lin, Y.W. Probing the Effects and Mechanisms of Electroacupuncture at Ipsilateral or Contralateral ST36-ST37 Acupoints on CFA-induced Inflammatory Pain. *Sci. Rep.* **2016**, *6*, 22123. [CrossRef]
31. Zhang, R.; Lao, L.; Ren, K.; Berman, B.M. Mechanisms of acupuncture-electroacupuncture on persistent pain. *Anesthesiology* **2014**, *120*, 482–503. [CrossRef] [PubMed]
32. Liu, X.; Zhu, B.; Zhang, S.X. Relationship between electroacupuncture analgesia and descending pain inhibitory mechanism of nucleus raphe magnus. *Pain* **1986**, *24*, 383–396. [CrossRef]
33. De Medeiros, M.A.; Canteras, N.S.; Suchecki, D.; Mello, L.E. Analgesia and c-Fos expression in the periaqueductal gray induced by electroacupuncture at the Zusanli point in rats. *Brain Res.* **2003**, *973*, 196–204. [CrossRef]
34. Yang, J.; Liu, W.Y.; Song, C.Y.; Lin, B.C. Only arginine vasopressin, not oxytocin and endogenous opiate peptides, in hypothalamic paraventricular nucleus play a role in acupuncture analgesia in the rat. *Brain Res. Bull.* **2006**, *68*, 453–458. [CrossRef] [PubMed]
35. Dempsey, C.E. The actions of melittin on membranes. *Biochim. Biophys. Acta* **1990**, *1031*, 143–161. [CrossRef]
36. Park, J.W.; Jeon, J.H.; Yoon, J.; Jung, T.Y.; Kwon, K.R.; Cho, C.K.; Lee, Y.W.; Sagar, S.; Wong, R.; Yoo, H.S. Effects of sweet bee venom pharmacopuncture treatment for chemotherapy-induced peripheral neuropathy: a case series. *Integr. Cancer Ther.* **2012**, *11*, 166–171. [CrossRef]
37. Lee, C.; Bae, S.-J.S.; Joo, H.; Bae, H. Melittin suppresses tumor progression by regulating tumor-associated macrophages in a Lewis lung carcinoma mouse model. *Oncotarget* **2017**, *8*, 54951–54965. [CrossRef]
38. Zimmermann, M. Ethical guidelines for investigations of experimental pain in conscious animals. *Pain* **1983**, *16*, 109–110. [CrossRef]
39. Dixon, W.J. The Up-and-Down Method for Small Samples. *J. Am. Stat. Assoc.* **1965**, *60*, 967–978. [CrossRef]
40. Chaplan, S.R.; Bach, F.W.; Pogrel, J.W.; Chung, J.M.; Yaksh, T.L. Quantitative assessment of tactile allodynia in the rat paw. *J. Neurosci. Methods* **1994**, *53*, 55–63. [CrossRef]
41. Choi, Y.; Yoon, Y.W.; Na, H.S.; Kim, S.H.; Chung, J.M. Behavioral signs of ongoing pain and cold allodynia in a rat model of neuropathic pain. *Pain* **1994**, *59*, 369–376. [PubMed]
42. Flatters, S.J.; Bennett, G.J. Ethosuximide reverses paclitaxel- and vincristine-induced painful peripheral neuropathy. *Pain* **2004**, *109*, 150–161. [CrossRef] [PubMed]
43. Park, J.H.; Kim, S.K.; Kim, H.N.; Sun, B.; Koo, S.; Choi, S.M.; Bae, H.; Min, B.I. Spinal cholinergic mechanism of the relieving effects of electroacupuncture on cold and warm allodynia in a rat model of neuropathic pain. *J. Physiol. Sci. JPS* **2009**, *59*, 291–298. [CrossRef] [PubMed]
44. Kim, W.; Chung, Y.; Choi, S.; Min, B.I.; Kim, S.K. Duloxetine Protects against Oxaliplatin-Induced Neuropathic Pain and Spinal Neuron Hyperexcitability in Rodents. *Int. J. Mol. Sci.* **2017**, *18*. [CrossRef] [PubMed]
45. Chae, H.K.; Kim, W.; Kim, S.K. Phytochemicals of Cinnamomi Cortex: Cinnamic Acid, but not Cinnamaldehyde, Attenuates Oxaliplatin-Induced Cold and Mechanical Hypersensitivity in Rats. *Nutrients* **2019**, *11*, 432. [CrossRef]

toxins

MDPI

Article

Identification of *Aethina tumida* Kir Channels as Putative Targets of the Bee Venom Peptide Tertiapin Using Structure-Based Virtual Screening Methods

Craig A. Doupnik

Department of Molecular Pharmacology & Physiology, University of South Florida College of Medicine, Tampa, FL 33612, USA; cdoupnik@health.usf.edu

Received: 20 August 2019; Accepted: 18 September 2019; Published: 19 September 2019

check for updates

Abstract: Venoms are comprised of diverse mixtures of proteins, peptides, and small molecules. Identifying individual venom components and their target(s) with mechanism of action is now attainable to understand comprehensively the effectiveness of venom cocktails and how they collectively function in the defense and predation of an organism. Here, structure-based computational methods were used with bioinformatics tools to screen and identify potential biological targets of tertiapin (TPN), a venom peptide from *Apis mellifera* (European honey bee). The small hive beetle (*Aethina tumida* (*A. tumida*)) is a natural predator of the honey bee colony and was found to possess multiple inwardly rectifying K^+ (Kir) channel subunit genes from a genomic BLAST search analysis. Structure-based virtual screening of homology modelled *A. tumida* Kir (*at*Kir) channels found TPN to interact with a docking profile and interface "footprint" equivalent to known TPN-sensitive mammalian Kir channels. The results support the hypothesis that *at*Kir channels, and perhaps other insect Kir channels, are natural biological targets of TPN that help defend the bee colony from infestations by blocking K^+ transport via *at*Kir channels. From these in silico findings, this hypothesis can now be subsequently tested in vitro by validating *at*Kir channel block as well as in vivo TPN toxicity towards *A. tumida*. This study highlights the utility and potential benefits of screening in virtual space for venom peptide interactions and their biological targets, which otherwise would not be feasible.

Keywords: bee venom; bioinformatics; computational docking; homology modelling; ion channel structure; protein–peptide interactions; tertiapin; venom peptides; virtual screening; small hive beetle

Key Contribution: Using structure-based computational modelling techniques, Kir channels expressed in the small hive beetle were discovered as suitable targets for channel block by the *Apis mellifera* venom peptide tertiapin. This novel finding highlights the utilization of computational tools in setting new research directions, and potentially expands the repertoire of venom actions aiding in honeybee defense from natural insect predators.

1. Introduction

Venoms from *Hymenoptera* and other venomous species are comprised of diverse mixtures of proteins, peptides, and small molecules [1,2]. The composition of these "venom cocktails" are species-dependent, where the concentration of individual toxin components can vary by age, sex, diet, and different environmental conditions [3]. Envenomation efficacy is largely driven by the adaptive evolutionary pressures that select for certain venom genes based on their ability to either: (1) aid in predation, (2) aid in defense from predation, and/or (3) aid in reproductive health and survival (e.g., anti-microbial and anti-parasitic activity) [4].

One of the well-established molecular targets of venom-derived toxins are the ion channels expressed in natural prey and predators. As potent modulators of ion channel function during envenomation, venom-derived peptides contribute to the overall venom response by causing a variety of physiologic responses including paralysis for host capture and pain for defense from predators [5]. The atomic-level structural details that have emerged for both venom-derived peptides and several ion channels have enabled structure-based computational screening techniques to be deployed for identifying potential target effectors for venom components in silico [6]. These methods are also helping to guide rational peptide design efforts to re-engineer venom peptides for potential drug development purposes [7–9].

While most efforts have focused on molecular targets of venom components in laboratory mammals and human tissues, understanding the biological targets of venom-derived peptides encountered in nature is essential for providing a comprehensive understanding of the evolutionary adaptations that drive target selectivity and affinity, and thereby contribute to overall venom efficacy. Such an insight can also be valuable in identifying potential off-target effects in humans where venom-derived peptides are being developed for both therapeutic and non-therapeutic basic research applications [10].

Here, the use of structure-based virtual screening techniques was deployed to search and identify putative ion channel targets using a small venom peptide from *Apis mellifera* (*A. melliferra*) venom called tertiapin (TPN). Venom produced by female worker bees is used primarily for individual defensive purposes, and to protect the colony from various invertebrates as well as vertebrate predators and/or pests. The updated genome assembly of *A. melliferra* (Amel_4.5) with venom transcriptomic analysis indicates over 100 proteins and peptides are present in honey bee venom to collectively mediate these responses [11]. TPN is a 21-amino acid peptide that represents a relatively small fractional component (0.1%) of the total protein content of bee venom [12], and was serendipitously discovered in 1998 to bind and block a subset of mammalian Kir channels [13,14]. The evolution-driven biological target(s) of TPN encountered in nature, however, is currently not established. Here, a hypothesis-driven in silico screening strategy is presented that supports insect Kir channels as potential natural targets for TPN-mediated channel block for bee colony defense from the small hive beetle. This novel finding highlights how the application of structure-based computational tools such as molecular docking can create new research directions by demonstrating mechanistically feasible and testable hypotheses on the adaptive pressures that drive interaction of venom peptides with their natural biological targets.

2. Results

2.1. Reliability of Molecular Docking of TPN to Kir Channel-Modelled Structures

The rat Kir1.1 channel is the prototypical TPN-sensitive Kir channel, having an IC_{50} of ~2 nM for functional channel block [14]. Interestingly, however, the human Kir1.1 channel isoform is insensitive to TPN block due primarily to two key amino acid differences in the outer vestibule of the Kir1.1 channel where TPN is known to bind [15,16]. Previous computational docking studies of NMR-derived TPN ensemble conformers (PDB ID 1TER.pdb [17]) to a homology-modelled rat Kir1.1 channel identified a favored TPN conformer having a pore-blocking binding pose where the positively charged C-terminal lysine side chain of TPN inserts and occupies the S1 K^+ binding site in the channel selectivity filter [7]. Moreover, the computational docking scores reliably differentiate TPN interactions among homology-modelled Kir1.1 isoforms known to be sensitive (rat) and insensitive (human and zebrafish) to TPN_Q channel block [7]. Thus, structure-based interactions between TPN and rat Kir1.1, derived from computational docking methods and validated in vitro, are thought to represent the high-affinity bound and blocked state of the channel [13] (but also see Reference [18]).

To further test the reliability of this approach, the same molecular docking protocol used for the homology-modelled rat Kir1.1 channel was applied to crystal structures of the TPN-sensitive murine Kir3.2 channel homo-tetramer [19,20]. Mammalian Kir3.2 channel subunits are expressed in neuronal and endocrine cells and assemble primarily as hetero-tetrameric channels with different Kir3.x subunits, and function to inhibit membrane excitability [21]. When heterologously expressed in *Xenopus* oocytes, the homo-tetrameric Kir3.2 construct used for X-ray crystallography yields channels functionally blocked by the oxidation-resistant TPN_Q variant peptide in a manner similar to hetero-tetrameric Kir3.1/3.2 channels [20,22–24]. Thus, docking TPN to the Kir3.2 crystal structure precludes homology modelling of the Kir channel.

Shown in Figure 1, rigid-body docking of TPN conformers to the Kir3.2 channel crystal structures was dependent on the NMR-derived TPN conformer used for docking, similar to that observed with TPN docking to the homology-modelled rKir1.1 channel [7]. For the Kir3.2 channel, the TPN conformer that yielded the highest docking score for both the closed-state and pre-opened-state conformations was TPN-13.

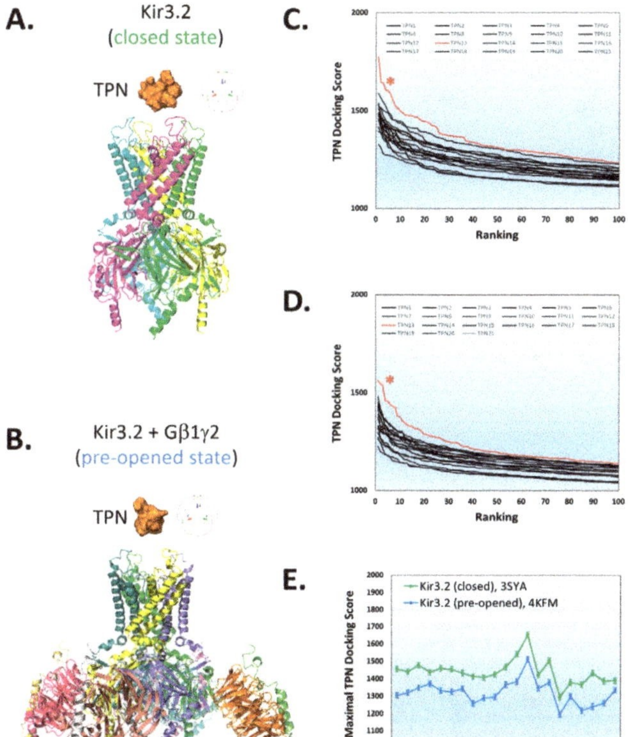

Figure 1. Preferential docking of the tertiapin (TPN)-13 conformer to mKir3.2 channel structures. **A.** Structural rendering of the Kir3.2 closed state (3SYA.pdb) (ribbon diagram) with TPN (orange, solid rendering) positioned above the outer vestibule. **B.** Structural rendering of the "pre-opened" conformation of Kir3.2 channel in complex with Gβγ dimers (4KFM.pdb) (ribbon diagram) with TPN (solid rendering) depicted above the outer vestibule of the channel. **C & D.** Plots of the top 100-ranked scores for all 21 TPN conformers docked to the Kir3.2 channel closed-state conformation (C) and pre-opened-state conformation (D). The data curves and asterisks indicated in red correspond to the TPN-13 conformer that yielded the highest score for each Kir3.2 channel conformation. **E.** Plot of the maximal docking scores (mean ± SD, top 5 complexes) for each TPN conformer docked to the Kir3.2 channel closed-state conformation (3SYA, green symbols) and pre-opened-state conformation (4KFM, blue symbols).

To further characterize the structural similarity among the 21 TPN conformers, hierarchical clustering analysis of the calculated pairwise alpha-carbon amino acid backbone RMSD values for the NMR ensemble structures was performed (Figure 2). The RMSD cluster analysis identified 4 distinct sub-conformations for TPN, where conformers TPN-12 and TPN-13 belonged to the same sub-conformation cluster group and were closest in structural similarity among the 21 conformers (Figure 2A). As previously reported, the TPN-12 conformer yielded the top-ranked docking score for the homology-modelled rat Kir1.1 channel [7] and represented the second best docking score for Kir3.2 (see Figure 1). Thus, the TPN docking results to Kir3.2 channels in both closed and pre-opened conformations are in good agreement with the previously characterized rat Kir1.1 docking study and support a favored role for the TPN sub-conformation state represented by the cluster group that includes TPN-12 and TPN-13 conformers. One of the major structural contributors mediating the different TPN sub-conformations was the orientation of the C3–C14 disulfide bond that contributes to the overall tertiary peptide structure and orientation of the surface exposed side chains (Figure 2B).

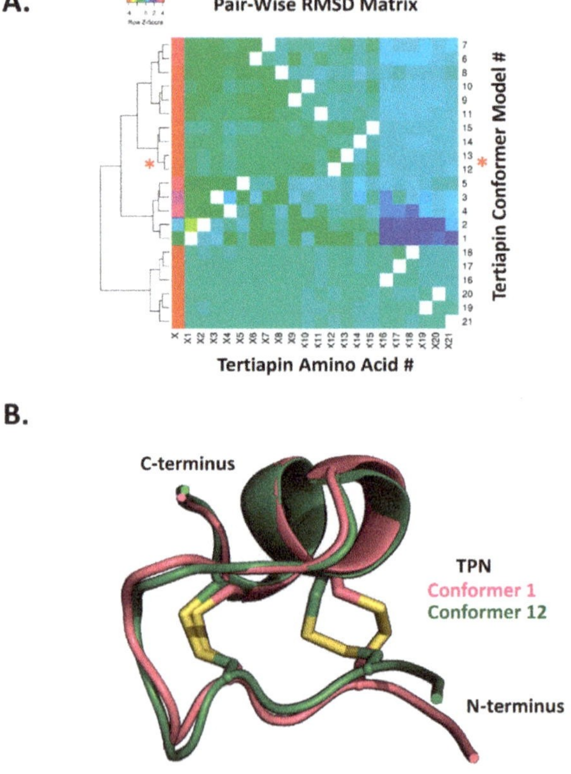

Figure 2. Hierarchical clustering of NMR-derived TPN structural conformers based on pairwise RMSD analysis. **A.** Heatmap and cluster analysis of the calculated pairwise RMSD along the TPN 21-amino acid alpha-carbon backbone. RMSD analysis was performed using VMD software, with the resulting 21 × 21 matrix (21 TPN conformers by 21 TPN amino acids) analyzed using Heatmapper (http://www.heatmapper.ca). The red asterisks denote the TPN-12 and TPN-13 conformer clusters that yield the top docking scores to Kir3.2 and are structurally similar. **B.** Structural alignment of TPN-1 and TPN-12 conformers, highlighting the different disulfide (Cys3–Cys14) bond configuration contributing to different peptide conformations.

Surface renderings of TPN-13 docked to the Kir3.2 channel are shown in Figure 3 where the entire TPN peptide structure is shown to be bound deep within the channel outer vestibule and plugs the channel like a "cork in a bottle". The TPN peptide interacts in an asymmetric manner making different contacts with the four identical Kir3.2 subunits. However, similar to the modelled Kir1.1 channel, the C-terminal TPN K21 side chain occupies the central channel pore with other TPN residues making contact with Kir3.2 vestibule residues including the Kir3.2 turret structures.

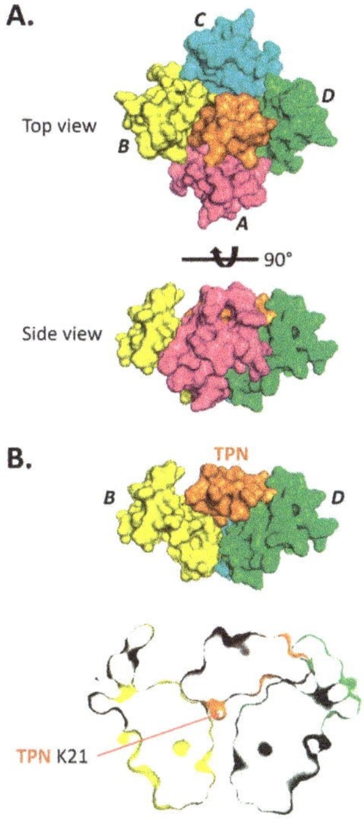

Figure 3. Binding pose of TPN docked to the Kir3.2 channel. **A.** Surface renderings of the TPN-13 conformer (shown in orange) docked to the Kir3.2 channel (subunits A, B, C, and D color-coded). TPN-13 was docked to the Kir3.2 channel closed state (3SYA.pdb) using Cluspro 2.0. Shown are a top view (upper image) from an extracellular vantage point, and a side view (lower image) where the TPN peptide is mostly occluded from the view by Kir3.2 subunit A (magenta). **B.** Solid side-view rendering (upper image) of the TPN-docked Kir3.2 channel with subunit A removed to expose for viewing the docked TPN-13 conformer (in orange) within the channel vestibule. The lower image is a "sectioned" side-view rendering that exposes the location of the C-terminal TPN lysine (K21) located at the mouth of the channel pore. Also visible is the juxtaposed TPN peptide with the Kir3.2 turret domain from subunit D.

2.2. Virtual Screening for TPN-Interacting Kir Channels

Given the reproducible outcomes for TPN docking to homology-modelled rKir1.1 channel and the two mKir3.2 channel crystal structures, homology models for 14 different mouse Kir channel isoforms (Figure 4A) were constructed analogous to rKir1.1 and then screened in silico for docking interactions with the TPN-12 conformer. The homology-modelled Kir channels were all homo-tetramers, and the only Kir channel not examined was Kir2.3 which contained a significantly larger extracellular turret loop region that precluded reliable modelling and assembly of the Kir2.3 homo-tetramer using the Swiss-Model homology-modelling program (see Materials and Methods section).

The ranked TPN-12 docking score profile obtained from the virtual screen of mouse Kir channel structures is shown in Figure 4B, where the scoring algorithm is weighted for receptor–ligand shape complementarity, electrostatic contacts, and van der Waal forces [25]. As reported previously, the top-ranked docking scores begin to rapidly diminish within the top ten scored complexes. The average score for the top 5 complexes for each Kir channel is shown in Figure 4C. In agreement with functional studies, three mouse Kir channels with the highest docking scores were channels known to be sensitive to functional TPN_Q block, namely Kir1.1, Kir3.2, and Kir3.4. Unexpectedly, however, the Kir channel having the second highest docking score was Kir4.1. When examining the top-ranked docking scores, the order for energetically favored interactions with TPN-12 was Kir1.1 > Kir4.1 > Kir3.4 > Kir3.2 > Kir3.1. The Kir3.1 docking scores were comparable to the TPN-insensitive Kir2.1 channel, which is in agreement with the insensitivity of homomeric mutant Kir3.1 channels to TPN_Q block [26]. Moreover, the other seven Kir channels with lowest TPN docking scores are also known to be insensitive to TPN_Q block (i.e., Kir2.x, Kir6.2, and Kir7.1) and therefore establish a baseline profile for Kir channels insensitive to TPN [27]. These initial findings from the virtual screen across mouse Kir channels largely agree with known Kir channel TPN sensitivities, but suggest the modelled Kir4.1 channel outer vestibule structure presents a viable receptor target for TPN interactions comparable to known TPN-sensitive Kir channels.

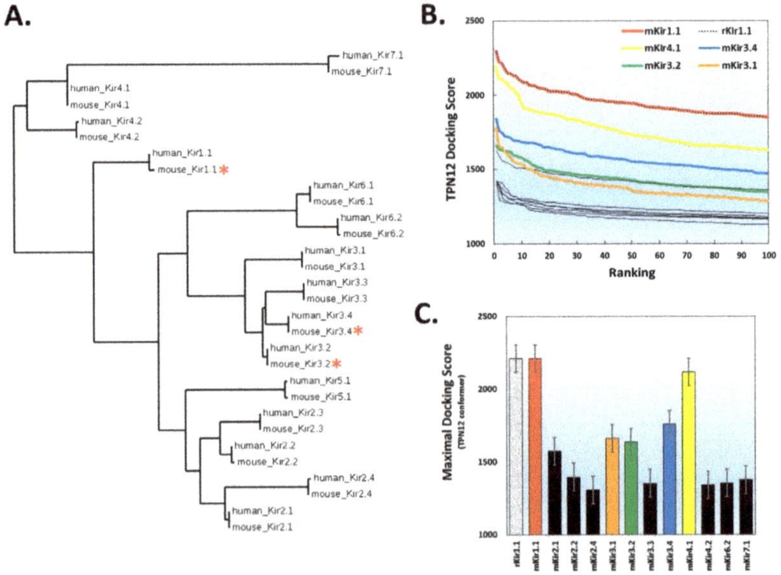

Figure 4. TPN docking profile to mammalian Kir channels. **A.** Dendrogram illustrating the amino acid sequence similarity of mouse and human Kir channel isoforms. A multiple sequence alignment was performed using the Constraint-based Multiple Alignment Tool (COBALT, National Center for Biotechnology Information). The tree function was used to generate the dendrogram illustrating the clustering of Kir channel subunit isoforms into their different gene subfamilies [21]. The red asterisks denote Kir channels known to be functionally blocked by TPN. **B.** Top-ranked docking scores for the TPN-12 conformer to the outer vestibule of 12 different homology-modelled mouse Kir channels. The rat Kir1.1 profile previously reported is also shown for comparison, and is identical to mKir1.1. The five Kir channels with the highest docking scores are color-coded; mKir1.1 (red), mKir4.1 (yellow), mKir3.4 (blue), Kir3.2 (green), and mKir3.1 (orange). **C.** Comparison of maximal docking scores for the TPN–Kir channel complexes. Bars represent the mean ± SD for the top five-ranked complexes for each TPN12-docked Kir channel complex. Colored bars correspond to the Kir channels color labelled in panel B.

2.3. Interface Analysis of TPN-Docked Kir Channels

Given the unexpected high TPN docking score to the homology-modelled Kir4.1 channel, refined docking of TPN to Kir4.1 was performed next to compare the predicted Kir channel–TPN interface contacts using PISA [28]. Shown in Figure 5, the TPN interface "footprint" on the Kir4.1 channel vestibule was similar to those on both the TPN-sensitive rat Kir1.1 and mouse Kir3.2 channels, where three major subunit contact sites within the Kir channel vestibule were observed. These interface "hot spots" corresponded to: (1) the turret region, (2) a "ring" region located along the wall of the channel vestibule, and (3) the pore entry region. Most of the exposed residue side chains of TPN participate in the predicted asymmetric binding interface in a Kir subunit-dependent manner. For mKir4.1, the predicted formations of hydrogen bonds were fewer, sharing some conserved sites in the channel turret and pore regions but absent in the mid-level ring region where mKir4.1 lacks an equivalent acidic reside present in rat Kir1.1 and mouse Kir3.2. The docking pose for TPN-12 within the Kir4.1 vestibule is shown in Figure 6, indicating a similar general orientation where the TPN C-terminal K21 side chain was positioned and inserts into the channel pore.

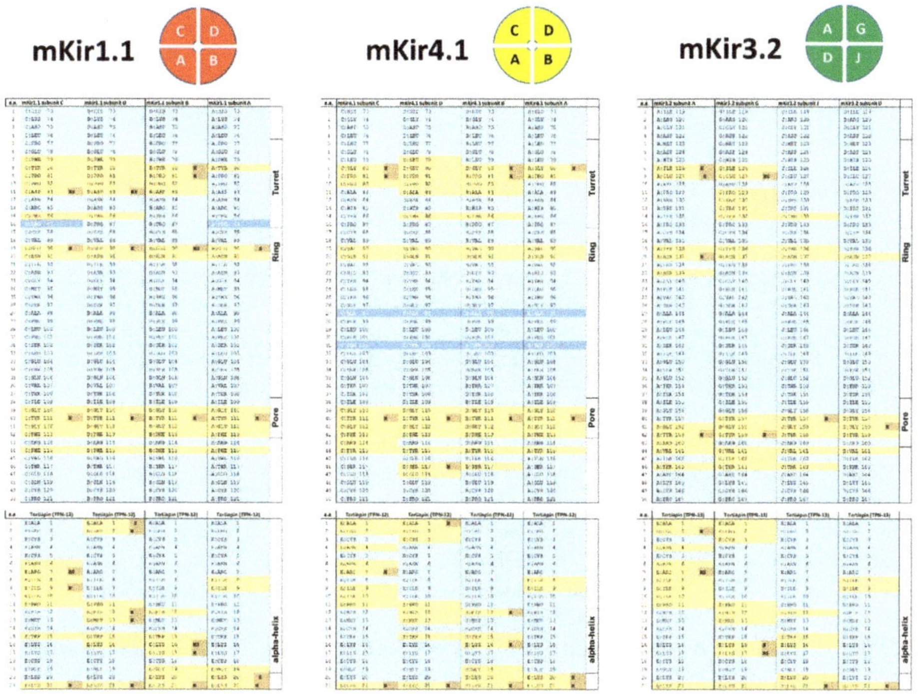

Figure 5. Comparative analysis of the docked tertiapin "footprint" among 3 of the highest scored Kir channel outer vestibules. Diagrams for the subunit assembled Kir channel tetramer arrangements (top view) for the homology-modelled mKir1.1 (red) and mKir4.1 (yellow) channels, and the mKir3.2 (green) homo-tetrameric channel. The predicted amino acid contacts between TPN and each Kir channel subunit are listed in each diagram below, with interfacing residues indicated in yellow and residues making hydrogen bonds or salt bridge link indicated in orange. Inaccessible residues are shown in dark blue, and solvent-accessible residues not involved in the TPN–Kir channel inferface are shown in light blue. TPN–Kir channel Interface analysis was performed using the PISA program on the top-scored docked complexes.

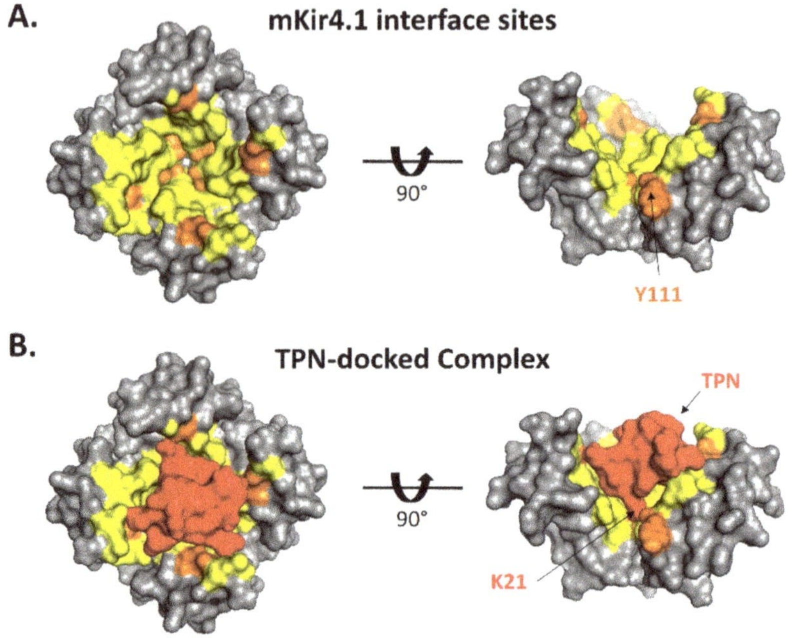

Figure 6. Surface interface and contact sites for the TPN-docked mKir4.1 channel complex. **A.** Surface rendering of the modelled outer vestibule of the mKir4.1 channel (top view, left; side view, right). Yellow residues depict PISA-predicted interface sites, with orange residues depicting sites with predicted H-bonds with the docked TPN peptide. For the side-view image, one of the channel subunits has been removed to expose the pore region of the vestibule. **B.** Surface rendering of TPN (red) docked to the outer vestibule of mKir4.1 channel (top view, left; side view, right). For the side-view image, the location of TPN K21 in the pore is exposed with one of the channel subunits removed.

2.4. Testing TPN_Q Block of Kir4.1 Channels Expressed in Xenopus Oocytes

To test whether TPN functionally blocks mKir4.1 channels, the mouse Kir4.1 isoform was expressed in *Xenopus* oocytes and K^+ currents recorded before and during 100 nM TPN_Q application. Shown in Figure 7, K^+ currents produced by expressed Kir4.1 channels were insensitive to 100 nM TPN_Q, a concentration that blocks nearly 100% of the rKir1.1 channel current [7,14]. The lack of mKir4.1 channel block by 100 nM TPN_Q is also consistent with a previous study that examined the blocking effects of a TPN_Q derivative on Kir4.1 channels [27]. Thus, despite the positive in silico docking scores demonstrating good shape complementarity between the receptor (mKir4.1) and ligand (TPN), the affinity for TPN_Q block of functional Kir4.1 channels is sufficiently low, indicating the virtual screening finding represents a "false positive" that is likely due to fewer and/or weaker interaction hotspots. This structure-based result may nevertheless serve as a useful guide for re-engineering the TPN_Q peptide scaffold to produce stronger interactions that yield a higher-affinity TPN variant that can functionally block the Kir4.1 channel receptor given its demonstrated shape complementarity.

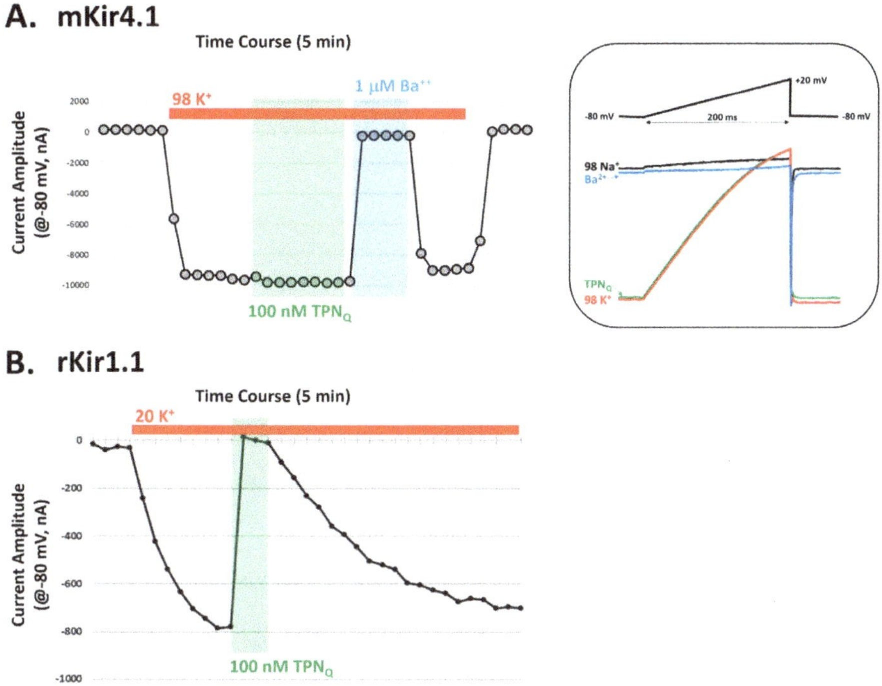

Figure 7. Validation testing for functional block of mKir4.1 channels by TPN_Q. **A.** Electrophysiological recordings of mKir4.1 channel currents before and during application of TPN_Q in *Xenopus* oocytes. The time-course plot shows the amplitude of membrane currents at −80 mV during 2-electrode voltage clamp recording. Indicated by the red bar, high K^+ (98 mM) application evokes inward mKir4.1-mediated K^+ currents. Application of either 100 nM TPN_Q (green) or 1 μM $BaCl_2$ (blue) demonstrates TPN_Q insensitivity and Ba^{2+} sensitivity of mKir4.1 currents. Right panel: Membrane currents evoked by the voltage-ramp protocol display the inward rectification properties of the mKir4.1 channel currents in the absence and presence of either 100 nM TPN_Q (green) or 1 μM $BaCl_2$ (blue). The results are representative of 7 different oocytes. **B.** Positive control comparison, showing similar electrophysiological recordings of rat Kir1.1 channel currents before and during application of 100 nM TPN_Q in *Xenopus* oocytes. High K^+ (20 mM) was applied to evoke inward rKir1.1-mediated K^+ currents (red bar), where application of 100 nM TPN_Q (green) blocked all the Kir1.1-mediated inward currents. The results are representative of 5 different oocytes.

2.5. *Hypothesis Testing with Structure-Based Virtual Screening*

The natural biological target of TPN as an active component of bee venom is currently not known. The venom produced by stinging female worker bees is used primarily for defensive purposes from individual predation and to protect the colony from a variety of different predators and pests encountered in nature. The ability to produce an effective and deterring noxious stimulus following a sting is the result of several venom components that work in concert on diverse molecular targets expressed across a wide range of predatory species encountered in nature [12,29]. How TPN specifically might contribute towards the bee defense response is not clear, while blocking renal Kir1.1 channels and/or neuronal and cardiac Kir3.x channels in mammals seems implausible. Insects are among the many natural predators and pests that bees encounter in nature, and therefore a testable hypothesis is that certain insect Kir channels are the natural targets of TPN in bee venom.

To begin to test this hypothesis, the TPN virtual screening protocol was applied to Kir channels identified from a BLAST search of the recently reported small hive beetle genome (*Aethina tumida*, assembly Atum_1.0, NW_017852934.1) [30]. The small hive beetle is a natural parasite of *A. mellifera* and is normally maintained by guard bee aggression towards adult and beetle larva that includes envenomation [31,32]. Eight predicted *Aethina tumida* (*A. tumida*) Kir (*at*Kir) channel subunits in the genomic Reference Sequence database were identified from the BLAST search using the mouse Kir3.2 subunit sequence, with six having full-length sequence similarity to that of the TPN-sensitive mouse Kir3.2 channel (Figure 8). A multiple sequence comparison with the family of mouse Kir channel subunits indicated the *at*Kir channel subunits were most similar to each other, clustering as a distinct *at*Kir channel gene family that was closest to the mammalian Kir channel gene subfamily expressed predominantly in epithelial cells and involved in K^+ homeostasis (i.e., Kir1.1, Kir4.x, and Kir7.1) (Figure 9B).

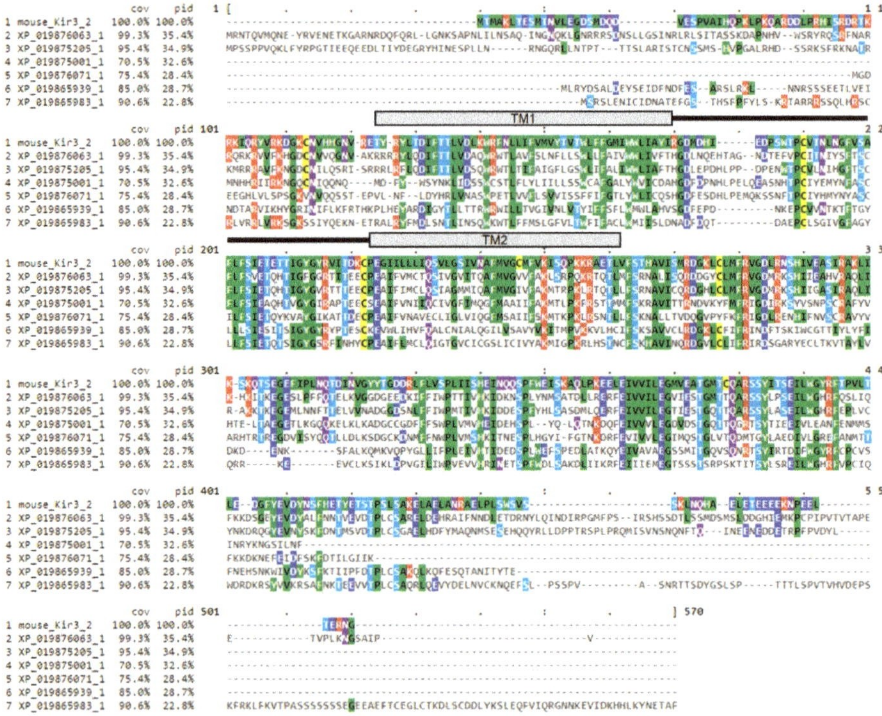

Figure 8. Multiple sequence alignment of six Kir channel subunit proteins identified in a BLAST search of the *Aethina tumida* (*A. tumida*) genome. The TPN-sensitive mouse Kir3.2 channel sequence was included for comparison, where the percentages of coverage (cov) and identity (pid) are shown for each *A. tumida* Kir (*at*Kir) channel subunit referenced to Kir3.2. The location of the 2 transmembrane domains (TM1 and TM2) are indicated, connected by the amino acid sequence of the the outer vestibule region that forms the receptor for TPN binding and block.

Structural models of the six *at*Kir channels were next constructed with homology modelling limited to the outer vestibule region as described for the mouse Kir channels. Molecular docking of TPN (conformer 13) identified two *at*Kir channels (XP_019865983.1 and XP_019865939.1) that displayed TPN docking profiles nearly equivalent to the TPN-sensitive mKir3.2 channel (3SYA.pdb) (Figure 9C,D). The interface and putative hot spots for TPN interactions with each of these *at*Kir channels were then further analyzed.

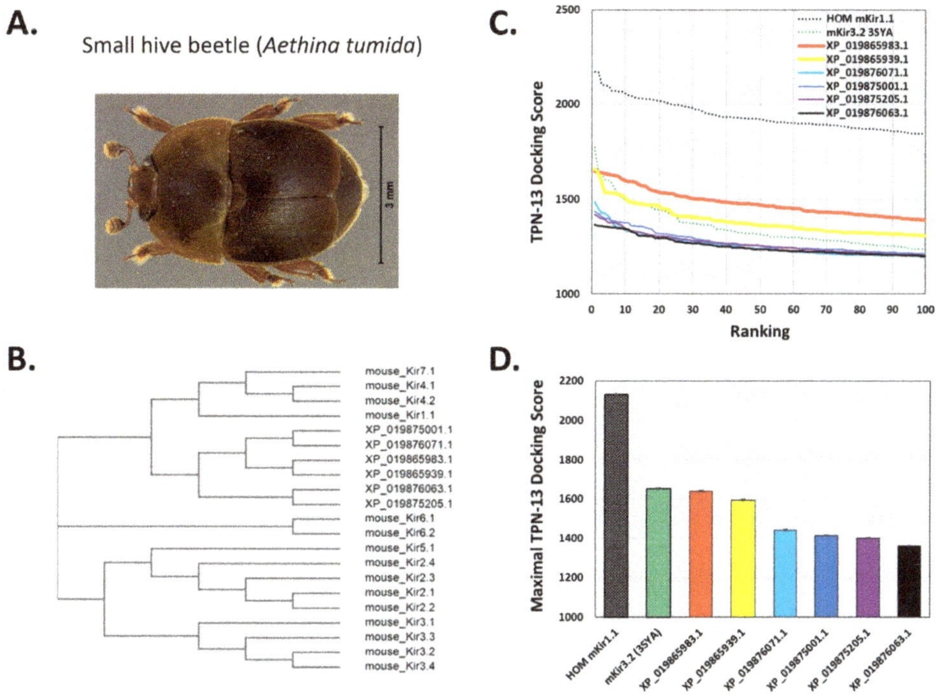

Figure 9. Docking TPN to homology-modelled *at*Kir channels. **A.** Photograph of the small hive beetle, *A. tumida*, courtesy of the University of Florida, Entomology and Nematology Department. **B.** Cladogram tree from a multiple sequence alignment depicting the pairwise similarity and associated clustering among mouse Kir channel subunit protein sequences and the six identified *at*Kir channel subunits. The neighbor-joining tree was created using the Clustal Omega program at the European Bioinformatics Institute (EMBL-EBI) without distance corrections. **C.** TPN docking scores for each homology-modelled *at*Kir channel. TPN docking scores to the TPN-sensitive mouse Kir1.1 (black dotted line) and Kir3.2 channels (green dotted line) were included for benchmark comparisons. The two *at*Kir channels having TPN docking scores similar to Kir3.2 are XP_019865983.1 (red line) and XP_019865939.1 (yellow line). Molecular docking was performed using ZDOCK and the TPN-13 conformer as described in Methods. **D.** Maximal TPN docking scores from the plots in panel C are shown for comparisons in descending order. The top 5 docking scores (mean ± SD) are plotted for each homology-modelled *at*Kir channel with comparisons to those for mKir1.1 and mKir3.2.

As shown in Figure 10, the predicted interface contacts between TPN and the *at*Kir channel (XP_019865983.1) outer vestibule were analogous to those between TPN-blocked mouse Kir1.1 and Kir3.2 channels, with electrostatic contacts occurring at two adjacent subunit aspartic acid residues (D113) located in the channel turret region, as well as the central "GYG" K^+ selectivity filter at the pore entry region. Moreover, the most favored docking pose of TPN to the *at*Kir channels was comparable to the rat Kir1.1 and mouse Kir3.2 channels (cf. Figure 3), where the side chain of TPN K21 occupied the pore selectivity filter (Figure 9). Sequence comparison of the outer vestibules of TPN-sensitive mouse Kir channels with the 2 *at*Kir channels (Figure 9A) highlight the common presence of critical acidic residues in the turret region that are necessary for high-affinity TPN binding [15,26]. These in silico findings therefore support the hypothesis that TPN targets insect Kir channels, where two *at*Kir channels were identified as putative natural targets that can next be functionally tested with expression in the *Xenopus* oocyte system.

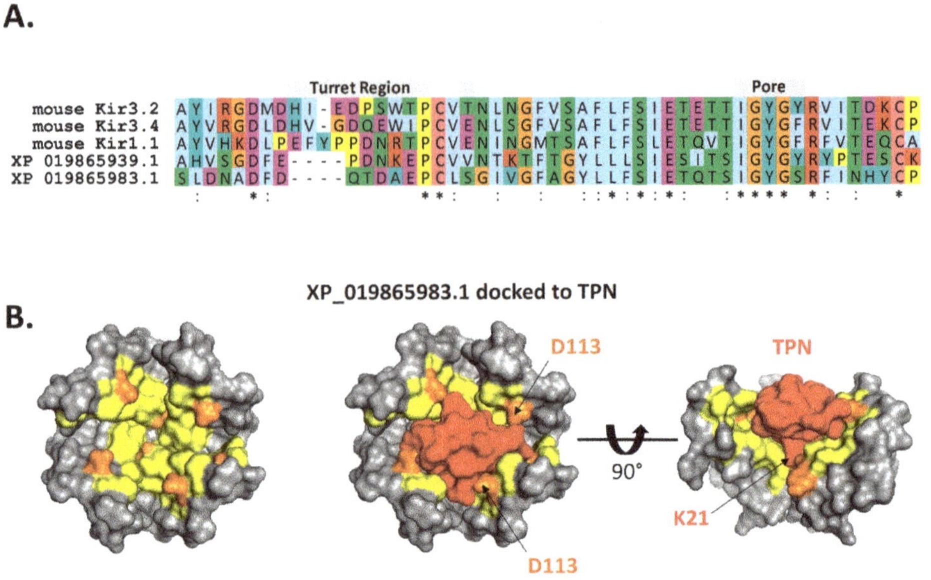

Figure 10. TPN docked to a homology-modelled *at*Kir channel. **A.** Sequence alignment of the outer vestibule region of TPN-sensitive mouse Kir channels and the two identified *at*Kir channels with high TPN docking scores (see Figure 8). The turret and pore regions are indicated and highlight the variable turret sequences containing acidic residues that are necessary for electrostatic contacts in TPN binding. **B.** Surface renderings of the outer vestibule of the homology-modelled *at*Kir channel XP_019865983.1. Left panel: top view where PISA-predicted TPN interface sites are indicated in yellow, and sites with predicted electrostatic contacts with the docked TPN peptide indicated in orange. Center panel: top view with the docked TPN peptide shown in red, and *at*Kir subunit turret residues (D113) indicated. Right panel: side view of the docked TPN with one *at*Kir channel subunit removed to expose the pore region where TPN K21 is predicted to make electrostatic contacts within the *at*Kir channel "GYG" K^+ selectivity filter.

3. Discussion

The results of this study highlighted both the utility and the limitations of structure-based virtual screening for venom peptides and their biological targets. The similar TPN docking and interface profiles of TPN-sensitive Kir3.2 and homology-modelled Kir1.1 channels provide further evidence for the reliability of molecular docking as a first-line screening tool for TPN-sensitive Kir channels. The unexpected docking results that predicted TPN block of mKir4.1 channels indicated the virtual screening methods are sufficiently sensitive to generate "false positive" interactions, and thus have the potential to identify novel venom targets in silico for subsequent validation testing in vitro. Moreover, these finding indicated mKir4.1 channels form a favorable outer vestibule receptor for TPN interactions (i.e., shape complementarity), but lack key interface contact sites necessary for high-affinity TPN binding and channel block. This observation may aid future peptide re-engineering efforts, taking into account the unique surface chemistry of the Kir4.1 outer vestibule as either a homo-tetramer or a hetero-tetramer assembled with other Kir channel subunits (e.g., Kir4.2 or Kir5.1).

The primary discovery deploying this computational approach is the novel finding that insect Kir channels, specifically certain Kir channels expressed in *A. tumida* that are distantly related to mammalian epithelial Kir channels, may be the natural targets of the TPN venom peptide that aid in honeybee defense by lethally blocking K^+ transport processes in insect predators. This hypothesis, assessed initially and supported using the virtual screening approach, can now focus on validation testing of the 2 specific *at*Kir channels that were identified as potentially TPN-sensitive using heterologous expression systems and functional assays. This role in bee defense would seemingly be more favorable to drive adaptive evolution of the TPN gene in *A. mellifera*, given insect predator encounters are expected to significantly outnumber encounters with mammalian predators. Other insect predators and their Kir channels of interest, including wasps and hornets, could similarly be screened using the structure-based molecular docking approach described here. Six putative *at*Kir channels were identified in this study, of those by comparison, five Kir channel subunit genes have been reported for the *Aedes aegypti* genome and three in *Drosophila melanogaster* [33,34]. The *Aedes* Kir channels are important for regulating secretion of K^+ in Malpighian tubules and have emerged as new targets for insecticide development and mosquito control [35]. The role of *at*Kir channels in the physiology of the small hive beetle is not currently known, but may similarly regulate transepithelial secretion of K^+ from hemolymph to urine for fluid homeostasis.

There are inherent assumptions with the in silico structural modelling of *at*Kir channels that should be acknowledged, including less structural conservation in the transmembrane domains and large C-terminal domain and how this may affect the outer vestibule structure and TPN docking results. There also is the possible scenario that native *at*Kir channels are hetero-tetramers and would similarly impact the TPN binding landscape. The TPN conformer used for rigid-body docking was also selected based on optimal conformer docking to the mammalian Kir channels (i.e., TPN-13). It remains possible that other TPN conformations preferentially dock to insect Kir channels, where incorporating NMR ensemble docking protocols and scoring would help obviate this current bias [36]. However, despite the absence of a high-resolution TPN–Kir channel complex, the virtual screening and docking results for TPN-sensitive Kir channels consistently point to a conserved mechanism for channel block, where key electrostatic contacts with multiple channel turrets and the vestibule ring region positions the C-terminal lysine side chain of TPN to occupy the channel pore and block conduction with high-affinity binding. The novel in silico results described here establish a solid rationale for follow-up of in vitro validation assays that otherwise would not have been considered or tested. This new research direction will further address the reliability of the structural models, where future refinements to the virtual screening protocol can be introduced along with any emergent or new structural details of a high-resolution TPN–Kir channel complex.

Screening and testing venom peptide interactions in vitro with other insect ion channel targets encountered in nature is impractical and an unlikely undertaking. The computational screening approach described here for hypothesis testing of TPN interactions with the *at*Kir channels highlights a more practical approach to identifying potential targets in silico that can then be tested in vitro. Applying this approach to a wider range of homology-modelled K^+ channels, both homo- and hetero-tetrameric assemblies, is very feasible and could accelerate the discovery process of venom peptide targets encountered in nature.

4. Materials and Methods

4.1. Ion Channel Structures and Homology Modelling

Three high-resolution crystal structures of Kir channels were used for computationally screening venom peptide interactions: the *Gallus gallus* Kir2.2 channel (3JYC.pdb), and the *Mus musculus* Kir3.2 channel in both closed-state and pre-opened conformations (3SYA.pdb and 4KFM.pdb, respectively). For homology-modelled Kir channels, the Kir2.2 channel served as the structural template where domain modelling was restricted to the outer vestibule region (~50 amino acids) to produce a chimeric Kir channel structure using the Swiss-Model homology-modelling server as described previously [7]. The homology-modelled Kir channel subunit was then assembled as a tetramer based on the macromolecular I4 space group determined for the assembled cKir2.2 tetramer using the PDBe PISA program (Protein Interfaces, Surfaces, and Assemblies: http://pdbe.org/pisa/). All structural renderings were performed using PyMol (v1.6, Schrödinger, New York, NY, USA).

4.2. *Computational Docking of TPN to Kir Channel Structures*

All NMR solution structures of TPN (1TER.pdb) [17] were initially used for in silico docking to the Kir3.2 channel outer vestibule structures using ZDOCK 3.0.2 [25]. ZDOCK performs rigid-body searches of docking orientations between the TPN conformer and the Kir channel outer vestibule, generating 2000 complexes for each Kir channel ranked by an initial-stage scoring function that computes optimized pairwise shape complementarity, electrostatic energies, and a pairwise statistical energy potential for interface atomic contacts energies [37]. The calculated and ranked TPN docking scores were then quantitatively compared among each Kir channel tested as previously reported [7].

4.3. *Kir Channel–TPN Interface Analysis*

To evaluate the predicted molecular contacts between the docked TPN peptide and Kir channels, the Cluspro2.0 program was used for refined docking and RMSD greedy clustering to identify the energetically-favored complex for subsequent interface analysis [38]. The predicted interface contacts were then determined using the PDBePISA program [28,39]. PISA identifies interface contacts based on physical–chemical models of macromolecular interactions and chemical thermodynamics identified within the docked structural complexes.

4.4. *Kir Channel Expression in Xenopus Oocytes*

To test TPN_Q sensitivity of the Kir4.1 channel in vitro, *Xenopus* oocytes were injected with cRNA transcribed in vitro by T7 RNA polymerase (mMessage mMachine, Ambion, Austin, TX, USA) from a linearized pCMV6 vector with the mouse Kir4.1 cDNA containing a Myc-DDK tag at the C-terminus (NM_001039484, Origene Technologies, Inc., Rockville, MD, USA). For a positive assay control, some oocytes were injected with cRNA encoding the rat Kir1.1 channel of which >95% was blocked by 100 nM TPN_Q. Oocytes were maintained for 3–5 days at 17–19 °C prior to electrophysiological recording in the following solution (in mM): 82.5 NaCl, 2.5 KCl, 1.0 $CaCl_2$, 1.0 $MgCl_2$, 1.0 $NaHPO_4$, 5.0 HEPES, 2.5 Na pyruvate, at pH 7.5 (NaOH), with 5% heat-inactivated horse serum. Single-stage V–VI oocytes were isolated as described previously by collagenase digestion of ovarian lobes (Xenopus 1, Dexter, MI, USA) [40].

4.5. *Two-Electrode Voltage Clamp Recording from Xenopus Oocytes*

Macroscopic mKir4.1 and rKir1.1 channel currents were recorded by two-electrode voltage clamp recording techniques where oocytes were initially superfused with the following bath solution (in mM): 98 NaCl, 1 $MgCl_2$, and 5 HEPES at pH 7.5 (NaOH). Glass electrodes having tip resistances of 0.8–1.0 MΩ were used to clamp oocytes at a holding membrane potential of −80 mV. After establishing a baseline holding current, the bath solution was changed to a "high K^+ solution" that was comprised of an equal molar substitution of NaCl for KCl. For mKir4.1 recordings, the extracellular K^+ concentration was 98 mM, and for rKir1.1 recordings, the concentration was 20 mM K^+. These concentrations were determined empirically to control for peak K^+ current amplitudes, and were attributed to differences in Kir4.1 vs Kir1.1 channel expression, single-channel conductance, and single-channel open time probability. From the −80 mV holding potential, large inward K^+ currents were evoked and were due to the expressed Kir channels, as un-injected oocytes yielded inward currents of <100 nA (data not shown).

Rapid application and washout of 100 nM TPN_Q or 1 mM $BaCl_2$ (dissolved in high K^+ solutions) was performed as described previously [40]. TPN_Q (lyophilized solid, Tocris Bioscience, Bristol, UK) was initially dissolved in water as a 100 μM stock solution, then aliquoted and stored at −23 °C until used on the day of the experiment by diluting in the high K^+ electrophysiological recording solution. Voltage ramps from −80 to +20 mV (200 ms in duration) were evoked periodically to assess the inward rectification characteristics of Kir channel currents during changes in the recording solutions. All recordings were performed at room temperature (21–23 °C). The membrane currents were digitized, stored, and later analyzed using an Analog-to-Digital acquisition board and PC computer (pCLAMP software, Digidata 1200 acquisition system, Axon Instruments, Foster City, CA, USA). Experiments were replicated in 7 oocytes.

Funding: This research received no external funding. The Article Processing Charges were funded by the University of South Florida Morsani College of Medicine.

Conflicts of Interest: The author declares no conflicts of interest.

References

1. Daly, N.L.; Wilson, D. Structural diversity of arthropod venom toxins. *Toxicon Off. J. Int. Soc. Toxinol.* **2018**, *152*, 46–56. [CrossRef] [PubMed]
2. de Graaf, D.C.; Aerts, M.; Danneels, E.; Devreese, B. Bee, wasp and ant venomics pave the way for a component-resolved diagnosis of sting allergy. *J. Proteom.* **2009**, *72*, 145–154. [CrossRef] [PubMed]
3. Casewell, N.R.; Wuster, W.; Vonk, F.J.; Harrison, R.A.; Fry, B.G. Complex cocktails: The evolutionary novelty of venoms. *Trends Ecol. Evol.* **2013**, *28*, 219–229. [CrossRef] [PubMed]
4. Fry, B.G.; Roelants, K.; Champagne, D.E.; Scheib, H.; Tyndall, J.D.; King, G.F.; Nevalainen, T.J.; Norman, J.A.; Lewis, R.J.; Norton, R.S.; et al. The toxicogenomic multiverse: Convergent recruitment of proteins into animal venoms. *Annu. Rev. Genom. Hum. Genet.* **2009**, *10*, 483–511. [CrossRef] [PubMed]
5. Kalia, J.; Milescu, M.; Salvatierra, J.; Wagner, J.; Klint, J.K.; King, G.F.; Olivera, B.M.; Bosmans, F. From foe to friend: Using animal toxins to investigate ion channel function. *J. Mol. Biol.* **2015**, *427*, 158–175. [CrossRef] [PubMed]
6. Gordon, D.; Chen, R.; Chung, S.H. Computational methods of studying the binding of toxins from venomous animals to biological ion channels: Theory and applications. *Physiol. Rev.* **2013**, *93*, 767–802. [CrossRef] [PubMed]
7. Doupnik, C.A.; Parra, K.C.; Guida, W.C. A computational design approach for virtual screening of peptide interactions across K(+) channel families. *Comput. Struct. Biotechnol. J.* **2015**, *13*, 85–94. [CrossRef] [PubMed]
8. Rashid, M.H.; Huq, R.; Tanner, M.R.; Chhabra, S.; Khoo, K.K.; Estrada, R.; Dhawan, V.; Chauhan, S.; Pennington, M.W.; Beeton, C.; et al. A potent and Kv1.3-selective analogue of the scorpion toxin HsTX1 as a potential therapeutic for autoimmune diseases. *Sci. Rep.* **2014**, *4*, 4509. [CrossRef] [PubMed]
9. Pennington, M.W.; Harunur Rashid, M.; Tajhya, R.B.; Beeton, C.; Kuyucak, S.; Norton, R.S. A C-terminally amidated analogue of ShK is a potent and selective blocker of the voltage-gated potassium channel Kv1.3. *FEBS Lett.* **2012**, *586*, 3996–4001. [CrossRef]
10. Lewis, R.J.; Garcia, M.L. Therapeutic potential of venom peptides. *Nat. Rev. Drug Discov.* **2003**, *2*, 790–802. [CrossRef]
11. Elsik, C.G.; Worley, K.C.; Bennett, A.K.; Beye, M.; Camara, F.; Childers, C.P.; de Graaf, D.C.; Debyser, G.; Deng, J.; Devreese, B.; et al. Finding the missing honey bee genes: Lessons learned from a genome upgrade. *BMC Genom.* **2014**, *15*, 86. [CrossRef] [PubMed]
12. Gauldie, J.; Hanson, J.M.; Rumjanek, F.D.; Shipolini, R.A.; Vernon, C.A. The peptide components of bee venom. *Eur. J. Biochem.* **1976**, *61*, 369–376. [CrossRef] [PubMed]
13. Doupnik, C.A. Venom-derived peptides inhibiting Kir channels: Past, present, and future. *Neuropharmacology* **2017**, *127*, 161–172. [CrossRef] [PubMed]
14. Jin, W.; Lu, Z. A novel high-affinity inhibitor for inward-rectifier K+ channels. *Biochemistry* **1998**, *37*, 13291–13299. [CrossRef] [PubMed]
15. Felix, J.P.; Liu, J.; Schmalhofer, W.A.; Bailey, T.; Bednarek, M.A.; Kinkel, S.; Weinglass, A.B.; Kohler, M.; Kaczorowski, G.J.; Priest, B.T.; et al. Characterization of Kir1.1 channels with the use of a radiolabeled derivative of tertiapin. *Biochemistry* **2006**, *45*, 10129–10139. [CrossRef] [PubMed]
16. Jin, W.; Klem, A.M.; Lewis, J.H.; Lu, Z. Mechanisms of inward-rectifier K+ channel inhibition by tertiapin-Q. *Biochemistry* **1999**, *38*, 14294–14301. [CrossRef] [PubMed]
17. Xu, X.; Nelson, J.W. Solution structure of tertiapin determined using nuclear magnetic resonance and distance geometry. *Proteins* **1993**, *17*, 124–137. [CrossRef] [PubMed]

18. Hu, J.; Qiu, S.; Yang, F.; Cao, Z.; Li, W.; Wu, Y. Unique mechanism of the interaction between honey bee toxin TPNQ and rKir1.1 potassium channel explored by computational simulations: Insights into the relative insensitivity of channel towards animal toxins. *PLoS ONE* **2013**, *8*, e67213. [CrossRef] [PubMed]
19. Whorton, M.R.; MacKinnon, R. X-ray structure of the mammalian GIRK2-betagamma G-protein complex. *Nature* **2013**, *498*, 190–197. [CrossRef]
20. Whorton, M.R.; MacKinnon, R. Crystal structure of the mammalian GIRK2 K+ channel and gating regulation by G proteins, PIP2, and sodium. *Cell* **2011**, *147*, 199–208. [CrossRef]
21. Hibino, H.; Inanobe, A.; Furutani, K.; Murakami, S.; Findlay, I.; Kurachi, Y. Inwardly rectifying potassium channels: Their structure, function, and physiological roles. *Physiol. Rev.* **2010**, *90*, 291–366. [CrossRef] [PubMed]
22. Lesage, F.; Guillemare, E.; Fink, M.; Duprat, F.; Heurteaux, C.; Fosset, M.; Romey, G.; Barhanin, J.; Lazdunski, M. Molecular properties of neuronal G-protein-activated inwardly rectifying K+ channels. *J. Biol. Chem.* **1995**, *270*, 28660–28667. [CrossRef] [PubMed]
23. Duprat, F.; Lesage, F.; Guillemare, E.; Fink, M.; Hugnot, J.P.; Bigay, J.; Lazdunski, M.; Romey, G.; Barhanin, J. Heterologous multimeric assembly is essential for K+ channel activity of neuronal and cardiac G-protein-activated inward rectifiers. *Biochem. Biophys. Res. Commun.* **1995**, *212*, 657–663. [CrossRef] [PubMed]
24. Kofuji, P.; Davidson, N.; Lester, H.A. Evidence that neuronal G-protein-gated inwardly rectifying K+ channels are activated by G beta gamma subunits and function as heteromultimers. *Proc. Natl. Acad. Sci. USA* **1995**, *92*, 6542–6546. [CrossRef] [PubMed]
25. Pierce, B.G.; Wiehe, K.; Hwang, H.; Kim, B.H.; Vreven, T.; Weng, Z. ZDOCK server: Interactive docking prediction of protein-protein complexes and symmetric multimers. *Bioinformatics* **2014**, *30*, 1771–1773. [CrossRef] [PubMed]
26. Ramu, Y.; Klem, A.M.; Lu, Z. Short variable sequence acquired in evolution enables selective inhibition of various inward-rectifier K+ channels. *Biochemistry* **2004**, *43*, 10701–10709. [CrossRef] [PubMed]
27. Ramu, Y.; Xu, Y.; Lu, Z. Engineered specific and high-affinity inhibitor for a subtype of inward-rectifier K+ channels. *Proc. Natl. Acad. Sci. USA* **2008**, *105*, 10774–10778. [CrossRef]
28. Krissinel, E.; Henrick, K. Inference of macromolecular assemblies from crystalline state. *J. Mol. Biol.* **2007**, *372*, 774–797. [CrossRef]
29. Santos, L.D.; Pieroni, M.; Menegasso, A.R.S.; Pinto, J.R.A.S.; Palma, M.S. A new scenario of bioprospecting of Hymenoptera venoms through proteomic approach. *J. Venom. Anim. Toxins* **2011**, *17*, 364–377.
30. Evans, J.D.; McKenna, D.; Scully, E.; Cook, S.C.; Dainat, B.; Egekwu, N.; Grubbs, N.; Lopez, D.; Lorenzen, M.D.; Reyna, S.M.; et al. Genome of the small hive beetle (Aethina tumida, Coleoptera: Nitidulidae), a worldwide parasite of social bee colonies, provides insights into detoxification and herbivory. *GigaScience* **2018**, *7*, giy138. [CrossRef]
31. Tarver, M.R.; Huang, Q.; de Guzman, L.; Rinderer, T.; Holloway, B.; Reese, J.; Weaver, D.; Evans, J.D. Transcriptomic and functional resources for the small hive beetle Aethina tumida, a worldwide parasite of honey bees. *Genom. Data* **2016**, *9*, 97–99. [CrossRef] [PubMed]
32. Neumann, P.; Pettis, J.S.; Schazfer, M.O. Quo vadis Aethina tumida? Biology and control of small hive beetles. *Apidologie* **2016**, *47*, 427–466. [CrossRef]
33. Nene, V.; Wortman, J.R.; Lawson, D.; Haas, B.; Kodira, C.; Tu, Z.J.; Loftus, B.; Xi, Z.; Megy, K.; Grabherr, M.; et al. Genome sequence of Aedes aegypti, a major arbovirus vector. *Science* **2007**, *316*, 1718–1723. [CrossRef] [PubMed]
34. Luan, Z.; Li, H.S. Inwardly rectifying potassium channels in Drosophila. *Sheng Li Xue Bao [Acta Physiol. Sin.]* **2012**, *64*, 515–519. [PubMed]
35. Beyenbach, K.W.; Yu, Y.; Piermarini, P.M.; Denton, J. Targeting renal epithelial channels for the control of insect vectors. *Tissue Barriers* **2015**, *3*, e1081861. [CrossRef] [PubMed]
36. Geng, C.; Narasimhan, S.; Rodrigues, J.P.; Bonvin, A.M. Information-Driven, Ensemble Flexible Peptide Docking Using HADDOCK. *Methods Mol. Biol.* **2017**, *1561*, 109–138. [CrossRef]
37. Mintseris, J.; Pierce, B.; Wiehe, K.; Anderson, R.; Chen, R.; Weng, Z. Integrating statistical pair potentials into protein complex prediction. *Proteins* **2007**, *69*, 511–520. [CrossRef]
38. Comeau, S.R.; Gatchell, D.W.; Vajda, S.; Camacho, C.J. ClusPro: A fully automated algorithm for protein-protein docking. *Nucleic Acids Res.* **2004**, *32*, W96–W99. [CrossRef]

39. Krissinel, E. Crystal contacts as nature's docking solutions. *J. Comput. Chem.* **2010**, *31*, 133–143. [CrossRef]
40. Doupnik, C.A.; Jaen, C.; Zhang, Q. Measuring the modulatory effects of RGS proteins on GIRK channels. *Methods Enzymol.* **2004**, *389*, 131–154. [CrossRef]

toxins

MDPI

Review

Spider Knottin Pharmacology at Voltage-Gated Sodium Channels and Their Potential to Modulate Pain Pathways

Yashad Dongol, Fernanda C. Cardoso and Richard J. Lewis *

Division of Chemistry and Structural Biology/Centre for Pain Research, Institute for Molecular Bioscience, The University of Queensland, Brisbane 4072, Australia; y.dongol@imb.uq.edu.au (Y.D.); f.caldascardoso@imb.uq.edu.au (F.C.C.)

* Correspondence: r.lewis@imb.uq.edu.au; Tel.: +61-7-3346-2984

Received: 24 September 2019; Accepted: 24 October 2019; Published: 29 October 2019

check for updates

Abstract: Voltage-gated sodium channels (Na_Vs) are a key determinant of neuronal signalling. Neurotoxins from diverse taxa that selectively activate or inhibit Na_V channels have helped unravel the role of Na_V channels in diseases, including chronic pain. Spider venoms contain the most diverse array of inhibitor cystine knot (ICK) toxins (knottins). This review provides an overview on how spider knottins modulate Na_V channels and describes the structural features and molecular determinants that influence their affinity and subtype selectivity. Genetic and functional evidence support a major involvement of Na_V subtypes in various chronic pain conditions. The exquisite inhibitory properties of spider knottins over key Na_V subtypes make them the best venom peptide leads for the development of novel analgesics to treat chronic pain.

Keywords: chronic pain; ICK peptide; knottins; Na_V; spider venom; voltage-gated sodium channel

Key Contribution: Spider venoms are a rich source of Na_V-modulating knottins. This review discusses how spider knottins modulate Na_V channels, the structural determinants that defines their affinity, potency and subtype selectivity and their potential to target Na_V subtypes involved in chronic pain conditions.

1. Introduction

Spiders are considered the most speciose and successful terrestrial venomous predators [1]. They comprise 119 families, 4141 genera and 48,255 species at the time of writing [2], with over 150,000 species estimated to exist [3,4]. They form the seventh most diverse order Araneae and completely rely on predation [3,5]. Their venoms comprise highly evolved venom peptides that facilitate both predatory behaviour by killing or paralysing the prey and defence against predation [6]. Medically significant cases of spider envenomation are less common and usually associated with intrusion in the spider's natural habitat or threatening encounters [7]. Spider venoms are highly specialized in targeting the molecular receptors, especially the neuronal system, of insects to immobilize or kill their preys. However, their venoms also impart noxious effects to higher organisms such as mammals. The conserved structure and function of targeted receptors from evolutionarily distant prey species, such as insects and threatening species, including mammals, likely explains the ability of spider venom peptides to potently modulate human receptors [8,9].

Recent advances in analytical technologies have made comprehensive biochemical and functional investigations of spider venoms feasible [10]. In addition, high-throughput technologies, such as fluorescence imaging and automated electrophysiology, have sped up the screening and discovery of novel bioactive venom peptides. Chemically, spider venoms comprise a highly complex cocktail of enzymatic and non-enzymatic protein and peptide toxins and low molecular weight organic compounds, such as nucleotides, free amino acids, biogenic amines, neurotransmitters, acylpolyamines, inorganic ions and salts [11–13]. Spider venom peptides modulate an array of ion channels and receptor proteins, including transient receptor potential (TRP) channels, acid sensing ion channels (ASICs), mechanosensitive ion channels (MSICs), ionotropic glutamate receptors (GluRs), G-protein coupled receptors (GPCRs), voltage-gated sodium (Na_V) channels, voltage-gated potassium (K_V) channels, voltage-gated calcium (Ca_V) channels and calcium-activated potassium channels (KCa) [4,14]. Interestingly, approximately one-third of the then described spider venom ion channel modulators targeted Na_V channels [15].

Venom peptides from spiders have been important tools in defining the function and pharmacology of Na_V channels and in elucidating binding sites in these channels [16–18]. For example, the hNa_V activator spider knottin Hm1a from *Heteroscodra maculata* recently elucidated the role of $Na_V1.1$ in mechanical hypersensitivity and chronic visceral pain [19,20], while other Na_V inhibitor spider knottins continue to be developed as novel analgesics [21]. Thus, spider venoms provide a rich source of bioactive peptides to probe the function and pharmacology of Na_V channels as well as being leads to new therapeutics. In this review, we provide an overview of spider knottin pharmacology at Na_V channels, describe the structural determinants driving their potency and selectivity and discuss the potential of spider knottins to target Na_V subtypes involved in chronic pain conditions.

2. Voltage-Gated Sodium Channel Function and Structure

Voltage-gated sodium channels ($Na_V1.1$–1.9) are transmembrane channel proteins selective to Na^+ ions. They open upon depolarization of the membrane to allow the influx of Na^+ ions and inactivate rapidly through a process named fast inactivation before returning to the closed state upon membrane hyperpolarization. Such rapid influx of Na^+ ions is key to generation and propagation of action potential and underlies transmission of a wide array of somatosensory signals, including touch, smell, temperature, proprioception and pain [21]. A range of molecules discovered from natural sources (e.g., venomous animals) interact with Na_V channels to activate or inhibit the influx of Na^+ ions [16,22]. Na_V channels are also expressed in non-excitable cells where they contribute to non-canonical functions [23], such as catecholamine release [24], angiogenesis [25], phagocytosis, endosomal acidification and podosome formation [26,27], production of pro-inflammatory mediators [28] and are key regulators in various human pathologies, such as cancer progression [29], multiple sclerosis [30], epilepsy [31] and pain syndromes [32,33]. In addition, mutations of Na_V channel-encoding genes contribute to diseases such as epilepsy, pain-related syndromes (e.g., inherited primary erythromelalgia (IEM), congenital insensitivity to pain (CIP) and paroxysmal extreme pain disorder (PEPD)) and cardiac arrhythmias, such as Brugada syndrome, atrial fibrillation and slow ventricular conduction [34–38].

Structurally, eukaryotic Na_V channels are complex transmembrane glycosylated proteins composed of a large pore-forming core protein (α-subunit, approximately 260 kDa) associated with one or more regulatory proteins (β-subunits, approximately 35 kDa) [39]. The α-subunit is primarily involved in Na^+ conductance, whereas β-subunits modulate the Na^+ current kinetics and α-subunit expression [40]. Four regulatory β-subunits (β1–β4) have been identified so far with a soluble splice variant β1B [41]. The β1 and β3 subunits make non-covalent interactions, while the β2 and β4 subunits make covalent interactions with the α-subunit to form a heteromeric protein [42].

The α-subunit comprises 24 transmembrane segments organized into four homologous, non-identical domains DI–DIV, each containing six transmembrane segments S1–S6 (Figure 1A,B) [43–45]. The S1–S4 segments of each domain contribute to the voltage sensing domain (VSD), and the S5 and S6 segments along with the extracellular connecting loop (P-loop) form the pore domain (PD) and selectivity filter. Conserved positively charged residues (arginine) at every third position in the S4 segment sense voltage changes across the membrane and regulate the gating kinetics of the Na_V channel [46] through a "sliding helix" or "helical screw" mechanism [47–49]. At resting membrane potentials, the S4 segments (voltage sensors) are drawn into the membrane where their positively charged residues form ion pairs with negatively charged adjacent residues from S1, S2 and/or S3 segments [50]. However, when the negative membrane potential becomes more positive during membrane depolarization, the S4 segments of DI–DIII move outward, resulting in a conformational change that opens the channel pore followed by the outward movement of DIV S4 that inactivates (blocks) the channel pore intracellularly [50,51]. Channel inactivation is the third cardinal feature of Na_V channels in addition to voltage sensing across the membrane and the selective Na^+ filter [52]. Structurally, the cytoplasmic DIII–DIV linker forms a hinge that facilitates the inactivation and is key to the fast inactivation mechanism. A cluster of hydrophobic amino acids (i.e., Ile, Phe, and Met (IFM motif)) function as a hydrophobic latch to stabilize the inactivated state, and mutations in these residues individually and together alter the kinetics of fast inactivation [53]. Besides this motif, residues in the S4–S5 linkers of DIII (e.g., A1329) and DIV (e.g., N1662) are crucial for the fast inactivation as they form the docking site for IFM motif [54].

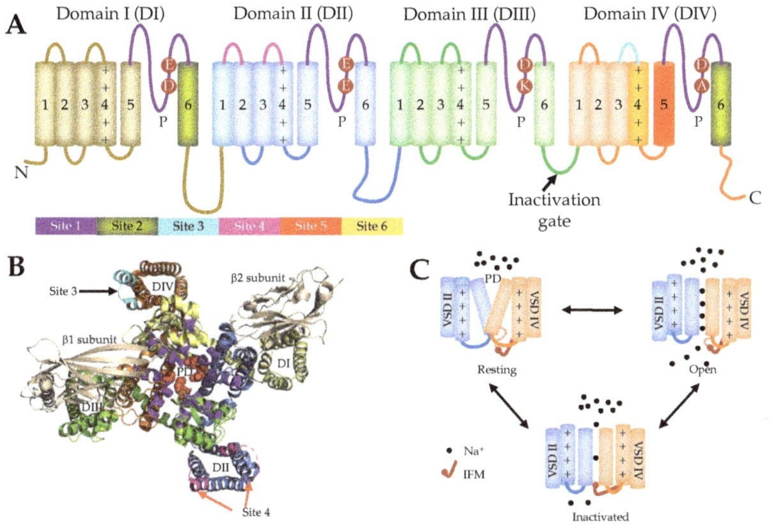

Figure 1. (**A**) Schematic representation of the α-subunit of voltage-gated sodium (Na_V) channel. Four non-identical domains (DI–DIV) feature six neurotoxin receptor sites (Sites 1–6) and key residues contributing to the outer Na^+ ion selectivity filter (EEDD) and inner selectivity filter (DEKA). The connecting S5–S6 linker is called P-loop (P) which together with S5 and S6 segments from each domain contributes in forming a Na^+ ion selective channel pore. (**B**) Three-dimensional NMR structure of the Na_V1.7 channel (PDB 6J8G) [55]. Four voltage sensing domains (VSDs), DI (yellow), DII (blue), DIII (green), and DIV (orange), are shown with their corresponding pore-forming segments (S5 and S6) arranged to form the pore domain (PD) selective to Na^+ ions. The P-loop that contributes to forming the inner selectivity filter is coloured in red spheres (DEKA) and outer selectivity filter (EEDD) is coloured in purple. The S6 segments of all the four domains contribute to form the intracellular region of the pore. Site 3 (cyan) and Site 4 (pink) are the major binding sites for spider knottins. The β1 and β2 subunits which interact with DIII and DI, respectively, are highlighted in beige colour. (**C**) Schematic of the gating cycle of Na_V channels. At polarized potentials, the DI–DIV S4 segments are drawn towards the intracellular side due to the positive gating charges to render the closed conformation (down state). Upon depolarization, the forces holding the down state are relieved and DI–DIII S4 segments are rapidly released extracellularly to open the S6 channel gate in the open conformation (up state). The DIV S4 moves up slowly compared to DI–DIII S4 and drives the fast inactivation, where the channel is occluded intracellularly by the Ile, Phe, and Met (IFM) motif. After cell repolarization, the channel returns to a closed (resting) state [56–58].

Although the Na_V channel gating has multiple kinetic states [59,60], it can be simplified into three distinct physiological states, the resting (closed), open, and inactivated, which develop from the voltage-sensitive conformational changes that occur within the α-subunit (Figure 1C) [57,61]. Toxins and drugs that interact with Na_V channels often bind preferentially to one of these conformational states to alter Na^+ conductance or the gating properties of the channel. Six neurotoxin receptor sites (Sites 1–6) have been identified on the Na_V channel. Site 1 neurotoxin physically occludes the channel pore, whereas neurotoxins acting at Sites 2–6 affect the gating mechanisms of the channel. Venom peptides target four neurotoxin receptor sites in human Na_V channels, namely, Site 1 (e.g., μ-conotoxins), Site 3 (e.g., scorpion α-toxins, sea anemone toxins and spider toxins), Site 4 (e.g., scorpion β-toxins, spider toxins) and Site 6 (e.g., δ-conotoxins) [16,62]. Given their physico-chemical properties, it is not surprising that Na_V modulatory venom peptides preferentially target the extracellular side of VSDII (Site 4) and VSDIV (Site 3) [14,63].

3. Spider-Venom ICK Peptides

Inhibitor cystine knot (ICK) peptides have a disulphide-rich structural motif that forms a "knot" that confers high structural, thermal and proteolytic stability, making them attractive starting points for structure–function studies and clinical lead development [64]. This structural motif comprises at least three disulphide bonds with connections between C1–C4, C2–C5 and C3–C6, where two disulphide bonds form a ring threaded by the third (C3–C6) disulphide bond to form the knot. These scaffolds were first described as "knottins" in 1980s [65] and later identified as a "cystine knot" in the crystal structure of nerve growth factor [66,67]. Pallaghy et al. [68], in 1994, coined the term "inhibitor cystine knot" to identify the cystine knot motif with a triple-stranded anti-parallel β-sheet topology. Craik et al. [69] further categorized these disulphide-rich structural motifs as (i) growth factor cystine knots (GFCKs), (ii) inhibitor cystine knots (ICKs) and (iii) cyclic cystine knots (CCKs). ICKs and CCKs have the same disulphide connectivity, but the disulphide connectivity in GFCK differs where C1–C2 threads the ring formed by C2–C4 and C3–C6. ICKs and CCKs are referred to as knottins and cyclotides, respectively [70]. Animal toxin cystine knots have an ICK structural motif [69].

Spider venoms are a rich source of disulphide-rich peptides, including knottins [4]. With few exceptions, such as the atracotoxins, they display the ICK features comprising three disulphide bonds (Figure 2A). However, certain variations are observed within the β-sheet topology (Figure 2B,C). Unlike the triple-stranded anti-parallel β-sheet topology defined in knottins, spider venom knottins typically comprise two β-strands with a few exceptions displaying a third strand at the N-terminal [71]. Besides the disulphide bridge connectivity, another conserved structural feature of spider venom knottins is the hydrophobic patch surrounded by charged amino acids on the toxin's surface [72,73] that contributes to potency and selectivity [74–83]. The UniProt database lists 747 entries on search term "spider venom ICK toxin" (23 September 2019) that are further categorized into their ion channel targets (Figure 3) which shows approximately 43% of the thus far described ion channel-impairing spider knottins targeted Na_V channel [84].

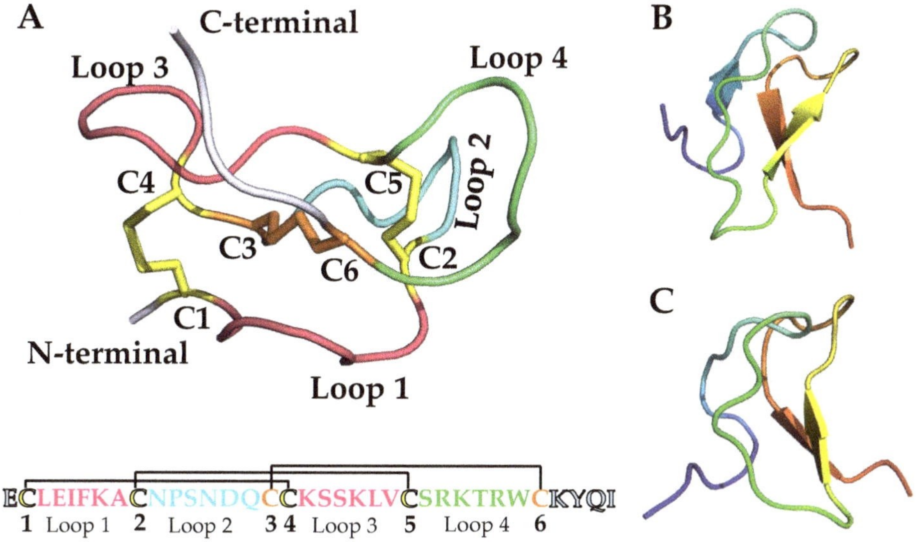

Figure 2. (**A**) **Top:** Spider venom knottin HwTx-IV (PDB: 2m50) [83] demonstrating the cystine knot motif with three disulphide bridges. A ring structure made up of two disulphide bridges, C1–C4 and C2–C5 (yellow), and the intervening peptide backbone (pink) penetrated by a third disulphide bridge, C3–C6 (orange), to form a pseudo-knot. The three-disulphide bonds form four loops (pink, green and cyan). **Below:** The primary structure of HwTx-IV with three disulphide bridges and four loops. (**B**,**C**) Spider venom knottins with varying β-sheet topology. The colour from the N-terminal to the C-terminal follows the rainbow spectrum from blue to red. (**B**) HnTx-IV (PDB: 1NIY) [85] comprises three β-sheets, whereas (**C**) CcoTx-I (PDB: 6BR0) [86] comprises two β-sheets.

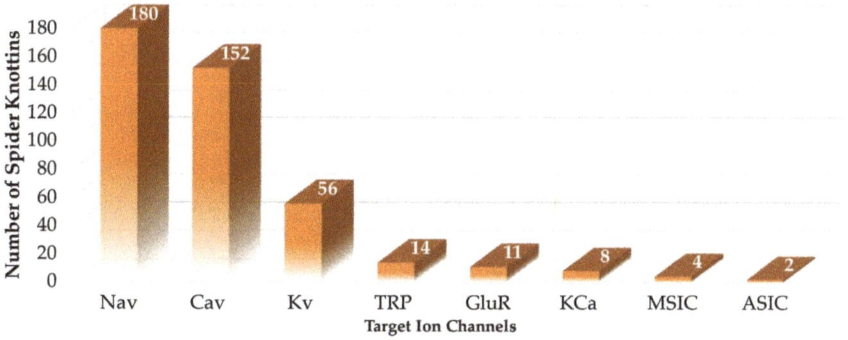

Figure 3. Number of spider venom knottins modulating ion channels. The data were collected from the UniProt database on 23 September 2019 using the following search descriptors: "voltage gated sodium channel impairing spider ICK toxin" for Na_V channel targeting spider knottins, "voltage gated calcium channel impairing spider ICK toxin" for voltage-gated calcium (Ca_V) channel targeting spider knottins, "voltage gated potassium channel impairing spider ICK toxin" for voltage-gated potassium (K_V) channel targeting spider knottins, "TRP impairing spider ICK toxin" for transient receptor potential (TRP) channel targeting spider knottins, "ionotropic glutamate receptor impairing spider ICK toxin" for ionotropic glutamate receptor (GluR) targeting spider knottins, "calcium-activated potassium channel impairing spider ICK toxin" for calcium-activated potassium (KCa) channel targeting spider knottins, "mechanosensitive ion channel impairing spider ICK toxin" for mechanosensitive ion channel (MSIC) targeting spider knottins and "ASIC impairing spider ICK toxin" for acid-sensing ion channel (ASIC) targeting spider knottins [84].

The first discovery of Na_V-modulating spider venom peptides was in the mid-1980s, when Fontana and Vital-Brazil [87] demonstrated that the crude venom of *Phoneutria nigriventer* is capable of activating Na_V channels in muscle and nerve cells. Later in 1991, Rezende et al. [88] isolated three neurotoxic fractions (PhTx1, PhTx2 and PhTx3) from *P. nigriventer* venom, and the most toxic fraction (PhTx2) was later shown by Araújo et al. [89] in 1992 to inhibit the Na_V channel inactivation. In 1989, Adams et al. [90] isolated μ-agatoxins (I–VI) from *Agelenopsis aperta* which became the first spider venom with disulphide-rich peptides (8 cysteines arranged into 4 disulphide bridges) targeting Na_V channels to induce repetitive firing in the neurons. Since then, a journey of three decades of research on spider venom peptides modulating Na_V channels resulted in the discovery of a number of venom peptides which have been applied into research on the mechanisms of Na_V channel modulation and potential therapeutics. Based upon the level of sequence identity and inter-cysteine spacing, these Na_V channel-targeting spider toxins were classified into 12 families (NaSpTx1–12) [15].

3.1. Pharmacology of NaSpTx

The spider knottins' interaction with Sites 3 and 4 displayed diverse pharmacological phenotypes (Tables 1 and 2). Broadly, they either (i) prevent channel opening in response to membrane depolarization by trapping the VSD II in the closed state; (ii) facilitate channel opening by trapping VSD II in open state or (iii) prevent channel inactivation by binding DIV S4 in the closed state to impair the movement of the inactivation gate [15,18,63]. Curiously, an integrated pharmacology of Site 3 and Site 4 indicates multiple binding site interactions by the same toxin [91,92]. For example, the toxic fraction PhTx2 from the venom of *P. nigriventer* not only prolonged the inactivation and deactivation (Site 3 phenotype) of the Na_V channel but also shifted the voltage dependence of activation (Site 4 phenotype) and steady-state inactivation towards negative potentials (Site 3 phenotype) [89]. Later, PnTx2–6 alone confirmed this complex pharmacology was achieved by a single toxin [93]. Further evidence of dual pharmacological profile includes versutoxin (VTX) from *Hadronyche versuta*, which besides the classical Site 3 features, such as delaying the channel inactivation and shifting the voltage dependence of inactivation towards more negative potential, also displayed the classical Site 4 feature of reducing the maximum (peak) sodium current [94].

Table 1. Pharmacological features of Site 3 interacting spider knottins resulting in delay of channel inactivation.

Features	Examples
Hyperpolarizing shift in voltage-dependence of activation	PhTx-2 [89], VTX [94], Hv1 [95], Ar1 [96], Hv1b [97], PnTx2-6 [93], JzTx-II [98]
Hyperpolarizing shift in steady-state inactivation	VTX [94,99], PhTx-2 [89], Ar1 [89], Hv1b [97], PnTx2-6 [93]
No significant effect in voltage-dependence of steady-state inactivation	JzTx-I [100,101], JzTx-II [98]
Reduced peak inward current amplitude	VTX [94], Ar1 [96], Hv1b [97], PnTx2-6 [93]
No change in peak inward current amplitude	JzTx-I [100]
Increased peak inward current amplitude	Hm1a [20]
Increased recovery rate from inactivation	VTX [94], Ar1 [96], JzTx-I [102], JzTx-II [98]
Decreased recovery rate from inactivation	PnTx2-6 [93]

Table 2. Pharmacological features of Site 4 interacting spider knottins resulting in reduction of peak inward current.

Features	Examples
Depolarizing shift in voltage-dependence of activation	ProTx-I [103], ProTx-II [77,103,104], JzTx-III [105,106], CcoTx-I [73], CcoTx-2 [73], CcoTx-3 [73], PaurTx-3 [73], JzTx-V [79,107], JzTx-IX [108], Hm-3 [109], Cd1a [110], Pre1a [111], Pn3a [61], Df1a [92], JxTx-XI [91], JzTx-35 [112]
No effect in voltage-dependence of activation	HwTx-IV [104,113–115], HnTx-III [116,117], JzTx-34 [118,119], Hm-1 [120], Hm-2 [120], Hd1a [121], GpTx-1 [122], Hl1a [123], PnTx1 [124], ProTx-III [80], Pre1a [111], JzTx-14 [125]
Hyperpolarizing shift in voltage-dependence of steady-state inactivation	HnTx-III [116], HnTx-IV [116], JzTx-V [79], Hm-1 [120], Hm-2 [120], JzTx-35 [112], PnTx4 (5-5) [126], Df1a [92], JzTx-34 [119]
Delay in channel inactivation	ProTx-II [104], JzTx-XI [91], Df1a [92], JzTx-14 [125]
Decreased channel recovery from inactivation	HnTx-III [116], JzTx-XI [91], Pn3a [61]
No effect in channel recovery from inactivation	HnTx-IV [116], JzTx-34 [118], HnTx-III [127], Hd1a [121]
Hyperpolarizing shift in voltage-dependence of activation	Df1a [92]
Depolarizing shift in voltage-dependence of steady-state inactivation	Df1a [92]

Detailed characterization of the dual effects of the spider knottin JzTx-XI from *Chilobrachys jingzhao* on $hNa_V1.5$ revealed a concentration dependence in the modulation of Na_V channels. At low concentrations (≤90 nM), JzTx-XI significantly reduced the peak currents (inhibition of channel activation; Site 4) but at higher concentrations (≥180 nM), besides reducing the peak currents, it also slowed the current decay (fast inactivation; Site 3) [91]. Further, these modulatory effects were demonstrated by Df1a from *Davus fasciatus* over hNa_V subtypes 1.1–1.7, where the toxin shifted the voltage-dependence of activation and steady-state fast inactivation of the hNa_V subtypes to more hyperpolarizing potentials, with exception of depolarizing shifts in activation of $hNa_V1.3$ and $hNa_V1.7$ and depolarizing shifts in the inactivation of $hNa_V1.3$ [92]. Furthermore, the toxin delayed the fast inactivation along with the reduction of peak currents in $hNa_V1.1$, $hNa_V1.3$ and $hNa_V1.5$ [92]. Such subtype-varying profiles have also recently been reported for Pn3a (*Pamphobeteus nigricolor*) [61], Pre1a (*Psalmopoeus reduncus*) [111] and JzTx-14 (*C. jingzhao*) [125]. These multi-site effects of spider knottins on Na_V channels need to be carefully considered when establishing their pharmacological profiles.

Another channel state modulated by spider knottins is channel inactivation [91,93,94,98,116]. For example, when tested over tetrodotoxin sensitive (TTX-S) Na_V channels on rat dorsal root ganglia (DRG) neurons, HnTx-III and HnTx-IV from *Selenocosmia hainana* differed in their channel repriming kinetics. More specifically, HnTx-III delayed channel recovery from inactivation, whereas HnTx-IV had no effects [116]. Similarly, steady-state inactivation can also be differently modulated by spider knottins. For example, JzTx-35 (*C. jingzhao*), which selectively targeted $hNa_V1.5$ similarly to JzTx-III (*C. jingzhao*), differed by shifting the steady-state inactivation of the channel towards more hyperpolarized potentials [112]. The hyperpolarizing shift in the voltage dependence of steady-state inactivation stabilizes the channel in the inactivated state [128]. However, potent inhibitor toxins like HwTx-IV (*Ornithoctonus huwena*), ProTx-III (*Thrixopelma pruriens*) and HnTx-IV showed no effect on steady-state inactivation [80,114,129]. Likewise, the excitatory JzTx-I (*C. jingzhao*) delayed the channel inactivation of other Site 3-acting spider knottins including δ-ACTXs, but the peak current amplitude, I–V relationship and steady-state inactivation remained unaltered [101]. Such characteristics among the spider knottins provide novel paths to modulate Na_V channels.

Spider knottins also inhibit Na_V channel activation. ProTx-I and ProTx-II from *T. pruriens* showed, for the first time, the depression of Na_V channel activation by shifting the voltage dependence of activation towards more depolarized potentials [103]. This is in contrast to typical scorpion β-toxins which, although reduced the peak current, shifted the voltage dependence of activation and inactivation to hyperpolarized potentials [130]. Its structural homology with hanatoxin isolated from *Grammostola spatulata* suggested interactions with the DII S3–S4 linker to inhibit the channel activation [103,131]. Later, residues critical for these interactions were identified in the domain II of the hNa_V channel [132]. Spider knottins include a growing number of depressant toxins, including JzTx-V (*C. jingzhao*), Df1a (*D. fasciatus*), Pre1a (*P. reduncus*), PnTx4(5-5) from *P. nigriventer*, CcoTx-1 (*Ceratogyrus cornuatus*), PaurTx (*Phrixotrichus auratus)* and Cd1a (*Ceratogyrus darlingi*) which induce a depolarizing shift in voltage-dependence of activation at specific Na_V subtypes [73,79,92,107,110,111]. However, a number of spider depressant knottins reduced the sodium currents without changing the activation or inactivation kinetics (e.g., HwTx-IV, HnTx-III, HnTx-IV) [114,116,129], by shifting activation and inactivation to hyperpolarizing potentials (e.g., Df1a) [92] or by inhibiting both activation and inactivation (e.g., JzTx-14) [125]. Spider knottins (e.g., JzTx-V) also altered the slope factor of activation and inactivation associated to shifts in their voltage dependence [79,91] suggesting cooperativity between the four S4 segments or multiple binding sites [9,91].

Spider knottins display distinct affinities and modes of action for insect and mammalian Na_V channels. Magi 5 from *Macrothele gigas* interacted with Site 3 on the insect Na_V channels and Site 4 on mammalian Na_V channels to induce Na^+ influx [133]. These observations support the concept of common binding "hot spots" proposed by Winterfield and Swartz (2000) [134], where binding sites in the voltage-gated ion channels are not independent structural sites. Recently, PnTx4(5-5) also showed a distinct affinity and mode of action on insect and mammalian Na_V channels [126]. On $BgNa_V$ from the cockroach *Blatella germanica*, PnTx4(5-5) strongly slowed channel inactivation (EC_{50} 213 nM) and increased current amplitude, while it inhibited sodium currents of the mammalian $Na_V1.2$–1.6 channels, with higher potency on $Na_V1.3$. This unique selectivity and species-dependent mode of action provides new insight into the molecular mechanisms of spider gating modifier toxins [126].

Cell background can also influence pharmacological profiles of spider knottins [116,117,129]. For example, hyperpolarizing shifts (10–11 mV) in voltage-dependence of steady-state inactivation imparted by HnTx-III and HnTx-IV in TTX-S Na^+ currents in rat DRG were not observed on heterologously expressed $hNa_V1.7$. Similarly, HnTX-III which delayed the recovery from inactivation of TTX-S Na^+ channels on rat DRG did not affect the repriming kinetics of heterologously expressed $hNa_V1.7$ [116,117]. Indeed, the difference in the relative proportion of Na_V subtypes in different DRG cell types (small and large diameter) [117], species and age [117,135], β-auxiliary subunit combinations [136] and difference in the membrane lipid composition [82] likely influence the biophysical and pharmacological properties of Na_V subtypes. The pharmacological and biophysical properties of Na_V channels are also influenced by the expression system and species differences. For example, Df1a was approximately 8.5 fold less potent at $hNa_V1.7$ expressed in *Xenopus* oocytes than at $hNa_V1.7$ expressed in HEK 293 cells [92]. Similarly, Pn3a was approximately 2 fold less potent at $rNa_V1.7$ and 5 fold less potent at $mNa_V1.7$ compared to $hNa_V1.7$ [61].

Interaction with membrane lipid is another important feature of spider knottins [14] that can influence affinity and potency [75,82,137]. The anionic charges in the polar head groups of the lipid surrounding Na_Vs probably increase the affinity of positively charged spider knottins, while hydrophobic residues in these toxins can make favourable electrostatic and hydrophobic interactions with the hydrophobic core of the lipid bilayer [138]. Although spider knottins like ProTx-I and ProTx-II exploit electrostatic interactions to increase their potency, HwTx-IV and Hd1a (*Haplopelma doriae*) rely less on membrane binding for potent inhibition [139,140]. Interestingly, a HwTx-IV analogue engineered to increase the affinity for lipid membrane showed improved inhibitory potency at $hNa_V1.7$ [137]. On the other hand, the most potent and selective analogues of GpTx-1 (*Grammostola porteri*) and ProTx-II had reduced affinity for lipid bilayer [75]. Thus, a direct correlation between the toxin–lipid interaction and the potency or the selectivity for Na_Vs could not be established [86] beyond facilitating the positioning of the toxin at the membrane surface proximal to exposed Na_V residues [75]. Indeed, the conserved amphipathicity of the spider knottins may be an evolutionary adaptation favouring toxin promiscuity [86].

3.2. Structure–Function of NaSpTx

Structure–function studies highlight the role of knottin residues in determining the toxin potency and selectivity [14]. For example, the distribution of Ser4 and Asp5 at N-terminus instead of cationic Lys4 and Arg5 of δ-ACTX-Hv1b (*H. versuta*) shifted selectivity for mammalian Na_V channels [97]. Similarly, CcoTx-2 (D32Y-CcoTx-1) potently inhibited $Na_V1.3$ (IC_{50} 88 nM), while CcoTx-1 was inactive at this subtype. Surprisingly, Asp32 or Tyr32 located on the side opposite the hydrophobic patch also influenced potency, suggesting that residues beyond the hydrophobic patch can also influence toxin–channel interactions [73]. In addition, the ICK fold retained by key mutants suggested that specific amino acid interactions between the toxin and channel are prime in Na_V channel modulation and subtype selectivity [83,85].

The NaSpTx family 1–3 incorporate most of the Na_V-modulating spider knottins with promising therapeutic lead potential, including ProTx-II [103,141], ProTx-I [132], ProTx-III [80], Df1a [92], Pn3a [61], HwTx-IV [83,137,142,143], GpTx-I [76] and CcoTx-I [144]. Sequence alignments of selected Na_V-modulating spider knottins targeting Sites 3 and 4 in Na_V channels are shown in Figure 4. Besides the shorter N-terminus and longer C-terminus in Site 3 and Site 4 targeting spider knottins, this alignment highlights conserved hydrophobic residues in loop 1 and positively charged residues in loop 4 of Site 4 targeting spider knottins. In contrast, negatively charged residues are distributed in loop 2 of NaSpTx1–3 spider knottins and in the N-terminal of NaSpTx families 1 and 2. The conserved Arg and Lys in loop 4 of NaSpTx1–3 appear to be crucial for inhibitory function of depressant spider toxins belonging to these families [145].

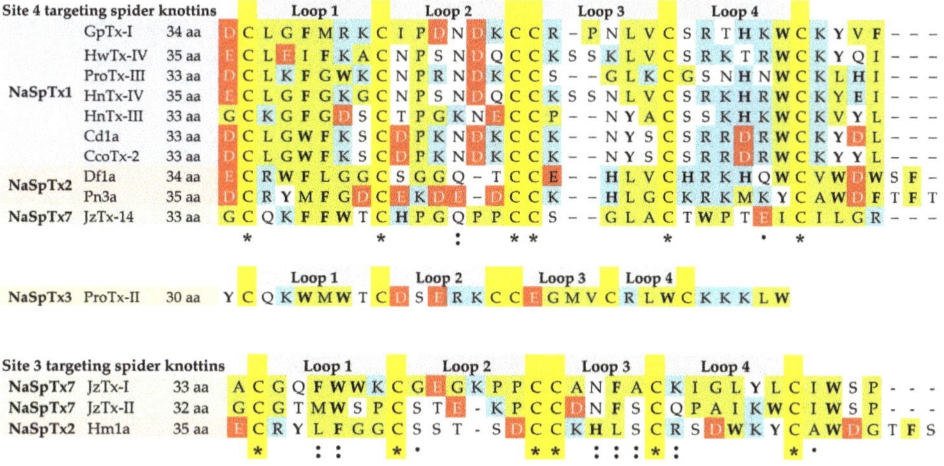

Figure 4. Multiple sequence alignment of spider knottins targeting Site 4 and Site 3 in Na_V channels. The NaSpTx family 1–3 generally target Site 4 to inhibit channel activity, except Hm1a which targets Site 3 to excite the channel [20]. JzTx-14 [125] from NaSpTx7 targets Site 4 and inhibits the channel, whereas JzTx-I [100] and JzTx-II [98] from NaSpTx7 targets Site 3 to excite the channel. Yellow highlights conserved cysteines, green highlights hydrophobic residues, cyan indicates positively charged residues, red indicates negatively charged residues and bold letter indicates the aromatic residues. The "*" indicates identical residues, ":" indicates strong conservation, "." indicates weak conservation.

The C-terminal WCK motif is also conserved across well-characterized sodium channel-blocking toxins from NaSpTx families 1 and 3, suggesting that these residues are key determinants of activity [83]. In the cryogenic electron microscopy (cryo-EM) structure of ProTx-II–hNav1.7 VSDII-Na_VAb complex, the corresponding Trp24 served as a hydrophobic anchor to stabilize ProTx-II interactions with $hNa_V1.7$ [58]. More specifically, the hydrophobic patch Trp5, Trp7, Trp24 and Trp30 stabilized binding by allowing deeper penetration into the membrane lipid [58]. In addition, the ProTx-II–hNa$_V$1.7 cryo-EM structure confirmed a key role of the C-terminal basic residues capped by hydrophobic residues in anchoring the toxin into the membrane [58]. In contrast, JzTx-14 belonging to NaSpTx7 has a loop 4 that lacks positively charged residues and Arg serving as a C-terminal cap, but still inhibits eight out of nine Na$_V$ channel subtypes at nanomolar concentrations [125]. It has additional hydrophobic residues in each of the four loops with only one acidic residue that suggest an alternative binding mode. Indeed, structure–function studies have shown that hydrophobic and aromatic residues in loop 1, loop 4 and C-terminus and positively charged residues distributed in loop 4 and C-terminus were critical for toxins' affinity [83,85,117]. Interestingly, the highly Na$_V$1.7-selective Pn3a, like other NaSpTx2 spider knottins, lacks positively charged residues in the C-terminus and instead contains hydrophobic and negatively charged Asp residues.

The overall net charge of the peptide also affects the toxin activity. For example, decreased net anionic charge in E1G, E4G, Y33W-HwTx-IV enhanced inhibition by 45 fold (IC_{50} 0.4 nM) compared to native HwTx-IV (IC_{50} 17 nM) [142], which was mostly driven by enhanced hydrophobic interactions associated to the Y33W mutation (IC_{50} 1.4 nM). Amidation of the C-terminus also has a direct influence on the potency of HwTx-IV [142]. While characterizing ProTx-III and Df1a interactions with Na$_V$ channels, Cardoso et al. [80,92] elucidated the significance of C-terminal amidation in enhancing potency and altering subtype selectivity of spider toxins.

The comparison of the potency of spider knottins over Na$_V$1.1–Na$_V$1.8 for Site 4 (Figure 5A) and Site 3 (Figure 5B) toxins highlights the limited pharmacological data for Site 3 spider knottins that are available mostly for Na$_V$1.3 and Na$_V$1.5. In contrast, Site 4 targeting spider knottins preferentially target hNa$_V$1.7 with Cd1a and CcoTx-2 having clear preference over hNa$_V$1.2, making this class an excellent starting point for the design of analgesic spider knottins. Indeed, the hNa$_V$1.7 selective spider knottin Pn3a confirms this potential [61,146] and shows analgesic effects in acute postsurgical pain [146]. A more complete list of spider knottins showing potency across different Na$_V$ channel subtypes and DRG are listed in Appendix A Tables A1 and A2.

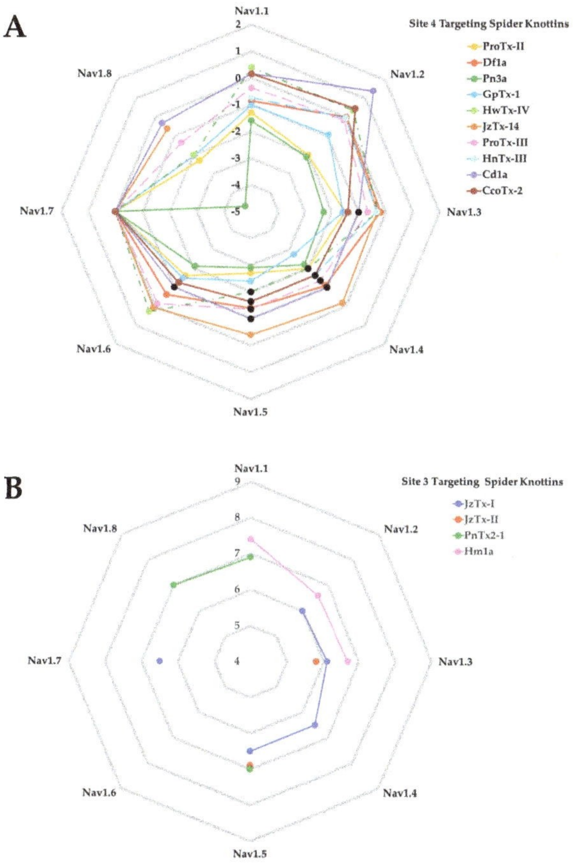

Figure 5. "Spider-plot" of Site 4 and Site 3 targeting spider knottins. (**A**) The pIC_{50} of Site 4 spider knottins normalized against $Na_V1.7$ are shown. These data are from assays performed on human Na_V subtypes, except JzTx-14 which was performed at mammalian Na_V subtypes. Data for GpTx-1 [122], ProTx-III [80], Cd1a [110], and CcoTx-2 [110] were obtained from Fluorescence Imaging Plate Reader (FLIPR) experiments, while the remainder were acquired using electrophysiology. Black dots indicate that the IC_{50} values for the corresponding knottins were less potent than the value indicated. (**B**) The pEC_{50} of Site 3 targeting spider knottins are shown. JzTx-I [100] was tested on rat $Na_V1.2$–1.4 and human $Na_V1.5$ and $Na_V1.7$. JzTx-II [98] was tested on rat $Na_V1.3$ and human $Na_V1.5$. PnTx2-1 [147] was tested on rat $Na_V1.1$ and $Na_V1.8$, and human $Na_V1.5$. Hm1a [20] was tested on human Na_V subtypes.

Mutagenesis and chimera studies of Na_V channels are typically used to determine critical residues for toxin binding on hNa_V channels [92,129,148]. These studies have revealed why the spider knottins HnTx-III, HnTx-IV, and HwTx-IV show Site 1-like channel inhibition (pore blocker) although they are gating modifiers [113,116,128]. Specifically, the Y326S mutation in $Na_V1.7$ decreased the channel sensitivity to tetrodotoxin (TTX) but not to HwTx-IV [114], while three residues (i.e., Glu753, Asp816 and especially Glu818) outside the pore were shown to be involved in the interactions of HnTx-IV with $hNa_V1.7$ (Figure 6A,B) [129]. $hNa_V1.7/rK_V2.1$ S3–S4 paddle chimera studies revealed that Df1a primarily interacted with the DII voltage sensor of $hNa_V1.7$ and had weaker interactions with VSDs of DIII and DIV [92]. Wingerd et al. [111] showed that the spider knottin Pre1a interacted with the DII and DIV S3–S4 loops of $Na_V1.7$ as well as the S1–S2 loop of DIV with the latter interaction likely conferring subtype selectivity. They also showed the role of the serine residue in the DIV S2 helix of $hNa_V1.1$

(Figure 6C) and rNa$_V$1.3 in inhibiting the fast inactivation process in these channel subtypes [111]. Spider knottin Hm1a also targets DIV S3b–S4 and S1–S2 loops that likely underlie its subtype selectivity for hNa$_V$1.1 [20].

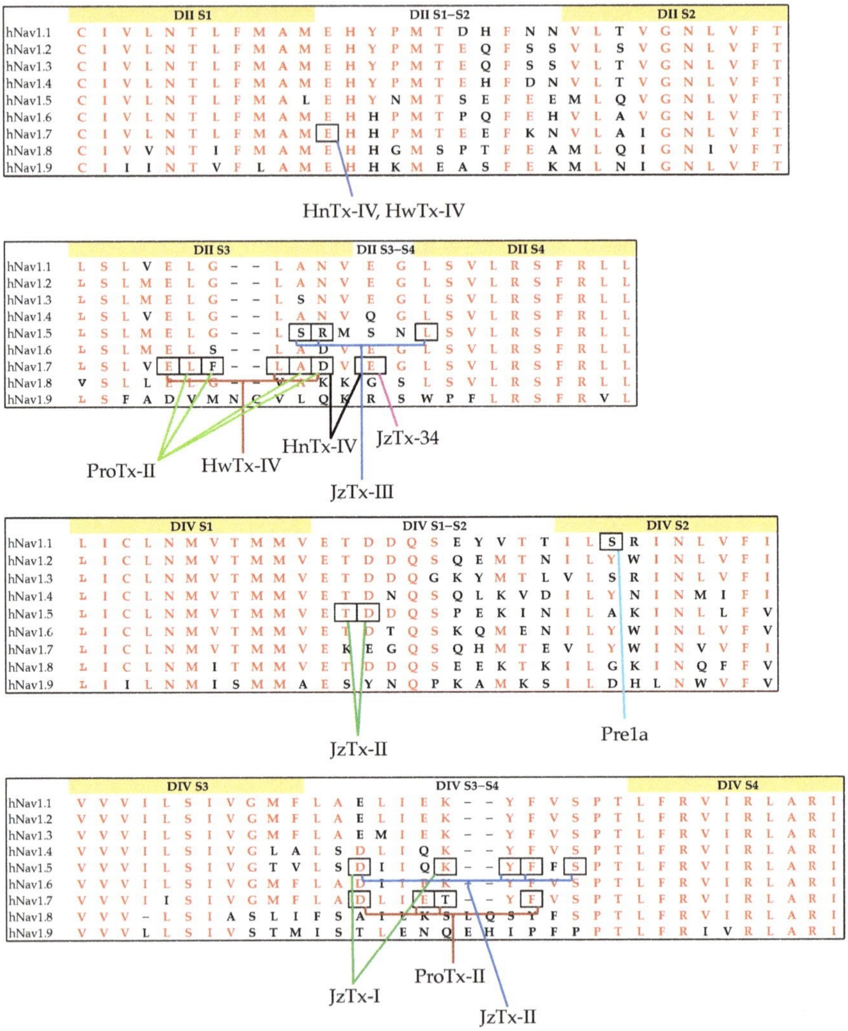

Figure 6. Sequence alignment of (**A**) DII S1–S2, (**B**) DII S3–S4, (**C**) DIV S1–S2 and (**D**) DIV S3–S4 of hNa$_V$1.1–1.9. Identical residues among hNa$_V$ subtypes are highlighted in red. hNa$_V$1.9 demonstrates the highest variation compared to other hNa$_V$ subtypes. Boxes highlights key residues in the interactions for the spider knottins HwTx-IV [149], HnTx-IV [129], ProTx-II [58,104], JzTx-III [106], JzTx-II [98], JzTx-I [100], JzTx-34 [119] and Pre1a [111].

Certain spider knottins can interact with multiple sites in the channel as demonstrated by ProTx-II's interactions at DII and DIV of hNa$_V$1.7 (Figure 6B,D) [55,104]. Furthermore, the DII residues, Glu753, Glu811, Leu814, Asp816 and Glu818, in hNa$_V$1.7 that are critical for inhibition of activation by HwTx-IV are partially conserved in hNa$_V$1.7 DIV. However, the partial conservation of DII residues in DIV (EgLDi) in wild-type hNa$_V$1.7 made HwTx-IV interact specifically with DII [149].

Mutational studies further identified that Asp1609 in $hNa_V1.5$ was crucial in determining the JzTx-II potency. However, $rNa_V1.8$ and $rNa_V1.9$ resistant to JzTx-II have Ala and Arg, respectively, instead of Asp1609 [98]. Similarly, Glu818 in $hNa_V1.7$ is conserved in HnTx-IV-sensitive Na_V channels $rNa_V1.2$ and $rNa_V1.3$ but is replaced by a neutral amino acid in HnTx-IV-resistant $rNa_V1.4$ and $hNa_V1.5$ [129]. In addition, Schmalhofer et al. [132] showed the crucial role of Phe813 in ProTx-II's selectivity for $hNa_V1.7$ over other Na_V subtypes. Finally, cysteine palmitoylation, which is a common reversible lipid modification process vital for Na_V channel biosynthesis, is also associated with the affinity of spider knottins to Na_V channels [150]. It regulates the gating and pharmacology of WT-$rNa_V1.2a$ as observed by the hyperpolarizing shift in steady-state inactivation and slowing in the channel recovery from fast inactivation upon depalmitoylation of intracellular cysteines on both WT-$rNa_V1.2a$ and G1097C-$rNa_V1.2a$ [150].

4. Knottins for Na_Vs in Pain Pathways

Pain allows direct perception of noxious stimuli to avoid actual or potential tissue damage. Primary sensory neuron (nociceptor) signals are transmitted to the brain through action potentials generated by ion channels and receptors. Genetic and molecular studies in animals and humans identified six Na_V channel subtypes (i.e., $Na_V1.1$, $Na_V1.3$, $Na_V1.6$, $Na_V1.7$, $Na_V1.8$ and $Na_V1.9$) critical for the generation and transmission of pain-related signals [20,21,36,151–158]. The $Na_V1.7$, $Na_V1.8$ and $Na_V1.9$ are preferentially expressed in the peripheral nervous system (PNS), while $Na_V1.1$ and $Na_V1.6$ are found in both the central nervous system (CNS) and PNS. The subtype $Na_V1.3$ is generally expressed in the CNS and absent in the adult PNS but is re-expressed in peripheral pain-signalling pathways upon neuronal injury [21,154,159]. The PNS localization of $Na_V1.3$, $Na_V1.7$, $Na_V1.8$ and $Na_V1.9$ avoids reaching the CNS and inducing associated off-target side effects. Besides these four major peripheral targets, there is evidence of the involvement of $Na_V1.6$ [160–162] and $Na_V1.1$ [20] in various peripheral pain pathways, which suggests these might also be drug targets in chronic pain types.

4.1. $Na_V1.1$

Votage-gated sodium channel subtype 1.1 ($Na_V1.1$) is a TTX-S sodium channel encoded by the *SCN1A* gene located on human chromosome 2q24.3 [163]. They initiate action potential and repetitive firing in neurons and are expressed in both the CNS and PNS and including the colonic myenteric plexus [17,164]. In the PNS, $Na_V1.1$ is predominantly expressed in medium-to-large diameter DRG neurons (A-fibres) but less expressed in small diameter unmyelinated neurons (i.e., C-fibres [165,166]) and has a smaller contribution in C-fibre-mediated nociceptive transmission [166,167]. However, in colonic afferents which predominantly comprise C-fibres, nearly 50% of the neurons are expressed $Na_V1.1$ [168]. The $hNa_V1.1$-selective activator Hm1a revealed its role in mechanical but not thermal hypersensitivity in the absence of neurogenic inflammation [20]. Recently, Salvatierra et al. [19] demonstrated the upregulation of $Na_V1.1$ in chronic visceral hypersensitivity (CVH) and its inhibition reducing the mechanical pain in an irritable bowel syndrome (IBS) rodent model. Furthermore, $Na_V1.1$ contributed to peripheral nerve injury-associated mechanical hypersensitivity [19].

Besides the role in nociception [19,20], $Na_V1.1$ participates in the familial hemiplegic migraine type 3 [169]. In addition, the anti-epileptic drug rufinamide, a $Na_V1.1$ inhibitor [170,171], alleviated spared nerve injury-evoked mechanical allodynia which also stabilizes $Na_V1.7$ in the inactivated state [172]. In addition to the $hNa_V1.1$-selective activator Hm1a, which identified a key role for this subtype in mechanosensitive pain, the spider knottins CcoTx-1, CcoTx-2, Df1a, ProTx-III, HwTx-IV and Pre1a inhibit $Na_V1.1$ in the nanomolar range and are thus potential leads to novel analgesics (Table A1).

4.2. $Na_V1.3$

Voltage-gated sodium channel subtype 1.3 ($Na_V1.3$) is a TTX-S sodium channel encoded by the *SCN3A* gene located on human chromosome 2q24.3 [163]. It produces fast activating and inactivating sodium currents and ramp currents due to the fact of its slow closed-state inactivation. These contribute to neuronal hyperexcitability by reducing thresholds and enhancing the repetitive and ectopic firing in injured neurons [17,154,173]. This channel is primarily expressed in embryonic DRG neurons and absent in adult DRG, but re-expressed during peripheral nerve injury and painful neuromas [166,174,175]. It is also expressed in enterochromaffin cells in the large and small intestine of humans and mice, where they participate in responses to chemical and mechanical stimuli [164,176,177].

Neuropathic pain models such as sciatic nerve transection [178], spinal nerve ligation (SNL) [179], SNI [180] and chronic constriction injury (CCI) confirmed the upregulation of $Na_V1.3$ [181]. Interestingly, this channel is upregulated only when peripheral projections are transected. The upregulation of $Na_V1.3$ is also associated to hyperexcitability of small DRG neurons [178]. Furthermore, infraorbital nerve-chronic constriction injury (ION-CCI) produced significant upregulation of $Na_V1.3$ and downregulation of $Na_V1.7$, $Na_V1.8$ and $Na_V1.9$ in trigeminal nerves [182].

Intrathecal administration of $Na_V1.3$-targeting antisense oligonucleotides attenuated $Na_V1.3$ upregulation and consequently reduced hyper-responsiveness of dorsal horn neurons and mitigated pain behaviours following CCI [181]. Chen et al. [156] also observed increased expression of $Na_V1.3$ in a CCI rat model in which neuropathic pain was alleviated by the intrathecal administration of MiR-96, a microRNA that inhibits $Na_V1.3$ expression. Another microRNA miR-30b attenuated SNL-evoked neuropathic pain by targeting *SCN3A* and downregulating the expression of $Na_V1.3$ mRNA and protein both in DRG neurons and the spinal cord [157].

The role of $Na_V1.3$ is also demonstrated in inflammatory pain [183], where its expression was upregulated in DRG neurons of rats with diabetic neuropathy and showing mechanical allodynia and thermal hyperalgesia [184]. In this same model, $Na_V1.3$ knockdown by adeno-associated virus (AAV)-shRNA-$Na_V1.3$ vector reduced neuropathic pain [185]. *Varicella zoster* virus (VZV) infection causing post-herpetic neuralgia (PHN) also showed upregulation of $Na_V1.3$ [186]. However, although $Na_V1.3$ was downregulated by antisense oligonucleotides in an SNI model, mechanical and cold allodynia were not attenuated [180]. Similarly, the mechanical allodynia remained unaltered following nerve injury in nociceptor specific and global $Na_V1.3$ knockout mouse models [187]. The druggability of $Na_V1.3$ in chronic pain management requires $Na_V1.3$-selective inhibitors [17]. Spider knottins ProTx-II, ProTx-III, HwTx-IV, HnTx-III, HnTx-IV and CcoTx-2 have nanomolar potency towards $Na_V1.3$ and rational engineering may generate $Na_V1.3$-selective leads (Table A1).

4.3. *$Na_V1.6$*

Voltage-gated sodium channel subtype 1.6 ($Na_V1.6$) is a TTX-S sodium channel encoded by the *SCN8A* gene which is located in human chromosome 12q13.13 [163]. They localize at the axon initial segment (AIS) and nodes of Ranvier in the CNS and PNS, including central projections and soma of the C-fibres [188–190]. It underlies persistent and resurgent sodium currents and repetitive neuronal excitability, with loss- or gain-of-function mutations reducing or increases the neuronal excitability, respectively [188]. Persson et al. [191] demonstrated the expression of $Na_V1.6$ in the axons of small nerve bundles beneath the epidermis and in the nerve terminals of nociceptors. Its increased expression is observed in complex regional pain syndrome Type 1 (CRPS1), post-herpetic neuralgia (PHN) patients [162,192] and in diabetic neuropathy in mice [193]. Recently, gain-of-function mutation M136V in $Na_V1.6$ was reported in trigeminal neuralgia with significantly increased peaks inward, resurgent currents and overall excitability of trigeminal nerves [194,195]. Deuis et al. [160] showed that oxaliplatin-induced cold allodynia is mediated by $Na_V1.6$ expressed in peripheral pathways, suggesting a key role in cold pain pathways. Finally, the selective inhibitor Cn2-E15R developed from the $Na_V1.6$ agonist Cn2 can be used to determine the extent of $Na_V1.6$ contributions to pain behaviours [196].

Local knockdown of $Na_V1.6$ alleviated spontaneous pain and mechanical allodynia imparted by the scorpion toxin BmK I [161]. Furthermore, local $Na_V1.6$ knockdown reversed mechanical pain in an SNL rat model by reducing sympathetic sprouting around $Na_V1.6$-positive neurons [197].

The $Na_V1.6$ expression was also upregulated in a pain model of DRG inflammation where $Na_V1.6$ knockdown reduced the pain behaviours and the abnormal bursting of the sensory neurons, including nociceptors [198]. Spider knottins modulating $Na_V1.6$ at nanomolar concentrations include ProTx-II, HwTx-IV, JZTx-14, Pre1a and Df1a (Table A1).

4.4. $Na_V1.7$

Voltage-gated sodium channel subtype 1.7 ($Na_V1.7$) is encoded by the *SCN9A* gene which is located in human chromosome 2q24.3 [163]. It is preferentially expressed in large-and-small diameter DRG neurons, visceral sensory neurons, olfactory sensory neurons, trigeminal ganglia and sympathetic neurons [151,152,199]. In DRG neurons, they are present from the peripheral to central terminals, with higher expression in small-diameter DRG neurons (C-fibres) [200]. This channel produces a rapidly activating and inactivating TTX-S sodium current that slowly recovers from inactivation and limits the frequency of firing. The slower onset of closed-state inactivation also limits inactivation during sub-threshold depolarizations and facilitates robust action potential generation that can amplify sub-threshold inputs [152,153,201,202]. Besides action potential generation and propagation, $Na_V1.7$ also contributes to neurotransmitter release in peripheral and central projections of sensory neurons [151,153].

Exclusive localization in the PNS and compelling genetic and functional evidences have centre-staged $Na_V1.7$ in pain research [153,158,203,204]. For example, mutations have been identified for various gain-of-function pain disorders, such as inherited erythromelalgia (IEM) [204], paroxysmal extreme pain disorder (PEPD) [203], small fibre neuropathy (SFN) [158] and painful diabetic peripheral neuropathy [205]. The gain-of-function mutations lead to hyperpolarizing shifts in activation, increased amplitude of ramp current, impaired inactivation, increased persistent currents and enhanced resurgent currents, all contributing to the hyperexcitability of DRG neurons [152]. Similarly, recessively inherited loss-of-function mutations are linked to congenital insensitivity to pain (CIP), with loss of olfaction being the only known side effect [36]. In addition, $Na_V1.7$ was upregulated in rodent models of visceral hypersensitivity [164]. These observations have supported $Na_V1.7$ as a promising therapeutic target for pain [153]. Considering the recent opportunities for spider knottins to unravel the mechanisms of Na_V modulation, the discovery and engineering of spider knottins selectively inhibiting $Na_V1.7$ provided exciting new opportunities for the development of novel pain therapeutics [135]. A number of spider knottins (Table A1) show nanomolar potency to inhibit $Na_V1.7$, with several undergoing optimization through saturation mutagenesis, directed evolution and/or rational engineering to enhance the potency and selectivity [14].

4.5. $Na_V1.8$

Voltage-gated sodium channel subtype 1.8 ($Na_V1.8$) is a TTX-R sodium channel encoded by the *SCN10A* gene in human chromosome 3p22.2 [163] and preferentially expressed in nociceptive DRG and trigeminal neurons (>90%) as well as in low-threshold mechanoreceptors [206,207], skin free nerve terminals [162], and corneal neurons [208]. It generates slowly inactivating rapidly repriming TTX-R sodium currents with a depolarized shift in the voltage dependence of activation and inactivation [154,209,210]. The channel also contributes to slow resurgent currents that probably underlie the excitability of nociceptors in DRG [211]. It also contributes significantly to the action potential upstroke and are sometimes referred to as overshoot channels [212].

The role of $Na_V1.8$ in inflammatory pain has been well documented. It had increased expression in DRG neurons when carrageenan was injected into rat hind paw [213] and in cultured DRG neurons treated with inflammatory mediators [214,215]. Similarly, Beyak et al. [216] showed increased $Na_V1.8$ currents in an animal model of colitis. Notably, inhibition of inflammatory pain induced by complete Freund's adjuvant (CFA) was observed in antisense-mediated $Na_V1.8$ knockdown in rats [217]. In addition, the upregulation of $Na_V1.8$ in a mouse model of bowel obstruction underpins its role in visceral hypersensitivity [218]. However, its role in neuropathic pain is not well defined with studies demonstrating downregulation of $Na_V1.8$ mRNA, protein and currents in the sciatic nerve after axonal transection [219–221]. On the other hand, increased $Na_V1.8$ levels were reported in spared axons and neuronal cell bodies of uninjured nerves [222,223]. This discrepancy is probably associated to the effects of inflammatory mediators in neuropathic pain models [154]. Finally, gain-of-function mutations of $Na_V1.8$ identified in painful neuropathy cases suggest its role in peripheral neuropathy [224]. Although a few spider toxins such as ProTx-I, ProTx-II and JxTx-14 targeted $Na_V1.8$ at nanomolar concentrations, only the spider knottin Hl1a shows selectivity towards $Na_V1.8$ (Table A1).

4.6. *$Na_V1.9$*

Voltage-gated sodium channel subtype 1.9 ($Na_V1.9$) is encoded by the *SCN11A* gene located in the human chromosome 3p22.2 [163]. These TTX-R channels are preferentially expressed in nociceptive DRG neurons, trigeminal ganglia and myenteric neurons [225,226], where they are activated only at hyperpolarized potentials near resting membrane potential to produce ultra-slow inactivating and persistent sodium currents [227]. These biophysical properties assist in amplifying subthreshold stimuli, lowering the threshold for single action potentials, and increasing repetitive firing [151,227,228].

The role of $Na_V1.9$ has been demonstrated in inflammatory pain with increased $Na_V1.9$ current density and lower thresholds for action potential generation that ultimately enhances neuronal excitability [151,214,229]. Indeed, $Na_V1.9$ knockout mice showed diminished mechanical hypersensitivity to formalin and CFA and failed to develop thermal hyperalgesia upon CFA or carrageenan injection [151,230–232]. Rare dominant gain-of-function mutations in *SCN11A* have been reported in a number of human pain disorders, such as familial episodic pain [233], painful small fibre neuropathy [234,235] and insensitivity to pain [155]. Despite the challenges in obtaining heterologous expression of $Na_V1.9$, chimeras $Na_V1.9/K_V2.1$ showed ProTx-I interacted with $Na_V1.9$ S3b–S4 paddle motif and potentiated $Na_V1.9$ currents in rat DRG [236].

5. Conclusions and Future Directions

In addition to a pivotal role of $Na_V1.7$ in pain processing, other Na_V subtypes including $Na_V1.1$, 1.3, 1.6, 1.8, and 1.9 are increasingly showing supportive and/or pivotal roles in various acute and chronic pain conditions. A large range of spider knottins modulate the Na_V function and continue to be developed as potential analgesic leads. In addition, spider knottins provide exquisite research tools to further explore the role of Na_V channels and how they can be modulated. Given that multiple sodium channels often contribute to chronic pain conditions, therapeutic leads targeting multiple Na_V channels could be advantageous; for example, chronic visceral pain may be best treated by a $Na_V1.1/Na_V1.7/Na_V1.8$ inhibitor, while diabetic neuropathy may be best treated by a $Na_V1.3/Na_V1.6/Na_V1.7$ inhibitor. However, despite Na_V-inhibiting spider knottin potential to target multiple subtypes, most have been optimized for potency and selectivity towards a single channel subtype $hNa_V1.7$ [14]. This review summarises spider knottin Na_V channel pharmacology that might be useful in guiding structure–function studies and the rational design of multi-valent spider knottin leads towards the development of therapeutic leads for chronic pain management.

Author Contributions: Conceptualization, F.C.C. and R.J.L.; data curation, Y.D.; writing—original draft preparation, Y.D.; writing—review and editing, F.C.C. and R.J.L.; supervision, F.C.C. and R.J.L.; project administration, R.J.L.; funding, R.J.L.

Funding: This research was funded by an Australian NHMRC Program Grant (APP1072113) and a Principal Research Fellowship to R.J.L.

Conflicts of Interest: The authors declare no conflict of interest.

Appendix A

Table A1. Inhibitory effects of spider knottins on Na_V channel subtypes. Values presented were obtained from electrophysiological experiments unless otherwise as stated.

Toxin	NaSpTx Family	Na_V1.1	Na_V1.2	Na_V1.3	Na_V1.4	Na_V1.5	Na_V1.6	Na_V1.7	Na_V1.8	Na_V1.9	Others
ProTx-I	2							51 nM (*n*, X, *h*); 72 nM (*s*, X, *h*); [103]	27 nM (*n*, X, *r*) [103]		
ProTx-II	3	15.8 nM (*s*, C, *h*) [141]	52.9 nM (*n*, H, *rNav1.2a*) [104] 41 nM (*n*, H, *h*) [132] 79.4 nM (*s*, H, *h*) [141]	109.9 nM (*n*, H, *r*) [104] 102 nM (*n*, C, *h*) [132] 25 nM (*s*, *h*) [141]	107.6 nM (*n*, H, *r*) [104] 39 nM (*n*, H, *h*) [132] 79.4 nM (*s*, H, *h*) [141]	29 nM (*s*, H, *h*) [103] 79.4 nM (*n*, H, *h*) [104] 79 nM (*n*, H, *h*) [132] 398 nM (*s*, H, *h*) [141]	26 nM (*n*, H, *h*) [132] 31.6 nM (*s*, C, *h*) [141]	0.7 nM (*n*, H, *h*) [104] 0.3 nM (*n*, H, *h*) [132] 0.8 nM (*s*, H, *h*) [141]	19 nM (*n*, X, *r*) [103] 146 nM (*n*, H, *h*) [132]		
GP-W7Q-W30L ProTx-II	3	6310 nM (*s*, C, *h*) [141]	794 nM (*s*, H, *h*) [141]		15,849 nM (*s*, H, *h*) [141]	>3162 nM (*s*, H, *h*) [141]	2512 nM (*s*, C, *h*) [141]	10 nM (*s*, H, *h*) [141]			
ProTx-III	1	60 nM, *rec-G*; 101 nM, *s-OH*; 11.3 nM, *s-NH*$_2$ (H, *h*) [80]		21.9 nM, *rec-G*; 41.3 nM, *s-OH*; 11.5 nM, *s-NH*$_2$ (H, *h*) [80]		>500 nM, *rec-G* and *s-OH*; >50 nM, *s-NH*$_2$ (H, *h*) [80]		9.5 nM, *rec-G*; 11.5 nM, *s-OH*; 2.5 nM, *s-NH*$_2$ (H, *h*) [80]			

Table A1. *Cont.*

Toxin	NaSpTx Family	Na$_V$1.1	Na$_V$1.2	Na$_V$1.3	Na$_V$1.4	Na$_V$1.5	Na$_V$1.6	Na$_V$1.7	Na$_V$1.8	Na$_V$1.9	Others
HwTX-IV	1	41 nM (*n*, H, *h*) [237]	150 nM (n, H, *r*) [114] 10 nM, *s-NH2*, 54 nM, *rec* (H, *h*) [83] 44 nM (*n*, H, *h*) [237]	338 nM (*n*, H, *r*) [114] 190 nM (*n*, H, *h*) [237]	400 nM (*n*, H, *r*) [114] >10,000 nM (*n*, H, *h*) [237]	>10,000 nM (*n*, H, *h*) [114] >10,000 nM (*n*, H, *h*) [237]	52 nM (*n*, H, *h*) [237] 83.3 nM (*n*, H, *h*) [237]	22.7 nM (*n*, H, *h*) [104] 26 nM (*n*, H, *r*) [114] 16 nM, *s-NH2*, 55 nM, *rec* (H, *h*) [83] 17 nM (*s*, H, *h*) [142] 32.4 nM (*s*, S, *h*, FLIPR) [137] 100 nM (*n*, H, *h*) [237] 32.6 nM (*n*, H, *h*, Manual ephys) [237]	>10,000 nM (*n*, H, *h*) [237]		30 nM (*n*, TTX-S currents, rat DRG) [113]

Table A1. *Cont.*

Toxin	NaSpTx Family	Nav1.1	Nav1.2	Nav1.3	Nav1.4	Nav1.5	Nav1.6	Nav1.7	Nav1.8	Nav1.9	Others
E1G-E4G-Y33W HwTx-IV	1	8.4 nM (*rec*, H, *h*) [143] 1100 nM (*rec*, H, *h*, FLIPR) [143]	11.9 nM (*rec*, H, *h*) [143] 540 nM (*rec*, H, *h*, FLIPR) [143]	7.2 nM (*rec*, H, *h*) [143] 1400 nM (*rec*, H, *h*, FLIPR) [143]	369 nM (*rec*, H, *h*) [143] >30,000 nM (*rec*, H, *h*, FLIPR) [143]	Insensitive up to 1000 nM (*rec*, H, *h*) [143] >30,000 nM (*rec*, H, *h*, FLIPR) [143]	6.8 nM (*rec*, C, *h*) [143] 600 nM (*rec*, H, *h*, FLIPR) [143]	0.4 nM (*s*, H, *h*) [142] 3.3 nM (*rec*, C, *h*) [143] 5100 nM (*rec*, H, *h*, FLIPR) [143]	Insensitive up to 1000 nM (*rec*, C, *h*) [143] >30,000 nM (*rec*, H, *h*, FLIPR) [143]		
E1G-E4G-F6W-Y33W HwTx-IV	1							7.55 nM (*s*, S, *h*, FLIPR) [137]			
HnTx-I	1		68,000 nM (*n*, X, *r*) [145]					>10,000 nM (*s*, H, *h*) [238]			No inhibition of TTX-S and TTX-R currents up to 100,000 nM [145]
G7W-N24S HnTx-I	1							440 nM (*rec*, C, *h*) [81]			
E1G-N23S-D26H-L32W HnTx-I	1							3.6 nM (*s*, H, *h*) [238]			
HnTx-III	1	1270 nM (*n*, H, *h*) [117]	275 nM (*n*, H, *h*) [117]	491 nM (*n*, H, *h*) [117]	No activity [117]	No activity [117]		232 nM (*n*, H, *h*) [117]			1.1 nM (TTX-S rat DRG); No inhibition in TTX-R currents [116]

Table A1. *Cont.*

Toxin	NaSpTx Family	$Na_V1.1$	$Na_V1.2$	$Na_V1.3$	$Na_V1.4$	$Na_V1.5$	$Na_V1.6$	$Na_V1.7$	$Na_V1.8$	$Na_V1.9$	Others
HnTx-IV	1		36.1 nM (*n*, H, *r*) [129]	375 nM (*n*, H, *r*) [129]	>10,000 nM (*n*, H, *r*) [129]	No inhibition up to 1000 nM [129]		21 nM (*s*, *n*, H, *h*) [127]			44.6 nM (TTX-S rat DRG) [116] 34 nm (TTX-S rat DRG) [85]
JzTx-III	7		No effect [106]	No effect [106]	No effect [106]	348 nM (*rec*, H, *h*) [106]	No effect [106]	No effect [106]			380 nM (*n*, rat cardiac myocytes) [105]
JzTx-V	3			292 nM (*s*, H, *h*) [79]	5.12 nM (*s*, H, *r*) [79]	2700 nM (*s*, H, *h*) [79]		61 nM (*s*, H, *h*) [79]			27.6 nM (*n*, TTX-R currents, rat DRG); 30.2 nM (*n*, TTX-S currents, rat DRG) [107]
JzTx-IX	2				5420 nM (*n*, H_T) [108]	450 nM (*n*, H_T) [108]					650 nM (*n*, TTX-R currents, rat DRG); 360 nM (*n*, TTX-S currents, rat DRG) [108]
JzTx-XI	2					124 nM (*n*, C) [91]					

Table A1. *Cont.*

Toxin	NaSpTx Family	Nav1.1	Nav1.2	Nav1.3	Nav1.4	Nav1.5	Nav1.6	Nav1.7	Nav1.8	Nav1.9	Others
JzTx-14	3		194 nM (*n*, H_T, *M*) [125]	426.3 nM (*n*, H_T, *M*) [125]	290.1 nM (*n*, H_T, *M*) [125]	478 nM (*n*, H_T, *M*) [125]	158.6 nM (*n*, H_T, *M*) [125]	188.9 nM (*n*, H_T, *M*) [125]	824 nM (*n*, H_T, *M*) [125]		
JzTx-34	2	No inhibition (*s*, H_T, *r*) [119]	No inhibition (*s*, H_T, *r*) [119]	7950 nM (*s*, H_T, *r*) [119]	No inhibition (*s*, H_T, *r*) [119]	No inhibition (*s*, H_T, *r*) [119]	No inhibition (*s*, H_T) [119]	610 nM (s, H_T, *h*) [119]	No inhibition (*s*, ND cells, *h*) [119]		85 nM (*rec*, TTX-S currents, rat DRG); No inhibition in TTX-R currents [118] 91 nM (*s*, TTX-S currents, rat DRG); No inhibition in TTX-R currents [119]
JzTx-35	2					1070 nM (*n*, H, *h*) [112]					
CcoTx-1	1	523 nM (*n*, X) [73] 1060 nM (*n*, H, *h*, FLIPR) [110]	3 nM (*n*, X) [73] 70 nM (*n*, H, *h*, FLIPR) [110]	No activity [73] >10,000 nM (*n*, H, *h*, FLIPR) [110]	888 nM (*n*, X) [73] >10,000 nM (*n*, H, *h*, FLIPR) [110]	323 nM (*n*, X) [73] >10,000 nM (*n*, H, *h*, FLIPR) [110]	>10,000 nM (*n*, H, *h*, FLIPR) [110]	5120 nM (*n*, H, *h*, FLIPR) [110]	55% block (*n*, X) [73] >10,000 nM (*n*, H, *h*, FLIPR) [110]		

Table A1. *Cont.*

Toxin	NaSpTx Family	Nav1.1	Nav1.2	Nav1.3	Nav1.4	Nav1.5	Nav1.6	Nav1.7	Nav1.8	Nav1.9	Others
CcoTx-2	1	407 nM (*n*, X) [73] 170 nM (*n*, H, *h*, FLIPR) [110]	8 nM (*n*, X) [73] 80 nM (*n*, H, *h*, FLIPR) [110]	88 nM (*n*, X) [73] 5570 nM (*n*, H, *h*, FLIPR) [110]	400 nM (*n*, X) [73] >10,000 nM (*n*, H, *h*, FLIPR) [110]	1634 nM (*n*, X) [73] >10,000 nM (*n*, H, *h*, FLIPR) [110]	3990 nM (*n*, H, *h*, FLIPR) [110]	230 nM (*n*, H, *h*, FLIPR) [110]	40% block (*n*, X) [73] >10,000 nM (*n*, H, *h*, FLIPR) [110]		
CcoTx-3	2	No activity [73]	No activity [73]	No activity [73]	No activity [73]	447 nM (*n*, X) [73]			45% block (*n*, X) [73]		
PaurTx3	1	610 nM (*n*, X) [73]	0.6 nM (*n*, X) [73]	42 nM (*n*, X) [73]	288 nM (*n*, X) [73]	72 nM (*n*, X) [73]			65% block (*n*, X) [73]		
Hm-1	9		32.4% block at 200 nM (*n*, X, *r*) [120]		336.4 nM (*n*, X, *r*) [120] 40% block at 200 nM (*n*, X, *r*) [120]	36.5% block at 200 nM (*n*, X, *h*) [120]	38.7% block at 200 nM (*n*, X, *m*) [120]				
Hm-2	9		64.6% block at 200 nM (*n*, X, *r*) [120]		154.8 nM (*n*, X, *r*) [120] 61.9% block at 200 nM (*n*, X, *r*) [120]	17.8% block at 200 nM (*n*, X, *h*) [120]	38.7% block at 200 nM (*n*, X, *m*) [120]				
GTx1-15	1			120 nM (*s*, H, *h*) [239]		No effect up to 2000 nM (*s*, H, *h*) [239]		7 nM (*s*, H, *h*) [239]	No effect up to 930 nM (*s*, H, *h*) [239]		

Table A1. *Cont.*

Toxin	NaSpTx Family	Nav1.1	Nav1.2	Nav1.3	Nav1.4	Nav1.5	Nav1.6	Nav1.7	Nav1.8	Nav1.9	Others
VSTx-3	1			190 nM (*s*, H, *h*) [239]		No effect up to 1000 nM (*s*, H, *h*) [239]		430 nM (*s*, H, *h*) [239]	770 nM (*s*, H, *h*) [239]		
Hd1a	1	87% block (*rec*, X, *h*) [121]	55% block (*rec*, X, *h*) [121]	23%–31% block (*rec*, X, *h*) [121]	23%–31% block (*rec*, X, *h*) [121]	No inhibition up to 1000 nM (*rec*, X, *h*) [121]	23%–31% block (*rec*, X, *h*) [121]	111 nM (*rec*, X, *h*) [121] 87% block (*rec*, X, *h*) [121]	No inhibition up to 1000 nM (*rec*, X, *h*) [121]		
Cd1a	1	2180 µM (*s*, H, *h*, FLIPR) [110]	130 µM (*s*, H, *h*, FLIPR) [110]	>30,000 nM (*s*, H, *h*, FLIPR) [110]	>30,000 nM (*s*, H, *h*, FLIPR) [110]	>30,000 nM (*s*, H, *h*, FLIPR) [110]	>30,000 nM (*s*, H, *h*, FLIPR) [110]	3340 nM (*s*, H, *h*, FLIPR) [110] 16 nM (*s*, H, *h*) [110]	6920 nM (*s*, H, *h*, FLIPR) [110]		
Pre1a	1	57.1 nM (*s*, H, *h*) [111]	189.6 nM (*s*, X, *r*) [111]	8000 nM (*s*, X, *r*) [111]	16.5% block at 1000 nM (*s*, X, *r*) [111]	8.6% block at 1000 nM (*s*, X, *r*) [111]	221.6 nM (*s*, H, *h*) [111]	114 nM (*s*, X, *r*) [111] 15 nM (*s*, H, *h*) [111]			
Pn3a	2	37 nM (*s*, H, *h*) [61]	124 nM (*s*, H, *h*) [61]	210 nM (*s*, H, *h*) [61] (	144 nM (*s*, H, *h*) [61]	800 nM (*s*, H, *h*) [61]	129 nM (*s*, H, *h*) [61])	0.9 nM (*s*, H, *h*) [61] 1.5 nM (*s*, H, *r*) [61] 4.4 nM (*s*, H, *m*) [61]	50,000 nM (*s*, H, *h*) [61]	2427 nM (*s*, H, *h*) [61]	

Table A1. *Cont.*

Toxin	NaSpTx Family	Nav1.1	Nav1.2	Nav1.3	Nav1.4	Nav1.5	Nav1.6	Nav1.7	Nav1.8	Nav1.9	Others
Hl1a	7	No inhibition (s, H_T, *h*) [123]	No inhibition (s, H_T, *h*) [123]	No inhibition (s, H_T, *h*) [123]	No inhibition (s, H_T, *h*) [123]	No inhibition (s, H_T, *h*) [123]	No inhibition (s, H_T, *h*) [123]	No inhibition (s, H_T, *h*) [123]	2190 nM (*s*, ND7/23 cell, *h*) [123]		3760 nM (*s*, rat DRG) [123]
GpTx-1	1	6000 nM (*s*, H, *h*, FLIPR) [122]	5000 nM (*s*, H, *h*, FLIPR) [122]	20 nM (*s*, C, *h*) [76] 22,000 nM (*s*, H, *h*, FLIPR) [122]	301 nM (*s*, H, *h*, Manual ephys) [76] 200 nM (HEK293, *h*, synthetic, PatchXpress) [76] 326,000 nM (*s*, H, *h*, FLIPR) [122]	4200 nM (*s*, H, *h*, Manual ephys) [76] >10,000 nM (*s*, H, *h*, PatchXpress) [76] 140,000 nM (*s*, H, *h*, FLIPR) [122]	17,000 nM (*s*, H, *h*, FLIPR) [122]	4.4 nM (*s*, H, *h*, Manual ephys) [76] 10 nM (*s*, H, *h*, PatchXpress) [76] 580 nM (*s*, H, *h*, FLIPR) [122] 8 nM, open/inactivated state; 13 nM, closed/resting state (*s*, C, *h*,) [122]	12,200 nM (*s*, C, *h*, Manual ephys) [76] 68,000 nM (*s*, H, *h*, FLIPR) [122]		
F5A-M6F-T26L-K28R-GpTx-1	1				1900 nM (*s*, H, *h*, PatchXpress) [76]	>10,000 nM (*s*, H, *h*, PatchXpress) [76]		1.6 nM (*s*, H, *h*, PatchXpress) [76]			

Table A1. *Cont.*

Toxin	NaSpTx Family	$Na_V1.1$	$Na_V1.2$	$Na_V1.3$	$Na_V1.4$	$Na_V1.5$	$Na_V1.6$	$Na_V1.7$	$Na_V1.8$	$Na_V1.9$	Others
Df1a	2	14.3 nM, *s-NH$_2$*; 30.7 nM, *s-OH*; (H, *h*) [92]	1.9 nM, *s-NH$_2$*; 3 nM, *s-OH*; (H, *h*) [92]	3 nM, *s-NH$_2$*; 10 nM, *s-OH*; (H, *h*) [92]	24 nM, *s-NH$_2$*; 53.6 nM, *s-OH*; (H, *h*) [92]	45.3 nM, *s-NH$_2$*; 125.6 nM, *s-OH*; (H, *h*) [92]	7.6 nM, *s-NH$_2$*; 23 nM, *s-OH*; (C, *h*) [92]	1.9 nM, *s-NH$_2$*; 60.5 nM, *s-OH*; (H, *h*) [92]			
Phlo1a	2							459 nM (*n*, X, *h*) [240]			
Phlo1b	2							360 nM (*n*, X, *h*) [240]			
Phlo2a	3		404 nM (*n*, X, *h*) [240]			218 nM (*n*, X, *h*) [240]		333 nM (*n*, X, *h*) [240]			
GrTx-1	3	630 nM (*n*, H, *h*) [241]	230 nM (*n*, H, *h*) [241]	770 nM (*n*, H, *h*) [241]	1290 nM (*n*, H_T, *h*) [241]	~22,000 nM (*n*, H, *h*) [241]	630 nM (*n*, H, *h*) [241]	370 nM (*n*, H_T, *h*) [241]			
GsAFII	3	5700 nM (*n*, H, *h*) [241]	12,000 nM (*n*, H, *h*) [241]	24,000 nM (*n*, H, *h*) [241]	4000 nM (*n*, H_T, *h*) [241]	~42,000 nM (*n*, H, *h*) [241]	6600 nM (*n*, H, *h*) [241]	1030 nM (*n*, H_T, *h*) [241]			

Note: *s*:- synthetic; *n*:- native; *rec*:- recombinantly expressed; *rec-G*:- recombinantly expressed with an extra N-terminal Glycine; *s-OH*:- synthetic free carboxyl end; *s-NH$_2$*:- synthetic C-terminal amidated; H:- HEK 293 cells; H_T:- transiently transfected HEK 293 cells; X:- *Xenopus* oocytes; C:- CHO cells; S:- SHSY5Y cells; *h*:- human Na_V; *r*:- rat Na_V; *m*:- mouse Na_V; *r*:- rat Na_V; *M*:- mammalian Na_V; FLIPR:- Fluorescence Imaging Plate Reader.

Table A2. Excitatory effects of spider knottins on Na_V channel subtypes. Values presented were obtained from electrophysiological experiments, unless otherwise as stated.

Toxin	NaSpTx Family	Na_V1.1	Na_V1.2	Na_V1.3	Na_V1.4	Na_V1.5	Na_V1.6	Na_V1.7	Na_V1.8	Na_V1.9	Others
JzTx-I	7		870 nM (*n*, H_T, *r*) [100]	845 nM (*n*, H_T, *r*) [100]	339 nM (*n*, H_T, *r*) [100]	335 nM (*n*, H_T, *h*) [100]		348 nM (*n*, H_T, *h*) [100]			130 nM (*n*, TTX-S currents, rat DRG); No inhibition in rat DRG TTX-R currents; 31 nM in rat cardiac myocytes) [101]
JzTx-II	7			1650 nM (*n*, H_T, *r*) [98]		125 nM (*n*, H_T, *h*) [98]					
Hm1a	2	38 nM (*s*, X, *h*) [20]	236 nM (*s*, X, *h*) [20]	220 nM (*s*, X, *h*) [20]	No inhibition up to 1000 nM (*s*, X, *h*) [20]	No inhibition up to 1000 nM (*s*, X, *h*) [20]	No inhibition up to 1000 nM (*s*, X, *h*) [20]	No inhibition up to 1000 nM (*s*, X, *h*) [20]	No inhibition up to 1000 nM (*s*, X, *h*) [20]		
PnTx2-1	6	122 nM (*n*, X, *r*) [147]	No inhibition up to 1000 nM (*n*, X, *r*) [147]	No inhibition up to 1000 nM (*n*, X, *r*) [147]	No inhibition up to 1000 nM (*n*, X, *r*) [147]	87 nM (*n*, X, *h*) [147]	No inhibition up to 1000 nM (*n*, X, *m*) [147]		101.1 nM (*n*, X, *r*) [147]		

Note: *s*:- synthetic; *n*:- native; H_T:- transiently transfected HEK 293 cells; X:- *Xenopus* oocytes; *h*:- human Na_V; *r*:- rat Na_V; *r*:- rat Na_V.

References

1. Nicholson, G.M. Spider Peptides. In *Handbook of Biologically Active Peptides*, 2nd ed.; Kastin, A.J., Ed.; Academic Press: Boston, MA, USA, 2013; pp. 461–472. [CrossRef]
2. Catalog, W.S. World Spider Catalog. Available online: https://wsc.nmbe.ch/statistics/ (accessed on 25 June 2019).
3. Caddington, J.; Levi, H. Systematic and evolution of spiders (Araenea). *Annu. Rev. Ecol. Syst.* **1991**, *22*, 565–592. [CrossRef]
4. King, G.F.; Hardy, M.C. Spider-venom peptides: Structure, pharmacology, and potential for control of insect pests. *Annu. Rev. Entomol.* **2013**, *58*, 475–496. [CrossRef] [PubMed]
5. Samiayyan, K. Spiders—The generalist super predators in agro-ecosystems. In *Integrated Pest Management*; Elsevier: San Diego, CA, USA, 2014; pp. 283–310. [CrossRef]
6. Cooper, A.M.; Nelsen, D.R.; Hayes, W.K. The Strategic Use of Venom by Spiders. In *Evolution of Venomous Animals and Their Toxins*; Malhotra, A., Ed.; Springer: Dordrecht, The Netherlands, 2017; pp. 145–166. [CrossRef]
7. Dongol, Y.; Dhananjaya, B.L.; Shrestha, R.K.; Aryal, G. Animal Venoms and Nephrotoxic Effects. In *Clinical Toxinology in Australia, Europe, and Americas. Toxinology*; Gopalakrishnakone, P., Vogel, C.-W., Seifert, S.A., Tambourgi, D.V., Eds.; Springer: Dordrecht, The Netherlands, 2018; pp. 539–556. [CrossRef]
8. Zlotkin, E. The insect voltage-gated sodium channel as target of insecticides. *Annu. Rev. Entomol.* **1999**, *44*, 429–455. [CrossRef] [PubMed]
9. Billen, B.; Vassilevski, A.; Nikolsky, A.; Debaveye, S.; Tytgat, J.; Grishin, E. Unique bell-shaped voltage-dependent modulation of Na^+ channel gating by novel insect-selective toxins from the spider *Agelena orientalis*. *J. Biol. Chem.* **2010**, *285*, 18545–18554. [CrossRef] [PubMed]
10. Escoubas, P.; Sollod, B.; King, G.F. Venom landscapes: Mining the complexity of spider venoms via a combined cDNA and mass spectrometric approach. *Toxicon* **2006**, *47*, 650–663. [CrossRef]
11. Sannaningaiah, D.; Subbaiah, G.K.; Kempaiah, K. Pharmacology of spider venom toxins. *Toxin Rev.* **2014**, *33*, 206–220. [CrossRef]
12. Pineda, S.S.; Undheim, E.A.; Rupasinghe, D.B.; Ikonomopoulou, M.P.; King, G.F. Spider venomics: Implications for drug discovery. *Future Med. Chem.* **2014**, *6*, 1699–1714. [CrossRef]
13. Escoubas, P.; Diochot, S.; Corzo, G. Structure and pharmacology of spider venom neurotoxins. *Biochimie* **2000**, *82*, 893–907. [CrossRef]
14. Cardoso, F.C.; Lewis, R.J. Structure–Function and therapeutic potential of spider venom-derived cysteine knot peptides targeting sodium channels. *Front. Pharmacol.* **2019**, *10*. [CrossRef]
15. Klint, J.K.; Senff, S.; Rupasinghe, D.B.; Er, S.Y.; Herzig, V.; Nicholson, G.M.; King, G.F. Spider-venom peptides that target voltage-gated sodium channels: Pharmacological tools and potential therapeutic leads. *Toxicon* **2012**, *60*, 478–491. [CrossRef]
16. Stevens, M.; Peigneur, S.; Tytgat, J. Neurotoxins and their binding areas on voltage-gated sodium channels. *Front. Pharmacol.* **2011**, *2*, 71. [CrossRef] [PubMed]
17. Wu, Y.; Ma, H.; Zhang, F.; Zhang, C.; Zou, X.; Cao, Z. Selective voltage-gated sodium channel peptide toxins from animal venom: Pharmacological probes and analgesic drug development. *ACS Chem. Neurosci.* **2018**, *9*, 187–197. [CrossRef] [PubMed]
18. Kalia, J.; Milescu, M.; Salvatierra, J.; Wagner, J.; Klint, J.K.; King, G.F.; Olivera, B.M.; Bosmans, F. From foe to friend: Using animal toxins to investigate ion channel function. *J. Mol. Biol.* **2015**, *427*, 158–175. [CrossRef] [PubMed]
19. Salvatierra, J.; Castro, J.; Erickson, A.; Li, Q.; Braz, J.; Gilchrist, J.; Grundy, L.; Rychkov, G.Y.; Deiteren, A.; Rais, R. $Na_V1.1$ inhibition can reduce visceral hypersensitivity. *JCI Insight* **2018**, *3*. [CrossRef]
20. Osteen, J.D.; Herzig, V.; Gilchrist, J.; Emrick, J.J.; Zhang, C.; Wang, X.; Castro, J.; Garcia-Caraballo, S.; Grundy, L.; Rychkov, G.Y.; et al. Selective spider toxins reveal a role for the $Na_V1.1$ channel in mechanical pain. *Nature* **2016**, *534*, 494–499. [CrossRef]
21. Cardoso, F.C.; Lewis, R.J. Sodium channels and pain: From toxins to therapies. *Br. J. Pharmacol.* **2018**, *175*, 2138–2157. [CrossRef]
22. Lukowski, A.L.; Narayan, A.R.H. Natural voltage-gated sodium channel ligands: Biosynthesis and Biology. *ChemBioChem* **2019**, *20*, 1231–1241. [CrossRef]

23. Black, J.A.; Waxman, S.G. Noncanonical roles of voltage-gated sodium channels. *Neuron* **2013**, *80*, 280–291. [CrossRef]
24. Yamamoto, R.; Yanagita, T.; Kobayashi, H.; Yokoo, H.; Wada, A. Up-regulation of sodium channel subunit mRNAs and their cell surface expression by antiepileptic valproic acid: Activation of calcium channel and catecholamine secretion in adrenal chromaffin cells. *J. Neurochem.* **1997**, *68*, 1655–1662. [CrossRef]
25. Andrikopoulos, P.; Fraser, S.P.; Patterson, L.; Ahmad, Z.; Burcu, H.; Ottaviani, D.; Diss, J.K.; Box, C.; Eccles, S.A.; Djamgoz, M.B. Angiogenic functions of voltage-gated Na^+ Channels in human endothelial cells: Modulation of vascular endothelial growth factor (VEGF) signaling. *J. Biol. Chem.* **2011**, *286*, 16846–16860. [CrossRef]
26. Carrithers, M.D.; Dib-Hajj, S.; Carrithers, L.M.; Tokmoulina, G.; Pypaert, M.; Jonas, E.A.; Waxman, S.G. Expression of the voltage-gated sodium channel $Na_V1.5$ in the macrophage late endosome regulates endosomal acidification. *J. Immunol.* **2007**, *178*, 7822–7832. [CrossRef] [PubMed]
27. Carrithers, M.D.; Chatterjee, G.; Carrithers, L.M.; Offoha, R.; Iheagwara, U.; Rahner, C.; Graham, M.; Waxman, S.G. Regulation of podosome formation in macrophages by a splice variant of the sodium channel SCN8A. *J. Biol. Chem.* **2009**, *284*, 8114–8126. [CrossRef] [PubMed]
28. Pucca, M.B.; Peigneur, S.; Cologna, C.T.; Cerni, F.A.; Zoccal, K.F.; Bordon, K.D.C.F.; Faccioli, L.H.; Tytgat, J.; Arantes, E.C. Electrophysiological characterization of the first *Tityus serrulatus* α-like toxin, Ts5: Evidence of a pro-inflammatory toxin on macrophages. *Biochimie* **2015**, *115*, 8–16. [CrossRef] [PubMed]
29. Fraser, S.P.; Ozerlat-Gunduz, I.; Brackenbury, W.J.; Fitzgerald, E.M.; Campbell, T.M.; Coombes, R.C.; Djamgoz, M.B.A. Regulation of voltage-gated sodium channel expression in cancer: Hormones, growth factors and auto-regulation. *Philos. Trans. R. Soc. B Biol. Sci.* **2014**, *369*. [CrossRef] [PubMed]
30. Waxman, S.G. Axonal conduction and injury in multiple sclerosis: The role of sodium channels. *Nat. Rev. Neurosci.* **2006**, *7*, 932–941. [CrossRef] [PubMed]
31. Kaplan, D.I.; Isom, L.; Petrou, S. 17. Role of Sodium Channels in Epilepsy. *Cold Spring Harb. Perspect. Med.* **2016**, *6*. [CrossRef]
32. Raouf, R.; Quick, K.; Wood, J.N. Pain as a channelopathy. *J. Clin. Investig.* **2010**, *120*, 3745–3752. [CrossRef]
33. Dib-Hajj, S.D.; Waxman, S.G. Sodium channels in human pain disorders: Genetics and pharmacogenomics. *Annu. Rev. Neurosci.* **2019**, *42*. [CrossRef]
34. Savio Galimberti, E.; Gollob, M.; Darbar, D. Voltage-gated sodium channels: Biophysics, pharmacology, and related channelopathies. *Front. Pharmacol.* **2012**, *3*. [CrossRef]
35. Probst, V.; Kyndt, F.; Potet, F.; Trochu, J.N.; Mialet, G.; Demolombe, S.; Schott, J.J.; Baro, I.; Escande, D.; Le Marec, H. Haploinsufficiency in combination with aging causes SCN5A-linked hereditary Lenegre disease. *J. Am. Coll. Cardiol.* **2003**, *41*, 643–652. [CrossRef]
36. Cox, J.J.; Reimann, F.; Nicholas, A.K.; Thornton, G.; Roberts, E.; Springell, K.; Karbani, G.; Jafri, H.; Mannan, J.; Raashid, Y. An SCN9A channelopathy causes congenital inability to experience pain. *Nature* **2006**, *444*, 894. [CrossRef]
37. Claes, L.; Del-Favero, J.; Ceulemans, B.; Lagae, L.; van Broeckhoven, C.; de Jonghe, P. De novo mutations in the sodium-channel gene SCN1A cause severe myoclonic epilepsy of infancy. *Am. J. Hum. Genet.* **2001**, *68*, 1327–1332. [CrossRef] [PubMed]
38. Mantegazza, M.; Gambardella, A.; Rusconi, R.; Schiavon, E.; Annesi, F.; Cassulini, R.R.; Labate, A.; Carrideo, S.; Chifari, R.; Canevini, M.P.; et al. Identification of an $Na_V1.1$ sodium channel (SCN1A) loss-of-function mutation associated with familial simple febrile seizures. *Proc. Natl. Acad. Sci. USA* **2005**, *102*, 18177–18182. [CrossRef] [PubMed]
39. Shen, H.; Zhou, Q.; Pan, X.; Li, Z.; Wu, J.; Yan, N. Structure of a eukaryotic voltage-gated sodium channel at near-atomic resolution. *Science* **2017**, *355*, eaal4326. [CrossRef] [PubMed]
40. Patino, G.A.; Brackenbury, W.J.; Bao, Y.; Lopez-Santiago, L.F.; O'Malley, H.A.; Chen, C.; Calhoun, J.D.; Lafrenière, R.G.; Cossette, P.; Rouleau, G.A. Voltage-gated Na+ channel β1B: A secreted cell adhesion molecule involved in human epilepsy. *J. Neurosci.* **2011**, *31*, 14577–14591. [CrossRef]
41. O'Malley, H.A.; Isom, L.L. Sodium channel β subunits: Emerging targets in channelopathies. *Annu. Rev. Physiol.* **2015**, *77*, 481–504. [CrossRef]
42. Patino, G.A.; Isom, L.L. Electrophysiology and beyond: Multiple roles of Na^+ channel β subunits in development and disease. *Neurosci. Lett.* **2010**, *486*, 53–59. [CrossRef]

43. Sato, C.; Ueno, Y.; Asai, K.; Takahashi, K.; Sato, M.; Engel, A.; Fujiyoshi, Y. The voltage-sensitive sodium channel is a bell-shaped molecule with several cavities. *Nature* **2001**, *409*, 1047. [CrossRef]
44. De Lera Ruiz, M.; Kraus, R.L. Voltage-Gated Sodium Channels: Structure, function, pharmacology, and clinical indications. *J. Med. Chem.* **2015**, *58*, 7093–7118. [CrossRef]
45. Yu, F.H.; Catterall, W.A. Overview of the voltage-gated sodium channel family. *Genome Biol.* **2003**, *4*, 207. [CrossRef]
46. Bezanilla, F. Gating currents. *J. Gen. Physiol.* **2018**, *150*, 911–932. [CrossRef] [PubMed]
47. Catterall, W.A. Molecular properties of voltage-sensitive sodium channels. *Annu. Rev. Biochem.* **1986**, *55*, 953–985. [CrossRef] [PubMed]
48. Guy, H.R.; Seetharamulu, P. Molecular model of the action potential sodium channel. *Proc. Natl. Acad. Sci. USA* **1986**, *83*, 508–512. [CrossRef] [PubMed]
49. Catterall, W.A. Forty Years of sodium channels: Structure, function, pharmacology, and epilepsy. *Neurochem. Res.* **2017**, *42*, 2495–2504. [CrossRef]
50. Catterall, W.A. Ion channel voltage sensors: Structure, function, and pathophysiology. *Neuron* **2010**, *67*, 915–928. [CrossRef]
51. Catterall, W.A. From ionic currents to molecular mechanisms: The structure and function of voltage-gated sodium channels. *Neuron* **2000**, *26*, 13–25. [CrossRef]
52. Clairfeuille, T.; Xu, H.; Koth, C.M.; Payandeh, J. Voltage-gated sodium channels viewed through a structural biology lens. *Curr. Opin. Struct. Biol.* **2017**, *45*, 74–84. [CrossRef]
53. West, J.W.; Patton, D.E.; Scheuer, T.; Wang, Y.; Goldin, A.L.; Catterall, W.A. A cluster of hydrophobic amino acid residues required for fast Na^+-channel inactivation. *Proc. Natl. Acad. Sci. USA* **1992**, *89*, 10910–10914. [CrossRef]
54. Goldin, A.L. Mechanisms of sodium channel inactivation. *Curr. Opin. Neurobiol.* **2003**, *13*, 284–290. [CrossRef]
55. Shen, H.; Liu, D.; Wu, K.; Lei, J.; Yan, N. Structures of human $Na_V1.7$ channel in complex with auxiliary subunits and animal toxins. *Science* **2019**, *363*, 1303–1308. [CrossRef]
56. Deuis, J.R.; Mueller, A.; Israel, M.R.; Vetter, I. The pharmacology of voltage-gated sodium channel activators. *Neuropharmacology* **2017**, *127*, 87–108. [CrossRef] [PubMed]
57. Zhang, A.H.; Sharma, G.; Undheim, E.A.B.; Jia, X.; Mobli, M. A complicated complex: Ion channels, voltage sensing, cell membranes and peptide inhibitors. *Neurosci. Lett.* **2018**. [CrossRef] [PubMed]
58. Xu, H.; Li, T.; Rohou, A.; Arthur, C.P.; Tzakoniati, F.; Wong, E.; Estevez, A.; Kugel, C.; Franke, Y.; Chen, J. Structural basis of $Na_V1.7$ inhibition by a gating-modifier spider toxin. *Cell* **2019**, *176*, 702–715. [CrossRef] [PubMed]
59. Schmidt-Hieber, C.; Bischofberger, J. Fast sodium channel gating supports localized and efficient axonal action potential initiation. *J. Neurosci.* **2010**, *30*, 10233–10242. [CrossRef] [PubMed]
60. Capes, D.L.; Goldschen-Ohm, M.P.; Arcisio-Miranda, M.; Bezanilla, F.; Chanda, B. Domain IV voltage-sensor movement is both sufficient and rate limiting for fast inactivation in sodium channels. *J. Gen. Physiol.* **2013**, *142*, 101–112. [CrossRef] [PubMed]
61. Deuis, J.R.; Dekan, Z.; Wingerd, J.S.; Smith, J.J.; Munasinghe, N.R.; Bhola, R.F.; Imlach, W.L.; Herzig, V.; Armstrong, D.A.; Rosengren, K.J. Pharmacological characterisation of the highly $Na_V1.7$ selective spider venom peptide Pn3a. *Sci. Rep.* **2017**, *7*, 40883. [CrossRef]
62. Kozlov, S. Animal toxins for channelopathy treatment. *Neuropharmacology* **2018**, *132*, 83–97. [CrossRef]
63. King, G.F. Tying pest insects in knots: The deployment of spider-venom-derived knottins as bioinsecticides. *Pest Manage. Sci.* **2019**, *75*, 2437–2445. [CrossRef]
64. Moore, S.J.; Leung, C.L.; Cochran, J.R. Knottins: Disulfide-bonded therapeutic and diagnostic peptides. *Drug Discov. Today Technol.* **2012**, *9*, e3–e11. [CrossRef]
65. Le Nguyen, D.; Heitz, A.; Chiche, L.; Castro, B.; Boigegrain, R.A.; Favel, A.; Coletti-Previero, M.A. Molecular recognition between serine proteases and new bioactive microproteins with a knotted structure. *Biochimie* **1990**, *72*, 431–435. [CrossRef]
66. McDonald, N.Q.; Lapatto, R.; Murray-Rust, J.; Gunning, J.; Wlodawer, A.; Blundell, T.L. New protein fold revealed by a 2.3-Å resolution crystal structure of nerve growth factor. *Nature* **1991**, *354*, 411–414. [CrossRef] [PubMed]
67. McDonald, N.Q.; Hendrickson, W.A. A structural superfamily of growth factors containing a cystine knot motif. *Cell* **1993**, *73*, 421–424. [CrossRef]

68. Pallaghy, P.K.; Nielsen, K.J.; Craik, D.J.; Norton, R.S. A common structural motif incorporating a cystine knot and a triple-stranded β-sheet in toxic and inhibitory polypeptides. *Protein Sci.* **1994**, *3*, 1833–1839. [CrossRef] [PubMed]
69. Postic, G.; Gracy, J.; Périn, C.; Chiche, L.; Gelly, J.-C. KNOTTIN: The database of inhibitor cystine knot scaffold after 10 years, toward a systematic structure modeling. *Nucleic Acids Res.* **2017**, *46*, D454–D458. [CrossRef] [PubMed]
70. Craik, D.J.; Daly, N.L.; Waine, C. The cystine knot motif in toxins and implications for drug design. *Toxicon* **2001**, *39*, 43–60. [CrossRef]
71. Saez, N.J.; Senff, S.; Jensen, J.E.; Er, S.Y.; Herzig, V.; Rash, L.D.; King, G.F. Spider-venom peptides as therapeutics. *Toxins* **2010**, *2*, 2851–2871. [CrossRef] [PubMed]
72. Agwa, A.J.; Huang, Y.H.; Craik, D.J.; Henriques, S.T.; Schroeder, C.I. Lengths of the C-terminus and interconnecting loops impact stability of spider-derived gating modifier toxins. *Toxins* **2017**, *9*, 248. [CrossRef]
73. Bosmans, F.; Rash, L.; Zhu, S.; Diochot, S.; Lazdunski, M.; Escoubas, P.; Tytgat, J. Four novel tarantula toxins as selective modulators of voltage-gated sodium channel subtypes. *Mol. Pharmacol.* **2006**, *69*, 419–429. [CrossRef]
74. Wang, J.M.; Roh, S.H.; Kim, S.; Lee, C.W.; Kim, J.I.; Swartz, K.J. Molecular surface of tarantula toxins interacting with voltage sensors in K_v channels. *J. Gen. Physiol.* **2004**, *123*, 455–467. [CrossRef]
75. Lawrence, N.; Wu, B.; Ligutti, J.; Cheneval, O.; Agwa, A.J.; Benfield, A.H.; Biswas, K.; Craik, D.J.; Miranda, L.P.; Henriques, S.T. Peptide-membrane interactions affect the inhibitory potency and selectivity of spider toxins ProTx-II and GpTx-1. *ACS Chem. Biol.* **2018**, *14*, 118–130. [CrossRef]
76. Murray, J.K.; Ligutti, J.; Liu, D.; Zou, A.; Poppe, L.; Li, H.; Andrews, K.L.; Moyer, B.D.; McDonough, S.I.; Favreau, P. Engineering potent and selective analogues of GpTx-1, a tarantula venom peptide antagonist of the $Na_V1.7$ sodium channel. *J. Med. Chem.* **2015**, *58*, 2299–2314. [CrossRef] [PubMed]
77. Smith, J.J.; Cummins, T.R.; Alphy, S.; Blumenthal, K.M. Molecular interactions of the gating modifier toxin, ProTx-II, with $Na_V1.5$: Implied existence of a novel toxin binding site coupled to activation. *J. Biol. Chem.* **2007**. [CrossRef] [PubMed]
78. Liu, Y.; Li, D.; Wu, Z.; Li, J.; Nie, D.; Xiang, Y.; Liu, Z. A positively charged surface patch is important for hainantoxin-IV binding to voltage-gated sodium channels. *J. Pept. Sci.* **2012**, *18*, 643–649. [CrossRef] [PubMed]
79. Luo, J.; Zhang, Y.; Gong, M.; Lu, S.; Ma, Y.; Zeng, X.; Liang, S. Molecular surface of JZTX-V (β-Theraphotoxin-Cj2a) interacting with voltage-gated sodium channel subtype $Na_V1.4$. *Toxins* **2014**, *6*, 2177–2193. [CrossRef] [PubMed]
80. Cardoso, F.C.; Dekan, Z.; Rosengren, K.J.; Erickson, A.; Vetter, I.; Deuis, J.; Herzig, V.; Alewood, P.; King, G.F.; Lewis, R.J. Identification and characterization of ProTx-III [μ-TRTX-Tp1a], a new voltage-gated sodium channel inhibitor from venom of the tarantula *Thrixopelma pruriens*. *Mol. Pharmacol.* **2015**, *88*, 291–303. [CrossRef]
81. Klint, J.K.; Chin, Y.K.; Mobli, M. Rational engineering defines a molecular switch that is essential for activity of spider-venom peptides against the analgesics target $Na_V1.7$. *Mol. Pharmacol.* **2015**, *88*, 1002–1010. [CrossRef]
82. Henriques, S.T.; Deplazes, E.; Lawrence, N.; Cheneval, O.; Chaousis, S.; Inserra, M.; Thongyoo, P.; King, G.F.; Mark, A.E.; Vetter, I.; et al. Interaction of tarantula venom peptide ProTx-II with lipid membranes is a prerequisite for its inhibition of human voltage-gated sodium channel $Na_V1.7$. *J. Biol. Chem.* **2016**, *291*, 17049–17065. [CrossRef]
83. Minassian, N.A.; Gibbs, A.; Shih, A.Y.; Liu, Y.; Neff, R.A.; Sutton, S.W.; Mirzadegan, T.; Connor, J.; Fellows, R.; Husovsky, M. Analysis of the structural and molecular basis of voltage-sensitive sodium channel inhibition by the spider toxin huwentoxin-IV (μ-TRTX-Hh2a). *J. Biol. Chem.* **2013**, *288*, 22707–22720. [CrossRef]
84. The UniProt Consortium. UniProt: A worldwide hub of protein knowledge. *Nucleic Acids Res.* **2018**, *47*, D506–D515. [CrossRef]
85. Li, D.; Xiao, Y.; Xu, X.; Xiong, X.; Lu, S.; Liu, Z.; Zhu, Q.; Wang, M.; Gu, X.; Liang, S. Structure-activity relationships of hainantoxin-IV and structure determination of active and inactive sodium channel blockers. *J. Biol. Chem.* **2004**, *279*, 37734–37740. [CrossRef]
86. Agwa, A.J.; Peigneur, S.; Chow, C.Y.; Lawrence, N.; Craik, D.J.; Tytgat, J.; King, G.F.; Henriques, S.T.; Schroeder, C.I. Gating modifier toxins isolated from spider venom: Modulation of voltage-gated sodium channels and the role of lipid membranes. *J. Biol. Chem.* **2018**, *293*, 9041–9052. [CrossRef] [PubMed]

87. Fontana, M.; Vital-Brazil, O. Mode of action of *Phoneutria nigriventer* spider venom at the isolated phrenic nerve-diaphragm of the rat. *Braz. J. Med. Biol. Res.* **1985**, *18*, 557–565. [PubMed]
88. Rezende, L., Jr.; Cordeiro, M.N.; Oliveira, E.B.; Diniz, C.R. Isolation of neurotoxic peptides from the venom of the 'armed'spider *Phoneutria nigriventer*. *Toxicon* **1991**, *29*, 1225–1233. [CrossRef]
89. Arújo, D.A.; Cordeiro, M.N.; Diniz, C.R.; Beirão, P.S. Effects of a toxic fraction, PhTx 2, from the spider *Phoneutria nigriventer* on the sodium current. *Naunyn Schmiedeberg's Arch. Pharmacol.* **1993**, *347*, 205–208. [CrossRef] [PubMed]
90. Adams, M.E.; Herold, E.E.; Venema, V.J. Two classes of channel-specific toxins from funnel web spider venom. *J. Comp. Physiol. A Neuroethol. Sen. Neural. Behav. Physiol.* **1989**, *164*, 333–342. [CrossRef] [PubMed]
91. Tang, C.; Zhou, X.; Huang, Y.; Zhang, Y.; Hu, Z.; Wang, M.; Chen, P.; Liu, Z.; Liang, S. The tarantula toxin jingzhaotoxin-XI (κ-theraphotoxin-Cj1a) regulates the activation and inactivation of the voltage-gated sodium channel $Na_V1.5$. *Toxicon* **2014**, *92*, 6–13. [CrossRef]
92. Cardoso, F.C.; Dekan, Z.; Smith, J.J.; Deuis, J.R.; Vetter, I.; Herzig, V.; Alewood, P.F.; King, G.F.; Lewis, R.J. Modulatory features of the novel spider toxin μ-TRTX-Df1a isolated from the venom of the spider *Davus fasciatus*. *Br. J. Pharmacol.* **2017**, *174*, 2528–2544. [CrossRef]
93. Matavel, A.; Cruz, J.S.; Penaforte, C.L.; Araújo, D.A.; Kalapothakis, E.; Prado, V.F.; Diniz, C.R.; Cordeiro, M.N.; Beirão, P.S. Electrophysiological characterization and molecular identification of the *Phoneutria nigriventer* peptide toxin PnTx2-6 1. *FEBS Lett.* **2002**, *523*, 219–223. [CrossRef]
94. Nicholson, G.M.; Little, M.J.; Tyler, M.; Narahashi, T. Selective alteration of sodium channel gating by Australian funnel-web spider toxins. *Toxicon* **1996**, *34*, 1443–1453. [CrossRef]
95. Little, M.J.; Zappia, C.; Gilles, N.; Connor, M.; Tyler, M.I.; Martin-Eauclaire, M.-F.; Gordon, D.; Nicholson, G.M. δ-Atracotoxins from Australian funnel-web spiders compete with scorpion α-toxin binding but differentially modulate alkaloid toxin activation of voltage-gated sodium channels. *J. Biol. Chem.* **1998**, *273*, 27076–27083. [CrossRef]
96. Nicholson, G.M.; Walsh, R.; Little, M.J.; Tyler, M.I. Characterisation of the effects of robustoxin, the lethal neurotoxin from the Sydney funnel-web spider *Atrax robustus*, on sodium channel activation and inactivation. *Pflügers Archiv* **1998**, *436*, 117–126. [CrossRef] [PubMed]
97. Szeto, T.H.; Birinyi-Strachan, L.C.; Smith, R.; Connor, M.; Christie, M.J.; King, G.F.; Nicholson, G.M. Isolation and pharmacological characterisation of δ-atracotoxin-Hv1b, a vertebrate-selective sodium channel toxin. *FEBS Lett.* **2000**, *470*, 293–299. [CrossRef]
98. Huang, Y.; Zhou, X.; Tang, C.; Zhang, Y.; Tao, H.; Chen, P.; Liu, Z. Molecular basis of the inhibition of the fast inactivation of voltage-gated sodium channel $Na_V1.5$ by tarantula toxin Jingzhaotoxin-II. *Peptides* **2015**, *68*, 175–182. [CrossRef] [PubMed]
99. Nicholson, G.M.; Willow, M.; Howden, M.E.; Narahashi, T. Modification of sodium channel gating and kinetics by versutoxin from the Australian funnel-web spider *Hadronyche versuta*. *Pflügers Archiv* **1994**, *428*, 400–409. [CrossRef] [PubMed]
100. Tao, H.; Chen, X.; Lu, M.; Wu, Y.; Deng, M.; Zeng, X.; Liu, Z.; Liang, S. Molecular determinant for the tarantula toxin Jingzhaotoxin-I slowing the fast inactivation of voltage-gated sodium channels. *Toxicon* **2016**, *111*, 13–21. [CrossRef] [PubMed]
101. Xiao, Y.; Tang, J.; Hu, W.; Xie, J.; Maertens, C.; Tytgat, J.; Liang, S. Jingzhaotoxin-I, a novel spider neurotoxin preferentially inhibiting cardiac sodium channel inactivation. *J. Biol. Chem.* **2005**, *280*, 12069–12076. [CrossRef] [PubMed]
102. Xiao, Y.; Li, J.; Deng, M.; Dai, C.; Liang, S. Characterization of the excitatory mechanism induced by Jingzhaotoxin-I inhibiting sodium channel inactivation. *Toxicon* **2007**, *50*, 507–517. [CrossRef]
103. Middleton, R.E.; Warren, V.A.; Kraus, R.L.; Hwang, J.C.; Liu, C.J.; Dai, G.; Brochu, R.M.; Kohler, M.G.; Gao, Y.-D.; Garsky, V.M. Two tarantula peptides inhibit activation of multiple sodium channels. *Biochemistry* **2002**, *41*, 14734–14747. [CrossRef]
104. Xiao, Y.; Blumenthal, K.M.; Jackson, J.O.; Liang, S.; Cummins, T.R. The tarantula toxins ProTx-II and HwTX-IV differentially interact with human $Na_V1.7$ voltage-sensors to inhibit channel activation and inactivation. *Mol. Pharmacol.* **2010**, *78*, 1124–1134. [CrossRef]
105. Xiao, Y.; Tang, J.; Yang, Y.; Wang, M.; Hu, W.; Xie, J.; Zeng, X.; Liang, S. Jingzhaotoxin-III, a novel spider toxin inhibiting activation of voltage-gated sodium channel in rat cardiac myocytes. *J. Biol. Chem.* **2004**, *279*, 26220–26226. [CrossRef]

106. Rong, M.; Chen, J.; Tao, H.; Wu, Y.; Jiang, P.; Lu, M.; Su, H.; Chi, Y.; Cai, T.; Zhao, L. Molecular basis of the tarantula toxin jingzhaotoxin-III (β-TRTX-Cj1α) interacting with voltage sensors in sodium channel subtype $Na_V1.5$. *FASEB J.* **2011**, *25*, 3177–3185. [CrossRef] [PubMed]
107. Zeng, X.; Deng, M.; Lin, Y.; Yuan, C.; Pi, J.; Liang, S. Isolation and characterization of Jingzhaotoxin-V, a novel neurotoxin from the venom of the spider *Chilobrachys jingzhao*. *Toxicon* **2007**, *49*, 388–399. [CrossRef] [PubMed]
108. Deng, M.; Kuang, F.; Sun, Z.; Tao, H.; Cai, T.; Zhong, L.; Chen, Z.; Xiao, Y.; Liang, S. Jingzhaotoxin-IX, a novel gating modifier of both sodium and potassium channels from Chinese tarantula *Chilobrachys jingzhao*. *Neuropharmacology* **2009**, *57*, 77–87. [CrossRef] [PubMed]
109. Nikolsky, A.; Billen, B.; Vassilevski, A.; Filkin, S.Y.; Tytgat, J.; Grishin, E. Voltage-gated sodium channels are targets for toxins from the venom of the spider *Heriaeus melloteei*. *Biochem. Moscow Suppl. Ser. A* **2009**, *3*, 245–253. [CrossRef]
110. Sousa, S.R.; Wingerd, J.S.; Brust, A.; Bladen, C.; Ragnarsson, L.; Herzig, V.; Deuis, J.R.; Dutertre, S.; Vetter, I.; Zamponi, G.W. Discovery and mode of action of a novel analgesic β-toxin from the African spider *Ceratogyrus darlingi*. *PLoS ONE* **2017**, *12*, e0182848. [CrossRef] [PubMed]
111. Wingerd, J.S.; Mozar, C.A.; Ussing, C.A.; Murali, S.S.; Chin, Y.K.; Cristofori-Armstrong, B.; Durek, T.; Gilchrist, J.; Vaughan, C.W.; Bosmans, F.; et al. The tarantula toxin β/δ-TRTX-Pre1a highlights the importance of the S1-S2 voltage-sensor region for sodium channel subtype selectivity. *Sci. Rep.* **2017**, *7*, 974. [CrossRef]
112. Wei, P.; Xu, C.; Wu, Q.; Huang, L.; Liang, S.; Yuan, C. Jingzhaotoxin-35, a novel gating-modifier toxin targeting both $Na_V1.5$ and $K_V2.1$ channels. *Toxicon* **2014**, *92*, 90–96. [CrossRef]
113. Peng, K.; Shu, Q.; Liu, Z.; Liang, S. Function and solution structure of huwentoxin-IV, a potent neuronal tetrodotoxin (TTX)-sensitive sodium channel antagonist from Chinese bird spider *Selenocosmia huwena*. *J. Biol. Chem.* **2002**, *277*, 47564–47571. [CrossRef]
114. Xiao, Y.; Bingham, J.-P.; Zhu, W.; Moczydlowski, E.; Liang, S.; Cummins, T.R. Tarantula huwentoxin-IV inhibits neuronal sodium channels by binding to receptor site 4 and trapping the domain II voltage sensor in the closed configuration. *J. Biol. Chem.* **2008**, *283*, 27300–27313. [CrossRef]
115. Deng, M.; Luo, X.; Jiang, L.; Chen, H.; Wang, J.; He, H.; Liang, S. Synthesis and biological characterization of synthetic analogs of Huwentoxin-IV (μ-theraphotoxin-Hh2a), a neuronal tetrodotoxin-sensitive sodium channel inhibitor. *Toxicon* **2013**, *71*, 57–65. [CrossRef]
116. Xiao, Y.; Liang, S. Inhibition of neuronal tetrodotoxin-sensitive Na^+ channels by two spider toxins: Hainantoxin-III and hainantoxin-IV. *Eur. J. Pharmacol.* **2003**, *477*, 1–7. [CrossRef]
117. Liu, Z.; Cai, T.; Zhu, Q.; Deng, M.; Li, J.; Zhou, X.; Zhang, F.; Li, D.; Li, J.; Liu, Y. Structure and function of Hainantoxin-III-a selective antagonist of neuronal tetrodotoxin-sensitive voltage-gated sodium channels isolated from the Chinese bird spider *Ornithoctonus hainana*. *J. Biol. Chem.* **2013**, *288*, 20392–20403. [CrossRef] [PubMed]
118. Chen, J.; Zhang, Y.; Rong, M.; Zhao, L.; Jiang, L.; Zhang, D.; Wang, M.; Xiao, Y.; Liang, S. Expression and characterization of jingzhaotoxin-34, a novel neurotoxin from the venom of the tarantula *Chilobrachys jingzhao*. *Peptides* **2009**, *30*, 1042–1048. [CrossRef] [PubMed]
119. Zeng, X.; Li, P.; Chen, B.; Huang, J.; Lai, R.; Liu, J.; Rong, M. Selective closed-state $Na_V1.7$ blocker JZTX-34 exhibits analgesic effects against pain. *Toxins* **2018**, *10*, 64. [CrossRef] [PubMed]
120. Billen, B.; Vassilevski, A.; Nikolsky, A.; Tytgat, J.; Grishin, E. Two novel sodium channel inhibitors from *Heriaeus melloteei* spider venom differentially interacting with mammalian channel's isoforms. *Toxicon* **2008**, *52*, 309–317. [CrossRef] [PubMed]
121. Klint, J.K.; Smith, J.J.; Vetter, I.; Rupasinghe, D.B.; Er, S.Y.; Senff, S.; Herzig, V.; Mobli, M.; Lewis, R.J.; Bosmans, F. Seven novel modulators of the analgesic target $Na_V1.7$ uncovered using a high-throughput venom-based discovery approach. *Br. J. Pharmacol.* **2015**, *172*, 2445–2458. [CrossRef] [PubMed]
122. Deuis, J.R.; Wingerd, J.S.; Winter, Z.; Durek, T.; Dekan, Z.; Sousa, S.R.; Zimmermann, K.; Hoffmann, T.; Weidner, C.; Nassar, M.A. Analgesic effects of GpTx-1, PF-04856264 and CNV1014802 in a mouse model of $Na_V1.7$-mediated pain. *Toxins* **2016**, *8*, 78. [CrossRef]
123. Meng, P.; Huang, H.; Wang, G.; Yang, S.; Lu, Q.; Liu, J.; Lai, R.; Rong, M. A novel toxin from *Haplopelma lividum* selectively inhibits the $Na_V1.8$ channel and possesses potent analgesic efficacy. *Toxins* **2017**, *9*, 7. [CrossRef]

124. Martin-Moutot, N.; Mansuelle, P.; Alcaraz, G.; Gouvea dos Santos, R.; Cordeiro, M.N.; De Lima, M.E.; Seagar, M.; van Renterghem, C. *Phoneutria nigriventer* toxin 1: A novel, state-dependent inhibitor of neuronal sodium channels which interacts with micro conotoxin binding sites. *Mol. Pharmacol.* **2006**, *69*, 1931–1937. [CrossRef]
125. Zhang, J.; Tang, D.; Liu, S.; Hu, H.; Liang, S.; Tang, C.; Liu, Z. Purification and characterization of JZTx-14, a potent antagonist of mammalian and prokaryotic voltage-gated sodium channels. *Toxins* **2018**, *10*, 408. [CrossRef]
126. Paiva, A.L.; Matavel, A.; Peigneur, S.; Cordeiro, M.N.; Tytgat, J.; Diniz, M.R.; de Lima, M.E. Differential effects of the recombinant toxin PnTx4(5-5) from the spider *Phoneutria nigriventer* on mammalian and insect sodium channels. *Biochimie* **2016**, *121*, 326–335. [CrossRef] [PubMed]
127. Liu, Y.; Tang, J.; Zhang, Y.; Xun, X.; Tang, D.; Peng, D.; Yi, J.; Liu, Z.; Shi, X. Synthesis and analgesic effects of μ-TRTX-Hhn1b on models of inflammatory and neuropathic pain. *Toxins* **2014**, *6*, 2363–2378. [CrossRef] [PubMed]
128. King, G.F.; Escoubas, P.; Nicholson, G.M. Peptide toxins that selectively target insect Na_V and Ca_V channels. *Channels* **2008**, *2*, 100–116. [CrossRef] [PubMed]
129. Cai, T.; Luo, J.; Meng, E.; Ding, J.; Liang, S.; Wang, S.; Liu, Z. Mapping the interaction site for the tarantula toxin hainantoxin-IV (β-TRTX-Hn2a) in the voltage sensor module of domain II of voltage-gated sodium channels. *Peptides* **2015**, *68*, 148–156. [CrossRef]
130. Cestele, S.; Qu, Y.; Rogers, J.C.; Rochat, H.; Scheuer, T.; Catterall, W.A. Voltage sensor-trapping: Enhanced activation of sodium channels by β-scorpion toxin bound to the S3-S4 loop in domain II. *Neuron* **1998**, *21*, 919–931. [CrossRef]
131. Swartz, K.J.; MacKinnon, R. Mapping the receptor site for hanatoxin, a gating modifier of voltage-dependent K^+ channels. *Neuron* **1997**, *18*, 675–682. [CrossRef]
132. Schmalhofer, W.; Calhoun, J.; Burrows, R.; Bailey, T.; Kohler, M.G.; Weinglass, A.B.; Kaczorowski, G.J.; Garcia, M.L.; Koltzenburg, M.; Priest, B.T. ProTx-II, a selective inhibitor of $Na_V1.7$ sodium channels, blocks action potential propagation in nociceptors. *Mol. Pharmacol.* **2008**, *74*, 1476–1484. [CrossRef]
133. Corzo, G.; Gilles, N.; Satake, H.; Villegas, E.; Dai, L.; Nakajima, T.; Haupt, J. Distinct primary structures of the major peptide toxins from the venom of the spider *Macrothele gigas* that bind to sites 3 and 4 in the sodium channel. *FEBS Lett.* **2003**, *547*, 43–50. [CrossRef]
134. Winterfield, J.R.; Swartz, K.J. A hot spot for the interaction of gating modifier toxins with voltage-dependent ion channels. *J. Gen. Physiol.* **2000**, *116*, 637–644. [CrossRef]
135. Gonçalves, T.C.; Benoit, E.; Partiseti, M.; Servent, D. The $Na_V1.7$ Channel subtype as an antinociceptive target for spider toxins in adult dorsal root ganglia neurons. *Front. Pharmacol.* **2018**, *9*. [CrossRef]
136. Shcherbatko, A.; Ono, F.; Mandel, G.; Brehm, P. Voltage-dependent sodium channel function is regulated through membrane mechanics. *Biophys. J.* **1999**, *77*, 1945–1959. [CrossRef]
137. Agwa, A.J.; Lawrence, N.; Deplazes, E.; Cheneval, O.; Chen, R.M.; Craik, D.J.; Schroeder, C.I.; Henriques, S.T. Spider peptide toxin HwTx-IV engineered to bind to lipid membranes has an increased inhibitory potency at human voltage-gated sodium channel $hNa_V1.7$. *Biochim. Biophys. Acta* **2017**, *1859*, 835–844. [CrossRef] [PubMed]
138. Hung, A.; Kuyucak, S.; Schroeder, C.I.; Kaas, Q. Modelling the interactions between animal venom peptides and membrane proteins. *Neuropharmacology* **2017**, *127*, 20–31. [CrossRef] [PubMed]
139. Agwa, A.J.; Henriques, S.T.; Schroeder, C.I. Gating modifier toxin interactions with ion channels and lipid bilayers: Is the trimolecular complex real? *Neuropharmacology* **2017**, *127*, 32–45. [CrossRef]
140. Deplazes, E.; Henriques, S.T.; Smith, J.J.; King, G.F.; Craik, D.J.; Mark, A.E.; Schroeder, C.I. Membrane-binding properties of gating modifier and pore-blocking toxins: Membrane interaction is not a prerequisite for modification of channel gating. *Biochim. Biophys. Acta* **2016**, *1858*, 872–882. [CrossRef]
141. Flinspach, M.; Xu, Q.; Piekarz, A.; Fellows, R.; Hagan, R.; Gibbs, A.; Liu, Y.; Neff, R.; Freedman, J.; Eckert, W. Insensitivity to pain induced by a potent selective closed-state $Na_V1.7$ inhibitor. *Sci. Rep.* **2017**, *7*, 39662. [CrossRef]
142. Revell, J.D.; Lund, P.-E.; Linley, J.E.; Metcalfe, J.; Burmeister, N.; Sridharan, S.; Jones, C.; Jermutus, L.; Bednarek, M.A. Potency optimization of Huwentoxin-IV on $hNa_V1.7$: A neurotoxin TTX-S sodium-channel antagonist from the venom of the Chinese bird-eating spider *Selenocosmia huwena*. *Peptides* **2013**, *44*, 40–46. [CrossRef]

143. Rahnama, S.; Deuis, J.R.; Cardoso, F.C.; Ramanujam, V.; Lewis, R.J.; Rash, L.D.; King, G.F.; Vetter, I.; Mobli, M. The structure, dynamics and selectivity profile of a $Na_V1.7$ potency-optimised huwentoxin-IV variant. *PLoS ONE* **2017**, *12*, e0173551. [CrossRef]
144. Shcherbatko, A.; Rossi, A.; Foletti, D.; Zhu, G.; Bogin, O.; Galindo Casas, M.; Rickert, M.; Hasa-Moreno, A.; Bartsevich, V.; Crameri, A.; et al. Engineering highly potent and selective microproteins against $Na_V1.7$ sodium channel for treatment of Pain. *J. Biol. Chem.* **2016**, *291*, 13974–13986. [CrossRef]
145. Li, D.; Xiao, Y.; Hu, W.; Xie, J.; Bosmans, F.; Tytgat, J.; Liang, S. Function and solution structure of hainantoxin-I, a novel insect sodium channel inhibitor from the Chinese bird spider *Selenocosmia hainana*. *FEBS Lett.* **2003**, *555*, 616–622. [CrossRef]
146. Mueller, A.; Starobova, H.; Morgan, M.; Dekan, Z.; Cheneval, O.; Schroeder, C.I.; Alewood, P.F.; Deuis, J.R.; Vetter, I. Anti-allodynic effects of the selective $Na_V1.7$ inhibitor Pn3a in a mouse model of acute post-surgical pain: Evidence for analgesic synergy with opioids and baclofen. *Pain* **2019**, *160*, 1766–1780. [CrossRef] [PubMed]
147. Peigneur, S.; Paiva, A.; Cordeiro, M.; Borges, M.; Diniz, M.; de Lima, M.; Tytgat, J. *Phoneutria nigriventer* Spider Toxin PnTx2-1 (δ-Ctenitoxin-Pn1a) Is a Modulator of Sodium Channel Gating. *Toxins* **2018**, *10*, 337. [CrossRef] [PubMed]
148. Bosmans, F.; Martin-Eauclaire, M.-F.; Swartz, K.J. Deconstructing voltage sensor function and pharmacology in sodium channels. *Nature* **2008**, *456*, 202–208. [CrossRef] [PubMed]
149. Xiao, Y.; Jackson, J.O.; Liang, S.; Cummins, T.R. Common molecular determinants of tarantula huwentoxin-IV inhibition of Na^+ channel voltage-sensors in domains II and IV. *J. Biol. Chem.* **2011**, *286*, 27301–27310. [CrossRef]
150. Bosmans, F.; Milescu, M.; Swartz, K.J. Palmitoylation influences the function and pharmacology of sodium channels. *Proc. Natl. Acad. Sci. USA* **2011**, *108*, 20213–20218. [CrossRef]
151. Kanellopoulos, A.H.; Matsuyama, A. Voltage-gated sodium channels and pain-related disorders. *Clin. Sci. (Lond.)* **2016**, *130*, 2257–2265. [CrossRef]
152. Dib-Hajj, S.D.; Geha, P.; Waxman, S.G. Sodium channels in pain disorders: Pathophysiology and prospects for treatment. *Pain* **2017**, *158* (Suppl. 1), s97–s107. [CrossRef]
153. Vetter, I.; Deuis, J.R.; Mueller, A.; Israel, M.R.; Starobova, H.; Zhang, A.; Rash, L.D.; Mobli, M. $Na_V1.7$ as a pain target–from gene to pharmacology. *Pharmacol. Ther.* **2017**, *172*, 73–100. [CrossRef]
154. Dib-Hajj, S.D.; Cummins, T.R.; Black, J.A.; Waxman, S.G. Sodium channels in normal and pathological pain. *Annu. Rev. Neurosci.* **2010**, *33*, 325–347. [CrossRef]
155. Leipold, E.; Liebmann, L.; Korenke, G.C.; Heinrich, T.; Giesselmann, S.; Baets, J.; Ebbinghaus, M.; Goral, R.O.; Stodberg, T.; Hennings, J.C.; et al. A *de novo* gain-of-function mutation in SCN11A causes loss of pain perception. *Nat. Genet.* **2013**, *45*, 1399–1404. [CrossRef]
156. Chen, H.P.; Zhou, W.; Kang, L.M.; Yan, H.; Zhang, L.; Xu, B.H.; Cai, W.H. Intrathecal miR-96 inhibits $Na_V1.3$ expression and alleviates neuropathic pain in rat following chronic construction injury. *Neurochem. Res.* **2014**, *39*, 76–83. [CrossRef] [PubMed]
157. Su, S.; Shao, J.; Zhao, Q.; Ren, X.; Cai, W.; Li, L.; Bai, Q.; Chen, X.; Xu, B.; Wang, J.; et al. MiR-30b Attenuates neuropathic pPain by regulating voltage-gated sodium channel $Na_V1.3$ in Rats. *Front. Mol. Neurosci.* **2017**, *10*, 126. [CrossRef] [PubMed]
158. Faber, C.G.; Hoeijmakers, J.G.; Ahn, H.S.; Cheng, X.; Han, C.; Choi, J.S.; Estacion, M.; Lauria, G.; Vanhoutte, E.K.; Gerrits, M.M.; et al. Gain of function $Na_V1.7$ mutations in idiopathic small fiber neuropathy. *Ann. Neurol.* **2012**, *71*, 26–39. [CrossRef] [PubMed]
159. Dib-Hajj, S.D.; Black, J.A.; Waxman, S.G. Voltage-gated sodium channels: Therapeutic targets for pain. *Pain Med.* **2009**, *10*, 1260–1269. [CrossRef]
160. Deuis, J.R.; Zimmermann, K.; Romanovsky, A.A.; Possani, L.D.; Cabot, P.J.; Lewis, R.J.; Vetter, I. An animal model of oxaliplatin-induced cold allodynia reveals a crucial role for $Na_V1.6$ in peripheral pain pathways. *Pain* **2013**, *154*, 1749–1757. [CrossRef]
161. Qin, S.; Jiang, F.; Zhou, Y.; Zhou, G.; Ye, P.; Ji, Y. Local knockdown of $Na_V1.6$ relieves pain behaviors induced by BmK I. *Acta Biochim. Biophys. Sin.* **2017**, *49*, 713–721. [CrossRef]
162. Zhao, P.; Barr, T.P.; Hou, Q.; Dib-Hajj, S.D.; Black, J.A.; Albrecht, P.J.; Petersen, K.; Eisenberg, E.; Wymer, J.P.; Rice, F.L.; et al. Voltage-gated sodium channel expression in rat and human epidermal keratinocytes: Evidence for a role in pain. *Pain* **2008**, *139*, 90–105. [CrossRef]

163. Catterall, W.A.; Goldin, A.L.; Waxman, S.G. International Union of Pharmacology. XLVII. Nomenclature and structure-function relationships of voltage-gated sodium channels. *Pharmacol. Rev.* **2005**, *57*, 397–409. [CrossRef]
164. Erickson, A.; Deiteren, A.; Harrington, A.M.; Garcia-Caraballo, S.; Castro, J.; Caldwell, A.; Grundy, L.; Brierley, S.M. Voltage-gated sodium channels: (Na_V)igating the field to determine their contribution to visceral nociception. *J. Physiol.* **2018**, *596*, 785–807. [CrossRef]
165. Black, J.A.; Dib-Hajj, S.; McNabola, K.; Jeste, S.; Rizzo, M.A.; Kocsis, J.D.; Waxman, S.G. Spinal sensory neurons express multiple sodium channel α-subunit mRNAs. *Brain Res. Mol. Brain Res.* **1996**, *43*, 117–131. [CrossRef]
166. Wang, W.; Gu, J.; Li, Y.Q.; Tao, Y.X. Are voltage-gated sodium channels on the dorsal root ganglion involved in the development of neuropathic pain? *Mol. Pain* **2011**, *7*, 16. [CrossRef] [PubMed]
167. Fukuoka, T.; Kobayashi, K.; Yamanaka, H.; Obata, K.; Dai, Y.; Noguchi, K. Comparative study of the distribution of the α-subunits of voltage-gated sodium channels in normal and axotomized rat dorsal root ganglion neurons. *J. Comp. Neurol.* **2008**, *510*, 188–206. [CrossRef] [PubMed]
168. Hockley, J.R.; González-Cano, R.; McMurray, S.; Tejada-Giraldez, M.A.; McGuire, C.; Torres, A.; Wilbrey, A.L.; Cibert-Goton, V.; Nieto, F.R.; Pitcher, T. Visceral and somatic pain modalities reveal Na_V1.7-independent visceral nociceptive pathways. *J. Physiol.* **2017**, *595*, 2661–2679. [CrossRef] [PubMed]
169. Jay Gargus, J.; Tournay, A. Novel mutation confirms seizure locus SCN1A is also FHM3 migraine locus. *Pediatr. Neurol.* **2007**, *37*, 407–410. [CrossRef] [PubMed]
170. Gilchrist, J.; Dutton, S.; Diaz-Bustamante, M.; McPherson, A.; Olivares, N.; Kalia, J.; Escayg, A.; Bosmans, F. Na_V1.1 modulation by a novel triazole compound attenuates epileptic seizures in rodents. *ACS Chem. Biol.* **2014**, *9*, 1204–1212. [CrossRef] [PubMed]
171. Bosmans, F.; Kalia, J. Derivatives of rufinamide and their use in inhibtion of the activation of human voltage-gated sodium channels. US Patent 9,771,335, 26 September 2017.
172. Suter, M.R.; Kirschmann, G.; Laedermann, C.J.; Abriel, H.; Decosterd, I. Rufinamide attenuates mechanical allodynia in a model of neuropathic pain in the mouse and stabilizes voltage-gated sodium channel inactivated state. *Anesthesiology* **2013**, *118*, 160–172. [CrossRef]
173. Cummins, T.R.; Aglieco, F.; Renganathan, M.; Herzog, R.I.; Dib-Hajj, S.D.; Waxman, S.G. Na_V1.3 sodium channels: Rapid repriming and slow closed-state inactivation display quantitative differences after expression in a mammalian cell line and in spinal sensory neurons. *J. Neurosci.* **2001**, *21*, 5952–5961. [CrossRef]
174. Waxman, S.G.; Kocsis, J.D.; Black, J.A. Type III sodium channel mRNA is expressed in embryonic but not adult spinal sensory neurons, and is reexpressed following axotomy. *J. Neurophysiol.* **1994**, *72*, 466–470. [CrossRef]
175. Black, J.A.; Nikolajsen, L.; Kroner, K.; Jensen, T.S.; Waxman, S.G. Multiple sodium channel isoforms and mitogen-activated protein kinases are present in painful human neuromas. *Ann. Neurol.* **2008**, *64*, 644–653. [CrossRef]
176. Strege, P.R.; Knutson, K.; Eggers, S.J.; Li, J.H.; Wang, F.; Linden, D.; Szurszewski, J.H.; Milescu, L.; Leiter, A.B.; Farrugia, G.; et al. Sodium channel Na_V1.3 is important for enterochromaffin cell excitability and serotonin release. *Sci. Rep.* **2017**, *7*, 15650. [CrossRef]
177. Bellono, N.W.; Bayrer, J.R.; Leitch, D.B.; Castro, J.; Zhang, C.; O'Donnell, T.A.; Brierley, S.M.; Ingraham, H.A.; Julius, D. Enterochromaffin cells are gut chemosensors that couple to sensory neural pathways. *Cell* **2017**, *170*, 185–198. [CrossRef] [PubMed]
178. Black, J.A.; Cummins, T.R.; Plumpton, C.; Chen, Y.H.; Hormuzdiar, W.; Clare, J.J.; Waxman, S.G. Upregulation of a silent sodium channel after peripheral, but not central, nerve injury in DRG neurons. *J. Neurophysiol.* **1999**, *82*, 2776–2785. [CrossRef] [PubMed]
179. Kim, C.H.; Oh, Y.; Chung, J.M.; Chung, K. The changes in expression of three subtypes of TTX sensitive sodium channels in sensory neurons after spinal nerve ligation. *Mol. Brain Res.* **2001**, *95*, 153–161. [CrossRef]
180. Lindia, J.A.; Kohler, M.G.; Martin, W.J.; Abbadie, C. Relationship between sodium channel Na_V1.3 expression and neuropathic pain behavior in rats. *Pain* **2005**, *117*, 145–153. [CrossRef]
181. Hains, B.C.; Saab, C.Y.; Klein, J.P.; Craner, M.J.; Waxman, S.G. Altered sodium channel expression in second-order spinal sensory neurons contributes to pain after peripheral nerve injury. *J. Neurosci.* **2004**, *24*, 4832–4839. [CrossRef]

182. Xu, W.; Zhang, J.; Wang, Y.; Wang, L.; Wang, X. Changes in the expression of voltage-gated sodium channels $Na_V1.3$, $Na_V1.7$, $Na_V1.8$, and $Na_V1.9$ in rat trigeminal ganglia following chronic constriction injury. *Neuroreport* **2016**, *27*, 929–934. [CrossRef]
183. Black, J.A.; Liu, S.; Tanaka, M.; Cummins, T.R.; Waxman, S.G. Changes in the expression of tetrodotoxin-sensitive sodium channels within dorsal root ganglia neurons in inflammatory pain. *Pain* **2004**, *108*, 237–247. [CrossRef]
184. Hong, S.; Morrow, T.J.; Paulson, P.E.; Isom, L.L.; Wiley, J.W. Early painful diabetic neuropathy is associated with differential changes in tetrodotoxin-sensitive and -resistant sodium channels in dorsal root ganglion neurons in the rat. *J. Biol. Chem.* **2004**, *279*, 29341–29350. [CrossRef]
185. Tan, A.M.; Samad, O.A.; Dib-Hajj, S.D.; Waxman, S.G. Virus-mediated knockdown of $Na_V1.3$ in dorsal root ganglia of STZ-induced diabetic rats alleviates tactile allodynia. *Mol. Med.* **2015**, *21*, 544–552. [CrossRef]
186. Garry, E.M.; Delaney, A.; Anderson, H.A.; Sirinathsinghji, E.C.; Clapp, R.H.; Martin, W.J.; Kinchington, P.R.; Krah, D.L.; Abbadie, C.; Fleetwood-Walker, S.M. Varicella zoster virus induces neuropathic changes in rat dorsal root ganglia and behavioral reflex sensitisation that is attenuated by gabapentin or sodium channel blocking drugs. *Pain* **2005**, *118*, 97–111. [CrossRef]
187. Nassar, M.A.; Baker, M.D.; Levato, A.; Ingram, R.; Mallucci, G.; McMahon, S.B.; Wood, J.N. Nerve injury induces robust allodynia and ectopic discharges in $Na_V1.3$ null mutant mice. *Mol. Pain* **2006**, *2*, 33. [CrossRef] [PubMed]
188. O'Brien, J.E.; Meisler, M.H. Sodium channel SCN8A ($Na_V1.6$): Properties and *de novo* mutations in epileptic encephalopathy and intellectual disability. *Front. Genet.* **2013**, *4*, 213. [CrossRef] [PubMed]
189. Black, J.A.; Renganathan, M.; Waxman, S.G. Sodium channel $Na_V1.6$ is expressed along nonmyelinated axons and it contributes to conduction. *Brain Res. Mol. Brain Res.* **2002**, *105*, 19–28. [CrossRef]
190. Ramachandra, R.; Elmslie, K.S. EXPRESS: Voltage-dependent sodium (Na_V) channels in group IV sensory afferents. *Mol. Pain* **2016**, *12*. [CrossRef]
191. Persson, A.K.; Black, J.A.; Gasser, A.; Cheng, X.; Fischer, T.Z.; Waxman, S.G. Sodium-calcium exchanger and multiple sodium channel isoforms in intra-epidermal nerve terminals. *Mol. Pain* **2010**, *6*, 84. [CrossRef]
192. Kennedy, P.G.; Montague, P.; Scott, F.; Grinfeld, E.; Ashrafi, G.H.; Breuer, J.; Rowan, E.G. *Varicella-zoster* viruses associated with post-herpetic neuralgia induce sodium current density increases in the ND7-23 Na_V-1.8 neuroblastoma cell line. *PLoS ONE* **2013**, *8*, e51570. [CrossRef]
193. Ren, Y.-S.; Qian, N.-S.; Tang, Y.; Liao, Y.-H.; Yang, Y.-L.; Dou, K.-F.; Toi, M. Sodium channel $Na_V1.6$ is up-regulated in the dorsal root ganglia in a mouse model of type 2 diabetes. *Brain Res. Bull.* **2012**, *87*, 244–249. [CrossRef]
194. Grasso, G.; Landi, A.; Alafaci, C. A novel pathophysiological mechanism contributing to trigeminal neuralgia. *Mol. Med.* **2016**, *22*, 452–454. [CrossRef]
195. Tanaka, B.S.; Zhao, P.; Dib-Hajj, F.B.; Morisset, V.; Tate, S.; Waxman, S.G.; Dib-Hajj, S.D. A gain-of-function mutation in $Na_V1.6$ in a case of trigeminal neuralgia. *Mol. Med.* **2016**, *22*, 338–348. [CrossRef]
196. Israel, M.R.; Thongyoo, P.; Deuis, J.R.; Craik, D.J.; Vetter, I.; Durek, T. The E15R point mutation in scorpion toxin Cn2 uncouples its depressant and excitatory activities on human $Na_V1.6$. *J. Med. Chem.* **2018**, *61*, 1730–1736. [CrossRef]
197. Xie, W.; Strong, J.A.; Zhang, J.M. Local knockdown of the $Na_V1.6$ sodium channel reduces pain behaviors, sensory neuron excitability, and sympathetic sprouting in rat models of neuropathic pain. *Neuroscience* **2015**, *291*, 317–330. [CrossRef] [PubMed]
198. Xie, W.; Strong, J.A.; Ye, L.; Mao, J.X.; Zhang, J.M. Knockdown of sodium channel $Na_V1.6$ blocks mechanical pain and abnormal bursting activity of afferent neurons in inflamed sensory ganglia. *Pain* **2013**, *154*, 1170–1180. [CrossRef] [PubMed]
199. Dib-Hajj, S.D.; Yang, Y.; Black, J.A.; Waxman, S.G. The $Na_V1.7$ sodium channel: From molecule to man. *Nat. Rev. Neurosci.* **2013**, *14*, 49–62. [CrossRef] [PubMed]
200. Black, J.A.; Frézel, N.; Dib-Hajj, S.D.; Waxman, S.G. Expression of $Na_V1.7$ in DRG neurons extends from peripheral terminals in the skin to central preterminal branches and terminals in the dorsal horn. *Mol. Pain* **2012**, *8*, 82. [CrossRef] [PubMed]
201. Rush, A.M.; Cummins, T.R.; Waxman, S.G. Multiple sodium channels and their roles in electrogenesis within dorsal root ganglion neurons. *J. Physiol.* **2007**, *579*, 1–14. [CrossRef]

202. Herzog, R.I.; Cummins, T.R.; Ghassemi, F.; Dib-Hajj, S.D.; Waxman, S.G. Distinct repriming and closed-state inactivation kinetics of $Na_V1.6$ and $Na_V1.7$ sodium channels in mouse spinal sensory neurons. *J. Physiol.* **2003**, *551*, 741–750. [CrossRef]
203. Fertleman, C.R.; Baker, M.D.; Parker, K.A.; Moffatt, S.; Elmslie, F.V.; Abrahamsen, B.; Ostman, J.; Klugbauer, N.; Wood, J.N.; Gardiner, R.M.; et al. SCN9A mutations in paroxysmal extreme pain disorder: Allelic variants underlie distinct channel defects and phenotypes. *Neuron* **2006**, *52*, 767–774. [CrossRef]
204. Yang, Y.; Wang, Y.; Li, S.; Xu, Z.; Li, H.; Ma, L.; Fan, J.; Bu, D.; Liu, B.; Fan, Z.; et al. Mutations in SCN9A, encoding a sodium channel α subunit, in patients with primary erythermalgia. *J. Med. Genet.* **2004**, *41*, 171–174. [CrossRef]
205. Blesneac, I.; Themistocleous, A.C.; Fratter, C.; Conrad, L.J.; Ramirez, J.D.; Cox, J.J.; Tesfaye, S.; Shillo, P.R.; Rice, A.S.; Tucker, S.J. Rare $Na_V1.7$ variants associated with painful diabetic peripheral neuropathy. *Pain* **2018**, *159*, 469–480. [CrossRef]
206. Shields, S.D.; Ahn, H.S.; Yang, Y.; Han, C.; Seal, R.P.; Wood, J.N.; Waxman, S.G.; Dib-Hajj, S.D. $Na_V1.8$ expression is not restricted to nociceptors in mouse peripheral nervous system. *Pain* **2012**, *153*, 2017–2030. [CrossRef]
207. Akopian, A.N.; Sivilotti, L.; Wood, J.N. A tetrodotoxin-resistant voltage-gated sodium channel expressed by sensory neurons. *Nature* **1996**, *379*, 257–262. [CrossRef] [PubMed]
208. Black, J.A.; Waxman, S.G. Molecular identities of two tetrodotoxin-resistant sodium channels in corneal axons. *Exp. Eye Res.* **2002**, *75*, 193–199. [CrossRef] [PubMed]
209. Dib-Hajj, S.D.; Tyrrell, L.; Cummins, T.R.; Black, J.A.; Wood, P.M.; Waxman, S.G. Two tetrodotoxin-resistant sodium channels in human dorsal root ganglion neurons. *FEBS Lett.* **1999**, *462*, 117–120. [CrossRef]
210. Akopian, A.N.; Souslova, V.; England, S.; Okuse, K.; Ogata, N.; Ure, J.; Smith, A.; Kerr, B.J.; McMahon, S.B.; Boyce, S.; et al. The tetrodotoxin-resistant sodium channel SNS has a specialized function in pain pathways. *Nat. Neurosci.* **1999**, *2*, 541–548. [CrossRef] [PubMed]
211. Tan, Z.-Y.; Piekarz, A.D.; Priest, B.T.; Knopp, K.L.; Krajewski, J.L.; McDermott, J.S.; Nisenbaum, E.S.; Cummins, T.R. Tetrodotoxin-resistant sodium channels in sensory neurons generate slow resurgent currents that are enhanced by inflammatory mediators. *J. Neurosci.* **2014**, *34*, 7190–7197. [CrossRef] [PubMed]
212. Blair, N.T.; Bean, B.P. Roles of tetrodotoxin (TTX)-sensitive Na+ current, TTX-resistant Na^+ current, and Ca^{2+} current in the action potentials of nociceptive sensory neurons. *J. Neurosci.* **2002**, *22*, 10277–10290. [CrossRef]
213. Tanaka, M.; Cummins, T.R.; Ishikawa, K.; Dib-Hajj, S.D.; Black, J.A.; Waxman, S.G. SNS Na^+ channel expression increases in dorsal root ganglion neurons in the carrageenan inflammatory pain model. *Neuroreport* **1998**, *9*, 967–972. [CrossRef]
214. Binshtok, A.M.; Wang, H.; Zimmermann, K.; Amaya, F.; Vardeh, D.; Shi, L.; Brenner, G.J.; Ji, R.-R.; Bean, B.P.; Woolf, C.J. Nociceptors are interleukin-1β sensors. *J. Neurosci.* **2008**, *28*, 14062–14073. [CrossRef]
215. Gold, M.S.; Reichling, D.B.; Shuster, M.J.; Levine, J.D. Hyperalgesic agents increase a tetrodotoxin-resistant Na+ current in nociceptors. *Proc. Natl. Acad. Sci. USA* **1996**, *93*, 1108–1112. [CrossRef]
216. Beyak, M.J.; Ramji, N.; Krol, K.M.; Kawaja, M.D.; Vanner, S.J. Two TTX-resistant Na^+ currents in mouse colonic dorsal root ganglia neurons and their role in colitis-induced hyperexcitability. *Am. J. Physiol. Gastrointest. Liver Physiol.* **2004**, *287*, G845–G855. [CrossRef]
217. Yu, Y.-Q.; Zhao, F.; Guan, S.-M.; Chen, J. Antisense-mediated knockdown of $Na_V1.8$, but not $Na_V1.9$, generates inhibitory effects on complete Freund's adjuvant-induced inflammatory pain in rat. *PLoS ONE* **2011**, *6*, e19865. [CrossRef] [PubMed]
218. Lin, Y.-M.; Fu, Y.; Winston, J.; Radhakrishnan, R.; Sarna, S.K.; Huang, L.-Y.M.; Shi, X.-Z. Pathogenesis of abdominal pain in bowel obstruction: Role of mechanical stress-induced upregulation of nerve growth factor in gut smooth muscle cells. *Pain* **2017**, *158*, 583–592. [CrossRef] [PubMed]
219. Dib-Hajj, S.; Black, J.; Felts, P.; Waxman, S. Down-regulation of transcripts for Na channel α-SNS in spinal sensory neurons following axotomy. *Proc. Natl. Acad. Sci. USA* **1996**, *93*, 14950–14954. [CrossRef] [PubMed]
220. Cummins, T.R.; Waxman, S.G. Downregulation of tetrodotoxin-resistant sodium currents and upregulation of a rapidly repriming tetrodotoxin-sensitive sodium current in small spinal sensory neurons after nerve injury. *J. Neurosci.* **1997**, *17*, 3503–3514. [CrossRef]
221. Decosterd, I.; Ji, R.-R.; Abdi, S.; Tate, S.; Woolf, C.J. The pattern of expression of the voltage-gated sodium channels $Na_V1.8$ and $Na_V1.9$ does not change in uninjured primary sensory neurons in experimental neuropathic pain models. *Pain* **2002**, *96*, 269–277. [CrossRef]

222. Gold, M.S.; Weinreich, D.; Kim, C.-S.; Wang, R.; Treanor, J.; Porreca, F.; Lai, J. Redistribution of $Na_V1.8$ in uninjured axons enables neuropathic pain. *J. Neurosci.* **2003**, *23*, 158–166. [CrossRef]
223. Zhang, X.-F.; Zhu, C.Z.; Thimmapaya, R.; Choi, W.S.; Honore, P.; Scott, V.E.; Kroeger, P.E.; Sullivan, J.P.; Faltynek, C.R.; Gopalakrishnan, M. Differential action potentials and firing patterns in injured and uninjured small dorsal root ganglion neurons after nerve injury. *Brain Res.* **2004**, *1009*, 147–158. [CrossRef]
224. Faber, C.G.; Lauria, G.; Merkies, I.S.; Cheng, X.; Han, C.; Ahn, H.S.; Persson, A.K.; Hoeijmakers, J.G.; Gerrits, M.M.; Pierro, T.; et al. Gain-of-function $Na_V1.8$ mutations in painful neuropathy. *Proc. Natl. Acad. Sci. USA* **2012**, *109*, 19444–19449. [CrossRef]
225. Dib-Hajj, S.D.; Tyrrell, L.; Black, J.A.; Waxman, S.G. NaN, a novel voltage-gated Na channel, is expressed preferentially in peripheral sensory neurons and down-regulated after axotomy. *Proc. Natl. Acad. Sci. USA* **1998**, *95*, 8963–8968. [CrossRef]
226. Rugiero, F.; Mistry, M.; Sage, D.; Black, J.A.; Waxman, S.G.; Crest, M.; Clerc, N.; Delmas, P.; Gola, M. Selective expression of a persistent tetrodotoxin-resistant Na^+ current and $Na_V1.9$ subunit in myenteric sensory neurons. *J. Neurosci.* **2003**, *23*, 2715–2725. [CrossRef]
227. Cummins, T.R.; Dib-Hajj, S.D.; Black, J.A.; Akopian, A.N.; Wood, J.N.; Waxman, S.G. A novel persistent tetrodotoxin-resistant sodium current in SNS-null and wild-type small primary sensory neurons. *J. Neurosci.* **1999**, *19*, RC43. [CrossRef] [PubMed]
228. Herzog, R.; Cummins, T.; Waxman, S. Persistent TTX-resistant Na^+ current affects resting potential and response to depolarization in simulated spinal sensory neurons. *J. Neurophysiol.* **2001**, *86*, 1351–1364. [CrossRef] [PubMed]
229. Maingret, F.; Coste, B.; Padilla, F.; Clerc, N.; Crest, M.; Korogod, S.M.; Delmas, P. Inflammatory mediators increase $Na_V1.9$ current and excitability in nociceptors through a coincident detection mechanism. *J. Gen. Physiol.* **2008**, *131*, 211–225. [CrossRef] [PubMed]
230. Priest, B.T.; Murphy, B.A.; Lindia, J.A.; Diaz, C.; Abbadie, C.; Ritter, A.M.; Liberator, P.; Iyer, L.M.; Kash, S.F.; Kohler, M.G.; et al. Contribution of the tetrodotoxin-resistant voltage-gated sodium channel $Na_V1.9$ to sensory transmission and nociceptive behavior. *Proc. Natl. Acad. Sci. USA* **2005**, *102*, 9382–9387. [CrossRef] [PubMed]
231. Amaya, F.; Wang, H.; Costigan, M.; Allchorne, A.J.; Hatcher, J.P.; Egerton, J.; Stean, T.; Morisset, V.; Grose, D.; Gunthorpe, M.J.; et al. The voltage-gated sodium channel $Na_V1.9$ is an effector of peripheral inflammatory pain hypersensitivity. *J. Neurosci.* **2006**, *26*, 12852–12860. [CrossRef] [PubMed]
232. Lolignier, S.; Amsalem, M.; Maingret, F.; Padilla, F.; Gabriac, M.; Chapuy, E.; Eschalier, A.; Delmas, P.; Busserolles, J. $Na_V1.9$ channel contributes to mechanical and heat pain hypersensitivity induced by subacute and chronic inflammation. *PLoS ONE* **2011**, *6*, e23083. [CrossRef]
233. Zhang, X.Y.; Wen, J.; Yang, W.; Wang, C.; Gao, L.; Zheng, L.H.; Wang, T.; Ran, K.; Li, Y.; Li, X.; et al. Gain-of-function mutations in SCN11A cause familial episodic pain. *Am. J. Hum. Genet.* **2013**, *93*, 957–966. [CrossRef]
234. Han, C.; Yang, Y.; de Greef, B.T.A.; Hoeijmakers, J.G.J.; Gerrits, M.M.; Verhamme, C.; Qu, J.; Lauria, G.; Merkies, I.S.J.; Faber, C.G.; et al. The domain II S4-S5 linker in $Na_V1.9$: A missense mutation enhances activation, impairs fast inactivation, and produces human painful neuropathy. *Neuromol. Med.* **2015**, *17*, 158–169. [CrossRef]
235. Huang, J.; Han, C.; Estacion, M.; Vasylyev, D.; Hoeijmakers, J.G.; Gerrits, M.M.; Tyrrell, L.; Lauria, G.; Faber, C.G.; Dib-Hajj, S.D.; et al. Gain-of-function mutations in sodium channel $Na_V1.9$ in painful neuropathy. *Brain* **2014**, *137*, 1627–1642. [CrossRef]
236. Bosmans, F.; Puopolo, M.; Martin-Eauclaire, M.F.; Bean, B.P.; Swartz, K.J. Functional properties and toxin pharmacology of a dorsal root ganglion sodium channel viewed through its voltage sensors. *J. Gen. Physiol.* **2011**, *138*, 59–72. [CrossRef]
237. Gonçalves, T.C.; Boukaiba, R.; Molgó, J.; Amar, M.; Partiseti, M.; Servent, D.; Benoit, E. Direct evidence for high affinity blockade of $Na_V1.6$ channel subtype by huwentoxin-IV spider peptide, using multiscale functional approaches. *Neuropharmacology* **2018**, *133*, 404–414. [CrossRef] [PubMed]
238. Zhang, Y.; Yang, Q.; Zhang, Q.; Peng, D.; Chen, M.; Liang, S.; Zhou, X.; Liu, Z. Engineering gain-of-function analogues of the spider venom peptide HNTX-I, a potent blocker of the $hNa_V1.7$ sodium channel. *Toxins* **2018**, *10*, 358. [CrossRef] [PubMed]

239. Cherki, R.S.; Kolb, E.; Langut, Y.; Tsveyer, L.; Bajayo, N.; Meir, A. Two tarantula venom peptides as potent and differential Na_V channels blockers. *Toxicon* **2014**, *77*, 58–67. [CrossRef] [PubMed]
240. Chow, C.Y.; Cristofori-Armstrong, B.; Undheim, E.A.; King, G.F.; Rash, L.D. Three peptide modulators of the human voltage-gated sodium channel 1.7, an important analgesic target, from the venom of an Australian tarantula. *Toxins* **2015**, *7*, 2494–2513. [CrossRef]
241. Redaelli, E.; Cassulini, R.R.; Silva, D.F.; Clement, H.; Schiavon, E.; Zamudio, F.Z.; Odell, G.; Arcangeli, A.; Clare, J.J.; Alagón, A. Target promiscuity and heterogeneous effects of tarantula venom peptides affecting Na^+ and K^+ ion channels. *J. Biol. Chem.* **2010**, *285*, 4130–4142. [CrossRef]

toxins MDPI

Review

Brown Spider (*Loxosceles*) Venom Toxins as Potential Biotools for the Development of Novel Therapeutics

Daniele Chaves-Moreira [1], Fernando Hitomi Matsubara [1], Zelinda Schemczssen-Graeff [1], Elidiana De Bona [1], Vanessa Ribeiro Heidemann [1], Clara Guerra-Duarte [2], Luiza Helena Gremski [1], Carlos Chávez-Olórtegui [2], Andrea Senff-Ribeiro [1], Olga Meiri Chaim [1], Raghuvir Krishnaswamy Arni [3] and Silvio Sanches Veiga [1,*]

1. Departamento de Biologia Celular, Universidade Federal do Paraná (UFPR), Curitiba 81531-970, PR, Brazil; moreirad@pennmedicine.upenn.edu (D.C.-M.); fernando_matsubara@hotmail.com (F.H.M.); zelinda1985@hotmail.com (Z.S.-G.); lidibona@gmail.com (E.D.B.); vane.biomed@gmail.com (V.R.H.); luiza_hg@yahoo.com.br (L.H.G.); senffribeiro@gmail.com (A.S.-R.); olgachaim@gmail.com (O.M.C.)
2. Departamento de Bioquímica e Imunologia, Universidade Federal de Minas Gerais (UFMG), Belo Horizonte 31270-901, MG, Brazil; claragd@gmail.com (C.G.-D.); olortegi@icb.ufmg.br (C.C.-O.)
3. Centro Multiusuário de Inovação Biomolecular, Departamento de Física, Universidade Estadual Paulista (UNESP), São José do Rio Preto 15054-000, SP, Brazil; arni@sjrp.unesp.br

* Correspondence: veigass@ufpr.br; Tel.: +55-(41)-3361-1776

Received: 6 May 2019; Accepted: 4 June 2019; Published: 19 June 2019

Abstract: Brown spider envenomation results in dermonecrosis with gravitational spreading characterized by a marked inflammatory reaction and with lower prevalence of systemic manifestations such as renal failure and hematological disturbances. Several toxins make up the venom of these species, and they are mainly peptides and proteins ranging from 5–40 kDa. The venoms have three major families of toxins: phospholipases-D, astacin-like metalloproteases, and the inhibitor cystine knot (ICK) peptides. Serine proteases, serpins, hyaluronidases, venom allergens, and a translationally controlled tumor protein (TCTP) are also present. Toxins hold essential biological properties that enable interactions with a range of distinct molecular targets. Therefore, the application of toxins as research tools and clinical products motivates repurposing their uses of interest. This review aims to discuss possibilities for brown spider venom toxins as putative models for designing molecules likely for therapeutics based on the status quo of brown spider venoms. Herein, we explore new possibilities for the venom components in the context of their biochemical and biological features, likewise their cellular targets, three-dimensional structures, and mechanisms of action.

Keywords: brown spider; venom; Loxosceles; toxins; biotools; drug targets; novel therapeutics

Key Contribution: The functional diversity of biological toxins and the often-unique selectivity of their effects coupled with high potency inspire their application or repurposing as research tools and clinical products. This review discusses the chemistry, biology, and clinical effects of some toxins found in brown spider venom that point to potential biotechnological and drug discovery.

1. Introduction: Venom Contents and Cellular Targets

Spider venoms are mixtures of biologically active peptides, proteins, glycoproteins, and small organic molecules which interact with cellular and molecular targets to trigger severe, sometimes fatal effects. However, the spider venom could be particularly interesting for the treatment of general diseases as a scaffold for toxin-based drug research. Several venom-based drugs or venom-derived molecules have found extensive use as tools for therapies. For instance, "Captopril", a competitive inhibitor of angiotensin-converting enzyme, is broadly used and well-established antihypertensive drug developed from a polypeptide toxin isolated from the venom of *Bothrops jararaca*; "Conotoxin" from the sea cone snail *Conus magus* used as an analgesic for severe chronic pain and "exendins"; and, recently, proteins obtained from the saliva of the Gila monster *Heloderma suspectum* benefited the treatment of type II diabetes [1–3].

Brown spiders (genus *Loxosceles*) has a worldwide distribution of approximately 130 species. Accidents caused by Loxosceles spider envenomation, Loxoscelism, are characterized by dermonecrotic lesions with gravitational spreading, and hence, these accidents are often referred to as necrotic or gangrenous arachnidism. In minor cases, it unveils systemic manifestations, including renal problems and hematological disturbances such as hemolysis, thrombocytopenia, and intravascular coagulation have been observed [4]. Based on proteomic and transcriptomic analysis, the venoms are mainly composed of low molecular mass peptides, proteins, and glycoproteins enriched in molecules in the 5–40 kDa range. There are three classes of "highly expressed molecules" that comprise approximately 95% of the toxin-encoding transcripts in the venom gland [4,5], biochemically characterized as belonging to the family of phospholipases-D, astacin-like proteases and low molecular mass peptides (ICK peptides or Knottins) [5–8]. Other toxins with low levels of expression have also been identified and include venom allergens, TCTP, hyaluronidases, serine proteases, and serine protease inhibitor [9,10].

Brown spider venom toxins are associated with many cellular changes followed by envenomation, either in humans or in animal-based models for experimental exposure. Rabbit skin exposed to crude venom or human biopsies indicated massive infiltration of inflammatory cells with predominantly polymorphonuclear leukocytes into the dermis, an event associated with dermonecrosis and histologically characterized as aseptic coagulative necrosis [11,12].

Brown spider venom toxins also exhibit indirect and robust activity on blood vessel endothelial cells that cause deregulated activation of leukocytes. The venom activity on endothelial cells was confirmed by experiments performed with umbilical vein endothelial cells, which after venom treatment increased expression and secretion of E-selectin, interleukin-8, and granulocyte macrophage colony-stimulating factor. Additionally, endothelial cells exposed to venom also overexpressed a growth-related oncogene and the monocyte chemoattractant protein-1 [13]. Human keratinocytes treated with venom increased the expression of vascular endothelial growth factor and rabbit aorta endothelial cells treated with venom bound venom toxins on cell surfaces, suffered morphological changes, detached from culture substratum, and their heparan-sulfate proteoglycans were degraded [14,15]. In vivo experiments of animals exposed to venoms indicated endothelial-leukocyte adhesion, transmigration of leukocytes across the blood vessel endothelium and degeneration of blood vessels [15,16]. Other cells targeted by venom toxins are fibroblasts that after exposure deregulated the expression of cytokines genes CXCL1, CXCL2, IL-6, and IL-8 mediators of inflammatory response activation [17]. Erythrocytes represent an additional cell target model of venom toxins. Venom exposure causes hemolysis and morphological changes that seem to depend on a mechanism reflecting a direct effect on cell surface phospholipids such as sphingomyelin and lysophosphatidylcholine leading to the influx of a calcium-mediated pathway by an L-type channel [18–20]; and another complement-dependent pathway with the activation of an endogenous metalloprotease, which degrades glycophorins and activates complement and lysis [21].

Platelets are also targets of brown spider venoms. Venom toxin treatment of human platelet-rich plasma induced in vitro platelet aggregation, an event that depends on the generation of lipids derived from platelet membranes [22–24]. Additionally, histopathological findings highlighted the marrow depression of megakaryocytes and thrombocytopenia in the peripheral blood after rabbit venom exposure and the generation of thrombus into blood vessels [25,26]. Finally, the cell surface of renal epithelial cells is also targeted by brown spider venom toxins and suffer direct cytotoxicity [27,28].

2. Recombinant Toxins: Biotools and Drug Targets

Brown spider venoms are obtained either by electrically stimulating the cephalothorax, which causes the venom glands to extrude the venom, or by gentle compression of the isolated venom glands to produce a venom gland extract. Both methods yield only a few microliters and micrograms of proteins from the venom with similar compositions and biological and biochemical properties [29,30]. Spider lethality following electrical stimulation or in the case of gland extract, the fact that they must be sacrificed, are drawbacks [4,5,31]. Molecular biology techniques for studying brown spider venom toxins have helped to overcome these limitations. At least two venom gland cDNA libraries have been constructed from venom glands of *L. laeta* [32] and *L. intermedia* [27]. Additionally, phospholipase-D family members of different brown spider species have been expressed in bacterial systems [22–24,27,32–36]. Site-directed mutant homologs of phospholipase-D have been obtained [18,19,28] and together with recombinant wild-type isoforms have been instrumental for studies on catalysis and determination of the crystal structures of phospholipase-D toxins to provide a better understanding about toxin biology and pharmacology [37–41]. Other recombinant brown spider venom toxins were reported for the astacin-member family [42,43] and an Inhibitor Cystine Knot peptide [44] have also been cloned, expressed and used for studies on the insecticide activities of venoms. A TCTP member-family toxin [10] and a recombinant hyaluronidase from *L. intermedia* venom were heterologously produced and in the case of hyaluronidase used to evaluate its role in dermonecrosis as a spreading factor [6] (see Table 1).

Table 1. Characteristics of recombinant toxins of *Loxosceles* spider venoms.

Toxin Family	MM (kDa)	Species	Biological Characteristics	N° of Sequences	PDB
PLD	30–35	*L. arizonica* [45] *L. boneti* [36] *L. gaucho* [46] *L. intermedia* [28] *L. laeta* [32] *L. reclusa* [34] *L. similis* [35]	-Hydrolysis of phospholipids; -Transphosphatidylation; -Dermonecrosis; -Inflammatory response; -Lethality; -Hemolysis; -Platelet aggregation; -Edema; -Nephrotoxicity; -Cytotoxicity; -Cytokine activation; -Complement activation.	199	1XX1 2F9R 3RLH 3RLG 4RW5 4RW3
Metalloprotease	30	*L. intermedia* [42]	-Hydrolysis of Gelatin, Fibronectin and Fibrinogen; -Cytotoxicity.	3	N.A.
ICK peptides	12	*L. intermedia* [44]	-Insecticidal activity.	1	N.A.
Hyaluronidase	45	*L. intermedia* [6]	-Hydrolysis of hyaluronic acid and chondroitin sulfate; -Dermonecrosis spreading.	1	N.A.
TCTP	22	*L. intermedia* [10]	-Edema; -Vascular permeability.	1	N.A.

N.A: not applied.

Finally, to surpass problems of expressing recombinant molecules using bacterial systems, such as inability to perform post-translational modifications or production of unfolded/insoluble proteins, brown spider recombinant toxins also have been produced using additional expression models as *Spodoptera frugiperda* insect cells [47,48]. The recombinant toxins produced in invertebrate systems might not only be useful for obtaining additional insights into Loxoscelism, but also serve as important tools for future pharmaceutical studies of prospection for drug discovery, serum therapy, and biotechnological applications (see Figure 1).

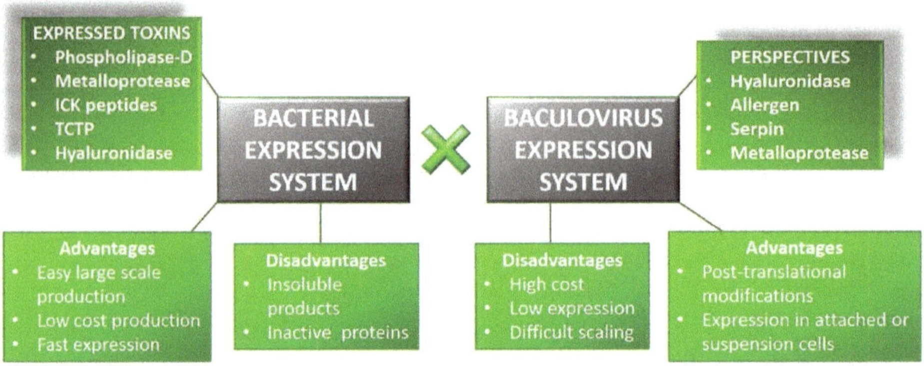

Figure 1. The different systems used for recombinant expression of *Loxosceles* toxins.

3. ICK Peptides: Analgesic Drug, Neuroprotective Effector and Bioinsecticide

Transcriptome analysis of *Loxosceles intermedia* venom glands revealed that 55.9% of the annotated transcripts encoding toxins are related to ICK peptides, also known as knottins, corresponding to the most representative group of identified toxins in this species [9]. ICK peptides contain the inhibitor cystine knot motif, which is an antiparallel β-sheet structured by a pseudo knot formed by two disulfide bonds and the intervening regions of the peptide backbone that is crossed by a third disulfide bond [49]. The ICK motif provides remarkable thermal, chemical, and biological stability and the peptides are overly stable in human serum for several days, conferring high half-life in gastric fluids and are likely relevant in the development of new drugs and therapies [50,51]. The ICK peptides exert their effects on voltage-gated ion channels expressed in the nervous system of animals [49].

For mammals, by acting on these molecular targets, the ICK peptides may be explored for use as analgesics. One example of this potential is the ICK toxin μ-TRTX-Tp1a from the Peruvian green-velvet tarantula *Thrixopelma pruriens* [52]. This toxin is an inhibitor of the $Na_v1.7$ sodium voltage-gated channel subtype, which is considered a relevant target for therapeutic solutions related to pathophysiological status such as pain. Recombinant μ-TRTX-Tp1a can revert, in a concentration-dependent manner, spontaneous pain induced in mice by intraplantar co-injection with OD1, a scorpion-venom peptide that is a potent activator of $Na_V1.6$ and $Na_V1.7$ channels [52,53]. Through in vitro assays, the toxin μ-TRTX-Hd1a, an ICK peptide present in the venom of the spider *Haplopelma doriae*, also activates $Na_V1.7$ channels. This toxin, at a concentration of 1 μM, was able to almost completely inhibit $Na_V1.7$-mediated currents recorded from oocytes expressing Na_V channel subunits [54]. Some authors hypothesized that the molecular targets of the peptide LiTx3 from *L. intermedia* are Na_V channels, which were also shown to be the target for the recombinant peptide U2-SCTX-Li1b encountered in *L. intermedia* venom [7,44]. Na_V or Ca_V channels may be the targets of the peptides LiTx1 and LiTx2 (see Figure 2). Different authors identified and sequenced several peptides that belong to the LiTx family encoded in the venom gland of *L. intermedia* [9]. Thus, the *L. intermedia* venom contains an impressive arsenal of molecules potentially important as an analgesic against acute and chronic pain conditions [9]. In a recent review, Netirojjanakil and Miranda [55] affirm that the challenge of venom-derived peptide therapeutic development remains in improving selectivity to the target and in the delivery of these peptides to the sites of action in the nervous system.

Other putative targets for spider ICK peptides are the acid-sensing ion channels (ASIC) encountered in the human central and peripheral nervous system, mainly in neurons [56]. These channels are specifically pH-modulated (low pH) in the extracellular environment. Depending on the decreasing pH that the neuronal cells are exposed to, the channel can be activated, which initiates sodium transport. The ASIC1a, a subunit of some ASIC channels, has been reported as a target that can be modulated, thus influencing pain or stroke clinical conditions [50]. The ICK peptide PcTx1 from the tarantula spider *Psalmopoeus cambridgei*, a known ASIC1a specific blocker, is a potent analgesic when intrathecal and intracerebroventricular injected in mice, producing effects similar to morphine [57].

Furthermore, PcTx1 toxin was neuroprotective in focal ischemia studies conducted in adult mouse: intracerebroventricular administration of this ICK peptide was able to reduce the percentage of the ipsilateral hemisphere infarct by more than 50% after 1 h of transient middle cerebral artery occlusion [58]. The authors also demonstrated the PcTx1 neuroprotective effects when this peptide was intracerebroventricular-injected in newborn piglets subjected to hypoxia-ischemia [59]. The ICK structural motif confers increased resistance to proteolysis, unlike the linear peptides that are highly susceptible to this process. Thus, ICK peptides and their respective biological properties possess significant potential for use in basic and applied research. The identification and characterization of these peptides in venoms from *Loxosceles* spiders may lead to the development of important appliances for the therapy of diseases affecting millions of people worldwide.

Studies of ICK peptides PnTx2-6 and PnTx2-5 identified in the venom of *Phoneutria nigreventer* spider shows that these toxins may be applied in the treatment of erectile dysfunction [60]. PnTx2-6 induces priapism in mice even after cavernosal denervation and increases relaxation in rat cavernous strips and in vivo, but induces significant side effects [61]. These unwanted effects and the difficulty to obtain this peptide in large amounts led to the design of a smaller peptide based on PnTx2-6 sequence, which showed promising features for erectile dysfunction treatment [62].

Another application for ICK peptides is the use as bioinsecticides. These peptides act upon targets in the peripheral or central nervous system of the insect inducing paralysis or lethality. The target may be sodium or calcium voltage-dependent channels, as well as calcium-activated potassium channels, presynaptic nerve terminals, or N-methyl-D-aspartate (NMDA) receptors [63]. Concerning to peptides from *L. intermedia*, after chromatography steps, the fraction containing LiTx1, LiTx2, and LiTx3 peptides proved to be toxic for the lepidopteran larvae of *S. frugiperda* resulting in flaccid paralysis or even death [7]. By studying *Loxosceles intermedia* venom gland, a cDNA of a 53 amino acid ICK peptide was obtained, heterologously expressed in the periplasm of *Escherichia coli*, and after purification caused irreversible flaccid paralysis in sheep blowflies. Such ICK peptide is biologically conserved in two other species: *L. laeta* and *L. gaucho* [64]. This biological activity of ICK peptides has an important biotechnological significance since it can lead to the development of effective bioinsecticides against pests of economic interest.

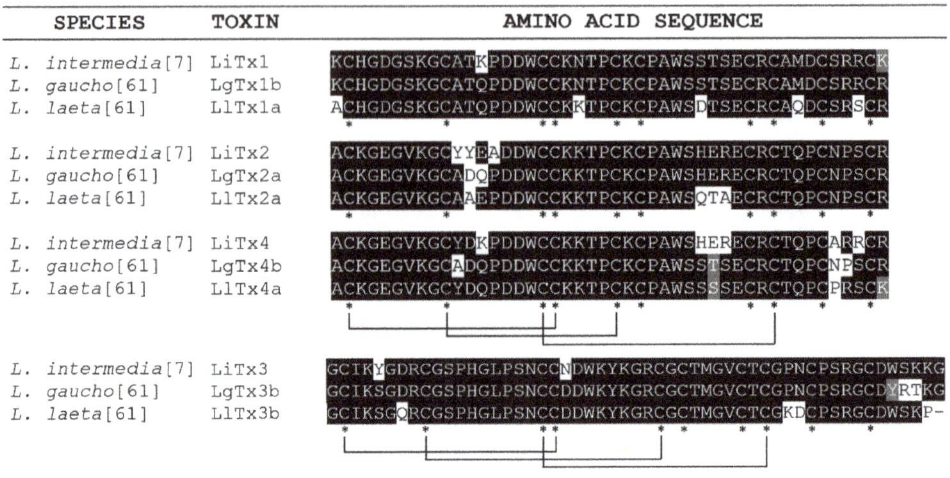

Figure 2. Predicted amino acid sequences of representative sequences of ICK peptides screened in RNA extracts from *L. intermedia, L. gaucho* and *L. laeta*. A fraction of *L. intermedia* containing LiTx1, LiTx2 and LiTx3 proved to be toxic against a lepidopteran larva [7]. A LiTx3 orthologue (Li1b) was heterologously expressed and also showed toxic activity in sheep blowflies [64]. Asterisks indicate conserved cysteine residues and the lines below the alignments indicate the pattern of disulphide bonds that form the inhibitor cystine knot motif [64].

4. Phospholipase-D: Treatment of Loxoscelism, Chemotherapy Drugs, and Anti-Inflammatory Drugs

The phospholipase-D (PLD) family of toxins, also known as dermonecrotic toxins, are the most studied and well-characterized components in *Loxosceles* venoms. These molecules catalyze the degradation of cell membrane phospholipids, such as sphingomyelin (SM), at a terminal phosphodiester bond to release choline and produce ceramide 1-phosphate (C1P) [65]. Also, PLDs can degrade lysophosphatidylcholine (LPC) in an Mg+2 dependent-manner and release lysophosphatidic acid (LPA) [66]. The PLD toxins also catalyze transphosphatidylation of the phosphodiester linkage between the phosphate and head groups of some phospholipids, forming alcohol, and a cyclic ceramide phosphate (CCP) when using SM or cyclic phosphatidic acid (CPA) when using LPC [44]. More than 20% of the transcripts from the *L. intermedia* venom glands corresponded to PLDs [9]. Moreover, the *L. intermedia* transcriptome analysis criteria for bioinformatics screening provided new putative isoforms of PLD, which can be included as new groups in the LoxTox family [67]. These data corroborate the identification of eleven PLD isoforms in the venom of *L. gaucho* and at least twenty-five in the *L. intermedia* venom [68,69]. The PLDs are responsible for a large variety of disturbances in Loxoscelism. Both native and recombinant forms of PLDs have been reported to trigger dermonecrotic lesions, cause an increase in vascular permeability, produce an intense inflammatory response at the inoculation site and at a systemic level, promote platelet aggregation, hemolysis, nephrotoxicity, and even lethality in controlled experiments [18,19,22,28].

The crystal structures of phospholipases-D from *L. laeta, L. intermedia, and L. gaucho* brought to light several insights about the overall conformation and catalytic mechanism and will direct the inhibitor design [37–40]. The single chain PLDs fold to form a distorted (α/β)8 barrel where the inner barrel surface lines with eight parallel β-strands linked by short flexible loops to eight α-helices that form the outer surface of the barrel (Figure 3). The catalytic loop is stabilized by a disulfide bridge (Cys51 and Cys57) in phospholipases-D class I (*L. laeta*) and a second disulfide bridge (Cys53 and Cys201) is present only in the phospholipases-D class II (*L. intermedia*), which links the catalytic loop to the flexible loop to significantly reduce the flexibility of the latter loop, as evidenced by the mean temperature factors [38–40]. Because the α-helices, β-strands, and loops vary in length and character, the barrel is significantly distorted. The interior of the barrel is densely packed with hydrophobic amino acids, and the short N-terminal section and the C-terminal extension, which contains a short α-helix, a β-strand, and a random coiled region serve to cap the torus of the far side of the barrel. The surface loops forming the near side of the barrel are mainly hydrophobic, and a narrow cavity provides access to the catalytic site, which is characterized by a ring of negatively charged amino acids [38–40]. This ring is considered to be the choline-binding site that interacts with Tyr228. The catalytic and Mg2+ binding sites are located in a shallow depression and contain His12, Glu32, Asp34, Asp91, His47, Asp52, Trp230, Asp233, Tyr228, and Asn252, which are fully conserved in *Loxosceles* PLDs. Recent site-directed mutagenesis studies of PLDs indicated the involvement of two histidines that are close to the metal ion-binding site in the acid-base catalytic mechanism. Based on the structural results, His12 and His47 of PLD have been identified as the key residues for catalysis and are assisted by a hydrogen bond network that involves Asp52, Asn252, and Asp233. The metal ion is coordinated by Glu32, Asp34, Asp91, and solvent molecules. The substrate is stabilized by Tyr228, and Lys93 [70].

In order to achieve an inhibitor prototype, we searched for possible inhibitors of the PLD from *L. intermedia*, and we discovered that halopemide derivatives could bind and inhibit the recombinant toxin [71]. These molecules, developed to target human PLD and treat cancer, could serve as a prototype for the design of new molecules to specifically treat Loxoscelism [72]. PLDs inhibitors exhibit anti-inflammatory activity and significantly reduce oxidative burst, leukocyte migration, degranulation, and inflammatory cytokine production [73].

Another interesting industrial application of the brown spider recombinant PLD is in the production of diverse beneficial endogenous bioactive lipids such as palmitoylethanolamide (PEA) that have anti-inflammatory and anti-neurodegenerative properties [74]. PEA was shown to reduce tumor necrosis factor alpha, pro-inflammatory cytokines, and prostaglandin E2 in the plasma. The neuroprotective effects of PEA are in part the result of its effects on downregulating the inflammatory cascade. Indeed, many neurodegenerative diseases are associated with a strong inflammatory component, such as Alzheimer's disease, Parkinson's disease or multiple sclerosis.

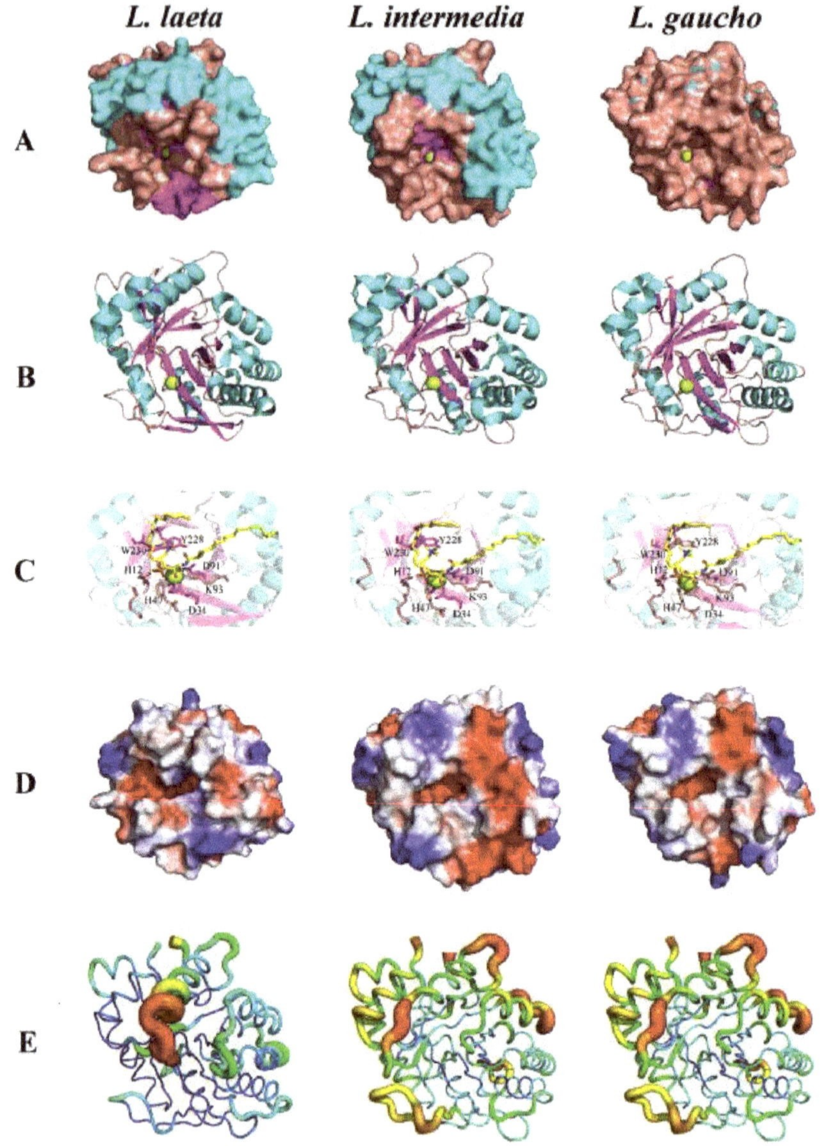

Figure 3. Structural comparison of venom phospholipase-D from *Loxosceles gaucho*, *Loxosceles intermedia* and *Loxosceles laeta*. (**A**) Surface view and (**B**) Ribbon view showing regions of α-helix (cyan), β-Sheet (magenta), Loop (salmon) and Magnesium ion (green sphere). (**C**) Zoom view of the catalytic site showing conserved amino acid residues (H12, H47, E32, D34, K93, Y228 and W230), Magnesium ion (green sphere), and the sphingomyelin (yellow stick). (**D**) Electrostatic surface colored by charge, from red (-2 kV) to blue (+2 kV). (**E**) Flexibility representation generated by b-factor putty, from more rigid regions in blue and green to more flexible regions yellow and red. Models are generated according to PDB codes: 1XX1 (*Loxosceles laeta*) and 3RLH (*Loxosceles intermedia*). Model for *Loxosceles gaucho* was generated using Modeller Program with the LgRec1 sequence from GenBank code: JX866729. PyMOL originated in all figures.

5. Proteases: Matrix Modulator and Thrombolytic Agent

Proteolysis on both the extracellular matrix (ECM) and cell surface modulates symptoms of envenomation by *Loxosceles* spiders [9,75,76]. Studies have revealed the proteolytic activity of the venom obtained directly from gland extracts of *L. rufescens and L. intermedia* (thus excluding potential contaminants with oral egesta) [30,77]. Also, transcriptome analyses from venom glands have encountered toxin-coding transcripts for serine-proteases and metalloproteases [9,78]. Proteases were considered highly expressed toxins in the venom glands, reaching about 23% in *L. intermedia*. Notably, metalloproteases were already reported in the whole venom of several species of *Loxosceles* genus [29,42].

Metalloproteases of *Loxosceles* venom are zinc-dependent endopeptidases that hydrolyze a variety of ECM molecules. For instance, two metalloproteases were characterized in the *L. intermedia* venom: Loxolysin A (20-28 kDa) and Loxolysin B (32–35 kDa), which hydrolyzes fibronectin, fibrinogen and denatured type I collagen [29]. Moreover, cDNA library of *L. intermedia* venom gland showed metalloprotease toxin-related sequences identified as astacin-like proteases due to the presence of enzymatic catalytic domain and structural motifs (HEXXHXXGFXHE "catalytic domain" and MXY "methionine-turn"). The recombinant form of LALP was able to induce morphological changes, such as loss of adhesion of muscular aorta cells in vitro, and hydrolyzed purified fibrinogen and fibronectin [29,30]. Furthermore, the relevance and conservation of metalloproteases for *Loxosceles* genus was also reported as a gene family by the identification of other four different LALP isoforms in the gland venoms of three *Loxosceles* species [43]. Recently, the whole venom complexity of the same species was analyzed using subproteomic and proteomic approaches for LALPs [8]. The majority of LALP-related molecules showed basic or neutral isoelectric points ranging between 24kDa and 29kDa for the three *Loxosceles* venoms.

Nevertheless, the venom toxins revealed different patterns of proteolytic activity upon gelatin and fibrinogen as substrates. These findings corroborate to the existence of a larger group of LALPs and propose the idea of a more intricate role for *Loxosceles* metalloproteases than previously suggested in Loxoscelism [41].

The enzymatic activities of brown spider proteases upon ECM, cell surface, and different proteins highlight these molecules as useful biotools [32]. Considering the physiopathological events related to ECM degradation, these proteases could be used for the establishment of protocol in pharmaceutical research for example as matrix modulator in healing processes, mostly in wound debridement removing the dead or damaged tissue. Theses proteases can also assist in antibiotic therapy, once some pathogenic bacteria produce biofilms, which in some cases help bacterial adhesion to host tissue and makes the penetration of the antibiotics administered difficult. Another possible application of brown spider proteases are as thrombolytic agents, due to their fibrinolytic activity and anticoagulant property. Although, further studies are necessary to investigate their potential as a therapeutic agent for thrombosis. Besides that, these proteases could participate as biotools in cleaner solutions for denture and contact lenses by removing impregnated proteinaceous materials and prolonging their viability [31,79,80].

6. Serine Protease Inhibitors: Anti-Proliferative and Anti-Metastatic Activities, Adjuvants in the Proteolytic Inhibition and Agricultural Pest Regulators

Inhibitors of serine proteases are grouped in three superfamilies according to their mechanism of action: canonical inhibitors, non-canonical inhibitors and serpins [81,82]. More than 1500 serpin sequences have been identified in the genomes of living organisms, and although they are serine protease inhibitors, several have additional functions as inhibitors of members of the cysteine protease family, caspase, and cathepsin [83,84]. Rather than being considered promiscuous, they appear selective in the sense that the targeted enzymes are often part of a conserved biological mechanism [85]. Human serpins are the most well-characterized serine protease inhibitors because they have a central role in several physiologic processes such as coagulation, fibrinolysis, development, malignancy, inflammation, and fertilization. Serpins inhibit a variety of circulating proteases as well as proteases that are activated or released in tissue, the reason why these molecules are involved in different pathologies and dysfunctions [86–88]. For instance, serpinopathies can occur due to genetic mutations that lead to inactivation of serpins by protein aggregation with loss of function [89].

Mammal serpins and serpin-derived peptides have been used in preclinical tests as a treatment option for serpinopathies, such as alpha-1 antitrypsin deficiency with emphysema, inflammatory vascular diseases from transplant, inflammatory vasculitic syndromes, and even sepsis with disseminated intravascular coagulation. Serpin-derived peptides are also in development as a new approach to block the adverse effects of serpins upregulated in cancer or inflammation [89].

Serpins are present in animal venoms from snakes, snails, sea anemones, wasps, scorpions, spiders and in ticks' saliva [9,90,91]. The transcriptome analyses of venom glands of *Loxosceles* genus spiders revealed transcripts encoding serine protease inhibitors. The cDNA library of the *L. intermedia* venom gland showed the presence of one serine protease inhibitor-related transcript [9]. In the *L. laeta* transcriptome, 0.6% of the transcripts were related to this same function [78]. The reasons for the presence of protease inhibitors in animal venoms and the physiological targets of these molecules are poorly understood. It has been proposed that these serine protease inhibitors would protect venom toxins from the protease actions of the prey body and manipulate host defenses [92,93]. These inhibitor sequences found in *L. intermedia* and *L. laeta* transcriptome analyses are similar to some tick and mammal serpins. *L. intermedia* serpin shows higher similarity to tick saliva serpins, such as from *Amblyomma americanum*, which is also an arachnid. It is known that arthropod serpins mediate several hemostatic and anti-inflammatory effects in mammalian blood [94]. The saliva serpin 6 and 19 from *A. americanum* contribute to hemostasis dysregulation of the host, facilitating blood feeding. At high molecular excess, recombinant Serpin 19 inhibits several serine proteinases of the blood-clotting cascade and forms inhibitory complexes with Factor Xa, Xia, and trypsin [95,96]. The best-characterized tick saliva serpin is the *Ixodes ricinus* immunosuppressor, Iris, which acts as an anticoagulant and inhibits the secretion of pro-inflammatory cytokines [97].

Inflammation-related complications are already focus of studies using serpins with therapeutic potential: C1 Esterase Inhibitor (C1NH) has been investigated toward many inflammation-related complications, and experimental treatment with this serpin showed decreased tissue complement activation and attenuated renal, intestinal and lung injury in a porcine model for hemorrhage [98]. Recombinant Alpha 1 antitrypsin-Pittsburgh has been investigated as a therapy for sepsis, attenuating the characteristic decreases in the functional concentrations of antithrombin, FXI, and fibrinogen [99].

Another putative biotechnological application for the serine protease inhibitors from *Loxosceles* venoms could be in the oncology field as antitumoral drugs focusing on the prevention of invasion and metastasis. A particular member of the serpin family, maspin, has been previously studied because of its inhibitory potential in breast and prostate cancer development [100]. Recently, the designing novel maspin-based chemotherapeutic agents with improved anti-cancer potency was suggested [101]. Katsukawa and co-workers [102] suggested that serpin 5 secreted by epithelial cells acts as a component of the extracellular surveillance system that facilitates the clearance of premalignant epithelial cells. Scabies mite serine protease inhibitors (SMSs) of the serpin superfamily were reported to interfere with all three pathways of the human complement system at different stages of their activation [103].

Another use of protease inhibitors from the *Loxosceles* spider venom could be the insertion of genes encoding serpins in cultivars, as previously described for some serine protease inhibitors applied in alfalfa, potato, cotton, and tobacco crops, which significantly incremented their resistance to attack by insects and predators [104].

Overall, the advantages of exploring the biotechnological potentials of serpins benefit from modulating serine protease activity by the introduction of serpin, as a therapeutic, or the blockade of serpins (serpin inhibitors). Several drugs currently in use or in development aim to replace dysfunctional serpins and to block adverse effects induced by aberrant protease or serpin actions [89].

7. Hyaluronidases: Adjuvant for Drug Absorption, Diagnostic Allergy Tests, Delivery of Chemotherapy and Contraceptive Molecules

Hyaluronidases (HAases) were reported in *L. deserta*, *L. rufescens*, *L. gaucho*, *L. intermedia*, *L. laeta* and *L. reclusa* venom. Proteomic and transcriptomic studies corroborated these data [9,78,105]. *L. intermedia* HAases were described as endo-β-*N*-acetyl-D-hexosaminidases. The first and unique *Loxosceles* HAase produced in a recombinant form is the Dietrich's HAase from *L. intermedia*, which presents 45 kDa and in vitro activity on hyaluronic acid (HA) and chondroitin sulfate (CS) degradation [6]. This study using the recombinant isoform confirmed the participation of the HAase as a spreading factor of the dermonecrotic lesion and the inoculated venom. A conserved cystinyl scaffold in the venom HAases suggests a structural similarity with other HAases. Mapping of the sequences of venom HAases on the crystal structure of *Apis mellifera* HAase supported this. Many venom HAases have been found to share a sequence homology of about 36% with that of spermatozoan PH-20, the testicular HAase that participates in fertilization [106]. In contrast to mammalian and microbial HAases, which are extensively studied for their physiological significances, the venom enzymes have received less attention [107].

Enzymes such as HAases have several biomedical applications by cleaving HA in tissues, they render tissues more permeable to injected fluids (spreading effect), increase membrane permeability, and reduce viscosity [108]. HAases have been used to reduce the extent of tissue damage following extravasation of parental infusions as electrolytes, chemotherapeutic agents, and antibiotics. HAases can be used therapeutically to promote resorption of excess fluids, to increase the effectiveness of local anesthesia. Some clinical studies reported that HAases could increase the speed of absorption of other substances, such as a human HAase (rHuPH20) increased insulin dispersion and accelerated its absorption [108].

Venom HAase of arthropods is a major allergen that can induce severe and occasionally fatal systemic IgE-mediated anaphylactic reactions in humans [106]. Determination of structural moieties responsible for the observed allergic potency will have great importance in clinical implications. Recently, the immunogenic potential of the HAase recombinant protein from social wasp (Vespidae) was suggested to its use for developing a diagnostic allergy test, as well as for specific immunotherapy [106,108].

The inhibition of the hydrolytic activities of HAases is also a very promising biotechnological output. Inhibitors of HAase are potent regulating-agents, which play a role in the maintenance of balance between the anabolism and catabolism of HA. The brown spider HAase action during the envenomation contributes to the local effects of the whole venom on the skin as well as potentiating systemic endeavors [106]. Antiserum and inhibitors for the spider HAase are potential agents to attenuate both local and systemic effects of Loxoscelism, as it was already demonstrated for other venom HAase [107]. The blockage of HAase activity would widen the time gap between the bite and the antivenom administration by limiting the diffusion of venom components, and it would reduce the antivenom load to achieve effective neutralization and, therefore, to reduce the collateral effects of the serum therapy [107].

8. TCTP: Antiparasitic Effect, Dental Restoration and Drug Delivery

The translationally controlled tumor protein (TCTP), also known as histamine-releasing factor (HRF), is a highly conserved, ubiquitous protein that has both intracellular and extracellular functions [109]. TCTP promotes allergic response in mammalian tissues by inducing the release of histamine from basophiles or mast cells. TCTP family proteins have already been described in the gland secretion of other arthropods, as ixodid ticks [110]. In *Loxosceles* venoms, it was encountered in *L. intermedia* and *L. laeta* transcriptome studies, and immunological cross-reaction studies suggest the presence of this toxin in *L. gaucho* venom [111]. Recombinant *L. intermedia* TCTP (LiRecTCTP) causes edema, increases vascular permeability, and is related to the inflammatory activity of the venom [10]. A TCTP protein was described in tarantula *Grammostola rosea* venom gland [112] and *Scytodes* spiders [113].

It is suggested that TCTP may play a crucial role in the establishment, maintenance, and pathogenesis of parasite infections. In a mice trial evaluating *Plasmodium* TCTP (42.2% of similarity with LiRecTCTP using EMBOSS Needle tool) as a malaria vaccine, a significant reduction of parasitemia in the early stages of the infection was seen [114,115]. TCTP from worms were also suggested as a putative filarial protein for diagnostic purposes [116]. In *Plasmodium*, TCTP has been shown to bind directly the anti-malarial drug artemisinin and to have higher expression levels on increased drug resistance conditions [117].

Furthermore, TCTP was detected in the biological fluid of asthmatic and parasitized patients [109]. Human TCTP (54.9% of similarity with LiRecTCTP using EMBOSS Needle tool) was described as a therapeutic target in asthma and allergy [109,118]. The N-terminal residues of TCTP (residues 1-10, MIIYRDLISH) form a protein transduction domain (PTD); these domains are recognized as promising vehicles for the delivery of macromolecular drugs. Different studies had already pointed out the TCTP PTD and some derivatives as efficient vehicle for drug delivery [119,120]. Recombinant TCTP from the prawn *Penaeus merguiensis* (57.2% of similarity with LiRecTCTP using EMBOSS Needle tool) has been studied as a supplement in dental restorative materials [121]. Recently, this TCTP was shown to promote osteoblast cells proliferation and differentiation, which improve restoration materials and their properties of inducing bone cell proliferation [114].

TCTP is described as a multifunctional protein involved in several cellular processes and is highly conserved [122]. In summary, LiTCTP is a promising toxin and potential target model with regards to its broad biotechnological applications for general biology fields (toxinology, parasitology, allergy, and oncology), and biomaterial research (dental restoration and drug delivery).

9. Brown Spider Venom Toxins: New Immunotherapies

Spider envenoming treatment by antivenom injection is controversial and no adequate clinical trials have been conducted so far. Besides, the best treatment protocol, which involves a combination of serum therapy and other drugs, remains to be established. Nonetheless, this treatment has the best therapeutic potential for treating loxoscelism as it has been shown to be efficient when initiated in time. In 2009, it was demonstrated that the equine-derived polyvalent loxoscelic antivenom produced against an equal proportion mixture of *L. intermedia, L. gaucho* and *L. laeta* venoms was efficient in reducing the envenoming effects of twice the minimum necrotizing dose of *L. intermedia* venom when administered to rabbits up until 12 h after venom injection [123]. Loxoscelic antivenom was also able to reduce the necrotic area caused by the venom even 48 h post-envenoming [123].

Traditional antivenom production is highly inefficient since it is difficult to obtain the necessary amount of venom to perform the immunization program. Each spider produces only a few microliters of venom. Taking Brazil as an example: there is a demand for 22,000 ampoules of antiloxoscelic serum per year. To produce this amount, 1,800 mg of venom is needed and requires venom extraction from approximately 36,000 spiders. Another important consideration is the toxic effect that crude venom exerts in the producer animal, commonly leading to the development of ulcers and abscesses, compromising the animal's health [124].

The availability of such a diverse group of recombinant PLDs represents an alternative source of immunogens for antivenom production. Recombinant PLDs showed to be active and was used to immunize mice, leading to the production of cross-reactive antibodies, which were also able to protect the animals against lethal effects of the whole venom [124]. In addition, horses immunized with this recombinant PLD developed antibodies that were able to cross-react and neutralize the lethal and dermonecrotic effects of *L. laeta* whole venom from Peru [125]. Antivenom produced using a combination of recombinant PLDs from *L. laeta* and *L. intermedia* as immunogens was tested. The antibodies showed cross-reactivity with the three main species of *Loxosceles* in Brazil and could neutralize their toxics effects more efficiently than an anti-arachnidic commercial antivenom, produced using a combination of *L. gaucho, Phoneutria nigriventer,* and *Tityus serrulatus* venom [126]. A combinational approach was also used with recombinant PLDs from *L. reclusa* and *L. bonetti* spiders (from North American origin), and also *L. laeta*, to immunize horses [127]. Individual immunization was also performed in rabbits. The monovalent antivenoms showed no cross-neutralization between North and South American species. The F(ab)2-based horse polyvalent antivenom showed high neutralizing potency, indicating a possible path for the development of a pan-american anti-loxoscelic antivenom. From *L. gaucho,* only one recombinant PLD has been produced, named LgRec1, which was also able to elicit neutralizing antibodies against the toxic effects of the analogous crude venom [46].

Other approaches for improving production of antiloxoscelic antivenom include the use of synthetic peptides mimicking mapped epitopes within the sequence of the main toxins from these venoms. The authors mapped epitopes from rLiD1 by SPOT assay using anti-rLiD1 antibodies [124]. Six regions were mapped, and the corresponding peptides were synthesized and used to develop an immunization protocol in combination with rLiD1, in different proportions. Although a mixture of six peptides was used, one of them appeared to be immunodominant. All of the used proportions between recombinant PLD and peptides were able to elicit antibodies that recognized rLiD1 by ELISA and neutralized the noxious effects of rLiD1 both in vitro and in vivo. Neutralizing antirLiD1 antibodies mapped an immunodominant epitope in a SPOT assay [124]. This epitope has 27 residues and is related to the active site of the enzyme. When used as an immunogen, the 27-mer peptide induces protective antibodies in mice and rabbit, protecting them from lethal and dermonecrotic effects of the venom respectively [128].

A neutralizing monoclonal antibody against *L. intermedia* was produced and its corresponding epitope was mapped by Phage Display techniques [129]. Synthetic peptides corresponding to the mapped epitopes were used as immunogens in rabbits, and the elicited antibodies were able to neutralize 60% of the dermonecrotic activity and 80% of the hemorrhage caused by *L. intermedia* crude venom [130]. To improve the use of molecules mimicking epitopes, chimeric recombinant proteins combining mapped epitopes in the same molecule was conducted with promising results. This approach was used to express in *E. coli* a chimeric non-toxic protein containing three rLiD1epitopes. These epitopes were previously identified, characterized and validated as potentially neutralizing regions [128–130]. The immunogenicity of the chimeric protein was assessed in rabbits and the developed antibodies neutralized the toxic effects of rLiD1 [131]. The chimeric protein was used in an immunization protocol either alone or combined with crude venom (a mixture of *L. intermedia, L. gaucho* and *L. laeta*). The three initial doses of the immunization schedule were composed of the venom, and the subsequent dose was composed of the chimeric protein. Compared to the traditional production of antivenom, this combined protocol was able to induce a similar ELISA and Western Blot serum reactivity towards the venoms of the three *Loxosceles* species. In neutralization assays, the sera produced by immunization with the combination of crude venom and chimeric protein met the necessary potency requirements for the actual production of antivenom for therapeutic use in humans. Although the immunization protocol using only the chimeric protein was not completely successful, the combined protocol used 67% less venom when compared to the traditional one, which is significant [132].

Finally, a multi-epitopic chimera containing linear and conformational sequences of the phospholipase-D (dermonecrotic) toxins from the *Loxosceles intermedia* and *L. laeta* venoms, hyaluronidases, and astacins (spreading factors), from the *L. intermedia* venom was produced and used as antigen to generate a polyvalent serum in rabbits. This serum was able to recognize the venoms of three different species of *Loxosceles* involved in accidents in South America (*L. intermedia, L. gaucho,* and *L. laeta*), besides neutralizing in vitro the enzymatic effects of crude venoms and lethality and dermonecrotic activities in vivo [133]. These results open the possibility of using this synthetic antigen as a tool to obtain new antivenom sera or as antigens for the production of anti-*Loxosceles* vaccines.

10. Conclusions

For most people, spiders often evoke fear and repulsion; however, their venoms form an extensive repertoire of novel molecules, which result in a wide range of biological processes. Several molecules have therapeutic and biotechnological potential and serve as the motif for the development of new molecules with industrial and medicinal applications (Table 2).

Table 2. Overview of potential biotechnological and pharmacological applications of toxins from *Loxosceles* spider venoms.

Toxin Family	Potential Uses as Biotools	Potential Uses for Drugs Design
Phospholipase-D [22–24,27,33,69,105]	-Antigens for a specific serum production for serum therapy; -Antigens for putative laboratory diagnosis tests; -Production of lipids for industrial interest; -Emulsification-free degumming of oil;	-Treatment of Loxoscelism; -Anti-inflammatory drugs, -Neuroprotective drugs; -Adjuvant drugs for cancer chemotherapy;
Metalloprotease [41–43]	-Trombolytic agents	Treatment of atherosclerosis
ICK peptides [7,44,64]	-Use as Bioinsecticide -Neuroprotective effect	Analgesic drugs
Hyaluronidase [6,9,78]	-Adjuvant for drugs absorption -Resorption of fluids -Diagnostic allergy test -Delivery of chemotherapy	Contraceptive method
Serpin [9,78]	-Inflammatory modulation -Agricultural pest regulators	Antitumoral drugs
TCTP [9,10,78]	-Antiparasitic effect -Dental restoration -Drug delivery	-N.A

N.A: not applied.

After analyses of the brown spider venom glands transcriptome, an expansion of the number of biotechnologically and pharmacologically relevant molecules and drug targets occurred and inspired the identification of a significant number of potential drug targets that can lead to the synthesis of new inhibitors. Moreover, some of these toxins could be used by themselves, as biotools in biological science projects, pharmaceutical industry or serum therapy, corroborating the high impact of the brown spider venom molecules for biotechnological development. Recent advances in the expression of recombinant toxins have overcome the necessity of obtaining them from a large number of spiders, as they have a very tiny amount of venom (Figure 4). Phospholipases-D, Astacin-like metalloproteases, Inhibitor Cystine Knot peptides, Hyaluronidase and TCTP have been successfully expressed in prokaryote system. The current goal is to promote their biochemical, biological and structural characterization for use them as models for novel therapeutics. All these potential uses and applications for the brown spider toxins are very encouraging. This could appear somewhat remote from the goal of treating diseases, but the challenge of studying the pharmacological properties of the toxins contained in the brown spider venoms can be very surprising. Once these toxins are prove to be versatile, they could be the missing key to discovery an important new drug for a major sickness.

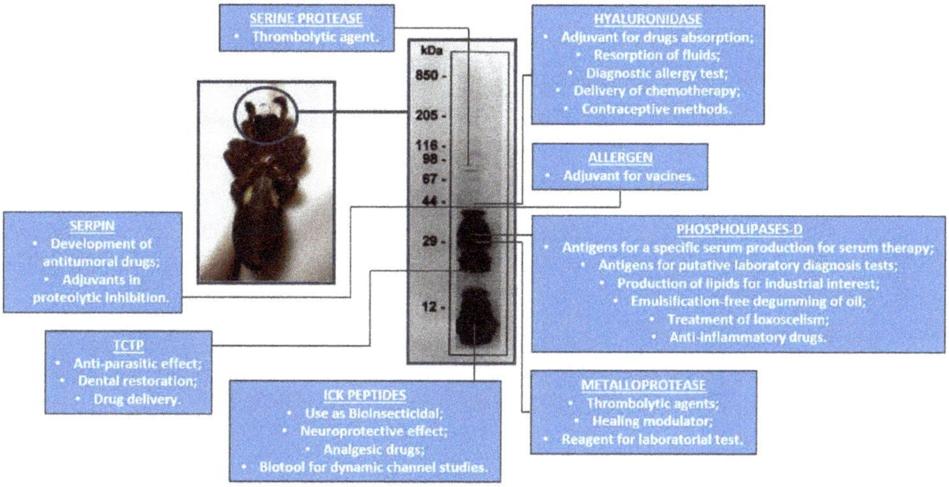

Figure 4. A summary of the *Loxosceles* spider venom toxins and their potential biotechnological and pharmacological applications.

Author Contributions: Conceptualization, D.C.-M. and S.S.V.; Methodology, D.C.-M., and R.K.A.; Resources, C.C.-O., R.K.A. and S.S.V.; Writing-Original Draft Preparation, D.C.-M., F.H.M., Z.S.-G., E.D.B., C.G.-D., A.S.-R. and O.M.C.; Writing-Review & Editing, V.R.H., L.H.G., and A.S.-R.; Visualization, L.H.G.; Supervision, C.C.-O., R.K.A. and S.S.V.; Project Administration, S.S.V.; Funding Acquisition, S.S.V.

Funding: This work was supported by grants from CAPES, CNPq, FAPESP, FAPEMIG, INCTTOX, FUNDAÇÃO ARAUCÁRIA-PR/SETI-PR/SESA-PR/MS-Decit/PPSUS, Brazil.

Conflicts of Interest: The authors declare no conflict of interest. The funders had no role in the design of the study; in the collection, analyses, or interpretation of data; in the writing of the manuscript, or in the decision to publish the results.

References

1. Eng, J.; Kleinman, W.A.; Singh, L.; Singh, G.; Raufman, J.P. Isolation and characterization of exendin-4, an exendin-3 analogue, from *Heloderma suspectum* venom. Further evidence for an exendin receptor on dispersed acini from guinea pig pancreas. *J. Biol. Chem.* **1992**, *267*, 7402–7405. [PubMed]
2. Smith, C.G.; Vane, J.R. The discovery of captopril. *FASEB J.* **2003**, *17*, 788–789. [CrossRef] [PubMed]
3. Prommer, E. Ziconotide: A new option for refractory pain. *Drugs Today* **2006**, *42*, 369–378. [CrossRef] [PubMed]
4. da Silva, P.H.; da Silveira, R.B.; Appel, M.H.; Mangili, O.C.; Gremski, W.; Veiga, S.S. Brown spiders and loxoscelism. *Toxicon* **2004**, *44*, 693–709. [CrossRef] [PubMed]
5. Gremski, L.H.; Trevisan-Silva, D.; Ferrer, V.P.; Matsubara, F.H.; Meissner, G.O.; Wille, A.C.; Vuitika, L.; Dias-Lopes, C.; Ullah, A.; de Moraes, F.R.; et al. Recent advances in the understanding of brown spider venoms: From the biology of spiders to the molecular mechanisms of toxins. *Toxicon* **2014**, *83*, 91–120. [CrossRef]
6. Ferrer, V.P.; de Mari, T.L.; Gremski, L.H.; Trevisan-Silva, D.; da Silveira, R.B.; Gremski, W.; Chaim, O.M.; Senff-Ribeiro, A.; Nader, H.B.; Veiga, S.S. A novel hyaluronidase from brown spider (*Loxosceles intermedia*) venom (Dietrich's Hyaluronidase): From cloning to functional characterization. *PLoS Negl. Trop. Dis.* **2013**, *7*, e2206. [CrossRef] [PubMed]
7. de Castro, C.S.; Silvestre, F.G.; Araujo, S.C.; Gabriel, M.Y.; Mangili, O.C.; Cruz, I.; Chávez-Olórtegui, C.; Kalapothakis, E. Identification and molecular cloning of insecticidal toxins from the venom of the brown spider *Loxosceles intermedia*. *Toxicon* **2004**, *44*, 273–280. [CrossRef]

8. Trevisan-Silva, D.; Bednaski, A.V.; Fischer, J.S.G.; Veiga, S.S.; Bandeira, N.; Guthals, A.; Marchini, F.K.; Leprevost, F.V.; Barbosa, V.C.; Senff-Ribeiro, A.; et al. A multi-protease, multi-dissociation, bottom-up-to-top-down proteomic view of the *Loxosceles intermedia* venom. *Sci. Data* **2017**, *4*, 170090. [CrossRef]
9. Gremski, L.H.; da Silveira, R.B.; Chaim, O.M.; Probst, C.M.; Ferrer, V.P.; Nowatzki, J.; Weinschutz, H.C.; Madeira, H.M.; Gremski, W.; Nader, H.B.; et al. A novel expression profile of the *Loxosceles intermedia* spider venomous gland revealed by transcriptome analysis. *Mol. Biosyst.* **2010**, *19*, 2403–2416. [CrossRef]
10. Sade, Y.B.; Boia-Ferreira, M.; Gremski, L.H.; da Silveira, R.B.; Gremski, W.; Senff-Ribeiro, A.; Chaim, O.M.; Veiga, S.S. Molecular cloning, heterologous expression and functional characterization of a novel translationally-controlled tumor protein (TCTP) family member from *Loxosceles intermedia* (brown spider) venom. *Int. J. Biochem. Cell Biol.* **2012**, *44*, 170–177. [CrossRef]
11. Ospedal, K.Z.; Appel, M.H.; Fillus-Neto, J.; Mangili, O.C.; Veiga, S.S.; Gremski, W. Histopathological findings in rabbits after experimental acute exposure to the Loxosceles intermedia (brown spider) venom. *Int. J. Exp. Pathol.* **2002**, *83*, 287–294. [CrossRef] [PubMed]
12. Barbaro, K.C.; Lira, M.S.; Araujo, C.A.; Pareja-Santos, A.; Tavora, B.C.; Prezotto-Neto, J.P.; Kimura, L.F.; Lima, C.; Lopes-Ferreira, M.; Santoro, M.L. Inflammatory mediators generated at the site of inoculation of Loxosceles gaucho spider venom. *Toxicon* **2010**, *56*, 972–979. [CrossRef] [PubMed]
13. Desai, A.; Lankford, H.A.; Warren, J.S. *Loxosceles deserta* spider venom induces the expression of vascular endothelial growth factor (VEGF) in keratinocytes. *Inflammation* **2000**, *24*, 1–9. [CrossRef] [PubMed]
14. Veiga, S.S.; Zanetti, V.C.; Braz, A.; Mangili, O.C.; Gremski, W. Extracellular matrix molecules as targets for brown spider venom toxins. *Braz. J. Med. Biol. Res.* **2001**, *34*, 843–850. [CrossRef] [PubMed]
15. Paludo, K.S.; Gremski, L.H.; Veiga, S.S.; Chaim, O.M.; Gremski, W.; de Freitas Buchi, D.; Nader, H.B.; Dietrich, C.P.; Franco, C.R. The effect of brown spider venom on endothelial cell morphology and adhesive structures. *Toxicon* **2006**, *47*, 844–853. [CrossRef] [PubMed]
16. Veiga, S.S.; Zanetti, V.C.; Franco, C.R.; Trindade, E.S.; Porcionatto, M.A.; Mangili, O.C.; Gremski, W.; Dietrich, C.P.; Nader, H.B. In vivo and in vitro cytotoxicity of brown spider venom for blood vessel endothelial cells. *Thromb. Res.* **2001**, *102*, 229–237. [CrossRef]
17. Dragulev, B.; Bao, Y.; Ramos-Cerrillo, B.; Vazquez, H.; Olvera, A.; Stock, R.; Algaron, A.; Fox, J.W. Upregulation of IL-6, IL-8, CXCL1, and CXCL2 dominates gene expression in human fibroblast cells exposed to *Loxosceles reclusa* sphingomyelinase D: Insights into spider venom dermonecrosis. *J. Investig. Dermatol.* **2007**, *127*, 1264–1266. [CrossRef] [PubMed]
18. Chaim, O.M.; da Silveira, R.B.; Trevisan-Silva, D.; Ferrer, V.P.; Sade, Y.B.; Boia-Ferreira, M.; Gremski, L.H.; Gremski, W.; Senff-Ribeiro, A.; Takahashi, H.K.; et al. Phospholipase-D activity and inflammatory response induced by brown spider dermonecrotic toxin: Endothelial cell membrane phospholipids as targets for toxicity. *Biochim. Biophys. Acta* **2011**, *1811*, 84–96. [CrossRef] [PubMed]
19. Chaves-Moreira, D.; Chaim, O.M.; Sade, Y.B.; Paludo, K.S.; Gremski, L.H.; Donatti, L.; de Moura, J.; Mangili, O.C.; Gremski, W.; da Silveira, R.B.; et al. Identification of a direct hemolytic effect dependent on the catalytic activity induced by phospholipase-D (dermonecrotic toxin) from brown spider venom. *J. Cell. Biochem.* **2009**, *107*, 655–666. [CrossRef] [PubMed]
20. Chaves-Moreira, D.; Souza, F.N.; Fogaça, R.T.; Mangili, O.C.; Gremski, W.; Senff-Ribeiro, A.; Chaim, O.M.; Veiga, S.S. The relationship between calcium and the metabolism of plasma membrane phospholipids in hemolysis induced by brown spider venom phospholipase-D toxin. *J. Cell. Biochem.* **2011**, *112*, 2529–2540. [CrossRef]
21. Tambourgi, D.V.; Da Silva, M.S.; Billington, S.J.; Goncalves De Andrade, R.M.; Magnoli, F.C.; Songer, J.G.; Van Den Berg, C.W. Mechanism of induction of complement susceptibility of erythrocytes by spider and bacterial sphingomyelinases. *Immunology* **2002**, *107*, 93–101. [CrossRef]
22. Appel, M.H.; da Silveira, R.B.; Chaim, O.M.; Paludo, K.S.; Silva, D.T.; Chaves-Moreira, D.; da Silva, P.H.; Mangili, O.C.; Senff-Ribeiro, A.; Gremski, W.; et al. Identification, cloning and functional characterization of a novel dermonecrotic toxin (phospholipase D) from brown spider (*Loxosceles intermedia*) venom. *Biochim. Biophys. Acta* **2008**, *1780*, 167–178. [CrossRef]
23. da Silveira, R.B.; Pigozzo, R.B.; Chaim, O.M.; Appel, M.H.; Dreyfuss, J.L.; Toma, L.; Mangili, O.C.; Gremski, W.; Dietrich, C.P.; Nader, H.B.; et al. Molecular cloning and functional characterization of two isoforms of

dermonecrotic toxin from *Loxosceles intermedia* (brown spider) venom gland. *Biochimie* **2006**, *88*, 1241–1253. [CrossRef]

24. da Silveira, R.B.; Pigozzo, R.B.; Chaim, O.M.; Appel, M.H.; Silva, D.T.; Dreyfuss, J.L.; Toma, L.; Dietrich, C.P.; Nader, H.B.; Veiga, S.S.; et al. Two novel dermonecrotic toxins LiRecDT4 and LiRecDT5 from brown spider (*Loxosceles intermedia*) venom: From cloning to functional characterization. *Biochimie* **2007**, *89*, 289–300. [CrossRef]
25. Tavares, F.L.; Peichoto, M.E.; Rangel Dde, M.; Barbaro, K.C.; Cirillo, M.C.; Santoro, M.L.; Sano-Martins, I.S. *Loxosceles gaucho* spider venom and its sphingomyelinase fraction trigger the main functions of human and rabbit platelets. *Hum. Exp. Toxicol.* **2011**, *30*, 1567–1574. [CrossRef]
26. da Silva, P.H.; Hashimoto, Y.; dos Santos, F.A.; Mangili, O.C.; Gremski, W.; Veiga, S.S. Hematological cell findings in bone marrow and peripheral blood of rabbits after experimental acute exposure to *Loxosceles intermedia* (brown spider) venom. *Toxicon* **2003**, *42*, 155–161. [CrossRef]
27. Chaim, O.M.; Sade, Y.B.; da Silveira, R.B.; Toma, L.; Kalapothakis, E.; Chavez-Olortegui, C.; Mangili, O.C.; Gremski, W.; von Dietrich, C.P.; Nader, H.B.; et al. Brown spider dermonecrotic toxin directly induces nephrotoxicity. *Toxicol. Appl. Pharmacol.* **2006**, *211*, 64–77. [CrossRef]
28. Kusma, J.; Chaim, O.M.; Wille, A.C.; Ferrer, V.P.; Sade, Y.B.; Donatti, L.; Gremski, W.; Mangili, O.C.; Veiga, S.S. Nephrotoxicity caused by brown spider venom phospholipase-D (dermonecrotic toxin) depends on catalytic activity. *Biochimie* **2008**, *90*, 1722–1736. [CrossRef]
29. Feitosa, L.; Gremski, W.; Veiga, S.S.; Elias, M.C.; Graner, E.; Mangili, O.C.; Brentani, R.R. Detection and characterization of metalloproteinases with gelatinolytic, fibronectinolytic and fibrinogenolytic activities in brown spider (*Loxosceles intermedia*) venom. *Toxicon* **1998**, *36*, 1039–1051. [CrossRef]
30. da Silveira, R.B.; Filho, J.F.S.; Mangili, O.C.; Veiga, S.S.; Gremski, W.; Nader, H.B. Identification of proteases in the extract of venom glands from brown spider. *Toxicon* **2002**, *40*, 815–822. [CrossRef]
31. Senff-Ribeiro, A.; Henrique da Silva, P.; Chaim, O.M.; Gremski, L.H.; Paludo, K.S.; da Silveira, R.B.; Gremski, W.; Mangili, O.C.; Veiga, S.S. Biotechnological applications of brown spider (*Loxosceles* genus) venom toxins. *Biotechnol. Adv.* **2008**, *26*, 210–218. [CrossRef]
32. Fernandes-Pedrosa, F.; Junqueira de Azevedo, I.L.; Goncalves-de-Andrade, R.M.; van den Berg, C.W.; Ramos, C.R.; Ho, P.L.; Tambourgi, D.V. Molecular cloning and expression of a functional dermonecrotic and haemolytic factor from *Loxosceles laeta* venom. *Biochem. Biophys. Res. Commun.* **2002**, *298*, 638–645. [CrossRef]
33. Vuitika, L.; Gremski, L.H.; Belisario-Ferrari, M.R.; Chaves-Moreira, D.; Ferrer, V.P.; Senff-Ribeiro, A.; Chaim, O.M.; Veiga, S.S. Brown spider phospholipase-D containing a conservative mutation (D233E) in the catalytic site: Identification and functional characterization. *J. Cell. Biochem.* **2013**, *114*, 2479–2492. [CrossRef]
34. Lee, S.; Lynch, K.R. Brown recluse spider (*Loxosceles reclusa*) venom phospholipase D (PLD) generates lysophosphatidic acid (LPA). *Biochem. J.* **2005**, *391 Pt 2*, 317–323. [CrossRef]
35. Silvestre, F.G.; de Castro, C.S.; de Moura, J.F.; Giusta, M.S.; De Maria, M.; Alvares, E.S.; Lobato, F.C.; Assis, R.A.; Goncalves, L.A.; Gubert, I.C.; et al. Characterization of the venom from the Brazilian Brown Spider *Loxosceles similis* Moenkhaus, 1898 (Araneae, Sicariidae). *Toxicon* **2005**, *46*, 927–936. [CrossRef]
36. Ramos-Cerrillo, B.; Olvera, A.; Odell, G.V.; Zamudio, F.; Paniagua-Solis, J.; Alagon, A.; Stock, R.P. Genetic and enzymatic characterization of sphingomyelinase D isoforms from the North American fiddleback spiders *Loxosceles boneti* and *Loxosceles reclusa*. *Toxicon* **2004**, *44*, 507–514. [CrossRef]
37. Coronado, M.A.; Ullah, A.; da Silva, L.S.; Chaves-Moreira, D.; Vuitika, L.; Chaim, O.M.; Veiga, S.S.; Chahine, J.; Murakami, M.T.; Arni, R.K. Structural Insights into Substrate Binding of Brown Spider Venom Class II Phospholipases D. *Curr. Protein Pept. Sci.* **2015**, *16*, 768–774. [CrossRef]
38. de Giuseppe, P.O.; Ullah, A.; Trevisan-Silva, D.; Gremski, L.H.; Wille, A.C.; Chaves Moreira, D.; Ribeiro, A.S.; Chaim, O.M.; Murakami, M.T.; Veiga, S.S.; et al. Structure of a novel class II phospholipase D: Catalytic cleft is modified by a disulphide bridge. *Biochem. Biophys. Res. Commun.* **2011**, *409*, 622–627. [CrossRef]
39. Murakami, M.T.; Fernandes-Pedrosa, M.F.; de Andrade, S.A.; Gabdoulkhakov, A.; Betzel, C.; Tambourgi, D.V.; Arni, R.K. Structural insights into the catalytic mechanism of sphingomyelinases D and evolutionary relationship to glycerophosphodiester phosphodiesterases. *Biochem. Biophys. Res. Commun.* **2006**, *342*, 323–329. [CrossRef]
40. Murakami, M.T.; Fernandes-Pedrosa, M.F.; Tambourgi, D.V.; Arni, R.K. Structural basis for metal ion coordination and the catalytic mechanism of sphingomyelinases D. *J. Biol. Chem.* **2005**, *280*, 13658–13664. [CrossRef]

41. Trevisan-Silva, D.; Bednaski, A.V.; Gremski, L.H.; Chaim, O.M.; Veiga, S.S.; Senff-Ribeiro, A. Differential metalloprotease content and activity of three *Loxosceles* spider venoms revealed using two-dimensional electrophoresis approaches. *Toxicon* **2013**, *76*, 11–22. [CrossRef]
42. da Silveira, R.B.; Wille, A.C.; Chaim, O.M.; Appel, M.H.; Silva, D.T.; Franco, C.R.; Toma, L.; Mangili, O.C.; Gremski, W.; Dietrich, C.P.; et al. Identification, cloning, expression and functional characterization of an astacin-like metalloprotease toxin from *Loxosceles intermedia* (brown spider) venom. *Biochem. J.* **2007**, *406*, 355–363. [CrossRef]
43. Trevisan-Silva, D.; Gremski, L.H.; Chaim, O.M.; da Silveira, R.B.; Meissner, G.O.; Mangili, O.C.; Barbaro, K.C.; Gremski, W.; Veiga, S.S.; Senff-Ribeiro, A. Astacin-like metalloproteases are a gene family of toxins present in the venom of different species of the brown spider (genus *Loxosceles*). *Biochimie* **2010**, *92*, 21–32. [CrossRef]
44. Matsubara, F.H.; Gremski, L.H.; Meissner, G.O.; Constantino Lopes, E.S.; Gremski, W.; Senff-Ribeiro, A.; Chaim, O.M.; Veiga, S.S. A novel ICK peptide from the *Loxosceles intermedia* (brown spider) venom gland: Cloning, heterologous expression and immunological crossreactivity approaches. *Toxicon* **2013**, *71*, 147–158. [CrossRef]
45. Lajoie, D.M.; Zobel-Thropp, P.A.; Kumirov, V.K.; Bandarian, V.; Binford, G.J.; Cordes, M.H. Phospholipase D toxins of brown spider venom convert lysophosphatidylcholine and sphingomyelin to cyclic phosphates. *PLoS ONE* **2013**, *8*, e72372. [CrossRef]
46. Magalhães, G.S.; Caporrino, M.C.; Della-Casa, M.S.; Kimura, L.F.; Prezotto-Neto, J.P.; Fukuda, D.A.; Portes-Junior, J.A.; Neves-Ferreira, A.G.; Santoro, M.L.; Barbaro, K.C. Cloning, expression and characterization of a phospholipase D from *Loxosceles gaucho* venom gland. *Biochimie* **2013**, *95*, 1773–1783. [CrossRef]
47. De Bona, E.; (Federal University of Paraná, Curitiba, Paraná, Brazil). Personal communication, 2019.
48. Da Justa, H.C.; (Federal University of Paraná, Curitiba, Paraná, Brazil). Personal communication, 2019.
49. Norton, R.S.; Pallaghy, P.K. The cystine knot structure of ion channel toxins and related polypeptides. *Toxicon* **1998**, *36*, 1573–1583. [CrossRef]
50. Saez, N.J.; Senff, S.; Jensen, J.E.; Er, S.Y.; Herzig, V.; Rash, L.D.; King, G.F. Spider-venom peptides as therapeutics. *Toxins* **2010**, *2*, 2851–2871. [CrossRef]
51. Herzig, V.; King, G.F. The Cystine Knot Is Responsible for the Exceptional Stability of the Insecticidal Spider Toxin ω-Hexatoxin-Hv1a. *Toxins* **2015**, *7*, 4366–4380. [CrossRef]
52. Cardoso, F.C.; Dekan, Z.; Rosengren, K.J.; Erickson, A.; Vetter, I.; Deuis, J.R.; Herzig, V.; Alewood, P.F.; King, G.F.; Lewis, R.J. Identification and Characterization of ProTx-III [mu-TRTX-Tp1a], a New Voltage-Gated Sodium Channel Inhibitor from Venom of the Tarantula *Thrixopelma pruriens*. *Mol. Pharmacol.* **2015**, *88*, 291–303. [CrossRef]
53. Zimmermann, L.; Morado-Diaz, C.J.; Davis-Lopez de Carrizosa, M.A.; de la Cruz, R.R.; May, P.J.; Streicher, J.; Pastor, Á.M.; Blumer, R. Axons giving rise to the palisade endings of feline extraocular muscles display motor features. *J. Neurosci.* **2013**, *33*, 2784–2793. [CrossRef]
54. Klint, J.K.; Smith, J.J.; Vetter, I.; Rupasinghe, D.B.; Er, S.Y.; Senff, S.; Herzig, V.; Mobli, M.; Lewis, R.J.; Bosmans, F.; et al. Seven novel modulators of the analgesic target NaV 1.7 uncovered using a high-throughput venom-based discovery approach. *Br. J. Pharmacol.* **2015**, *172*, 2445–2458. [CrossRef]
55. Netirojjanakul, C.; Miranda, L.P. Progress and challenges in the optimization of toxin peptides for development as pain therapeutics. *Curr. Opin. Chem. Biol.* **2017**, *38*, 70–79. [CrossRef]
56. Baron, A.; Diochot, S.; Salinas, M.; Deval, E.; Noel, J.; Lingueglia, E. Venom toxins in the exploration of molecular, physiological and pathophysiological functions of acid-sensing ion channels. *Toxicon* **2013**, *75*, 187–204. [CrossRef]
57. Mazzuca, M.; Heurteaux, C.; Alloui, A.; Diochot, S.; Baron, A.; Voilley, N.; Blondeau, N.; Escoubas, P.; Gélot, A.; Cupo, A.; et al. A tarantula peptide against pain via ASIC1a channels and opioid mechanisms. *Nat. Neurosci.* **2007**, *10*, 943–945. [CrossRef]
58. Pignataro, G.; Simon, R.P.; Xiong, Z.G. Prolonged activation of ASIC1a and the time window for neuroprotection in cerebral ischaemia. *Brain* **2007**, *130 Pt 1*, 151–158. [CrossRef]
59. Yang, M.J.; Lin, W.Y.; Lu, K.H.; Tu, W.C. Evaluating antioxidative activities of amino acid substitutions on mastoparan-B. *Peptides* **2011**, *32*, 2037–2043. [CrossRef]
60. Nunes, K.P.; Torres, F.S.; Borges, M.H.; Matavel, A.; Pimenta, A.M.C.; De Lima, M.E. New insights on arthropod toxins that potentiate erectile function. *Toxicon* **2013**, *69*, 152–159. [CrossRef]

61. Ravelli, K.G.; Ramos, A.T.; Gonçalves, L.B.; Magnoli, F.C.; Troncone, L.R.P. *Phoneutria nigriventer* spider toxin Tx2-6 induces priapism in mice even after cavernosal denervation. *Toxicon* **2017**, *130*, 29–34. [CrossRef]
62. Nunes-Silva, C.; Nunes, K.P.; Torres, F.S.; Cassoli, J.S.; Santos, D.M.; Almeida, F.D.M.; Matavel, A.; Cruz, J.S.; Santos-Miranda, A.; Nunes, A.D.; et al. PnPP-19, a Synthetic and Nontoxic Peptide Designed from a *Phoneutria nigriventer* Toxin, Potentiates Erectile Function via NO/cGMP. *J. Urol.* **2015**, *194*, 1481–1490. [CrossRef]
63. Windley, M.J.; Herzig, V.; Dziemborowicz, S.A.; Hardy, M.C.; King, G.F.; Nicholson, G.M. Spider-venom peptides as bioinsecticides. *Toxins* **2012**, *4*, 191–227. [CrossRef]
64. Matsubara, F.H.; Meissner, G.O.; Herzig, V.; Justa, H.C.; Dias, B.C.L.; Trevisan-Silva, D.; Gremski, L.H.; Gremski, W.; Senff-Ribeiro, A.; Chaim, O.M.; et al. Insecticidal activity of a recombinant knottin peptide from *Loxosceles intermedia* venom and recognition of these peptides as conserved family in the genus. *Insect Mol. Biol.* **2017**, *26*, 25–34. [CrossRef]
65. Stock, R.P.; Brewer, J.; Wagner, K.; Ramos-Cerrillo, B.; Duelund, L.; Jernshoj, K.D.; Olsen, L.F.; Bagatolli, L.A. Sphingomyelinase D activity in model membranes: Structural effects of in situ generation of ceramide-1-phosphate. *PLoS ONE* **2012**, *7*, e36003. [CrossRef]
66. van Meeteren, L.A.; Frederiks, F.; Giepmans, B.N.; Pedrosa, M.F.; Billington, S.J.; Jost, B.H.; Tambourgi, D.V.; Moolenaar, W.H. Spider and bacterial sphingomyelinases D target cellular lysophosphatidic acid receptors by hydrolyzing lysophosphatidylcholine. *J. Biol. Chem.* **2004**, *279*, 10833–10836. [CrossRef]
67. Kalapothakis, E.; Chatzaki, M.; Goncalves-Dornelas, H.; de Castro, C.S.; Silvestre, F.G.; Laborne, F.V.; De Moura, J.F.; Veiga, S.S.; Chavez-Olortegui, C.; Granier, C.; et al. The Loxtox protein family in *Loxosceles intermedia* (Mello-Leitao) venom. *Toxicon* **2007**, *50*, 938–946. [CrossRef]
68. Wille, A.C.; Chaves-Moreira, D.; Trevisan-Silva, D.; Magnoni, M.G.; Boia-Ferreira, M.; Gremski, L.H.; Gremski, W.; Chaim, O.M.; Senff-Ribeiro, A.; Veiga, S.S. Modulation of membrane phospholipids, the cytosolic calcium influx and cell proliferation following treatment of B16-F10 cells with recombinant phospholipase-D from *Loxosceles intermedia* (brown spider) venom. *Toxicon* **2013**, *67*, 17–30. [CrossRef]
69. Machado, L.F.; Laugesen, S.; Botelho, E.D.; Ricart, C.A.; Fontes, W.; Barbaro, K.C.; Roepstorff, P.; Sousa, M.V. Proteome analysis of brown spider venom: Identification of loxnecrogin isoforms in *Loxosceles gaucho* venom. *Proteomics* **2005**, *5*, 2167–2176. [CrossRef]
70. Vuitika, L.; Chaves-Moreira, D.; Caruso, I.; Lima, M.A.; Matsubara, F.H.; Murakami, M.T.; Takahashi, H.K.; Toledo, M.S.; Coronado, M.A.; Nader, H.B.; et al. Active site mapping of *Loxosceles* phospholipases D: Biochemical and biological features. *Biochim. Biophys. Acta* **2016**, *1861*, 970–979. [CrossRef]
71. Chaves-Moreira, D.; Moraes, F.; Caruso, I.; Chaim, O.M.; Senff-Ribeiro, A.; Sussuchi, L.; Chahine, J.; Arni, R.K.; Veiga, S.S. Potential implications for drug design against phospholipase-D from Brown spider venom. *J. Cell. Biochem.* **2017**, *118*, 726–738. [CrossRef]
72. Selvy, P.E.; Lavieri, R.R.; Lindsley, C.W.; Brown, H.A. Phospholipase D: Enzymology, functionality, and chemical modulation. *Chem. Rev.* **2011**, *111*, 6064–6119. [CrossRef]
73. Issuree, P.D.; Pushparaj, P.N.; Pervaiz, S.; Melendez, A.J. Resveratrol attenuates C5ainduced inflammatory responses in vitro and in vivo by inhibiting phospholipase D and sphingosine kinase activities. *FASEB J.* **2009**, *23*, 2412–2424. [CrossRef]
74. Alhouayek, M.; Muccioli, G.G. Harnessing the anti-inflammatory potential of palmitoylethanolamide. *Drug Discov. Today* **2014**, *19*, 1632–1639. [CrossRef]
75. Veiga, S.S.; da Silveira, R.B.; Dreyfuss, J.L.; Haoach, J.; Pereira, A.M.; Mangili, O.C.; Gremski, W. Identification of high molecular weight serine-proteases in *Loxosceles intermedia* (brown spider) venom. *Toxicon* **2000**, *38*, 825–839. [CrossRef]
76. Veiga, S.S.; Feitosa, L.; dos Santos, V.L.; de Souza, G.A.; Ribeiro, A.S.; Mangili, O.C.; Porcionatto, M.A.; Nader, H.B.; Dietrich, C.P.; Brentani, R.R.; et al. Effect of brown spider venom on basement membrane structures. *Histochem. J.* **2000**, *32*, 397–408. [CrossRef]
77. Young, A.R.; Pincus, S.J. Comparison of enzymatic activity from three species of necrotising arachnids in Australia: *Loxosceles rufescens, Badumna insignis* and *Lampona cylindrata*. *Toxicon* **2001**, *39*, 391–400. [CrossRef]
78. Fernandes-Pedrosa, F.; Junqueira-de-Azevedo, L.; Goncalves-de-Andrade, R.M.; Kobashi, L.S.; Almeida, D.D.; Ho, P.L.; ambourgi, D.V. Transcriptome analysis of *Loxosceles laeta* (Araneae, Sicariidae) spider venomous gland using expressed sequence tags. *BMC Genom.* **2008**, *9*, 279. [CrossRef]

79. Chaim, O.M.; Trevisan-Silva, D.; Chaves-Moreira, D.; Wille, A.C.; Ferrer, V.P.; Matsubara, F.H.; Mangili, O.C.; Silveira, R.B.; Gremski, L.H.; Gremski, W.; et al. Brown spider (*Loxosceles* genus) venom toxins: Tools for biological purposes. *Toxins* **2011**, *3*, 309–344. [CrossRef]
80. Sawant, R.; Nagendran, S. Protease: An enzyme with multiple industrial applications. *J. Pharm. Pharm. Sci.* **2014**, *3*, 568–579.
81. Otlewski, J.; Krowarsch, D.; Apostoluk, W. Protein inhibitors of serine proteinases. *Acta Biochim. Pol.* **1999**, *46*, 531–565.
82. Krowarsch, D.; Cierpicki, T.; Jelen, F.; Otlewski, J. Canonical protein inhibitors of serine proteases. *Cell. Mol. Life Sci.* **2003**, *60*, 2427–2444. [CrossRef]
83. Huntington, J.A. Serpin structure, function and dysfunction. *J Thromb. Haemost.* **2011**, *9*, 26–34. [CrossRef] [PubMed]
84. Gatto, M.; Iaccarino, L.; Ghirardello, A.; Bassi, N.; Pontisso, P.; Punzi, L.; Shoenfeld, Y.; Doria, A. Serpins, immunity and autoimmunity: Old molecules, new functions. *Clin. Rev. Allergy Immunol.* **2013**, *45*, 267–280. [CrossRef] [PubMed]
85. Sanrattana, W.; Maas, C.; de Maat, S. SERPINs-From Trap to Treatment. *Front. Med.* **2019**, *6*, 25. [CrossRef] [PubMed]
86. Rubin, H. Serine protease inhibitors (SERPINS): Where mechanism meets medicine. *Nat. Med.* **1996**, *2*, 632–633. [CrossRef] [PubMed]
87. Davies, M.J.; Lomas, D.A. The molecular aetiology of the serpinopathies. *Int. J. Biochem. Cell Biol.* **2008**, *40*, 1273–1286. [CrossRef] [PubMed]
88. Lysvand, H.; Helland, R.; Hagen, L.; Slupphaug, G.; Iversen, O.J. Psoriasis pathogenesis–Pso p27 constitutes a compact structure forming large aggregates. *Biochem. Biophys. Rep.* **2015**, *2*, 132–136. [CrossRef]
89. Lucas, A.; Yaron, J.R.; Zhang, L.; Macaulay, C.; McFadden, G. Serpins: Development for Therapeutic Applications. In *Serpins Methods in Molecular Biology*; Humana Press: New York, NY, USA, 2018; Volume 1826, pp. 255–265.
90. Yuan, C.H.; He, Q.Y.; Peng, K.; Diao, J.B.; Jiang, L.P.; Tang, X.; Liang, S.P. Discovery of a distinct superfamily of Kunitz-type toxin (KTT) from tarantulas. *PLoS ONE* **2008**, *3*, e3414. [CrossRef]
91. Borges, M.H.; Figueiredo, S.G.; Leprevost, F.V.; De Lima, M.E.; Cordeiro, M.D.N.; Diniz, M.R.; Yates, J.R. Venomous extract protein profile of Brazilian tarantula *Grammostola iheringi*: Searching for potential biotechnological applications. *J. Proteom.* **2016**, *136*, 35–47. [CrossRef]
92. Zupunski, V.Z.; Kordis, D.; Gubensek, F. Adaptive evolution in the snake venom Kunitz/BPTI protein family. *FEBS Lett.* **2003**, *547*, 131–136. [CrossRef]
93. Mulenga, A.; Khumthong, R.; Chalaire, K.C. *Ixodes scapularis* tick serine proteinase inhibitor (serpin) gene family; annotation and transcriptional analysis. *BMC Genom.* **2009**, *10*, 217. [CrossRef]
94. Meekins, D.A.; Kanost, M.R.; Michel, A. Serpins in arthropod biology. *Semin. Cell Dev. Biol.* **2017**, *62*, 105–119. [CrossRef] [PubMed]
95. Mulenga, A.; Kim, T.; Ibelli, A.M. Amblyomma americanum tick saliva serine protease inhibitor 6 is a cross-class inhibitor of serine proteases and papain-like cysteine proteases that delays plasma clotting and inhibits platelet aggregation. *Insect Mol. Biol.* **2013**, *22*, 306–319. [CrossRef] [PubMed]
96. Kim, T.K.; Tirloni, L.; Radulovic, Z.; Lewis, L.; Bakshi, M.; Hill, C.; da Silva Vaz, I., Jr.; Logullo, C.; Termignoni, C.; Mulenga, A. Conserved *Amblyomma americanum* tick Serpin19, an inhibitor of blood clotting factors Xa and XIa, trypsin and plasmin, has anti-haemostatic functions. *Int. J. Parasitol.* **2015**, *45*, 613–627. [CrossRef] [PubMed]
97. Chmelar, J.; Oliveira, C.J.; Rezacova, P.; Francischetti, I.M.; Kovarova, Z.; Pejler, G.; Kopacek, P.; Ribeiro, J.M.; Mares, M.; Kopecky, J.; et al. A tick salivary protein targets cathepsin G and chymase and inhibits host inflammation and platelet aggregation. *Blood* **2011**, *117*, 736–744. [CrossRef] [PubMed]
98. Dalle Lucca, J.J.; Li, Y.; Simovic, M.; Pusateri, A.E.; Falabella, M.; Dubick, M.A.; Tsokos, G.C. Effects of C1 Inhibitor on Tissue Damage in a Porcine Model of Controlled Hemorrhage. *Shock* **2012**, *38*, 82–91. [CrossRef] [PubMed]
99. Colman, R.W.; Flores, D.N.; De La Cadena, R.A.; Scott, C.F.; Cousens, L.; Barr, P.J.; Hoffman, I.B.; Kueppers, F.; Fisher, D.; Idell, S.; et al. Recombinant alpha 1-antitrypsin Pittsburgh attenuates experimental gram-negative septicemia. *Am. J. Pathol.* **1988**, *130*, 418–426. [PubMed]

100. Schaefer, J.S.; Zhang, M. Hypoxia effects: Implications for maspin regulation of the uPA/uPAR complex. *Cancer Biol. Ther.* **2005**, *4*, 1033–1035. [CrossRef]
101. Bernardo, M.M.; Dzinic, S.H.; Matta, M.J.; Dean, I.; Saker, L.; Sheng, S. The Opportunity of Precision Medicine for Breast Cancer with Context-Sensitive Tumor Suppressor Maspin. *J. Cell. Biochem.* **2017**, *118*, 1639–1647. [CrossRef]
102. Katsukawa, M.; Ohsawa, S.; Zhang, L.; Yan, Y.; Igaki, T. Serpin Facilitates Tumor-Suppressive Cell Competition by Blocking Toll-Mediated Yki Activation in Drosophila. *Curr. Biol.* **2018**, *28*, 1756–1767. [CrossRef]
103. Mika, A.; Reynolds, S.L.; Mohlin, F.C.; Willis, C.; Swe, P.M.; Pickering, D.A.; Halilovic, V.; Wijeyewickrema, L.C.; Pike, R.N.; Blom, A.M.; et al. Novel scabies mite serpins inhibit the three pathways of the human complement system. *PLoS ONE* **2012**, *7*, e40489. [CrossRef]
104. Christeller, J.; Laing, W. Plant serine proteinase inhibitors. *Prot. Pept. Lett.* **2005**, *12*, 439–447. [CrossRef]
105. Ribeiro, R.O.; Chaim, O.M.; da Silveira, R.B.; Gremski, L.H.; Sade, Y.B.; Paludo, K.S.; Senff-Ribeiro, A.; de Moura, J.; Chávez-Olórtegui, C.; Gremski, W.; et al. Biological and structural comparison of recombinant phospholipase D toxins from *Loxosceles intermedia* (brown spider) venom. *Toxicon* **2007**, *50*, 1162–1174. [CrossRef] [PubMed]
106. Girish, K.S.; Kemparaju, K.; Nagaraju, S.; Vishwanath, B.S. Hyaluronidase inhibitors: A biological and therapeutic perspective. *Curr. Med. Chem.* **2009**, *16*, 2261–2288. [CrossRef] [PubMed]
107. Fox, J.W. A brief review of the scientific history of several lesser-known snake venom proteins: L-amino acid oxidases, hyaluronidases and phosphodiesterases. *Toxicon* **2013**, *62*, 75–82. [CrossRef] [PubMed]
108. Girish, K.S.; Kemparaju, K. The magic glue hyaluronan and its eraser hyaluronidase: A biological overview. *Life Sci* **2007**, *80*, 1921–1943. [CrossRef] [PubMed]
109. Macdonald, S.M. Potential role of histamine releasing factor (HRF) as a therapeutic target for treating asthma and allergy. *J. Asthma Allergy* **2012**, *5*, 51–59. [CrossRef] [PubMed]
110. Mulenga, A.; Azad, A.F. The molecular and biological analysis of ixodid ticks histamine release factors. *Exp. Appl. Acarol.* **2005**, *37*, 215–229. [CrossRef]
111. Buch, D.R.; Souza, F.N.; Meissner, G.O.; Morgon, A.M.; Gremski, L.H.; Ferrer, V.P.; Trevisan-Silva, D.; Matsubara, F.H.; Boia-Ferreira, M.; Sade, Y.B.; et al. Brown spider (*Loxosceles* genus) venom toxins: Evaluation of biological conservation by immune cross-reactivity. *Toxicon* **2015**, *108*, 154–166. [CrossRef]
112. Kimura, T.; Ono, S.; Kubo, T. Molecular Cloning and Sequence Analysis of the cDNAs Encoding Toxin-Like Peptides from the Venom Glands of *Tarantula Grammostola rosea*. *Int. J. Pept.* **2012**, 731293. [CrossRef]
113. Zobel-Thropp, P.A.; Correa, S.M.; Garb, J.E.; Binford, G.J. Spit and venom from scytodes spiders: A diverse and distinct cocktail. *J. Proteome Res.* **2014**, *13*, 817–835. [CrossRef]
114. Sangsuwan, J.; Wanichpakorn, S.; Kedjarune-Leggat, U. Translationally controlled tumor protein supplemented chitosan modified glass ionomer cement promotes osteoblast proliferation and function. *Mater. Sci. Eng. C Mater. Biol. Appl.* **2015**, *54*, 61–68. [CrossRef] [PubMed]
115. Taylor, K.J.; Van, T.T.; MacDonald, S.M.; Meshnick, S.R.; Fernley, R.T.; Macreadie, I.G.; Smooker, P.M. Immunization of mice with *Plasmodium* TCTP delays establishment of *Plasmodium* infection. *Parasite Immunol.* **2015**, *37*, 23–31. [CrossRef] [PubMed]
116. Fu, Y.; Lan, J.; Wu, X.; Yang, D.; Zhang, Z.; Nie, H.; Hou, R.; Zhang, R.; Zheng, W.; Xie, Y.; et al. Expression of translationally controlled tumor protein (TCTP) gene of *Dirofilaria immitis* guided by transcriptomic screening. *Korean J. Parasitol.* **2014**, *52*, 21–26. [CrossRef] [PubMed]
117. Bommer, U. Cellular Function and Regulation of the Translationally Controlled Tumour Protein TCTP. *Open Allergy J.* **2012**, *5*, 19–32. [CrossRef]
118. Kashiwakura, J.C.; Ando, T.; Matsumoto, K.; Kimura, M.; Kitaura, J.; Matho, M.H.; Zajonc, D.M.; Ozeki, T.; Ra, C.; MacDonald, S.M.; et al. Histamine-releasing factor has a proinflammatory role in mouse models of asthma and allergy. *J. Clin. Investig.* **2011**, *122*, 218–228. [CrossRef]
119. Bae, H.D.; Lee, K. On employing a translationally controlled tumor protein-derived protein transduction domain analog for transmucosal delivery of drugs. *J. Control. Release* **2013**, *170*, 358–364. [CrossRef]
120. Maeng, J.; Kim, H.Y.; Shin, D.H.; Lee, K. Transduction of translationally controlled tumor protein employing TCTP-derived protein transduction domain. *Anal. Biochem.* **2012**, *435*, 47–53. [CrossRef]
121. Wanachottrakul, N.; Chotigeat, W.; Kedjarune-Leggat, U. Translationally controlled tumor protein against apoptosis from 2-hydroxy-ethyl methacrylate in human dental pulp cells. *J. Mater. Sci. Mater. Med.* **2011**, *22*, 1479–1487. [CrossRef]

122. Amson, R.; Pece, S.; Marine, J.C.; Di Fiore, P.P.; Telerman, A. TPT1/TCTP-regulated pathways in phenotypic reprogramming. *Trends Cell Biol.* **2012**, *23*, 37–46. [CrossRef]
123. Pauli, I.; Minozzo, J.C.; da Silva, P.H.; Chaim, O.M.; Veiga, S.S. Analysis of therapeutic benefits of antivenin at different time intervals after experimental envenomation in rabbits by venom of the brown spider (*Loxosceles intermedia*). *Toxicon* **2009**, *53*, 660–671. [CrossRef]
124. Felicori, L.; Araujo, S.C.; de Avila, R.A.; Sanchez, E.F.; Granier, C.; Kalapothakis, E.; Chávez-Olórtegui, C. Functional characterization and epitope analysis of a recombinant dermonecrotic protein from *Loxosceles intermedia* spider. *Toxicon* **2006**, *48*, 509–519. [CrossRef]
125. Duarte, C.G.; Bonilla, C.; Guimarães, G.; Machado de Avila, R.A.; Mendes, T.M.; Silva, W.; Tintaya, B.; Yarleque, A.; Chávez-Olórtegui, C. Anti-loxoscelic horse serum produced against a recombinant dermonecrotic protein of Brazilian *Loxosceles intermedia* spider neutralize lethal effects of *Loxosceles laeta* venom from Peru. *Toxicon* **2014**, *93*, 37–40. [CrossRef] [PubMed]
126. de Almeida, D.M.; Fernandes-Pedrosa, M.F.; de Andrade, R.M.; Marcelino, J.R.; Gondo-Higashi, H.; de Azevedo Ide, L.; Ho, P.L.; van den Berg, C.; Tambourgi, D.V. A new anti-loxoscelic serum produced against recombinant sphingomyelinase D: Results of preclinical trials. *Am. J. Trop. Med. Hyg.* **2008**, *79*, 463–470. [CrossRef] [PubMed]
127. Olvera, A.; Ramos-Cerrillo, B.; Estevez, J.; Clement, H.; de Roodt, A.; Paniagua-Solis, J.; Vazquez, H.; Zavaleta, A.; Arruz, M.S.; Stock, R.P.; et al. North and South American *Loxosceles* spiders: Development of a polyvalent antivenom with recombinant sphingomyelinases D as antigens. *Toxicon* **2006**, *48*, 64–74. [CrossRef] [PubMed]
128. Dias-Lopes, C.; Guimarães, G.; Felicori, L.; Fernandes, P.; Emery, L.; Kalapothakis, E.; Nguyen, C.; Molina, F.; Granier, C.; Chavez-Olortegui, C. A protective immune response against lethal, dermonecrotic and hemorrhagic effects of *Loxosceles intermedia* venom elicited by a 27-residue peptide. *Toxicon* **2009**, *55*, 481–487. [CrossRef] [PubMed]
129. Alvarenga, L.M.; Martins, M.S.; Moura, J.F.; Kalapothakis, E.; Oliveira, J.C.; Mangili, O.C.; Granier, C.; Chávez-Olórtegui, C. Production of monoclonal antibodies capable of neutralizing dermonecrotic activity of *Loxosceles intermedia* spider venom and their use in a specific immunometric assay. *Toxicon* **2003**, *42*, 725–731. [CrossRef] [PubMed]
130. de Moura, J.; Felicori, L.; Moreau, V.; Guimaraes, G.; Dias-Lopes, C.; Molina, L.; Alvarenga, L.M.; Fernandes, P.; Frézard, F.; Ribeiro, R.R.; et al. Protection against the toxic effects of *Loxosceles intermedia* spider venom elicited by mimotope peptides. *Vaccine* **2011**, *29*, 7992–8001. [CrossRef]
131. Mendes, T.M.; Oliveira, D.; Figueiredo, L.F.; Machado-de-Avila, R.A.; Duarte, C.G.; Dias-Lopes, C.; Guimarães, G.; Felicori, L.; Minozzo, J.C.; Chávez-Olortegui, C. Generation and characterization of a recombinant chimeric protein (rCpLi) consisting of B-cell epitopes of a dermonecrotic protein from *Loxosceles intermedia* spider venom. *Vaccine* **2013**, *31*, 2749–2755. [CrossRef]
132. Figueiredo, L.F.; Dias-Lopes, C.; Alvarenga, L.M.; Mendes, T.M.; Machado-de-Avila, R.A.; McCormack, J.; Minozzo, J.C.; Kalapothakis, E.; Chávez-Olórtegui, C. Innovative immunization protocols using chimeric recombinant protein for the production of polyspecific loxoscelic antivenom in horses. *Toxicon* **2014**, *86*, 59–67. [CrossRef]
133. Almeida-Lima, S.; Guerra-Duarte, C.; Costal-Oliveira, F.; Mendes, T.M.; Figueiredo, L.F.M.; Oliveira, D.; Ávila, R.A.M.; Ferrer, V.P.; Trevisan-Silva, D.; Veiga, S.S.; et al. Recombinant protein containing B-cell epitopes of different *Loxosceles* spider toxins generates neutralizing antibodies in immunized rabbits. *Front. Immunol.* **2018**, *9*, 653. [CrossRef]

toxins

MDPI

Article

Chemical Synthesis, Proper Folding, Na_V Channel Selectivity Profile and Analgesic Properties of the Spider Peptide Phlotoxin 1

Sébastien Nicolas [1,†], Claude Zoukimian [2,3,†], Frank Bosmans [4,5,†], Jérôme Montnach [1], Sylvie Diochot [6], Eva Cuypers [5], Stephan De Waard [1], Rémy Béroud [2], Dietrich Mebs [7], David Craik [8], Didier Boturyn [3], Michel Lazdunski [6], Jan Tytgat [5] and Michel De Waard [1,2,*]

1. Institut du Thorax, Inserm UMR 1087/CNRS UMR 6291, LabEx "Ion Channels, Science & Therapeutics", F-44007 Nantes, France; sebastien.nicolas@univ-nantes.fr (S.N.); jerome.montnach@univ-nantes.fr (J.M.); stephan.de-waard@etu.univ-nantes.fr (S.D.W.)
2. Smartox Biotechnology, 6 rue des Platanes, F-38120 Saint-Egrève, France; Claude.Zoukimian@univ-grenoble-alpes.fr (C.Z.); remy.beroud@smartox-biotech.com (R.B.)
3. Department of Molecular Chemistry, Univ. Grenoble Alpes, CNRS, 570 rue de la chimie, CS 40700, 38000 Grenoble, France; didier.boturyn@univ-grenoble-alpes.fr
4. Faculty of Medicine and Health Sciences, Department of Basic and Applied Medical Sciences, 9000 Gent, Belgium; frank.bosmans@ugent.be
5. Toxicology and Pharmacology, University of Leuven, Campus Gasthuisberg, P.O. Box 922, Herestraat 49, 3000 Leuven, Belgium; eva.cuypers@kuleuven.be (E.C.); jan.tytgat@kuleuven.be (J.T.)
6. Université Côte d'Azur, CNRS UMR7275, Institut de Pharmacologie Moléculaire et Cellulaire, 660 route des lucioles, 6560 Valbonne, France; diochot@ipmc.cnrs.fr (S.D.); lazdunski@ipmc.cnrs.fr (M.L.)
7. Institute of Legal Medicine, University of Frankfurt, Kennedyallee 104, 60488 Frankfurt, Germany; mebs@em.uni-frankfurt.de
8. Institute for Molecular Bioscience, University of Queensland, Brisbane 4072, Australia; d.craik@imb.uq.edu.au

* Correspondence: michel.dewaard@univ-nantes.fr; Tel.: +33-228-080-076

† Contributed equally to this work.

Received: 16 May 2019; Accepted: 16 June 2019; Published: 21 June 2019

check for updates

Abstract: Phlotoxin-1 (PhlTx1) is a peptide previously identified in tarantula venom (*Phlogius* species) that belongs to the inhibitory cysteine-knot (ICK) toxin family. Like many ICK-based spider toxins, the synthesis of PhlTx1 appears particularly challenging, mostly for obtaining appropriate folding and concomitant suitable disulfide bridge formation. Herein, we describe a procedure for the chemical synthesis and the directed sequential disulfide bridge formation of PhlTx1 that allows for a straightforward production of this challenging peptide. We also performed extensive functional testing of PhlTx1 on 31 ion channel types and identified the voltage-gated sodium (Na_V) channel Na_V1.7 as the main target of this toxin. Moreover, we compared PhlTx1 activity to 10 other spider toxin activities on an automated patch-clamp system with Chinese Hamster Ovary (CHO) cells expressing human Na_V1.7. Performing these analyses in reproducible conditions allowed for classification according to the potency of the best natural Na_V1.7 peptide blockers. Finally, subsequent in vivo testing revealed that intrathecal injection of PhlTx1 reduces the response of mice to formalin in both the acute pain and inflammation phase without signs of neurotoxicity. PhlTx1 is thus an interesting toxin to investigate Na_V1.7 involvement in cellular excitability and pain.

Keywords: spider toxin; directed disulfide bond formation; Na_V channel activity; Na_V1.7; pain target; automated patch-clamp

Key Contribution: This manuscript describes the first complete chemical synthesis of phlotoxin 1 that uses a directed disulfide bond formation strategy. Thanks to the synthetic product, phlotoxin 1

activity could be fully characterized with regard to its selectivity profile on K_V and Na_V channels, and its potency could be ranked among other toxins active on $Na_V1.7$; an important pain target.

1. Introduction

Voltage-gated sodium (Na_V) channels are critical for the generation and propagation of action potentials [1–4]. They are composed of a pore-forming α-subunit and can be associated with β-subunits [5]. Nine isoforms of vertebrate α-subunits have been identified so far ($Na_V1.1$ to $Na_V1.9$), that can be further distinguished by their sensitivity to tetrodotoxin (TTX); a toxin from the Japanese Puffer fish. Indeed, $Na_V1.5$, 1.8 and 1.9 are TTX-resistant (TTX-r), whereas the other α-subunits are TTX-sensitive (TTX-s). These channels also differ by their distribution with $Na_V1.1$, 1.2 and 1.3 principally found in the central nervous system, whereas $Na_V1.6$, 1.7, 1.8 and 1.9 are predominantly, but not exclusively, expressed in the peripheral nervous system. In addition, $Na_V1.4$ is predominantly found within the skeletal muscle, whereas $Na_V1.5$ is chiefly present in cardiac muscle.

Na_V channels are involved in a wide array of physiological processes. In particular, $Na_V1.7$ was clearly identified as playing a crucial role in nociceptive pathways, which led to research into the development of novel therapeutics for pain treatment [6–18]. For examples, missense mutations of the *SCN9A* gene that encodes $Na_V1.7$ produces congenital indifference to pain [19]. Mice in which the *SCN9A* gene is inactivated produce a similar phenotype of pain resistance [20,21]. *A contrario*, gain of function mutations of *SCN9A* lead to the opposite spectra of clinical manifestations, including paroxysmal extreme pain disorder [22], painful small fiber neuropathy [23,24], iodiopathic small fiber neuropathy [2,25], or primary erythromelalgia with burning pain in extremities [26–28]. A set of biophysical alterations in $Na_V1.7$ channel properties accompanies these pathologies, including changes in fast inactivation, the induction of persistent currents, and lower voltage thresholds for activation. Upregulation of $Na_V1.7$ is also associated with metastatic potential in prostate cancer in vivo and could therefore be used as a putative functional diagnostic marker [29,30]. Finally, $Na_V1.7$ may (i) have a role in the migration and cytokine responses of human dendritic cells [31]; (ii) help regulate neural excitability in vagal afferent nerves [32]; and (iii) contribute to odor perception in humans [33]. Despite its therapeutic potential, the task of identifying selective $Na_V1.7$ channel inhibitors remain challenging given the high level of sequence homologies among Na_V channel isoforms, particularly in the structural loci governing ion conduction and selectivity. In spite of these difficulties, Xenome Pharmaceuticals successfully discovered XEN402, a compound that exhibits a voltage-dependent block of $Na_V1.7$ and is capable of alleviating pain in erythromelalgia patients [34]. Researchers at Merck reported the discovery of a novel benzazepinone compound that blocks $Na_V1.7$ and is orally effective in a rat model of neuropathic pain [35]. Finally, Genentech investigators found that aryl sulfonamide inhibitors selectively block $Na_V1.7$ by a voltage-sensor trapping mechanism [36]. Due to their physiological importance, Na_V channels are also one of the foremost targets of animal venoms or plant neurotoxins [37–39]. The binding properties of peptide toxins have characteristic features that facilitate the identification of new Na_V channel isoform-selective pharmacological entities. For example, many of the peptidic toxins identified so far do not target the conserved pore region but rather act as gating modifiers by influencing movements of the less-conserved voltage-sensing domain within Na_V channels [40,41]. This feature further enhances the success rate for identifying $Na_V1.7$ blockers with substantially improved selectivity over other Na_V isoforms. Reports on high affinity toxins for $Na_V1.7$ that are efficient to treat pain remain infrequent. For instance, the tarantula venom peptide protoxin II (ProTx-II) potently inhibits $Na_V1.7$ activation and abolishes C-fiber compound action potentials in desheathed cutaneous nerves [42]. However, ProTx-II application has little effect on action potential propagation of an intact nerve, an observation that may explain why ProTx-II is not efficacious in rodent models of acute and inflammatory pain. The scorpion toxin OD1 impairs $Na_V1.7$ fast inactivation at low nanomolar concentrations but lacks the required Na_V channel isoform selectivity [43]. Finally, μ-SLPTX-Ssm6a from centipede venom was reported to block $Na_V1.7$-mediated currents and produce favorable analgesic activity in a rodent model of chemical-induced, thermal, and acid-induced pain [44]; however, these data have yet to be reproduced. Part of the lack of efficacy of toxins on pain treatment can be explained by the fact that they require a concomitant activation of the opioid system to reveal their analgesic properties [45]. The theraphosidae family of spiders, belonging to the mygalomorph suborder, provided up to 20 analgesic peptides so far, all acting on $Na_V1.7$, and belong to one of three spider toxin families (NaSpTx-1, NaSpTx-2 and NaSpTx-3) [46]. All these peptides vary in size from 26 to 35 amino acid residues, and are folded according to an inhibitor cysteine knot architecture with three disulfide bridges organized in a Cys^1-Cys^4, Cys^2-Cys^5, and Cys^3-Cys^6 pattern. As a rule, these peptides are difficult to fold and require expert chemical techniques for synthetic production. Altogether, because analgesic peptides are difficult to identify, it remains important to further enlarge the repertoire of $Na_V1.7$-blocking toxins available to investigators interested in pain therapeutics.

Here, we report the chemical synthesis and the directed disulfide bridge formation of phlotoxin-1 (PhlTx1), a 34-residue and three disulfide-bridged toxin from the venom of a Papua New Guinea tarantula of a *Phlogiellus* genus spider species that was only scarcely characterized so far [47]. In addition, some synergistic effects were observed to occur between low doses of PhlTx1 and opioids for the treatment of inflammatory pain, suggesting an effect on $Na_V1.7$ channel [45,48]. Herein, PhlTx1 was tested on a large array of ion channels including voltage-gated potassium (K_V) channels, members of the two-pore domain potassium channel family (TASK1, TRAAK), inward-rectifying potassium channels, voltage-gated calcium (Ca_V) channels and Na_V channels expressed in either Xenopus *laevis* oocytes, COS or CHO cells. Remarkably, the principal effect was seen on Na_V channels. In particular, $Na_V1.7$ was found to represent the most sensitive isoform for PhlTx1 inhibition. We compared the $Na_V1.7$ blocking efficacy of PhlTx1 to 10 other-published $Na_V1.7$ blocking toxins that we chemically synthesized. Using an automated patch-clamp system with a single CHO expressing human $Na_V1.7$ cell line, we ranked the potency of PhlTx1 activity on human $Na_V1.7$ channel *versus* these other spider toxins in uniform experimental conditions. Finally, the analgesic potential of PhlTx1 was studied using the formalin pain test, indicating that it also represents an interesting lead compound for the development of an analgesic.

2. Results

2.1. PhlTx1 Description

PhlTx1 has been purified originally from the venom of *Phlogiellus* sp., *Theraphosidae Selenocosmiinae* (endemic to Papua New Guinea) and sequenced [47]. The peptide contains 34 amino acid residues, six cysteine residues bridged in an inhibitory cysteine-knot (ICK) architecture fold and is amidated at the C-terminus. The reported molecular weight of PhlTx1 is 4058.83 Da. Sequence alignment of PhlTx1 with other spider toxins illustrate that PhlTx1 has limited homology with previously identified peptides (sequence identities varying between 24 and 59% at best) (Figure 1). According to its sequence, PhlTx1 fits best within the NaSpTx-1 family with the following disulfide bridge organization: Cys^2-Cys^{17}, Cys^9-Cys^{22}, Cys^{16}-Cys^{29}. In contrast, it has very little homology with toxins from NaSpTx-2, NaSpTx-3 and NaSpTx-7 families (Figure 1). Several structural features of PhlTx1 hint at difficulties performing chemical synthesis. First, it contains three Pro residues (Pro^{11}, Pro^{18} and Pro^{27}) that are all susceptible to trans/cis isomerization and hence influence the proper induction of the secondary structures as well as the appropriate disulfide bridge pattern. Second, the immediate proximity of Cys^{16} and Cys^{17} is potentially a factor that could lead to disulfide bridge disarrangement, accompanied by inappropriate folding of the peptide and altered pharmacology. Finally, the lack of reporting on the chemical synthesis of PhlTx1, in spite of its potential interest ($Na_V1.7$ target for pain treatment) and its discovery dating back to 2005 is a sign that its chemical synthesis is not straightforward.

Name		Identity (%)	
Family 1: NaSpTx1			--CLG-F--C-P-N--CC---NRVCSR-----WCK-K---------
PhlTx1	**μ-theraphotoxin-Pspp-1**	100	-ACLGQWDSCDPKASKCCP--NYACEWKYP--WCRYKLF--------
TlTx1	κ-theraphotoxin-Tb1a	59	AACLGMFESCDPNNDKCCP--NRECNRKHK--WCKYKLW--------
TlTx2	κ-theraphotoxin-Tb1b	56	DDCLGMFSSCDPKNDKCCP--NRVCRSRDQ--WCKYKLW--------
CcoTx1	β-theraphotoxin-Cm1a	55	-DCLGWFKSCDPKNDKCCK--NYTCSRRDR--WCKYDL---------
CcoTx2	β-theraphotoxin-Cm1b	55	-DCLGWFKSCDPKNDKCCK--NYTCSRRDR--WCKYYL---------
TlTx3	κ-theraphotoxin-Tb1c	53	DDCLGMFSSCDPNNDKCCP--NRVCRVRDQ--WCKYKLW--------
HnTx-III	μ-theraphotoxin-Hhn2a	52	-GCKGFGDSCTPGKNECCP--NYACSSKHK--WCKVYL---------
HwTx-I	μ/ω-theraphotoxin-Hs1a	48	-ACKGVFDACTPGKNECCP--NRVCSDKHK--WCKWKL---------
PaurTx3	β-theraphotoxin-Ps1a	35	-DCLGFLWKCNPSNDKCCR-PNLVCSRKDK--WCKYQI---------
HnTx-V	μ-theraphotoxin-Hhn1a	29	-ECLGFGKGCNPSNDQCCKSANLVCSRKHR--WCKYEI---------
HnTx-IV	μ-theraphotoxin-Hhn1b	29	-ECLGFGKGCNPSNDQCCKSSNLVCSRKHR--WCKYEI---------
HnTx-I	μ-theraphotoxin-Hhn2b	29	-ECKGFGKSCVPGKNECCS--GYACNSRDK--WCKVLL---------
HwTx-IV	μ-theraphotoxin-Hs2a	23	-ECLEIFKACNPSNDQCCKSSKLVCSRKTR--WCKYQI---------
Family 2: NaSpTx2			-ECR--FGGC---DSDCC---HLGC---------CAWDGTF------
ProTx-I	β/ω-theraphotoxin-Tp1a	18	-ECRYWLGGCSAGQT-CCK--HLVCSRRHG--WCVWDGTFS------
Pn3a	μ-theraphotoxin-Pn3a	18	-DCRYMFGDCEKDED-CCK--HLGCKRKMK--YCAWDFTFT------
HaTx1	κ-theraphotoxin-Gr1a	15	-ECRYLFGGCKTTSD-CCK--HLGCKFRDK--YCAWDFTFSNSRDKW
Family 3: NaSpTx3			-YCQK-MWTCD--ERKCCE----VC------LWCK-----------
GrTx1	β-theraphotoxin-Gr1a	21	-DCVRFWGKCSQTSD-CCP--HLACKSKWPRNICVWDGSV-------
ProTx-II	β/ω-theraphotoxin-Tp2a	20	-YCQKWMWTCDSERK-CCE--GMVCR-----LWCKKKLW--------
GsAFI	β-theraphotoxin-Gr1b	17	-YCQKWLWTCDSERK-CCE--DMVCR-----LWCKKRL---------
GsAFII	κ-theraphotoxin-Gr2c	16	-YCQKWMWTCDEERK-CCE--GLVCR-----LWCKKKIEW-------
Family 7: NaSpTx7			-ECGGFWWKCG-GKP-CC---YVCSP--W---WC----P-------
VsTx-I	κ-theraphotoxin-Gr3a	18	-ECGKFMWKCKNSND-CCK--DLVCSSRWK--WCVLASPF-------

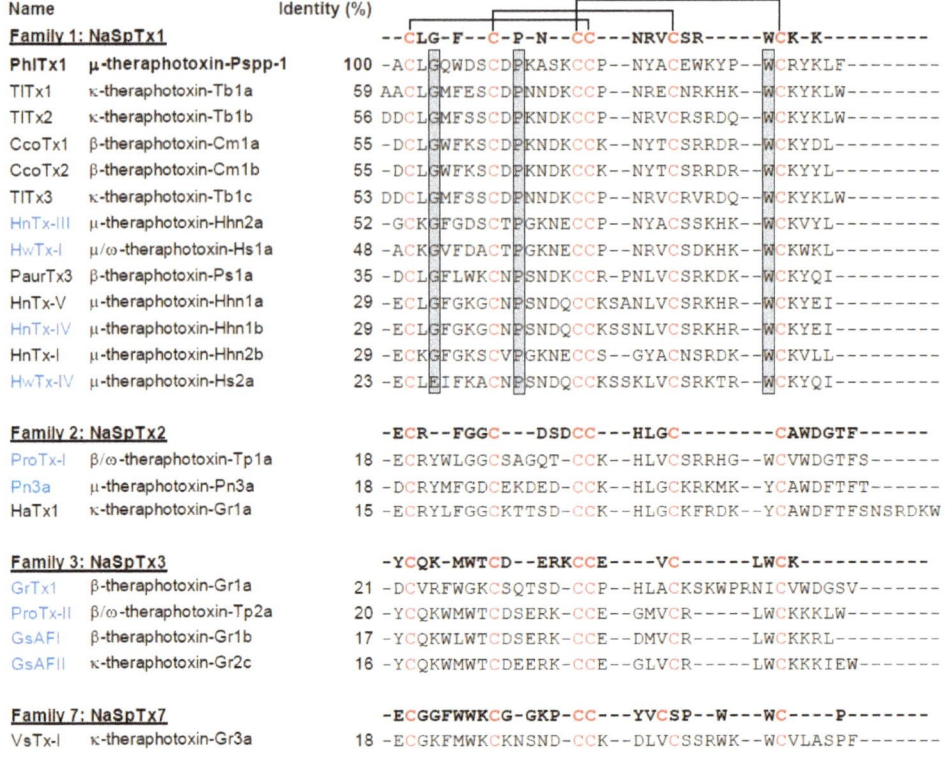

Figure 1. Sequence alignment of PhlTx1 with other spider toxins. Highly conserved cysteines are indicated in red and probable cysteine pairing, according to the inhibitory cysteine knot motif and the consensus sequence for NaSpTx-1 family of toxins, is indicated at the top with black lines. Percent conserved residues are indicated on the right. Shaded boxed residues correspond to the consensus residues of NaSpTx-1 toxin sequences. The lower homology with toxins from NaSpTx-2, NaSpTx-3 and NaSpTx-7 families are also shown. Toxins that are in blue have been compared in terms of activity on the $Na_V1.7$ channel with PhlTx1 (see Figure 7).

2.2. PhlTx1 Chemical Synthesis

In a first attempt to produce synthetic PhlTx1, the peptide was first stepwise assembled using fmoc chemistry, fully deprotected and purified from the crude synthetic products by preparative reversed-phase high pressure liquid chromatography (RP-HPLC) (Figure 2A). The purified linear peptide has the expected monoisotopic mass of 4061.79 (Figure 2A inset). Random oxidative folding of the peptide was performed at 0.1 mg/mL in a 100 mM Tris-HCl buffer at pH 8.4 with 5 mM reduced (GSH), 0.5 mM oxidized glutathione (GSSG) and 2 M Gn.HCl during 72 h at room temperature. According to the elution profile on RP-HPLC, the folding was (i) not straightforward, (ii) of very low yield and (iii) provided several peaks, possibly because of trans/cis isomerization properties of the Pro residues (data not shown). However, a dominant peak was purified as shown on the elution profile (Figure 2B). This purified peak resulted in the observation of two peaks in analytical RP-HPLC unless the column was heated, indicating the involvement of at least one Pro residue involved in trans/cis isomerization. Purifying either peak resulted in the production of the second peak demonstrating that the two forms (cis and trans) of the peptide are in equilibrium (data not shown). Other oxidative folded products may reflect misfolding of the peptide and inappropriate disulfide bridge arrangements. Purified folded/oxidized synthetic PhlTx1 was nevertheless shown to possess the proper monoisotopic mass of 4055.74 Da (Figure 2B inset). The 6 Da reduction in molecular weight of PhlTx1 is consistent with the formation of three disulfide bridges, but does not provide any indication about the favored pattern of disulfide bridges adopted by the toxin during this oxidative folding.

Because the random oxidative folding strategy and the final yield of production of PhlTx1 seemed problematic, we tried a directed disulfide bond formation strategy that ensures that the proper disulfide bridges are formed as expected for a NaSpTx-1 family toxin. Three different protecting groups were used for the lateral chains of Cys residues: Trt for Cys^9-Cys^{22}, Acm for both Cys^2 and Cys^{17}, and Mob for both Cys^{16} and Cys^{29}. The sequential order of disulfide bridge formation was thus Cys^9-Cys^{22} first after a classical deprotection of Trt groups with TFA, followed by Cys^2-Cys^{17} second and lastly Cys^{16}-Cys^{29} (Figure 2C). The two first disulfide bridges were sequentially formed in the same reaction buffer (one pot reaction), while the deprotection of Mob and the formation of the third disulfide bridge were done after purification of the two-disulfide-bridged PhlTx1. The synthetic crude PhlTx1 with the four remaining protecting groups (2 Acm and 2 Mob) after deprotection is shown on the RP-HPLC elution profile in Figure 2D, while the crude reaction mixture after formation of the first disulfide bridge is shown in Figure 2E. Formation of the first disulfide bridge is witnessed by the mass spectrometry analyses that illustrate a reduction in molecular weight (see insets; exact mass 4443.97 Da for the unfolded and 4441.96 Da for the one-disulfide bridged PhlTx1). The second disulfide bridge was formed after formation of the first one without intermediary purification in acidic conditions by the removal of the Acm protecting groups using iodine (see crude reaction mixture after formation of the second disulfide bridge in Figure 2F) and purified to homogeneity (Figure 2G). The acidic conditions were set to avoid disulfide bridge scrambling and secondary reactions with iodine such as iodine adducts on tyrosine or tryptophan residues. Next, the third disulfide bridge was formed in an oxidative and acidic buffer after removal of the Mob protecting groups with trifluoromethanesulfonic acid (TFMSA). Again, acidic conditions were used to avoid the risks of scrambling (see crude product in Figure 2H). The purified two-disulfide and three disulfide-bridged PhlTx1 are shown in Figure 2I. The large leftward shift observed in the retention time during elution is mainly due to the removal of the Mob protecting groups that are highly hydrophobic. All figure insets illustrating mass spectrometry profiles of the products indicate that each disulfide bridge has been formed properly with the appropriate removals of the protecting groups (exact mass of 4297.87 Da for the two disulfide-bridged PhlTx1 and 4055.73 Da for the fully-bridged disulfide PhlTx1). The overall yield of PhlTx1 production was 1.4%, which was 5 times better than that reached by random folding strategy. Nevertheless, the first strategy is expected to yield the same type of folding as both pure synthetic PhlTx1 coeluted perfectly (Figure 2J). This further illustrates that we purified the right peak within the random oxidative folding strategy, a fact that was not guaranteed in advance considering the presence of several peaks with the proper masses for oxidized PhlTx1. The directed disulfide bonding strategy we used should reveal itself to be very useful in experimental conditions where the random oxidative folding strategy turns to be inefficient (in SAR studies for example).

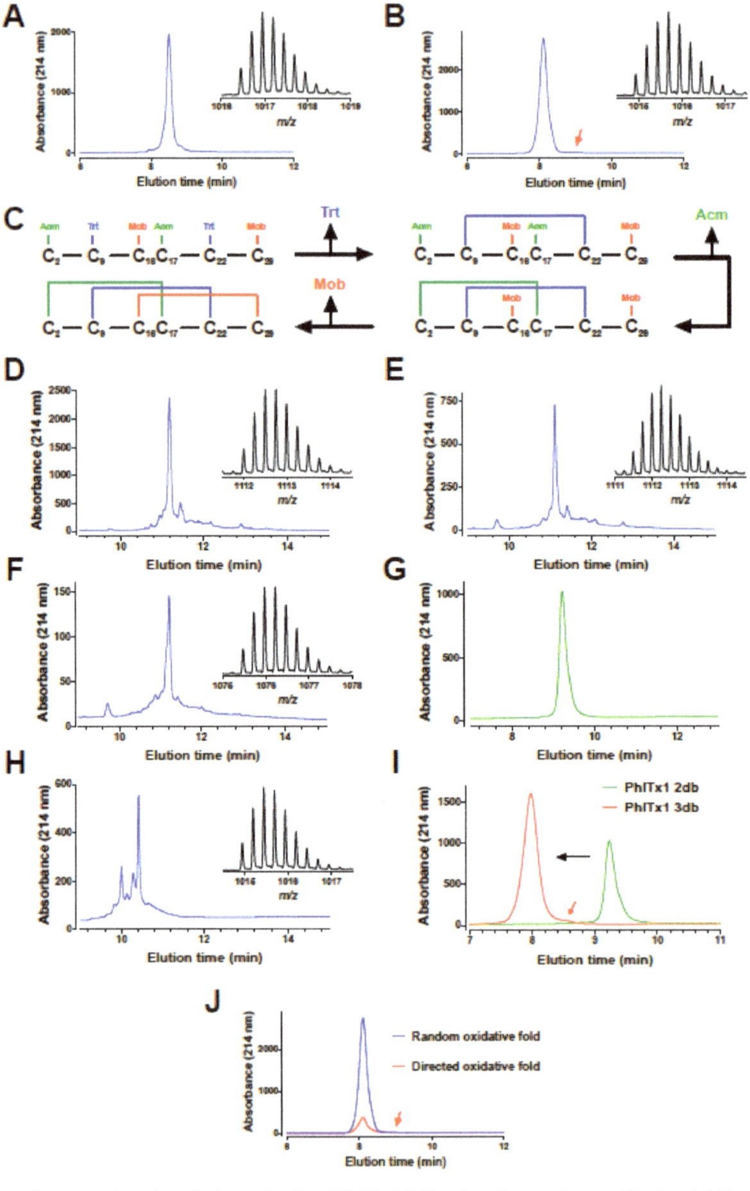

Figure 2. Comparative chemical synthesis of PhlTx1 following the random oxidative folding or the directed disulfide bond formation strategies. (**A**) Analytical RP-HPLC of the purified linear PhlTx1 meant to be produced by random oxidative folding (only Trt protecting groups for the 6 cysteine residues during chemical synthesis). Inset: MS spectrum of synthetic linear PhlTx1. $[M + 4H]^{4+}$ of 1016.45. (**B**) Analytical RP-HPLC of the folded oxidized PhlTx1. Red arrow possibly indicates the second conformer of PhlTx1 that is present. Inset: MS spectrum of purified PhlTx1. $[M+4H]^{4+}$ of 1014.94. (**C**) Schematic procedure employed for the directed disulfide bond formation strategy. (**D**) Analytical RP-HPLC of the crude linear PhlTx1 used for the directed disulfide bond formation strategy. Inset: MS spectrum of the synthetic compound with the Acm and Mob protecting groups. $[M + 4H]^{4+}$ of 1111.99. (**E**) Analytical RP-HPLC of crude PhlTx1 with its first disulfide bridge. Inset: corresponding MS

spectrum of the compound. $[M + 4H]^{4+}$ of 1111.50. (**F**) Analytical RP-HPLC of crude PhlTx1 with its two first disulfide bridges. Inset: corresponding MS spectrum of the compound. $[M + 4H]^{4+}$ of 1075.47. (**G**) Analytical RP-HPLC of purified PhlTx1 with its two first disulfide bridges. (**H**) Analytical RP-HPLC of crude PhlTx1 in its fully folded configuration. Inset: corresponding MS spectrum of the compound. $[M + 4H]^{4+}$ of 1014.94. (**I**) (**G**) Analytical RP-HPLC of purified two-disulfide bridged (2db) and three-disulfide-bridged (3db) PhlTx1 to illustrate the important reduction of hydrophobicity of the peptide upon removal of the Mob protecting groups. (**J**) Coelution of purified PhlTx1 produced by random oxidative folding with that produced by a directed disulfide bond formation strategy.

2.3. Ion Channel Selectivity of PhlTx1 and Preferential Activity on $Na_v1.7$

We tested the biological activity of PhlTx1 on a large selection of ion channels that comprise K_V channels, two members of the two-pore domain potassium channel family (TASK1, TREK2), inward-rectifying potassium channels, the acetylcholine receptor and Na_V channels (Figure 3). All tested targets were heterologously expressed in either *Xenopus laevis* oocytes and/or COS cells and the resulting ionic currents were measured using electrophysiological voltage-clamp techniques. When applying 1 μM PhlTx1 to all tested ion channels and measuring current inhibition at the voltage of maximum ion flux, $K_V3.4$ was the only non-Na_V channel impacted by the toxin (significant inhibition close to 20%). None of the channels tested were activated by the toxin.

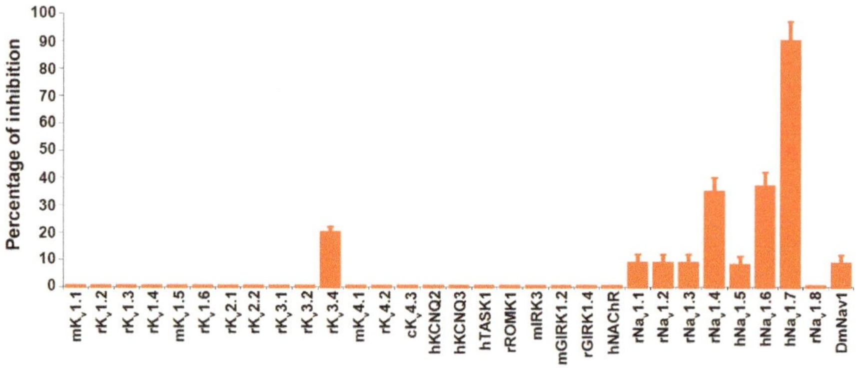

Figure 3. Overview of all tested channels indicating the percentage inhibition upon application of 1 μM PhlTx1. Expression system was either *Xenopus laevis* oocytes (all Na_V channels) and/or COS cells. Estimation of the effect on nicotinic acetylcholine receptor NAChR was achieved by ^{125}I-α-bungarotoxin binding as previously described [49]. Clones were from the following species: m, mouse; r, rat; c, canine; h, human; and Para/tipE, Fruit fly.

Using the two-electrode voltage-clamp technique on *Xenopus laevis* oocytes, the effect of PhlTx1 was also compared on eight different cloned vertebrate Na_V channels co-expressed with the β_1 subunit ($Na_V1.1$-$1.8/\beta_1$) and on the neuronal insect Na_V channel, para, co-expressed with the tipE subunit (Figures 3 and 4). When measured at the voltage of maximum sodium influx from a holding potential of −90 mV, 1 μM of PhlTx1 marginally decreased the sodium currents (10%) of most Na_V channel subtypes, while $Na_V1.8/\beta_1$ was not inhibited. Conversely, $Na_V1.4/\beta_1$ and $Na_V1.6/\beta_1$ currents revealed a maximum reduction of 35% when 1 μM PhlTx1 was applied (Figure 3). However, the inward currents of $Na_V1.7/\beta_1$ were almost completely inhibited (90 ± 7%) at 1 μM (Figure 3). Normalized current-voltage relationships (I-V curve) of $Na_V1.2/\beta_1$ and $Na_V1.3/\beta_1$ channels seemed to be shifted towards more negative potentials when PhlTx1 was applied, but shifts were not statistically significant ($p < 0.05$) (Figure 4). The activation phase of the other studied Na_V channel subtypes was not affected. No obvious alteration in channel availability was observed, except a 5-mV negative shift for $Na_V1.3/\beta_1$, although that was also non-significant ($p > 0.05$).

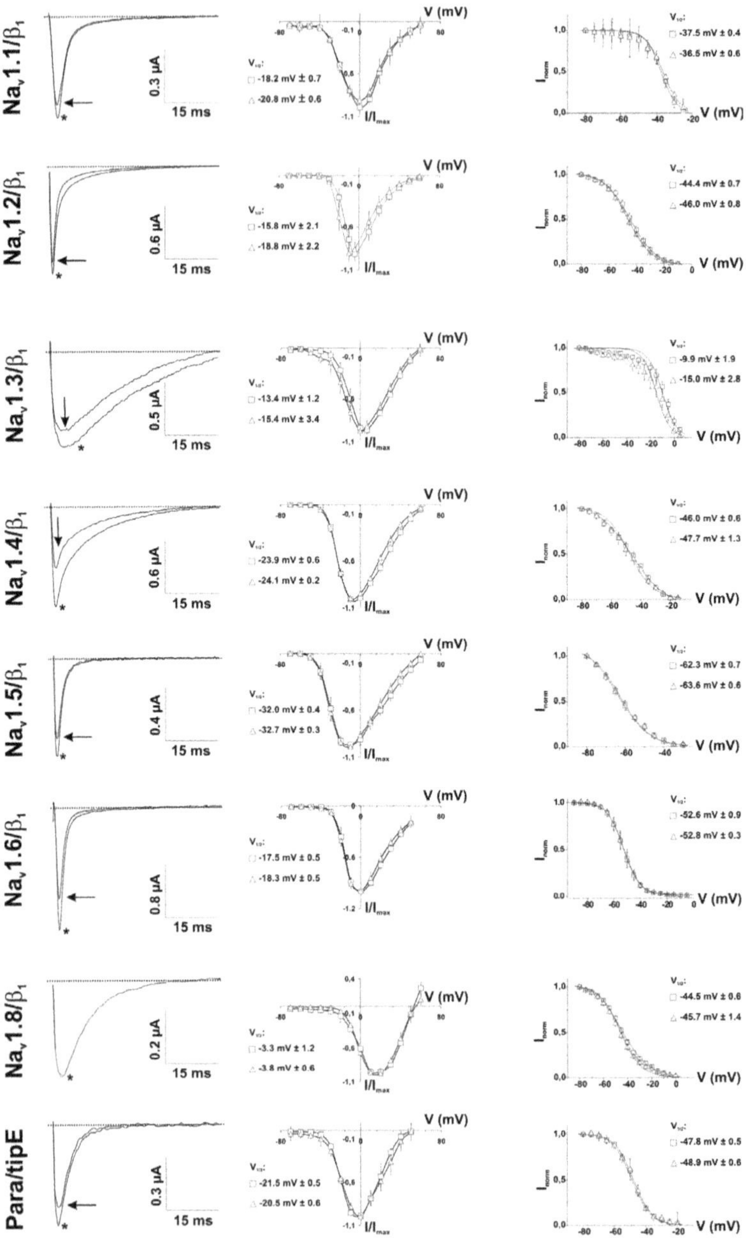

Figure 4. 1 µM of PhlTx1 was tested on Na$_V$1.1/β$_1$, Na$_V$1.2/β$_1$, Na$_V$1.3/β$_1$, Na$_V$1.4/β$_1$, Na$_V$1.5/β$_1$, Na$_V$1.6/β$_1$, Na$_V$1.8/β$_1$ and para/tipE ($n \geq 3$). Left column: current traces were evoked by a 50-ms depolarization to the voltage of maximum sodium influx, depending on the Na$_V$ studied, from a holding potential of −90 mV. At 1 µM PhlTx1, all studied Na$_V$ channels, except Na$_V$1.4/β$_1$, were blocked for about 10% (no toxin: *). The current of Na$_V$1.4/β$_1$ was reduced for about 35 ± 5%. Middle column: normalized I-V curves reveal no significant shift of the activation voltage ($p > 0.05$). Symbols: (□) before and (Δ) after addition of 1 µM PhlTx1. Right column: steady-state inactivation curves for all studied Na$_V$ isoforms. No significant shift was observed for any of the channels ($p < 0.05$).

We further characterized the inhibition of $Na_V1.7/\beta_1$ currents by PhlTx1. The residual inward current after at 1 μM PhlTx1 addition seems to occur without any alteration in channel kinetics (Figure 5A). Outward sodium currents at depolarizing voltages (+100 mV) were also blocked, as assayed with the help of tetrodotoxin (TTX; 50 nM) which physically occludes the pore (Figure 5B). Furthermore, $Na_V1.7/\beta_1$ inhibition did not seem to be very voltage-dependent, since the reduction of sodium currents at more hyperpolarized voltages (−70 to −30 mV) was similar to the reduction of sodium current at more depolarized potentials (−20 to 60 mV). The $Na_V1.7/\beta_1$ gating parameters, before and after addition of 1 μM PhlTx1 ($n = 4$; Figure 5C), are not affected ($p < 0.05$; see Figure 5D). Again, no alteration in steady-state inactivation or E_{rev} was seen (Figure 5B,E). In order to obtain the IC_{50} value of PhlTx1 on $Na_V1.7/\beta_1$, expressed in *Xenopus laevis* oocytes, the percentage of toxin-induced block obtained at a stimulus frequency of 0.3 Hz was plotted against the concentration of toxin used and a fit with the Hill equation yielded a value of 260 ± 46 nM with a Hill coefficient = 1.3 (Figure 5F).

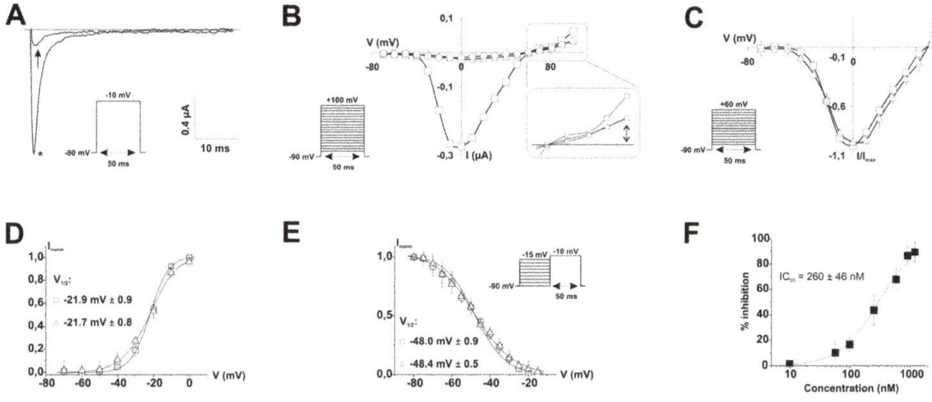

Figure 5. (**A**) Effect of 1 μM of PhlTx1 on $Na_V1.7/\beta_1$. Current trace was evoked by a 50-ms depolarization to −10 mV, from a holding potential of −90 mV. A nearly complete block of the inward sodium current is seen (no toxin: *). (**B**) I–V protocol to positive voltages (+100 mV). □ represents control conditions where no toxin was added. 50 nM of TTX was added (○) after maximum block was obtained with 1 μM of PhlTx1 (Δ). No further reduction of the outward current was seen (see inset). Therefore, the remaining outward current does not contain a $Na_V1.7/\beta_1$ component anymore. (**C**) Normalized I-V curve of $Na_V1.7/\beta_1$ before (□) and after addition of 1 μM PhlTx1 (Δ) (n = 5). (**D**) Normalized activation curves derived from (**C**). No change in activation voltages or $V_{1/2}$ was seen. (**E**) Steady-state inactivation curves before and after addition of 1 μM PhlTx1. No effect was seen. (**F**) In order to obtain the IC_{50} value of PhlTx1 on $Na_V1.7/\beta_1$, the percentage of toxin-induced block was plotted against the concentration of toxin used and a fit with the Hill equation yielded a value of 260 ± 46 nM (n = 4; Hill coefficient = 1.3). The stimulus frequency was 0.3 Hz.

2.4. *Refined Affinity of PhlTx1 for the $Na_v1.7$ Channel in Mammalian Cells*

Following our initial screen for the selectivity of synthetic PhlTx1 and the discovery that $Na_V1.7$ was the main target, we decided to further evaluate the activity of PhlTx1. We used a CHO mammalian cell line expressing the human $Na_V1.7$ instead of *Xenopus* oocytes for the pharmacological evaluation. To this end, we used an automated patch-clamp system, the Nanion syncropatch 384PE, and a standardized robotic method from Beckmann to apply PhlTx1 in the recording chambers and collect the kinetic information of $Na_V1.7$ current from a high number of $Na_V1.7$-expressing cells. The syncropatch 384PE has the potential to record from 384 cells at a time. 100-ms pulses from −100 mV to −10 mV were applied at a frequency of 0.2 Hz and various concentrations of PhlTx1 were applied to the cells. An example of a $Na_V1.7$ current recording is illustrated in Figure 6A along with the effect of 100 nM PhlTx1. It is of interest to note that current inhibition develops over time at this PhlTx1 concentration that is above 50% at the end of a 13-min application time. As in oocytes experiments, PhlTx1 does not affect the kinetics of $Na_V1.7$ currents (activation or inactivation). We illustrated the time course of current block by PhlTx1 at concentrations (33 nM, 100 nM, 333 nM and 1 μM) that best frame the inhibition of $Na_V1.7$-mediated currents (Figure 6B). Note that the highest achievable inhibition was 85%–92% for the two most efficient concentrations (333 nM and 1 μM). The time constant of inhibition was concentration-dependent as expected and could be fitted with decreasing mono-exponentials with time constants of 253 s (33 nM, n = 4), 159 s (100 nM, n = 8), 97 s (333 nM, n = 6) and 36 s (1 μM, n = 8). Reporting the maximally reached inhibition at the end of the PhlTx1 application as a function of PhlTx1 concentration indicates that PhlTx1 inhibits $Na_V1.7$ currents with an IC_{50} value of 39 ± 2 nM (Figure 6C). Using a manual patch clamp, which is better suited to investigate current recovery from block than an automated patch clamp that requires several washing steps, we investigated the reversibility properties of a PhlTx1 block. As shown, the toxin effect was partially and poorly reversible (Figure 6D). After 16 min of washout of 100 nM PhlTx1, we observed a maximum of 32% recovery of the blocked current that occurred with a time constant of 303 s. Since $Na_V1.4$ and $Na_V1.6$ were the two most sensitive channels to the PhlTx1 block, we also performed dose-response curves for these two channels with the automated patch clamp system. According to the fits of the data, the calculated IC_{50} values of PhlTx1 for $hNa_V1.4$ and $hNa_V1.6$ expressed in CHO and HEK293 cells, respectively, were above 3 μM, indicating that PhlTx1 was indeed quite selective for the human $Na_V1.7$ channel (Figure 6E,F).

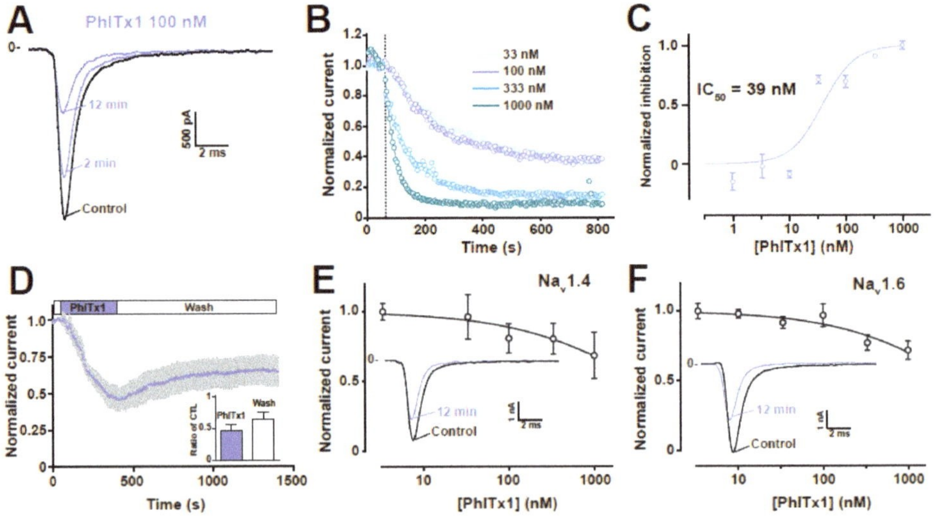

Figure 6. PhlTx1 inhibition of $Na_V1.7$ channels expressed in a mammalian cell line. (**A**) Representative current traces of $Na_V1.7$ current elicited at -10 mV (holding potential = −100 mV) before (Control) and at various times after application of 100 nM PhlTx1 (2 min and 12 min). (**B**) Average normalized current amplitudes before (left from vertical dotted line) and after application of various concentrations of PhlTx1 (right of dotted line). The average data points were fitted by mono-exponential decay equation y = 1-exp-t/τ + c with τ being the time. A c value of 0.09 at 1 μM PhlTx1 indicates that the block induced by PhlTx1 is not complete. A plateau of inhibition was reached for all concentrations. (**C**) Average dose-response curve of $hNa_V1.7$ current block by PhlTx1. A sigmoid Hill fit provides an IC_{50} value of 39 ± 2 nM and a Hill value of 1.53. Numbers of cells per concentration: 4 to 8. (**D**) Average kinetics of reversibility of PhlTx1 block of $hNa_V1.7$ currents (n = 5 cells). (**E**) Average dose-response curve of hNav1.4 block by PhlTx1. Numbers of cells per concentration: 4 to 13. (**F**) Average dose-response curve of hNav1.4 block by PhlTx1. Numbers of cells per concentration: 15 to 23.

2.5. Comparison of the $Na_v1.7$ Channel Blocking Efficience of PhlTx1 with That of Leading Toxins Active on $Na_v1.7$

PhlTx1 has two important properties underpinning its potential to be developed as analgesic: (i) a suitable selectivity profile, and (ii) a high affinity for $Na_v1.7$. Therefore, it was of interest to test how PhlTx1 ranks in terms of $Na_v1.7$ blocking activity compared to some leading peptides that are published as being active on this channel type [50–53]. Comparing data from published information is challenging as often the experiments are performed in different experimental conditions (including different cell lines, different species from which the $Na_v1.7$ clone originates, as well as differing application conditions and chemical synthesis quality, or even if the toxin is of natural or synthetic origin). Thus, we decided to chemically synthesize 10 additional toxins that are reported to block $Na_v1.7$ from various NaSpTx families (1, 2 and 3) and to test them in similar experimental conditions on the CHO cell line expressing $Na_v1.7$. Representative $Na_v1.7$-mediated currents traces are shown for each toxin type along with the extent of current block by 100 nM of this toxin at two time points (left panels of Figure 7A–J). Several observations can be made. ProTx-I, GsAFI, ProTx-II and HnTx-IV all lead to both relatively rapid and almost a complete block of $Na_v1.7$ current. The average time courses of inhibition are shown on the right panels for a concentration of 100 nM; a concentration set arbitrary that we consider as a good cut-off concentration to decide whether a toxin is an interesting lead blocker for $Na_v1.7$. At this concentration, all toxins block over 50% of the inward current with the exception of Pn3a; this toxin being fully insensitive at this concentration. The block by GrTx1 reached a plateau of inhibition of about 50% on average. The toxins differed also by their time course of block. At 100 nM, the fastest blocking toxins were ProTx-I (double exponential time course of inhibition with time constants of τ_1 = 4 s and τ_2 = 114 s), GsAF1 (τ = 21 s) and GrTx1 (τ = 18 s). Slower, but complete blocks, were observed for HwTx-IV (τ = 194 s), HnTx-III (τ = 149 s), HnTx-IV (τ = 62 s), GsAFII (τ = 98 s) and ProTx-II (τ = 72 s). The slowest blocking toxin was HwTx-I with an incomplete block even after 11 min 20 sec of application (τ = 492 s). The block by GrTx1 was accompanied by a slight current recovery at -10 mV test potential after it reached its maximal block. This is most likely due to a secondary alteration of the voltage-dependence of activation by the toxin, possibly by binding on a second site of lower affinity. This finding is in agreement with the concept of multimodal action of Tarentula toxins developed earlier, including for GrTx1 [54]. Finally, to fully characterize these peptides, we reported the blocking efficacies as a function of toxin concentrations (Figure 7K). The dose-response curves were illustrated for each NaSpTx families (NaSpTx-1: left panel; NaSpTx-2: middle panel; and NaSpTx-3: right panel). As illustrated, within the first family of toxins, PhlTx1 inhibition was most comparable to the inhibition by HnTx-III or HwTx-I (IC_{50} of 39 nM compared to 50.6 nM for HnTx-III or 25.1 nM for HwTx-I). Two toxins outperformed PhlTx1: HnTx-IV with an IC_{50} of 4.3 nM and HwTx-IV with an IC_{50} of 9.6 nM. Within the NaSpTx2 family, ProTx-I was 5.5-fold better than PhlTx1 with an IC_{50} of 7.1 nM, but Pn3a, reportedly very efficient, surprisingly had an estimated IC_{50} of 1457 nM. Within the NaSpTx3 family, all toxins were between 2.6- and 39-fold more active than PhlTx1 (IC_{50} values between 1 nM for GsAFI and 15 nM for GrTx1). The inhibition efficiency of GsAFI was unexpectedly even better than that of ProTx-II, the reference toxin in the literature for blocking $Na_v1.7$ channels. Several of these findings are in contrast with published reports demonstrating the importance of a standardized procedure to properly compare the potency of all these toxins (Table 1).

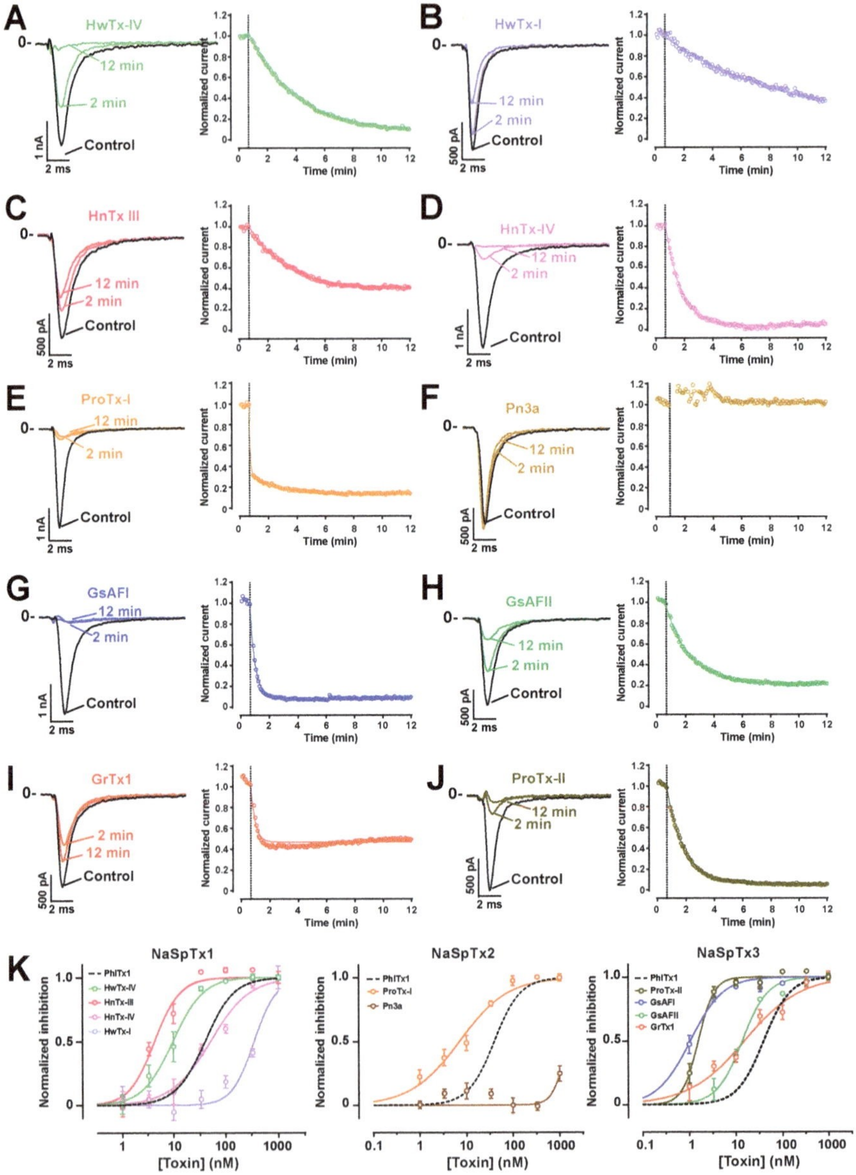

Figure 7. Comparison of PhlTx1-mediated inhibition of $Na_V1.7$ currents with the inhibition mediated by other reported $Na_V1.7$-blocking toxins. (**A–J**) Ten synthetic toxins, reportedly active on $Na_V1.7$ channel, from three families (NaSpTx1, NaSPTx2 and NaSpTx3) were tested for their blocking potency at 100 nM. Representative traces elicited from a holding potential of -100 mV and test pulse −10 mV in control condition and 2 and 12 min of toxin application time (left panels). All toxins were active at 100 nM with the exception of Pn3a. The kinetic of $Na_V1.7$ current block are shown in the right panels, thereby differentiating the fast and slow blocking toxins at this 100-nM concentration. (**K**) Normalized dose-response curves of current inhibition of each toxin compared to PhlTx1 for each NaSpTx family. Inhibitions were measured at end of a 12- or 15-min application time depending on toxin properties (fast or slow blocking). IC_{50} and Hill values obtained were 7.1 ± 1.2 nM and 0.84 (ProTx-I; n = 4–8 cells

per point), 1.0 ± 1.1 nM and 1.2 (GsAFI; n = 5–8 cells per point), 13.6 ± 1.2 nM and 1.6 (GsAFII; n = 2–8 cells per point), 1.5 ± 1.1 nM and 2.5 (ProTx-II; n = 5–8 cells per point), 4.3 ± 1.1 nM and 1.74 (HnTx-IV; n = 5–8 cells per point), 15.3 ± 1.2 nM and 0.73 (GrTx1; n = 5–8 cells per point), 1457 ± 169 nM and 3 (Pn3a; n = 3–7 cells per point), 50.6 ± 1.2 nM and 1.1 (HnTx-III; n = 5–8 cells per point), 25.1 ± 1.1 nM and 2.3 (HwTx-I; n = 2–7 cells per point), and 9.6 ± 1.2 nM and 1.5 (HwTx-IV; n = 6–8 cells per point). IC_{50} values of HwTx-IV, HwTx-I and HnTx-III are likely to be slightly under-evaluated because of incompletely reaching equilibrium at the lowest effective concentrations. The block by PhlTx1 is shown for comparison (dashed line).

Table 1. Comparison of IC_{50} values (in nM) for the human $Na_V1.7$ channel of toxins studied here or published (Publ.) as referenced (Ref.). Published data for GrTx1, GsAFI and GsAFII arise from purified peptides.

Family			NaSpTx1			NaSpTx2			NaSpTx3		
Toxin	PhlTx1	HnTx-III	HnTx-IV	HwTx-I	HwTx-IV	ProTx-I	Pn3a	GrTx1	ProTx-II	GsAFI	GsAFII
IC_{50}	39	50.6	4.3	25.1	9.6	7.1	1457	15.3	1.5	1.0	13.6
Publ.	250	232	21	630	26	72	0.9	370	1	40	1030
Ref.	[47]	[51]	[52]	[55]	[50]	[56]	[45]	[54]	[57]	[54]	[54]

With the exception of ProTx-II, none of the IC_{50} values we found matched those of the literature. We systematically found better values by an order of 2.7- (HwTx-IV) to 76-fold (GsAFI). The differences in affinity observed for GsAFI, GsAFII and GrTx1 are intriguing. In our analyses, these compounds were 40-, 76- and 25-fold more active in our hands than in an earlier report [54]. Here, two factors may explain the observed differences: (i) lack of use of BSA to avoid non-specific sticking of the peptides to the plastic tubes and dishes, and (ii) the fact that purified peptides were used and not synthetic ones. Quantifying native peptides is more difficult than quantifying synthetic ones because of limited quantities of material and is frequently a source of mistake in defining IC_{50} values. The 25-fold difference in IC_{50} value for HwTx-I also demonstrates the importance of standardized protocols for affinity measurements. *A contrario*, the most surprising finding was that Pn3a is far less active than expected [45]. The reason for this discrepancy is unclear, particularly since the chemical synthesis was straightforward. A more in-depth analysis of the disulfide bridge pattern acquired during the synthesis, possibly at odds with what was obtained earlier, may come as an explanation at a later stage.

2.6. Analgesic Potential of PhlTx1 In Vivo

Given the role of $Na_V1.7$ in nociception, we next evaluated the analgesic activity of PhlTx1 in an inflammatory pain assay on mice and compared the results to those obtained with morphine. Mice were injected intrathecally with vehicle solution only (0.9% NaCl, n = 11), morphine (0.25 mg in 10 μL vehicle, n = 6) or toxin-containing solution (100 pmoles PhlTx1 in 10 μL vehicle, 0.47 μg/mouse, n = 5). Rating of formalin-induced behavior was performed according to the time spent lifting, licking or biting the affected paw. In all cases, no neurotoxicity was observed after intrathecal injection. Strikingly, application of PhlTx1 substantially reduced the response of mice in both the acute pain (Phase I) and inflammation (Phase II) phases induced upon formalin injection into the paw, thereby demonstrating the analgesic effect of the toxin, possibly via a mechanism involving $Na_V1.7$ inhibition (Figure 8). This is the first formal description of the anti-nociceptive potential of PhlTx1. Although it appears to contradict a previous report suggesting a lack of effect of PhlTx1 on acute pain [45], it must be emphasized that the routes of administration differed (intrathecal here *versus* intraperitoneal in the previous study).

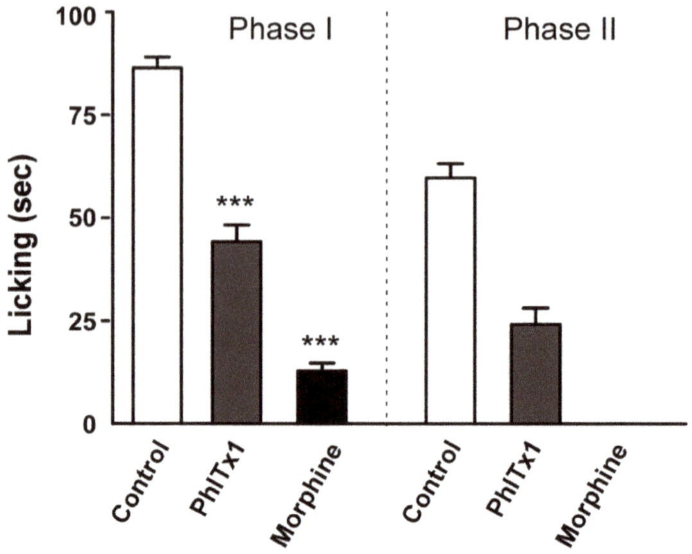

Figure 8. PhlTx1 is effective in a mouse model of acute and inflammatory pain. Effects of PhlTx1 (100 pmoles) and morphine (0.25 mg) on first (0–10 min) and second (10–45 min) phase of formalin-induced spontaneous pain behavior (n = 6–11) in mice. The licking value for morphine is 0 during phase II for all mice. Comparisons are *versus* vehicle unless specified. Mean ± s.e.m. *** = $p < 0.001$. This figure was presented in an earlier meeting in 2006 [47].

3. Discussion

In this report, we illustrated that PhlTx1 is a new member of the NaSpTx-1 family of toxins active on Na_V channels. Since its discovery in 2005, reports on the use of PhlTx1 have been scarce [45,47] and an extensive description of its pharmacology has been lacking. Part of the reason for this lack of published information, at a time where the $Na_V1.7$ has become a very interesting target for pain treatment, may lie in the difficulties linked to its chemical synthesis. Although the random oxidative folding strategy seems to work, the yields remain largely unsatisfactory to envision any kind of clinical future for this peptide or even to perform a complete Ala scan of the peptide to identify the pharmacophore of PhlTx1. Taking for granted that PhlTx1 folds according to the disulfide bridge motif of the NaSpTx-1 family, we decided to produce the toxin using a directed disulfide bond formation strategy. This strategy ensured that the disulfide bond pattern was respected and unique, led to a better yield of peptide production, and enforced the proper production of toxin variants that otherwise would fail to fold or oxidize properly. Concerning the wild-type sequence of PhlTx1, we do believe however that the random oxidative folding does yield the proper fold and disulfide bridges as both synthetic products coelute.

Although many new toxins are discovered each year, the same questioning regarding the natural target and the potential applications arises systematically. In many cases it is not sufficient to perform a blast search and find some homologous peptides, as this may be insufficient information to determine the target of the toxin. Here, PhlTx1 sequence is quite novel as its sequence barely matches other spider toxins. The fact that PhlTx1 belongs to the NaSpTx-1 family is also not sufficient information to indicate its potential cellular target. For this reason, we performed extensive testing of PhlTx1 activity on several voltage-dependent and one ligand-gated ion channels. Remarkably, we identified $Na_V1.7$ as the most sensitive ion channel for PhlTx1, with very few additional ion channels being sensitive to this toxin. Two other Na_V channels, $Na_V1.4$ and $Na_V1.6$, showed interesting sensitivities as well to PhlTx1, that were better evidenced using mammalian cells than oocytes. The discrepancy in

IC_{50} value for PhlTx1 blockage observed between oocytes and mammalian cells is a quite common phenomenon. It finds its origin in multiple factors such as lipid composition, the presence or absence of auxiliary subunits, or the fact that oocytes possess an extra vitelline membrane that peptides have to cross to reach their target. The rather narrow selectivity profile places PhlTx1 as an interesting lead candidate for the development of an analgesic. A careful reexamination of its affinity for the human $Na_V1.7$ channel isoform, expressed in mammalian cells, further reveals that its affinity is below 100-nM. This issue is particularly important if this toxin needs to be further investigated for its analgesic properties considering that its chemical synthesis is not straightforward. High affinity toxins may benefit from the fact that lower amounts need to be used in vivo to become efficient in their therapeutic task.

The modus operandi of channel block by PhlTx1 leads to some thoughts on its potential binding site. At face value, PhlTx1 activity resembles that of TTX that inhibits the pore. Other spider toxins such as HnTx-I, HnTx-III, HnTx-IV, HnTx-V and HwTx-IV also reduce the current amplitude of TTX-sensitive Na_V channels and have therefore been hypothesized to occlude the ion conduction pathway. HnTx-III, HnTx-IV and HnTx-V shift the voltage midpoint of steady-state inactivation to more hyperpolarized potentials, an effect that is not described with TTX when tested in rabbit purkinje fibers or here with PhlTx1. However, it is worth noting that most gating-modifier toxins interact with one or more voltage-sensing domains to inhibit or activate the channel [58]. Therefore, future work on PhlTx1 will include the determination of its binding site.

4. Conclusions

In summary, we successfully synthesized substantial quantities of the tarantula venom toxin PhlTx1 using two unrelated procedures that should greatly facilitate future SAR studies. The synthetic PhlTx1 is biologically active and was shown to predominantly inhibit $Na_V1.7$-mediated currents in two heterologous expression systems, whereas a large collection of other ion channels is not or only slightly influenced. When tested in a mouse model for inflammatory pain, PhlTx1 reduced the response of mice in the acute pain and inflammation phases, thereby supporting the role of $Na_V1.7$ in pain perception. Although PhlTx1 is not the most potent $Na_V1.7$ ligand isolated to date, it is not a weak affinity blocker according to our comparative analyses with leading $Na_V1.7$ acting toxins. In addition, it can reasonably be assumed that its affinity towards the channel may be improved further. For example, accumulating evidence suggests that defined peptide modifications can result in drastically increased toxin potencies [59–61]. The observation that $Na_V1.7$ loss-of-function in humans does not induce mortality offers tantalizing prospects for finding new routes of analgesia [19]. PhlTx1, as a selective antagonist of $Na_V1.7$, should therefore be considered as another exciting lead for novel pain treatments or as a potent pharmacological tool to dissect $Na_V1.7$ contribution to cellular excitability.

5. Materials and Methods

5.1. Chemicals and Peptides

The following toxins: ProTx-I, ProTx-II, GsAFI, GsAFII, GrTx1, Pn3a, HnTx-III, HnTx-IV, HwTx-I and HwTx-IV were all chemically assembled and provided by Smartox Biotechnology (Saint-Egrève, France).

5.2. Chemical Synthesis of PhlTx1

Linear PhlTx1 was assembled stepwise using fmoc solid-phase chemistry on a Symphony Synthesizer (Protein Technologies Inc., Tucson, AZ, USA) at a 0.1 mmol scale on 2-chlorotrityl chloride resin (substitution approx. 1.6 mmol/g). Fmoc protecting groups were removed using 20% piperidine in dimetilformamid (DMF) and free amine was coupled using tenfold excess of Fmoc amino acids and HCTU/DIEA activation in NMP/DMF (3 times 15 min). For the random oxidative folding strategy, all cysteine residues were introduced with trityl protecting groups. For the directed disulfide bond formation strategy, Cys^2 and Cys^{17} were introduced with Acm protecting groups, Cys^9 and Cys^{22} with trityl protecting groups, and Cys^{16} and Cys^{29} with Mob protecting groups. Linear peptides were deprotected and cleaved from the resin with TFA/H_2O/1,3-dimethoxybenzene/TIS 92.5/2.5/2.5/2.5 (vol.), then precipitated out in cold diethyl ether and the resulting white solids were washed twice with diethyl ether to afford crude linear peptides. Next, for random oxidative folding strategy, the fully deprotected PhlTx1 was purified by preparative reversed-phase (RP) HPLC prior to oxidative folding. Purification by RP-HPLC on a C18 (10 μm, 100 Å) Phenomenex Luna stationary phase on an Agilent Technologies preparative HPLC system (eluent system H_2O/MeCN + 0.1% TFA), afforded pure linear PhlTx1, which was folded by air oxidation at 0.1 mg/mL in a 100 mM Tris buffer at pH 8.4, containing 5 mM GSH, 0.5 mM GSSG and 2 M Gn.HCl. After 72 hrs at room temperature, the pH of the reaction mixture was adjusted to 3.0 and purified by preparative RP-HPLC. Two purifications, firstly by RP-HPLC on a C18 (10 μm, 100 Å) Phenomenex Luna stationary phase on an Agilent Technologies preparative HPLC system (eluent system H_2O/MeCN + 0.1% TFA), then secondly on a C12 (4 μm, 90 Å) Phenomenex Proteo Jupiter stationary phase on a semi-preparative HPLC system (eluent system H_2O/MeCN + 0.1% TFA), afforded pure synthetic PhlTx1 in a 0.25% overall yield. For the directed disulfide bond formation strategy, crude PhlTx1 was dissolved in H_2O/MeCN (1:1) at 10 mg/mL and added dropwise to a solution containing 0.1 M citric acid and 10% DMSO, at pH 7.8, to a final peptide concentration of 0.1 mg/mL. After one night under gentle stirring, pH was adjusted to 1–2, and 1 eq. of 50 mM iodine in MeCN was added every five minutes, for a total of five additions. Five minutes after the last addition, the excess of iodine was quenched with sodium ascorbate and the solution was filtered and purified by preparative RP-HPLC. Purification by RP-HPLC on a C18 (10 μm, 100 Å) Phenomenex Luna stationary phase on an Agilent Technologies preparative HPLC system (eluent system H_2O/MeCN + 0.1% TFA) afforded the pure two-disulfide bond PhlTx1. The freeze-dried peptide was dissolved in TFA/phenol at 0 °C and TFMSA was added to reach a concentration of 5 mg/mL of peptide in TFA/phenol/TFMSA (8:1:1). The mixture was stirred for 10 min at 0 °C and then the peptide was precipitated out in cold diethyl ether and the resulting white solid was washed twice with diethyl ether. The peptide was dissolved in H_2O/MeCN (1:1) at 10 mg/mL and added dropwise to a solution containing 0.1 M citric acid, 15% DMSO and 2 M Gn.HCl at pH 2.0, to a final peptide concentration of 0.1 mg/mL. After 48 h, the solution was purified by RP-HPLC on a C18 (4 μm, 90 Å) Phenomenex Proteo Jupiter stationary phase on an Agilent Technologies preparative HPLC system (eluent system H_2O/MeCN + 0.1% TFA) to afford pure synthetic PhlTx1 in a 1.4% overall yield.

5.3. Cell Culture

CHO cells stably expressing the human $Na_V1.7$ cells were cultured in Dulbecco's Modified Eagle's Medium (DMEM) supplemented with 10% fetal calf serum, 1 mM pyruvic acid, 4 mM glutamine, 10 IU/mL penicillin and 10 μg/mL streptomycin (Gibco, Grand Island, NY, USA), and incubated at 37 °C in a 5% CO_2 atmosphere. For automated patch-clamp recordings, cells were detached with trypsin and floating single cells were diluted (~300,000 cells/mL) in medium contained (in mM): 4 KCl, 140 NaCl, 5 Glucose, 10 HEPES (pH 7.4, osmolarity 290 mOsm).

5.4. *Xenopus* Oocyte Expression and Recording Experiments

For in vitro transcription, $Na_V1.5$/pSP64T and $Na_V1.8$/pSP64T were first linearized with *Xba*I and β_1/pSP64T with *Eco*RI. Capped cRNAs were synthesized from the linearized plasmid using the SP6 mMESSAGE-mMACHINE® transcription kit (Ambion, USA). The $Na_V1.1$/pLCT1, $Na_V1.2$/pLCT1, $Na_V1.3$/pNa3T, $Na_V1.4$/pUI-2, para/pG19-13-5 and tipE/pGH19 vector were linearized with *Not*I and $Na_V1.7$/pBSTA.rPN1 was linearized with *Sac*II. Transcriptions were performed with the T7 mMESSAGE-mMACHINE® kit (ThermoFisher Scientific, Illkirch, France). The harvesting of stage V-VI oocytes from the ovarian lobes of anaesthetized female *Xenopus laevis* frogs was carried out as previously described [62,63]. The use of *Xenopus laevis* was approved by the Animal Care Committee of the University of Leuven. Oocytes were injected with 50 nL of cRNA at a concentration of 1 ng nL^{-1}

using a Drummond (USA) micro-injector. The ND96 solution used for incubating the oocytes contained (in mM): NaCl 96, KCl 2, $CaCl_2$ 1.8, $MgCl_2$ 2 and HEPES 5 (pH 7.4), supplemented with 50 mg L^{-1} gentamycin sulfate and 180 mg L^{-1} theophyllin. Two-electrode voltage-clamp (TEVC) recordings were performed at room temperature (19–23 °C) using a GeneClamp 500 amplifier (Molecular Devices, USA) controlled by a pClamp data acquisition system (Molecular Devices, USA). Whole-cell currents from oocytes were recorded 2 to 4 days after injection. Voltage and current electrodes were filled with 3 M KCl. Resistances of both electrodes were kept as low as possible (<0.5 MΩ). Bath solution composition was (in mM): NaCl 96, KCl 2, $CaCl_2$ 1.8, $MgCl_2$ 2 and HEPES 5 (pH 7.4). Currents were filtered at 1 kHz with a four-pole low-pass Bessel filter, and sampled at 5 kHz. PhlTx1 was dissolved in ND96 containing 0.1% bovine serum albumin (BSA). This stock solution was added to the bath solution at the concentrations indicated. Data manipulation was performed in pClamp8 (Molecular Devices, USA) and Origin software (MVB Scientific, Nes-Ameland, The Netherlands). Averaged data are presented as mean ± SEM. In general, current-voltage relationships (I-V curves) were evoked in oocytes expressing the cloned Na_v channels by 50-ms depolarizations between −70 to +120 mV, using 5 or 10 mV increments from a holding potential of −90 mV. To avoid overestimation of a potential toxin-induced shift in the current-voltage relationship due to inadequate voltage control when measuring large sodium currents in oocytes, only results from cells with currents lower than 1.5 μA were considered. In order to obtain IC_{50} values, the percentage of toxin-induced block was plotted against the concentration of toxin used. A fit with the Hill equation yielded the IC_{50} values.

5.5. *Pharmacological Applications Using the Automated Patch-Clamp System*

PhlTx1 and other $Na_v1.7$-acting toxins were investigated on CHO cells expressing the human $Na_v1.7$ channel using the Automated patch-clamp system from Nanion (München, Germany), the SyncroPatch 384PE. Chips with single-hole and high-resistance (~6–7 MΩ) were used for CHO cell recordings. Voltage pulses and whole-cell recordings were achieved using the PatchControl384 v1.5.2 software (Nanion, Munich, Germany) and the Biomek v1.0 interface (Beckman Coulter). Prior recordings, dissociated cells were shaken at 60 RPM in a cell hotel reservoir at 10 °C. After cell catching, sealing, whole-cell formation, liquid application, recording, and data acquisition were all performed sequentially and automatically. The intracellular solution contained (in mM): 10 CsCl, 110 CsF, 10 NaCl, 1 $MgCl_2$, 1 $CaCl_2$, 10 EGTA and 10 HEPES (pH 7.2, osmolarity 280 mOsm), and the extracellular solution (in mM): 140 NaCl, 4 KCl, 2 $CaCl_2$, 1 $MgCl_2$, 5 Glucose and 10 HEPES (pH 7.4, osmolarity 298 mOsm). Whole-cell experiments were done at −100 mV holding potential and at room temperature (18–22 °C), while currents triggered at −10 mV test potential were sampled at 20 kHz. Stimulation frequency was set at 0.2 Hz. Toxins were prepared at various concentrations in the extracellular solution, itself supplemented with 0.3% BSA. The peptides were distributed in 384-well compound plates according to the number of toxins to be tested (generally four), the concentration range tested according to the assumed IC_{50} values, and the number of cells desired for each experimental condition. Compound solutions were diluted 3 times in the patch-clamp recording well by adding 30 μL to 60 μL external solution to reach the final reported concentration and the test volume of 90 μL. Percentages of current inhibitions were measured at the end of a 12- to 15-min application time (12-min for fast blocking toxins; 15-min for slow blocking ones). A single concentration of peptide was tested on each cell for building the full-inhibition curves.

5.6. *Formalin Pain Test*

Pain behavior experiments were performed in C57BL/6J mice with the formalin test which evaluates behavioral responses to subcutaneous injection of 10 μL of 5% formalin into the plantar surface of the right hindpaw. The total time spent in licking and biting the right hindpaw over the next 45 min and divided into two phases (acute phase I, from 0 to 10 min, and inflammatory phase II, from 10 to 45 min) was determined and used as "pain" parameter. The effects of drugs on acute and inflammatory pain were evaluated after intrathecal injection of PhlTx1 (10 μL at 10 μM), or vehicle

(NaCl 0.9%) (10 μL) or morphine-HCl (Cooper, 10 μL: 0.25 mg). Data were analyzed with GraphPad Prism 4. After testing the normality of data distribution, the statistical difference between different groups was analyzed using one way Anova followed by a Newman-Keuls multiple comparison test when $p < 0.05$. Mice procedures were approved by the Institutional Local Ethical Committee and authorized by the French Ministry of Research according to the European Union regulations and the Directive 2010/63/EU (Agreements C061525, NCE/2011-06 and 01550.03).

Author Contributions: Conceptualization, M.D.W., J.T., R.B. and D.B.; methodology, S.N., C.Z. and F.B.; software, S.N. and J.M.; validation, D.M., and D.C.; formal analysis, S.N., F.B. and J.M.; investigation, S.N., C.Z., F.B., J.M., S.D., E.C. and S.D.W.; resources, J.T.; data curation, J.T. and M.D.W.; writing—original draft preparation, M.D.W. and J.T.; writing—review and editing, M.D.W.; supervision, D.M., D.C., D.B., M.L., J.T. and M.D.W.; project administration, M.L.; funding acquisition, M.D.W.

Funding: M. De Waard thanks the Agence Nationale de la Recherche (ANR) for its financial support to the laboratory of excellence "Ion Channels, Science and Therapeutics" (grant N° ANR-11-LABX-0015). This work was supported by the Fondation Leducq in the frame of its program of ERPT equipment support (purchase of an automated patch-clamp system), by a grant "New Team" of the Région Pays de la Loire to M. De Waard, and by a European FEDER grant in support of the automated patch-clamp system of Nanion. The salary of S. Nicolas is supported by the Fondation Leducq, while the fellowship of J. Montnach is provided by an ANR Grant to M. De Waard entitled Bradycardia (grant N° ANR-15-CE14-0004-02).

Acknowledgments: We would like to thank the following persons: A.L. Goldin, Univ. of California, Irvine, USA for sharing $rNa_V1.1$, $rNa_V1.2$ and $rNa_V1.3$; G. Mandel, State Univ. of New York, USA for sharing $rNa_V1.4$; R.G. Kallen, Univ. of Pennsylvania, Philadelphia, USA for sharing $hNa_V1.5$, Roche (Palo Alto, CA, USA) for sharing $hNa_V1.6$ and $hNa_V1.7$; John N. Wood, Univ. College London, UK for sharing $rNa_V1.8$; S.H. Heinemann, Friedrich-Schiller-Universität Jena, Germany for sharing the $r\beta_1$ subunit; Martin S. Williamson, IACR-Rothamsted, UK for sharing the $DmNa_V1$ and tipE clone; and Nanion, Munich, Germany, for sharing the $hNa_V1.7$ cell line.

Conflicts of Interest: The authors Claude Zoukimian, Rémy Béroud and Michel De Waard declare the following competing interest: employee, CEO and consultant, respectively, of Smartox Biotechnology. The funders had no role in the design of the study; in the collection, analyses, or interpretation of data; in the writing of the manuscript, or in the decision to publish the results.

References

1. Dib-Hajj, S.D.; Cummins, T.R.; Black, J.A.; Waxman, S.G. Sodium channels in normal and pathological pain. *Annu. Rev. Neurosci.* **2010**, *33*, 325–347. [CrossRef] [PubMed]
2. Faber, C.G.; Lauria, G.; Merkies, I.S.; Cheng, X.; Han, C.; Ahn, H.S.; Persson, A.K.; Hoeijmakers, J.G.; Gerrits, M.M.; Pierro, T.; et al. Gain-of-function Nav1.8 mutations in painful neuropathy. *Proc. Natl. Acad. Sci. USA* **2012**, *109*, 19444–19449. [CrossRef] [PubMed]
3. Hille, B. *Ion Channels of Excitable Membranes*, 3rd ed.; Sinauer Associates Inc.: Sunderland, MA, USA, 2001; Volume 1.
4. Leipold, E.; Liebmann, L.; Korenke, G.C.; Heinrich, T.; Giesselmann, S.; Baets, J.; Ebbinghaus, M.; Goral, R.O.; Stodberg, T.; Hennings, J.C.; et al. A de novo gain-of-function mutation in SCN11A causes loss of pain perception. *Nat. Genet.* **2013**, *45*, 1399–1404. [CrossRef] [PubMed]
5. Ahern, C.A.; Payandeh, J.; Bosmans, F.; Chanda, B. The hitchhiker's guide to the voltage-gated sodium channel galaxy. *J. Gen. Physiol.* **2016**, *147*, 1–24. [CrossRef] [PubMed]
6. Bregman, H.; Berry, L.; Buchanan, J.L.; Chen, A.; Du, B.; Feric, E.; Hierl, M.; Huang, L.; Immke, D.; Janosky, B.; et al. Identification of a potent, state-dependent inhibitor of Nav1.7 with oral efficacy in the formalin model of persistent pain. *J. Med. Chem.* **2011**, *54*, 4427–4445. [CrossRef] [PubMed]
7. Chakka, N.; Bregman, H.; Du, B.; Nguyen, H.N.; Buchanan, J.L.; Feric, E.; Ligutti, J.; Liu, D.; McDermott, J.S.; Zou, A.; et al. Discovery and hit-to-lead optimization of pyrrolopyrimidines as potent, state-dependent Na(v)1.7 antagonists. *Bioorg. Med. Chem. Lett.* **2012**, *22*, 2052–2062. [CrossRef] [PubMed]
8. Focken, T.; Liu, S.; Chahal, N.; Dauphinais, M.; Grimwood, M.E.; Chowdhury, S.; Hemeon, I.; Bichler, P.; Bogucki, D.; Waldbrook, M.; et al. Discovery of Aryl Sulfonamides as Isoform-Selective Inhibitors of NaV1.7 with Efficacy in Rodent Pain Models. *ACS Med. Chem. Lett.* **2016**, *7*, 277–282. [CrossRef]
9. Frost, J.M.; DeGoey, D.A.; Shi, L.; Gum, R.J.; Fricano, M.M.; Lundgaard, G.L.; El-Kouhen, O.F.; Hsieh, G.C.; Neelands, T.; Matulenko, M.A.; et al. Substituted Indazoles as Nav1.7 Blockers for the Treatment of Pain. *J. Med. Chem.* **2016**, *59*, 3373–3391. [CrossRef]

10. Graceffa, R.F.; Boezio, A.A.; Able, J.; Altmann, S.; Berry, L.M.; Boezio, C.; Butler, J.R.; Chu-Moyer, M.; Cooke, M.; DiMauro, E.F.; et al. Sulfonamides as Selective NaV1.7 Inhibitors: Optimizing Potency, Pharmacokinetics, and Metabolic Properties to Obtain Atropisomeric Quinolinone (AM-0466) that Affords Robust in Vivo Activity. *J. Med. Chem.* **2017**, *60*, 5990–6017. [CrossRef]
11. Ho, G.D.; Tulshian, D.; Bercovici, A.; Tan, Z.; Hanisak, J.; Brumfield, S.; Matasi, J.; Heap, C.R.; Earley, W.G.; Courneya, B.; et al. Discovery of pyrrolo-benzo-1,4-diazines as potent Na(v)1.7 sodium channel blockers. *Bioorg. Med. Chem. Lett.* **2014**, *24*, 4110–4113. [CrossRef]
12. Macsari, I.; Besidski, Y.; Csjernyik, G.; Nilsson, L.I.; Sandberg, L.; Yngve, U.; Ahlin, K.; Bueters, T.; Eriksson, A.B.; Lund, P.E.; et al. 3-Oxoisoindoline-1-carboxamides: Potent, state-dependent blockers of voltage-gated sodium channel Na(V)1.7 with efficacy in rat pain models. *J. Med. Chem.* **2012**, *55*, 6866–6880. [CrossRef] [PubMed]
13. Marx, I.E.; Dineen, T.A.; Able, J.; Bode, C.; Bregman, H.; Chu-Moyer, M.; DiMauro, E.F.; Du, B.; Foti, R.S.; Fremeau, R.T., Jr.; et al. Sulfonamides as Selective NaV1.7 Inhibitors: Optimizing Potency and Pharmacokinetics to Enable in Vivo Target Engagement. *ACS Med. Chem. Lett.* **2016**, *7*, 1062–1067. [CrossRef] [PubMed]
14. Nguyen, H.N.; Bregman, H.; Buchanan, J.L.; Du, B.; Feric, E.; Huang, L.; Li, X.; Ligutti, J.; Liu, D.; Malmberg, A.B.; et al. Discovery and optimization of aminopyrimidinones as potent and state-dependent Nav1.7 antagonists. *Bioorg. Med. Chem. Lett.* **2012**, *22*, 1055–1060. [CrossRef] [PubMed]
15. Roecker, A.J.; Egbertson, M.; Jones, K.L.G.; Gomez, R.; Kraus, R.L.; Li, Y.; Koser, A.J.; Urban, M.O.; Klein, R.; Clements, M.; et al. Discovery of selective, orally bioavailable, N-linked arylsulfonamide Nav1.7 inhibitors with pain efficacy in mice. *Bioorg. Med. Chem. Lett.* **2017**, *27*, 2087–2093. [CrossRef] [PubMed]
16. Sun, S.; Jia, Q.; Zenova, A.Y.; Chafeev, M.; Zhang, Z.; Lin, S.; Kwan, R.; Grimwood, M.E.; Chowdhury, S.; Young, C.; et al. The discovery of benzenesulfonamide-based potent and selective inhibitors of voltage-gated sodium channel Na(v)1.7. *Bioorg. Med. Chem. Lett.* **2014**, *24*, 4397–4401. [CrossRef]
17. Suzuki, S.; Kuroda, T.; Kimoto, H.; Domon, Y.; Kubota, K.; Kitano, Y.; Yokoyama, T.; Shimizugawa, A.; Sugita, R.; Koishi, R.; et al. Discovery of (phenoxy-2-hydroxypropyl)piperidines as a novel class of voltage-gated sodium channel 1.7 inhibitors. *Bioorg. Med. Chem. Lett.* **2015**, *25*, 5419–5423. [CrossRef] [PubMed]
18. Wu, W.; Li, Z.; Yang, G.; Teng, M.; Qin, J.; Hu, Z.; Hou, L.; Shen, L.; Dong, H.; Zhang, Y.; et al. The discovery of tetrahydropyridine analogs as hNav1.7 selective inhibitors for analgesia. *Bioorg. Med. Chem. Lett.* **2017**, *27*, 2210–2215. [CrossRef]
19. Cox, J.J.; Reimann, F.; Nicholas, A.K.; Thornton, G.; Roberts, E.; Springell, K.; Karbani, G.; Jafri, H.; Mannan, J.; Raashid, Y.; et al. An SCN9A channelopathy causes congenital inability to experience pain. *Nature* **2006**, *444*, 894–898. [CrossRef]
20. Nassar, M.A.; Stirling, L.C.; Forlani, G.; Baker, M.D.; Matthews, E.A.; Dickenson, A.H.; Wood, J.N. Nociceptor-specific gene deletion reveals a major role for Nav1.7 (PN1) in acute and inflammatory pain. *Proc. Natl. Acad. Sci. USA* **2004**, *101*, 12706–12711. [CrossRef]
21. Gingras, J.; Smith, S.; Matson, D.J.; Johnson, D.; Nye, K.; Couture, L.; Feric, E.; Yin, R.; Moyer, B.D.; Peterson, M.L.; et al. Global Nav1.7 knockout mice recapitulate the phenotype of human congenital indifference to pain. *PLoS ONE* **2014**, *9*, e105895. [CrossRef]
22. Fertleman, C.R.; Baker, M.D.; Parker, K.A.; Moffatt, S.; Elmslie, F.V.; Abrahamsen, B.; Ostman, J.; Klugbauer, N.; Wood, J.N.; Gardiner, R.M.; et al. SCN9A mutations in paroxysmal extreme pain disorder: Allelic variants underlie distinct channel defects and phenotypes. *Neuron* **2006**, *52*, 767–774. [CrossRef] [PubMed]
23. Hoeijmakers, J.G.; Han, C.; Merkies, I.S.; Macala, L.J.; Lauria, G.; Gerrits, M.M.; Dib-Hajj, S.D.; Faber, C.G.; Waxman, S.G. Small nerve fibres, small hands and small feet: A new syndrome of pain, dysautonomia and acromesomelia in a kindred with a novel NaV1.7 mutation. *Brain* **2012**, *135*, 345–358. [CrossRef] [PubMed]
24. Bennett, D.L.; Clark, A.J.; Huang, J.; Waxman, S.G.; Dib-Hajj, S.D. The Role of Voltage-Gated Sodium Channels in Pain Signaling. *Physiol. Rev.* **2019**, *99*, 1079–1151. [CrossRef] [PubMed]
25. Faber, C.G.; Hoeijmakers, J.G.; Ahn, H.S.; Cheng, X.; Han, C.; Choi, J.S.; Estacion, M.; Lauria, G.; Vanhoutte, E.K.; Gerrits, M.M.; et al. Gain of function Nanu1.7 mutations in idiopathic small fiber neuropathy. *Ann. Neurol.* **2012**, *71*, 26–39. [CrossRef] [PubMed]
26. Cummins, T.R.; Dib-Hajj, S.D.; Waxman, S.G. Electrophysiological properties of mutant Nav1.7 sodium channels in a painful inherited neuropathy. *J. Neurosci.* **2004**, *24*, 8232–8236. [CrossRef]

27. Dib-Hajj, S.D.; Rush, A.M.; Cummins, T.R.; Hisama, F.M.; Novella, S.; Tyrrell, L.; Marshall, L.; Waxman, S.G. Gain-of-function mutation in Nav1.7 in familial erythromelalgia induces bursting of sensory neurons. *Brain* **2005**, *128*, 1847–1854. [CrossRef]
28. Fischer, T.Z.; Waxman, S.G. Familial pain syndromes from mutations of the NaV1.7 sodium channel. *Ann. N. Y. Acad. Sci.* **2010**, *1184*, 196–207. [CrossRef]
29. Chen, B.; Zhang, C.; Wang, Z.; Chen, Y.; Xie, H.; Li, S.; Liu, X.; Liu, Z.; Chen, P. Mechanistic insights into Nav1.7-dependent regulation of rat prostate cancer cell invasiveness revealed by toxin probes and proteomic analysis. *FEBS J.* **2019**. [CrossRef]
30. Yildirim, S.; Altun, S.; Gumushan, H.; Patel, A.; Djamgoz, M.B. Voltage-gated sodium channel activity promotes prostate cancer metastasis in vivo. *Cancer Lett.* **2012**, *323*, 58–61. [CrossRef]
31. Kis-Toth, K.; Hajdu, P.; Bacskai, I.; Szilagyi, O.; Papp, F.; Szanto, A.; Posta, E.; Gogolak, P.; Panyi, G.; Rajnavolgyi, E. Voltage-gated sodium channel Nav1.7 maintains the membrane potential and regulates the activation and chemokine-induced migration of a monocyte-derived dendritic cell subset. *J. Immunol.* **2011**, *187*, 1273–1280. [CrossRef]
32. Muroi, Y.; Ru, F.; Kollarik, M.; Canning, B.J.; Hughes, S.A.; Walsh, S.; Sigg, M.; Carr, M.J.; Undem, B.J. Selective silencing of Na(V)1.7 decreases excitability and conduction in vagal sensory neurons. *J. Physiol.* **2011**, *589*, 5663–5676. [CrossRef] [PubMed]
33. Weiss, J.; Pyrski, M.; Jacobi, E.; Bufe, B.; Willnecker, V.; Schick, B.; Zizzari, P.; Gossage, S.J.; Greer, C.A.; Leinders-Zufall, T.; et al. Loss-of-function mutations in sodium channel Nav1.7 cause anosmia. *Nature* **2011**, *472*, 186–190. [CrossRef] [PubMed]
34. Goldberg, Y.P.; Price, N.; Namdari, R.; Cohen, C.J.; Lamers, M.H.; Winters, C.; Price, J.; Young, C.E.; Verschoof, H.; Sherrington, R.; et al. Treatment of Na(v)1.7-mediated pain in inherited erythromelalgia using a novel sodium channel blocker. *Pain* **2012**, *153*, 80–85. [CrossRef] [PubMed]
35. Hoyt, S.B.; London, C.; Abbadie, C.; Felix, J.P.; Garcia, M.L.; Jochnowitz, N.; Karanam, B.V.; Li, X.; Lyons, K.A.; McGowan, E.; et al. A novel benzazepinone sodium channel blocker with oral efficacy in a rat model of neuropathic pain. *Bioorg. Med. Chem. Lett.* **2013**, *23*, 3640–3645. [CrossRef] [PubMed]
36. Ahuja, S.; Mukund, S.; Deng, L.; Khakh, K.; Chang, E.; Ho, H.; Shriver, S.; Young, C.; Lin, S.; Johnson, J.P., Jr.; et al. Structural basis of Nav1.7 inhibition by an isoform-selective small-molecule antagonist. *Science* **2015**, *350*, aac5464. [CrossRef] [PubMed]
37. Bosmans, F.; Swartz, K.J. Targeting voltage sensors in sodium channels with spider toxins. *Trends Pharmacol. Sci.* **2010**, *31*, 175–182. [CrossRef] [PubMed]
38. Catterall, W.A.; Cestele, S.; Yarov-Yarovoy, V.; Yu, F.H.; Konoki, K.; Scheuer, T. Voltage-gated ion channels and gating modifier toxins. *Toxicon* **2007**, *49*, 124–141. [CrossRef]
39. Gilchrist, J.; Bosmans, F. Animal toxins can alter the function of Nav1.8 and Nav1.9. *Toxins* **2012**, *4*, 620–632. [CrossRef]
40. Catterall, W.A.; Goldin, A.L.; Waxman, S.G. International Union of Pharmacology. XLVII. Nomenclature and structure-function relationships of voltage-gated sodium channels. *Pharmacol. Rev.* **2005**, *57*, 397–409. [CrossRef]
41. Payandeh, J.; Scheuer, T.; Zheng, N.; Catterall, W.A. The crystal structure of a voltage-gated sodium channel. *Nature* **2011**, *475*, 353–358. [CrossRef]
42. Schmalhofer, W.A.; Calhoun, J.; Burrows, R.; Bailey, T.; Kohler, M.G.; Weinglass, A.B.; Kaczorowski, G.J.; Garcia, M.L.; Koltzenburg, M.; Priest, B.T. ProTx-II, a selective inhibitor of NaV1.7 sodium channels, blocks action potential propagation in nociceptors. *Mol. Pharmacol.* **2008**, *74*, 1476–1484. [CrossRef] [PubMed]
43. Maertens, C.; Cuypers, E.; Amininasab, M.; Jalali, A.; Vatanpour, H.; Tytgat, J. Potent modulation of the voltage-gated sodium channel Nav1.7 by OD1, a toxin from the scorpion *Odonthobuthus doriae*. *Mol. Pharmacol.* **2006**, *70*, 405–414. [CrossRef]
44. Yang, S.; Xiao, Y.; Kang, D.; Liu, J.; Li, Y.; Undheim, E.A.; Klint, J.K.; Rong, M.; Lai, R.; King, G.F. Discovery of a selective NaV1.7 inhibitor from centipede venom with analgesic efficacy exceeding morphine in rodent pain models. *Proc. Natl. Acad. Sci. USA* **2013**, *110*, 17534–17539. [CrossRef] [PubMed]
45. Deuis, J.R.; Dekan, Z.; Wingerd, J.S.; Smith, J.J.; Munasinghe, N.R.; Bhola, R.F.; Imlach, W.L.; Herzig, V.; Armstrong, D.A.; Rosengren, K.J.; et al. Pharmacological characterisation of the highly NaV1.7 selective spider venom peptide Pn3a. *Sci. Rep.* **2017**, *7*, 40883. [CrossRef] [PubMed]

46. Goncalves, T.C.; Benoit, E.; Partiseti, M.; Servent, D. The NaV1.7 Channel Subtype as an Antinociceptive Target for Spider Toxins in Adult Dorsal Root Ganglia Neurons. *Front. Pharmacol.* **2018**, *9*, 1000. [CrossRef]
47. Bosmans, F.; Escoubas, P.; Diochot, S.; Mebs, D.; Craik, D.; Hill, J.; Nakajima, T.; Lazdunski, M.; Tytgat, J. Isolation and characterization of phlotoxin 1 (PhlTx1), a novel peptide active on voltage-gated sodium channels. In Proceedings of the 13ème Rencontres en Toxinologie "Toxines et douleur", Paris, France, 1–2 December 2005.
48. Emery, E.C.; Luiz, A.P.; Wood, J.N. Nav1.7 and other voltage-gated sodium channels as drug targets for pain relief. *Expert Opin. Ther. Targets* **2016**, *20*, 975–983. [CrossRef] [PubMed]
49. Blacklow, B.; Kornhauser, R.; Hains, P.G.; Loiacono, R.; Escoubas, P.; Graudins, A.; Nicholson, G.M. alpha-Elapitoxin-Aa2a, a long-chain snake alpha-neurotoxin with potent actions on muscle (alpha1)(2)betagammadelta nicotinic receptors, lacks the classical high affinity for neuronal alpha7 nicotinic receptors. *Biochem. Pharmacol.* **2011**, *81*, 314–325. [CrossRef]
50. Xiao, Y.; Bingham, J.P.; Zhu, W.; Moczydlowski, E.; Liang, S.; Cummins, T.R. Tarantula huwentoxin-IV inhibits neuronal sodium channels by binding to receptor site 4 and trapping the domain ii voltage sensor in the closed configuration. *J. Biol. Chem.* **2008**, *283*, 27300–27313. [CrossRef]
51. Liu, Z.; Cai, T.; Zhu, Q.; Deng, M.; Li, J.; Zhou, X.; Zhang, F.; Li, D.; Li, J.; Liu, Y.; et al. Structure and function of hainantoxin-III, a selective antagonist of neuronal tetrodotoxin-sensitive voltage-gated sodium channels isolated from the Chinese bird spider *Ornithoctonus hainana*. *J. Biol. Chem.* **2013**, *288*, 20392–20403. [CrossRef]
52. Liu, Y.; Tang, J.; Zhang, Y.; Xun, X.; Tang, D.; Peng, D.; Yi, J.; Liu, Z.; Shi, X. Synthesis and analgesic effects of mu-TRTX-Hhn1b on models of inflammatory and neuropathic pain. *Toxins* **2014**, *6*, 2363–2378. [CrossRef]
53. Klint, J.K.; Smith, J.J.; Vetter, I.; Rupasinghe, D.B.; Er, S.Y.; Senff, S.; Herzig, V.; Mobli, M.; Lewis, R.J.; Bosmans, F.; et al. Seven novel modulators of the analgesic target NaV 1.7 uncovered using a high-throughput venom-based discovery approach. *Br. J. Pharmacol.* **2015**, *172*, 2445–2458. [CrossRef]
54. Redaelli, E.; Cassulini, R.R.; Silva, D.F.; Clement, H.; Schiavon, E.; Zamudio, F.Z.; Odell, G.; Arcangeli, A.; Clare, J.J.; Alagon, A.; et al. Target promiscuity and heterogeneous effects of tarantula venom peptides affecting Na+ and K+ ion channels. *J. Biol. Chem.* **2010**, *285*, 4130–4142. [CrossRef] [PubMed]
55. Meng, E.; Cai, T.F.; Li, W.Y.; Zhang, H.; Liu, Y.B.; Peng, K.; Liang, S.; Zhang, D.Y. Functional expression of spider neurotoxic peptide huwentoxin-I in *E. coli*. *PLoS ONE* **2011**, *6*, e21608. [CrossRef]
56. Middleton, R.E.; Warren, V.A.; Kraus, R.L.; Hwang, J.C.; Liu, C.J.; Dai, G.; Brochu, R.M.; Kohler, M.G.; Gao, Y.D.; Garsky, V.M.; et al. Two tarantula peptides inhibit activation of multiple sodium channels. *Biochemistry* **2002**, *41*, 14734–14747. [CrossRef]
57. Park, J.H.; Carlin, K.P.; Wu, G.; Ilyin, V.I.; Musza, L.L.; Blake, P.R.; Kyle, D.J. Studies examining the relationship between the chemical structure of protoxin II and its activity on voltage gated sodium channels. *J. Med. Chem.* **2014**, *57*, 6623–6631. [CrossRef] [PubMed]
58. Bosmans, F.; Martin-Eauclaire, M.F.; Swartz, K.J. Deconstructing voltage sensor function and pharmacology in sodium channels. *Nature* **2008**, *456*, 202–208. [CrossRef] [PubMed]
59. Chi, V.; Pennington, M.W.; Norton, R.S.; Tarcha, E.J.; Londono, L.M.; Sims-Fahey, B.; Upadhyay, S.K.; Lakey, J.T.; Iadonato, S.; Wulff, H.; et al. Development of a sea anemone toxin as an immunomodulator for therapy of autoimmune diseases. *Toxicon* **2012**, *59*, 529–546. [CrossRef]
60. Craik, D.J.; Adams, D.J. Chemical modification of conotoxins to improve stability and activity. *ACS Chem. Biol.* **2007**, *2*, 457–468. [CrossRef]
61. Han, T.S.; Teichert, R.W.; Olivera, B.M.; Bulaj, G. Conus venoms—A rich source of peptide-based therapeutics. *Curr. Pharm. Des.* **2008**, *14*, 2462–2479. [CrossRef]
62. Altafaj, X.; Joux, N.; Ronjat, M.; De Waard, M. Oocyte expression with injection of purified T7 RNA polymerase. *Methods Mol. Biol.* **2006**, *322*, 55–67. [CrossRef]
63. Geib, S.; Sandoz, G.; Carlier, E.; Cornet, V.; Cheynet-Sauvion, V.; De Waard, M. A novel Xenopus oocyte expression system based on cytoplasmic coinjection of T7-driven plasmids and purified T7-RNA polymerase. *Recept. Channels* **2001**, *7*, 331–343. [PubMed]

toxins

MDPI

Article

Sa12b Peptide from Solitary Wasp Inhibits ASIC Currents in Rat Dorsal Root Ganglion Neurons

Carmen Hernández [1], Katsuhiro Konno [2], Emilio Salceda [1], Rosario Vega [1], André Junqueira Zaharenko [3] and Enrique Soto [1,*]

1 Instituto de Fisiología, Benemérita Universidad Autónoma de Puebla, Puebla 72570, Mexico; mary_car123@hotmail.com (C.H.); emilio.salceda@gmail.com (E.S.); axolotl_56@yahoo.com.mx (R.V.)
2 Institute of Natural Medicine, University of Toyama, Toyama 930-0194, Japan; kkgon@inm.u-toyama.ac.jp
3 Laboratório de Genética, Instituto Butantan, São Paulo 05503-900, Brazil; a.j.zaharenko@gmail.com
* Correspondence: enrique.soto@correo.buap.mx or esoto24@gmail.com

Received: 30 July 2019; Accepted: 4 October 2019; Published: 10 October 2019

check for updates

Abstract: In this work, we evaluate the effect of two peptides Sa12b (EDVDHVFLRF) and Sh5b (DVDHVFLRF-NH_2) on Acid-Sensing Ion Channels (ASIC). These peptides were purified from the venom of solitary wasps *Sphex argentatus argentatus* and *Isodontia harmandi*, respectively. Voltage clamp recordings of ASIC currents were performed in whole cell configuration in primary culture of dorsal root ganglion (DRG) neurons from (P7-P10) CII Long-Evans rats. The peptides were applied by preincubation for 25 s (20 s in pH 7.4 solution and 5 s in pH 6.1 solution) or by co-application (5 s in pH 6.1 solution). Sa12b inhibits ASIC current with an IC_{50} of 81 nM, in a concentration-dependent manner when preincubation application was used. While Sh5b did not show consistent results having both excitatory and inhibitory effects on the maximum ASIC currents, its complex effect suggests that it presents a selective action on some ASIC subunits. Despite the similarity in their sequences, the action of these peptides differs significantly. Sa12b is the first discovered wasp peptide with a significant ASIC inhibitory effect.

Keywords: venom peptides; FMRF-amide; insect neurotoxin; protons; pH regulation; acid-sensing ion channels; acid-gated currents

Key Contribution: Sa12b, a FMRF-amide like peptide obtained from solitary wasp venom potently inhibits acid-sensing ion channel currents in rat neurons with an IC_{50} of 81 nM.

---

1. Introduction

Acid-sensing ion channels (ASICs) are proton-gated Na^+ channels of the ENaC/Degenerin channel family characterized by their sodium permeability, sensitivity to amiloride, and voltage insensitivity [1–4]. ASICs are widely distributed in the central and peripheral nervous systems, as well as in sensory and non-neuronal tissue [5]. Most functions of these channels have been described using inhibitors of ASIC channels combined with the use of knockout or knockdown animals [6]. The most potent and selective modulators of ASICs described to date are animal venoms obtained from spiders, snakes, and sea anemones [7–9].

FMRFa (Phe-Met-Arg-Phe amide) is an abundant tetrapeptide in invertebrate nervous systems, where it acts as a neurotransmitter and neuromodulator. RFa-related peptides share with FMRFa the characteristic C-terminus motive Arg-Phe-NH_2 [10]. These neuropeptides are direct activators of two ion channels of the ENaC/Deg superfamily: the invertebrate FMRFa-gated Na^+ channel (FaNaC) and the Hydra-RFa-gated Na^+ channels (HyNaC) [11].

While FaNaC and HyNaC channels are activated by neuropeptides and modulated by acidic pH, ASICs are activated by pH and modulated by neuropeptides [12]. Several studies show that RFa-related peptides reduce desensitization and increase the sustained current and peak amplitude of ASIC currents [13–18]. These effects are pH-dependent, require the presence of the amide group, and are competitive with Ca^{2+}. Three possible binding sites to ASIC have been proposed: the acidic pocket, the bottom of the thumb domain, and the central vestibule [19–23].

In this work, we studied the effects of two FMRFa related peptides (Sa12b and Sh5b [24,25] extracted from the venom of solitary wasps *Sphex argentatus argentatus* and *Isodontia harmandi*) on ASIC currents of rat dorsal root ganglion (DRG) neurons using the voltage clamp technique. We found that Sa12b exerts a potent inhibitory action on ASIC currents in DRG neurons.

2. Results

Stable proton-gated currents were recorded from 123 DRG neurons obtained from 32 rats (about 30% of the cells registered expressed a stable proton-gated current). These neurons had a membrane capacitance (C_m) of 46.8 ± 1.45 pF (Gaussian fit shows a normal distribution of C_m $r^2 > 0.95$), a resting membrane potential (V_m) of −55.3 ± 1.4 mV, a membrane resistance (R_m) of 137.5 ± 13.6 MΩ, an access resistance (R_a) of 4 ± 0.3 MΩ and a membrane time constant (τ) of 131 ± 6.7 ms. Cell average diameter was 38.6 ± 6.8 μm, estimated from C_m, which corresponds to medium-size DRG neurons according to Petruska's classification [26].

2.1. ASIC Current in DRG Neurons

ASIC currents from isolated DRG neurons showed diverse characteristics, which result from the expression of ASIC heteromers and homomers of ASIC1–4 subunits in these neurons. The currents range from transient and rapid currents with partial or complete desensitization to currents with slow desensitization with a large sustained component (Figure 1). No clear groups could be formed to categorize the currents considering all the parameters analyzed, although according to their desensitization time constant (T_{des}), we found that 61% of the registered currents showed $T_{des} < 300$ ms, 29.5% $T_{des} > 300$ and < 600 ms, while only the remaining 9.5% had slow kinetics with $T_{des} > 600$ ms.

Under control conditions, the pH gated currents activated at pH 6.1 showed a maximal inward peak current (I_{peak}) of 4.5 ± 0.5 nA, a sustained component (I_{SS}) of 0.09 ± 0.01 nA, a T_{des} of 348 ± 22 ms, and an integral of the current (I_{int}) of 2.03 ± 0.171 nC. Current density had an average magnitude of 0.097 ± 0.009 nA/pF and a desensitization coefficient (I_{SS}/I_{peak}) of 0.04 ± 0.01 (mean ± ES, $n = 95$). None of the parameters obtained from the records show any correlation with the C_m, which is an indicator of cell size.

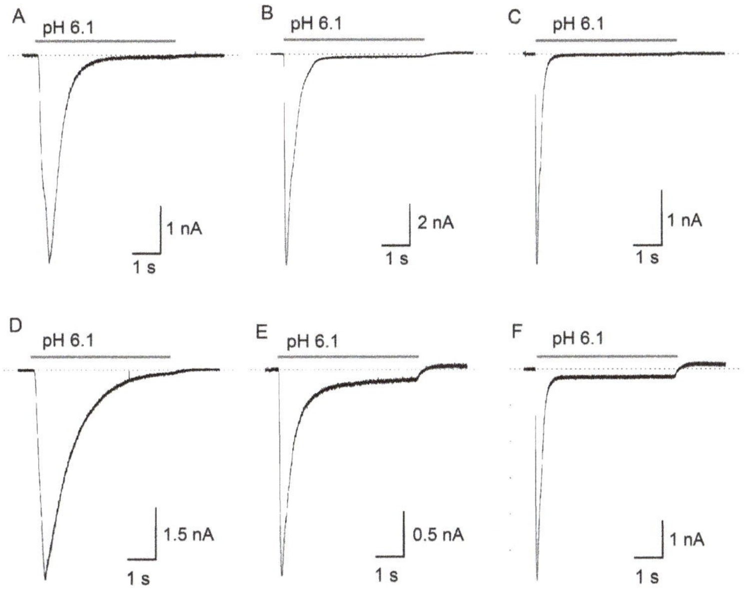

Figure 1. Diversity of acid-gated currents in dorsal root ganglion (DRG) neurons. The currents were elicited by a 5 s perfusion with a pH 6.1 solution. (**A**,**D**) depict currents with slow activation and slow desensitization (n = 9). (**B**,**E**), currents with rapid activation and intermediate desensitization (n = 28. C and F, currents with rapid activation and rapid desensitization (n = 58). (**A–C**) lack a sustained component (I_{SS}), whereas (**D–F**) present it.

2.2. *Sa12b Action on ASIC Currents*

The peptide was initially tested at 10 µM, this concentration was used because it is close to the EC_{50} of FMRFa. With application of 10 µM Sa12b in preincubation form (20 s before and 5 s during acid pulse), Sa12b inhibited ASIC currents 92.7 ± 7.3% ($p < 0.05$ paired Student's *t*-test, $n = 5$) (Figure 2A). In contrast, during co-application (toxin applied only during the 5 s of acid pulse) Sa12b produced a non-significant inhibition of ASIC currents of 12.9 ± 4.9% ($n = 4$) (Figure 2B).

The inhibitory action of Sa12b in I_{peak} was dose-dependent with preincubation application (Figures 2A–C and 3), it was adjusted with a dose-response function with an $IC_{50} = 81 \pm 29.4$ nM, H = 1.8 and $r^2 = 0.97$ ($n = 34$). All Sa12b effects were fully reversed after 1 min washout of the peptide. Other parameters of ASIC current were not significantly modified by Sa12b perfusion except for the T_{des}, which increased 28% with 300 nM Sa12b (Table 1).

To determine whether or not the effect of Sa12b was selective for some type of ASIC current, a correlation analysis between the current properties (I_{peak}, T_{des}, and I_{SS}) and the effect of Sa12b was performed. It was found that the inhibitory effect of Sa12b on ASIC currents does not depend on the C_m, the T_{des}, or the I_{SS}/I_{peak} of the control currents; regardless of the concentration tested either during preincubation or co-application of the peptide.

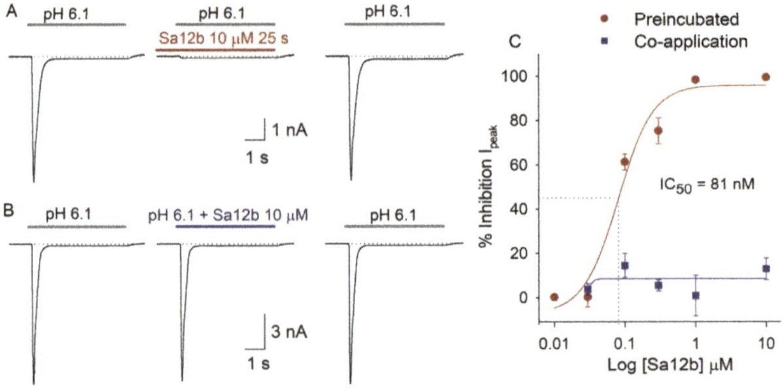

Figure 2. Effect of Sa12b on Acid-Sensing Ion Channels (ASIC) currents. In (**A**), recordings of ASIC current in dorsal root ganglion (DRG) neurons in control current, after 10 μM Sa12b preincubation application (20 s before and 5s during acid pulse) and after one recovery of 1 min washout. Sa12b inhibits the I_{peak} (98%) of ASIC current with 3% inhibition of I_{SS} component. In (**B**), 10 μM Sa12b co-application (peptide applied during 5 s along with acid pulse) inhibits I_{peak} 10% and increases I_{SS} by 18%. In (**C**), concentration-response relationship of Sa12b on ASIC I_{peak}. Sa12b concentrations used were: 10, 30, 100, and 300 nM and 1 and 10 μM. The red circles represent the effect produced by preincubation, and the blue squares represent the effect during co-application of Sa12b (n = 34).

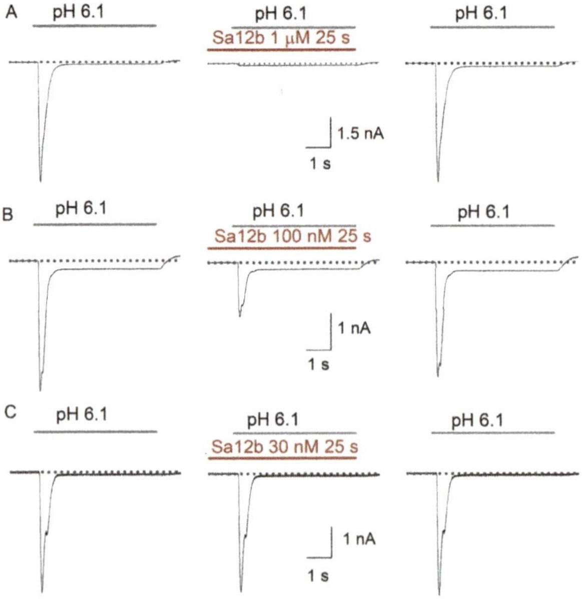

Figure 3. Typical traces of the effect of preincubation perfusion with Sa12b on the ASIC current at the different tested concentrations. In (**A**), the use of 1 μM Sa12b produced a reversible nearly total inhibition of the I_{peak} with no effect on the small I_{SS} component. In (**B**), 100 nM Sa12b caused an inhibition of I_{peak} and I_{SS} of 66% and 7%. In (**C**), 30 nM Sa12b produced an inhibition of I_{peak} and I_{SS} of 2% and 10%, respectively. The inhibitory effects of Sa12b were completely reversed after 1 min washout of the toxin. The dotted lines indicate the zero current, and the horizontal bars show Sa12b preincubation and pH 6.1 perfusion.

Table 1. Effect of Sa12b on macroscopic Acid-Sensing Ion Channels (ASIC) currents in dorsal root ganglion (DRG) neurons.

	[Sa12b]	*n*	% I_{peak}	% I_{SS}	% T_{des}
Co-application	30 nM	5	↑ 4 ± 3	↑ **39 ± 24** (p = 0.02)	↓ 4 ± 3
	100 nM	4	↓ 14 ± 5	↓ 21 ± 16	↑ 5 ± 1
	300 nM	6	↓ 5 ± 3	↓30 ± 14	↑ 3 ± 5
	1 μM	5	↑ 1 ± 9	↑ 15 ± 14	↑ 4 ± 4
	10 μM	4	↓ 13 ± 5	↓ 29 ± 19	↓ 2 ± 5
Preincubation Application	30 nM	6	↓ 0.2 ± 4	↑ 19 ± 22	↑ 0.03 ± 4
	100 nM	5	↓ **63 ± 4** (p = 0.003)	↑ 4 ± 21	↑ 17 ± 18
	300 nM	9	↓ **76 ± 5** (p = 0.0002)	↑ 81 ± 51	↑ **28 ± 12** (p = 0.048)
	1 μM	5	↓ **98 ± 1** (p = 0.03)	↓ 13 ± 27	
	10 μM	5	↓ **92 ± 7** (p = 0.04)	↓ 31 ± 20	

The effects that presented a significant difference are shown in red. The upward arrows indicate an increase and the downward arrows indicate a decrease. Student´s *t*-test.

2.3. *pH Activation Versus Sa12b Effect*

To determine whether or not Sa12b action is pH-dependent, the effect of Sa12b 100 nM (concentration close to IC_{50}) was analyzed as a function of pH used to activate the current (pH from 4.0 to 6.5). As previously described, the current amplitude increased as a function of proton concentration (Figure 4A,B). The pH which activated 50% of the ASIC current (pH_{50}) was about 6.1 as previously described for ASIC currents in DRG neurons [27]. The relationship between pH and proton-gated current amplitude in the presence of 100 nM Sa12b showed no significant difference with that found in control condition (Figure 4B). Analysis of percent inhibitory effect of 100 nM Sa12b as a function of pH showed that pH gating of the current did not significantly modify the inhibitory action of Sa12b (Figure 4C). These data indicate that Sa12b does not interact with the proton-gating mechanism of ASICs.

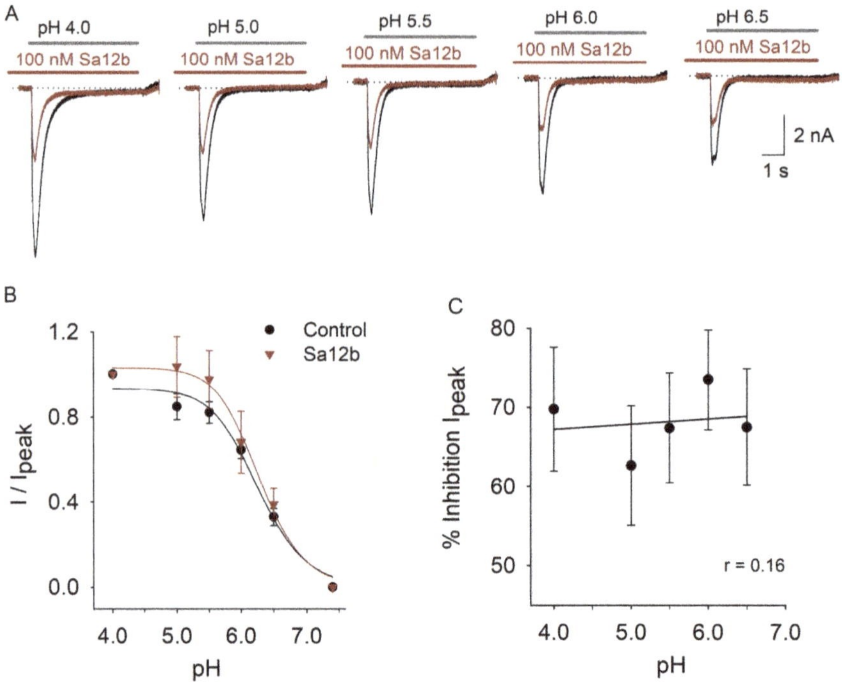

Figure 4. Effect of pH-gating the ASIC current on Sa12b action. In (**A**), recordings of ASIC current at different gating pHs in control (black traces) and after preincubation with 100 nM Sa12b (red traces). The inhibitory effect of Sa12b is similar regardless of the pH used to activate the current. All recordings are from the same cell, which desensitize nearly completely and shows small I_{SS} component. In (**B**), relation between the pH used to activate the current and the normalized I_{peak} in control (black) and after 100 nM Sa12b. Data were adjusted with a sigmoidal function, no significant difference between pH sensitivity of the current in control (pH_{50} = 6.26 ± 0.1) and with Sa12b (pH_{50} 6.27 ± 0.06) was found. The pHs used to activate the current were: pH 6.5, n = 15; pH 6.0, n = 15; pH 5.5, n = 16; pH 5.0, n = 17; pH 4.0, n = 14. In (**C**), plot of the percent I_{peak} inhibition produced by 100 nM Sa12b against pH. The data were adjusted with a linear function showing that inhibition produced by Sa12b is independent of the pH used to activate the ASIC current.

2.4. *Effect of Sh5b*

As with Sa12b peptide, the application of Sh5b peptide was carried out under co-application and preincubation. The concentrations at which the peptide was tested were: for co-application 100 nM, 3 µM, 10 µM, and 30 µM; for preincubation application, the concentrations were 100 nM, 1 and 10 µM.

In the co-application protocol, 100 nM Sh5b (n = 5) showed no consistent concentration-dependent effects on the analyzed parameters. At 3 µM Sh5b (n = 12) decreased the T_{des} by 7% (p = 0.046) with highly variable non-significant increase of the I_{SS}. Increasing Sh5b concentration to 10 µM produced an increase of the I_{peak} in some cells and a decrease in other group, but overall change was non-significant (Table 2). Other parameter changes were also non-significant. At 30 µM Sh5b (n = 6) increased the I_{SS} 78 ± 16% (p = 0.004) (Figure 5). However, the observed effects on ASIC current when using Sh5b in co-application were not dependent on concentration (Table 2).

Table 2. Effect of Sh5b on macroscopic ASIC currents in DRG neurons.

	[Sa12b]	n	% I_{peak}	% I_{SS}	% T_{des}
Co-application	100 nM	5	↓ 2 ± 4	↑ 85 ± 74	↓ 1 ± 2
	3 µM	12	↓6 ± 3	↑ 116 ± 104	↓ 7 ± 4
	10 µM	9	↑17 ± 15	↑ 1 ± 11	↓ 10 ± 5
	30 µM	6	↓1 ± 6	↑ 78 ± 16	↑ 9 ± 5
Preincubation application	100 nM	9	↓0.5 ± 6	↑ 53 ± 38	↑ 13 ± 15
	1 µM	5	↓9 ± 5	↑ 14 ± 41	↑ 3 ± 5
	10 µM	12	↓11 ± 4	↓ 8 ± 15	↓ 5 ± 4

The effects that presented a significant difference are shown in red. The upward arrows indicate an increase and the downward arrows indicate a decrease. Student´s *t*-test.

The use of 100 nM Sh5b in preincubation (n = 9) produced no effect on the analyzed parameters. Perfusion of 1 µM Sh5b (n = 5) produced a marginal decrease of the I_{peak} (9 ± 5%), and an increase of the I_{SS}, both effects were non-significant. 10 µM Sh5b (n = 12) did not produced significant effects on the studied parameters either (Figure 6, Table 2).

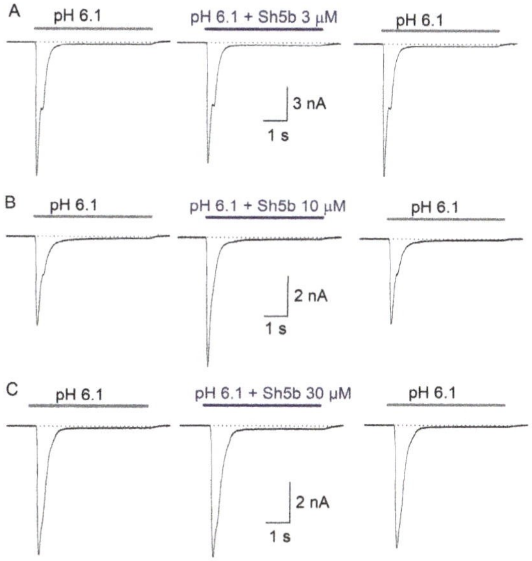

Figure 5. Effect of Sh5b peptide on ASIC currents of DRG neurons. Graphs show ASIC current in control, co-application, and after one minute of peptide washout. In (**A**), co-application of 3 µM Sh5b reduced I_{peak} of ASIC currents by 9.6%, while I_{SS} was increased by 30%. In (**B**), co-application of 10 µM Sh5b, increased I_{peak} by 44.6% and I_{SS} 14.6%. In (**C**), the co-application of 30 µM Sh5b caused an inhibition of 3.8% on I_{peak} and an increase of 102% on I_{SS} from 79 pA to 159 pA. Effects were reversed by 1 min peptide washout.

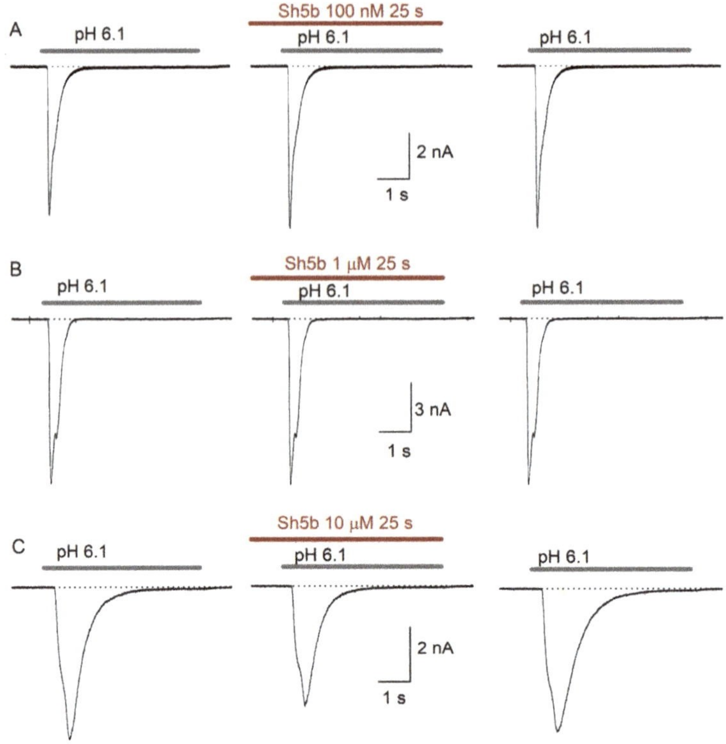

Figure 6. Graphs showing the effect of Sh5b preincubation on ASIC currents. Recordings show ASIC current under control conditions, after preincubation with Sh5b and after one-minute peptide washout. In (**A**), shows the effect of preincubation with 100 nM Sh5b, which produced a marginal increase of the I_{peak} and I_{SS} of 1% and 3% respectively, with no change in T_{des}. In (**B**), preincubation with 1 μM Sh5b inhibits I_{peak} and I_{SS} by 1% and 5% respectivley. In (**C**), use of 10 μM Sh5b inhibits the I_{peak} by 18% and increased the I_{SS} by 26%, with no change in T_{des}. The effect was reversed by 1 min washout of the peptide.

3. Discussion

3.1. Sa12b

Sa12b peptide, when applied by preincubation, reversibly inhibits the amplitude of the peak of ASIC currents (IC_{50} ~ 81 nM) in rat DRG neurons in a concentration-dependent manner without consistent action on the time course of desensitization or the sustained component of the current. Currents activated by H^+ in DRG neurons are heterogeneous due to the combination of two or more ASIC subunits with coexistence of multiple populations of channels in the same cell [28–31]. The inhibitory effect of Sa12b was similar in all cells regardless of the kinetics of currents, which indicates that Sa12b action is not specific to any particular ASIC subunit; however, this question requires further exploration on channels expressed in a heterologous system.

We found no effect on the I_{peak} during co-application of Sa12b and acidic pH. That the inhibitory effect of Sa12b was observed only after preincubation application suggests that the peptide needs to interact with the channel during its closed state; an alternative explanation would be that this effect is due to a slow interaction of the peptide with ASIC or a slow conformational change of the channel induced by Sa12b [21]. RFa-related peptides also seem to produce their modulating effect only when applied before acid gating of the channel [20].

The inhibitory potency of Sa12b (IC_{50} = 81 nM) on ASIC currents is comparable to the inhibition caused by peptides of vegetable and animal origin, such as chlorogenic acid (CGA, polyphenol) and the gastrodin (phenol) that inhibits ASIC currents in rat DRG neurons (IC_{50} ~ 230 nM and ~ 210 nM respectively) [32,33]. APETx2 (from the sea anemone *Anthopleura elegantissima*) inhibits the homomeric channels of rASIC3 (IC_{50} 37–63 nM) and hASIC3 (IC_{50} ~ 175 nM) [34]; mambalgines (from the black mamba and the green mamba) inhibit the homomers of ASIC1a and ASIC1b, and the heteromers containing ASIC1a with an IC_{50} ranging from 11 to 250 nM [35,36]; or PhcrTx1 peptide extracted from *Phymanthus crucifer* (IC_{50} ~ 100 nM) which inhibits ASIC currents ≅ 40% [37]. The inhibitory effect of Sa12b in ASIC currents is only surpassed in potency by two known ASIC1a inhibitors: PcTx1, from tarantula venom *Psalmopoeus cambridgei* (IC_{50} = 1 nM) [38] and Hi1a, from the venom of the Australian spider *Hadronyches infensa* (IC_{50} = 0.4–0.5 nM), however, PcTx1 behaves as an agonist of ASIC1b (EC_{50} ~ 100 nM), while Hi1a produces an incomplete current inhibition at saturating concentration (1 μM) [9]. It is worth note that Sa12b produces a close to 100% inhibition of I_{peak} at 1 μM. Which suggests that Sa12b exerts an unspecific action among ASIC subunits, although the lack of inhibition of I_{SS} suggest some kind of selectivity among ASIC subunits. To define this, it will be needed to perform experiments in a heterologous expression system studying the action of Sa12b on specific homomers of ASIC subunits.

It is speculated that modulation of ASIC channels by RFa-related peptides is due to direct interaction between the peptide and the extracellular domain of the channel having the lower region of the palmar domain of the channel as a probable binding site, specifically the region occupied by the central vestibule of the channel; furthermore, it has been suggested that RFa-related peptides bind to the channel in the closed state and dissociate very slowly from the desensitized state [22]. Since Sa12b has a very short amino acid sequence, binding in the central vestibule may plug the channel, decreasing the conductance instead of slowing inactivation and desensitization of ASIC currents, which is what RFa does.

Sa12b sequence (EDVDHVFLRF) suggests the presence of a hydrophobic patch provided by the amino acids: Val3, Val6, Phe7, Leu8, and Phe10; the Phe15 residue in APETx2 is of great importance for this toxin to inhibit the currents of ASIC3 [39]. Similarly, PcTx1 has a hydrophobic patch conferred by Trp7 and Trp24 which interacts with the thumb domain of the ASIC channel, while the basic group of PcTx1 (Arg26, Arg27, and Arg28) enters the acidic pocket to form strong hydrogen bonds [40]. Sa12b also possesses two residues with a positive charge (His5 and Arg9) that could be a binding site with ASIC channels.

3.2. *Sh5b*

Sh5b did not produce consistent, reproducible, effects on ASIC currents, it shows various effects on most of the analyzed parameters, including dual effects on the I_{peak} and T_{des}. The complex action of Sh5b suggests that this peptide presents selective action on some subunits of ASICs. As already mentioned, the macroscopic currents activated by H^+ in the DRG neurons present a morphological heterogeneity resulting from the combination of two or more ASIC subunits, so the inconsistent action of Sh5b could be given by selectivity of the peptide for some ASIC subunits. Future studies using heterologous expression of ASIC subunits could clarify whether Sh5b possesses any selectivity; if so, Sh5b can become a pharmacological tool that allows studying specific ASIC subunits.

Application of Sh5b by preincubation showed a tendency to inhibit the current peak. The I_{SS} component increased slightly after application of Sh5b, and the I_{SS}/I_{peak} relationship also increased; this last parameter was the one that had statistically significant effects in the greatest number of the tested concentrations, which suggests a modification on the desensitization process of ASICs. However, the T_{des} and the integral of the current show no consistent changes, exhibiting dual effects.

During co-application, the I_{SS}/I_{peak} relationship showed a tendency towards the increase, but the T_{des} did not show noticeable differences.

RFa-related peptides have an NH_2 group which is positively charged at pH 5 to 8 [21]. The effects of Sh5b could be due to the positive charge given by its amine group. Other inhibitors of ASICs, such as the PhcrTx1 peptide, which at pH 7.4 has a net charge of +5.03, APETx2 (net charge = +2.00), and PcTx1 (net charge = +3) [37] also have that particularity. Aminoglycosides are also positively-charged ASICs modulators [27].

Analysis of the structure of Sa12b (EDVDHVFLRF) and Sh5b (DVDHVFLRFa) showed that Sa12b has an extra Glu in its N-terminal, while Sh5b has an amide residue in its C-terminal. Sa12b has three negatively charged amino acids (Glu1, Asp2, and Asp4) and two positively charged ones (His5 and Arg9), which gives the peptide a negative net charge, besides it has four polar amino acids (Glu1, Asp2, Asp4, and Arg9) and six apolar ones (Val3, His5, Val6, Phe7, Leu8, Phe10). In contrast, Sh5b presents in its sequence two negatively charged amino acids (Asp1 and Asp3) and two positively charged ones (His4 and Arg8), which makes it a peptide with neutral charge. With respect to solubility, Sh5b consists of three polar amino acids (Asp1, Asp3, and Arg8) and six apolar ones (Val2, His4, Val5, Phe6, Leu7, Phe9). These structural differences, mainly the difference of net charges, could favor differences in the folding of the tertiary structure, which could produce the differences in the interaction of Sa12b and Sh5b with ASIC.

4. Conclusions

The results from this work show that the application of Sa12b exerts an inhibitory effect on ASIC currents from DRG neurons, this effect was concentration-dependent and reversed after washout of the peptide. Since the inhibition was close to 100% at 1 μM and all ASIC subunits are expressed in DRGs, it suggests that Sa12b inhibits different ASIC subunits without an apparent selectivity. Sa12b is the first discovered wasp peptide with a significant ASIC inhibitory action.

5. Material and Methods

5.1. Animals and Cell Culture

To study the effect of Sa12b and Sh5b on ASIC, DRG neurons were obtained from Long-Evans CII / ZV rats of 7 to 10 days of postnatal age, of either sex. Animals were provided by the laboratory animal facility 'Claude Bernard' of the Autonomous University of Puebla. The study was performed in accordance with the recommendations in the Guiding Principles in the Care and Use of Vertebrate Animals in Research and Training of the American Physiological Society, and with the regulations of the NOM-062-ZOO-1999 of the Mexican Ministry of Agriculture, Stockbreeding, Rural Development, Fishing and Food. The protocol was reviewed and approved by the Institutional Committee for Animal Care and Use (IACUC) of the Autonomous University of Puebla (VIEP-BUAP) on 17 July 2017. The ethical approval code is SOEE-UALVIEP-17-1. All efforts were made to minimize animal suffering and to reduce the number of animals used. DRG neurons were isolated and maintained in primary culture according to the methodology described previously [41]. The dissection and cell culture were performed within a level I biosafety laminar flow hood (Nuaire, Plymouth, MN, USA). Rats were anesthetized with sevoflurane and sacrificed by decapitation. Subsequently, the rat was placed in prone position to make a longitudinal incision through the vertebral bodies removing the spinal cord. Dorsal root ganglia were isolated (approximately 12 to 18 per rat) using conventional dissection under a stereoscopic microscope (American Optical, Southbridge, MA, USA). Once extracted, DRG neurons were placed in a disposable sterile centrifuge tube (Corning, Corning, NY, USA), in which they were incubated for 30 min at 37 °C in Leibovitz L15 medium (L15) (Invitrogen, Waltham, MA, USA), added with 1.25 mg/mL of trypsin and 1.25 mg/mL of collagenase (both from Sigma-Aldrich, St. Louis, MO, USA) for an enzymatic dissociation.

After the enzymatic treatment, the ganglia were washed 3 times with 100% L15 medium; after each wash, the cells were subjected to mechanical dissociation using glass three-gauge Pasteur pipettes; between each wash, a cell pellet was formed using a centrifuge at 5000 rpm. After the third wash, once the cell pellet was formed, the supernatant was discarded, and the cell suspension was placed in a 35 mm culture dish (Corning) on 12 × 10 mm glass plates (Corning) previously treated with poly-D-lysine (Sigma-Aldrich, St. Louis, MO, USA).

Dissociated neurons were incubated for a period of time ranging from 2 to 8 h in a humidified atmosphere (95% O_2, 5% CO_2, at 37 °C) using a water-jacketed CO_2 incubator (Nuaire, Plymouth, MN, USA) allowing for settlement and adhesion of isolated cells to the glass plates. The cells were cultured in modified L15 medium, supplemented with 10% fetal bovine serum (Gibco, Waltham, MA, USA), 100 IU penicillin (Lakeside, Hayward, CA USA), fungizone 2.5 µL/mL (Gibco), $NaHCO_3$ 15.7 mM (J.T. Baker, Radnor DE, USA) and 15.8 mM HEPES (Sigma-Aldrich, St. Louis, MO, USA).

5.2. Recording of ASIC Currents in DRG Neurons

After an incubation period of 2 to 8 h, the recording of ASIC currents in DRG neurons was performed. Cells were transferred to a recording chamber mounted in a phase-contrast inverted microscope (TMS, Nikon Co. Tokyo, Japan). Neurons that were not attached to other cells, and that had a round or ovoid shape (without dendritic or axonal extensions) with a delimited refringent membrane were chosen for recording.

The recording chamber was constantly perfused with extracellular solution (Table 3). Recordings were performed in whole-cell voltage-clamp mode using an Axopatch 1D amplifier (Molecular Devices, Union City, CA, USA). Data collection and generation of commands for the perfusion change were carried out by the pClamp 9.2 (Molecular Devices) software in a 16-bit data acquisition system (Digidata 1320, Molecular Devices). Microelectrodes were made from borosilicate glass capillaries (TW120-3; WPI, Sarasota, FL, USA) with a micropipette puller (80-PC; Sutter Instruments Company, San Rafael, CA, USA), which once filled with the intracellular solution (Table 3) had a resistance of 1.4 to 3.1 MΩ. The signals were digitized at 5 kHz. The series resistance was electronically compensated at 80%. Throughout the recording, access resistance and seal quality were monitored to ensure stable recording conditions. The records that showed a > 10% change in access resistance compared to the initial conditions were excluded from data analysis.

Table 3. Solutions used for electrophysiological recording.

	Extracellular [mM]	Acid Solution [mM]	Intracellular [mM]
NaCl	140	140	10
KCl	5.4	5.4	125
$CaCl_2$	1.8	1.8	0.134
$MgCl_2$	1.2	1.2	-
HEPES	10	-	5
MES	-	10	-
D-glucose	10	10	-
EGTA	-	-	10
ATP- Mg	-	-	2
GTP-Na	-	-	1
	adjusted to pH 7.4 with NaOH	adjusted to desired pH with NaOH	adjusted to pH 7.2 with KOH

Proton-gated currents were obtained with a holding potential of −60 mV. Cells were subjected to a test protocol with an acid solution of pH 6.1 for 5 s (Table 3). In all the experiments at least two control recordings were made before performing some type of experimental manipulation in order to guarantee that the cells expressed a stable proton-gated current; the margin of variation in the amplitude of the current between one control recording and another should be less than 10%.

5.3. Wasp Peptides

The peptides Sa12b (EDVDHVFLRF, molecular weight = 1276.4 g/mol) and Sh5b (DVDHVFLRF-NH2, molecular weight = 1146.3 g/mol) were purified from the venom extracts of solitary wasps *Sphex argentatus argentatus* and *Isodontia harmandi*, respectively, and the structure was determined by MALDI-TOF/TOF MS analysis (manuscript in preparation). The synthetic specimens of these peptides were used in this study.

5.4. Peptide Synthesis

The peptide was synthesized on an automated PSSM-8 peptide synthesizer (Shimadzu Corp., Kyoto, Japan) by a stepwise solid-phase method using N-9-fluorenylmethoxycarbonyl (Fmoc) chemistry. All the resins and Fmoc-L-amino acids were purchased from HiPep Laboratories (Kyoto, Japan). Cleavage of the peptide from the resin was achieved by treatment with a mixture of TFA/H_2O/triisopropylsilane (TIS) (95:2.5:2.5) at room temperature for 2 h. After removal of the resin by filtration and washing twice with trifluoroacetic acid (TFA), the combined filtrate was added dropwise to diethyl ether at 0 °C and then centrifuged at 3000 rpm for 10 min. Thus, obtained crude synthetic peptide was purified by semipreparative reverse-phase HPLC using CAPCELL PAK C_{18}, 10 × 250 mm with isocratic elution of 20–25% CH_3CN/H_2O/0.1% TFA at a flow rate of 3 mL/min. The homogeneity and the sequence were confirmed by MALDI-TOF MS and analytical HPLC.

5.5. Experimental Design and Data Analysis

ASIC currents were activated by micro-perfusion of the cell under recording with an acid solution (pH 6.1) through a square tube using a rapid perfusion exchange system (SF-77B, Warner Inst., Hamden, CT, USA). The pH-gated current was activated using a pH of 6.1 which coincides with the pH_{50} previously demonstrated for ASIC currents in DRG neurons [41]. Capsazepine 10 μM was added to the extracellular solution at pH 6.1 in order to limit the activation of TRPV1 receptors, which are also sensitive to acid and are expressed in DRG neurons [42]. To study the effect of Sa12b and Sh5b peptides on ASIC currents of DRG neurons two application protocols were used [41]. Peptides were applied by sustained application (preincubation) and by co-application. In the preincubation, the toxin was applied through the pH 7.4 extracellular solution for 20 s before the acid pulse and during the 5 s that the acid pulse lasted. In co-application, the compound was applied only during the 5-second acid pulse. The effects observed during preincubation result from channel exposure to the peptide during the closed, open, and desensitized states. During co-application the toxins interacts with the channel in the open and desensitized states.

The passive properties of the neurons were recorded in each experiment, including the membrane capacitance (C_m), cell-membrane voltage (V_m), membrane resistance (R_m), and access resistance (R_a). Solutions were prepared at the time of experiment; the peptides were kept frozen at −20 °C in aliquots at different concentrations in deionized water added with 1 mg/mL of albumin (Sigma-Aldrich) to prevent the peptides from adhering to the walls of the perfusion tubes.

The proton-gated currents were processed offline using the software Clampfit 9.2 (Molecular Devices), Microsoft Office Excel 2010 and SigmaPlot 12.0. For each experimental condition two control recordings were obtained, one recording with the application of the peptide, and two washout recordings. The problem currents were normalized with respect to the average of the control currents in order to obtain the percentage of change in the parameters measured in the presence of the toxins.

For the analysis of the toxin actions, the concentration-response curves were adjusted with a Hill equation:

$$Y = A_2 + (A_1 - A_2)/(1 + (x/E_{50})\ H)$$

where: Y = Pharmacological effect, x = Concentration tested, A_1 and A_2 = Maximum and minimum effect, E_{50} = Concentration in which 50% of the effect is obtained, H = Hill constant.

To study the desensitization of the current, a simple exponential function was adjusted, obtaining the decay constant of the current (T_{des}).

To determine the statistical significance of the data, a paired Student's *t*-test was used and *p* values reported; the experimental data are presented as the mean ± E.S.

Author Contributions: Conceptualization, K.K., A.J.Z. and E.S. (Enrique Soto); Methodology, K.K., E.S. (Emilio Salceda) and R.V.; Validation, E.S. (Enrique Soto) and R.V.; Investigation, C.H., E.S. (Enrique Soto), E.S. (Emilio Salceda); Writing—Review & Editing, C.H., E.S. (Enrique Soto), R.V. and K.K.

Funding: This study was supported by grant from Vicerrectoría de Investigación y Estudios de Posgrado (VIEP-BUAP grants to ES) and grant from Consejo Nacional de Ciencia y Tecnología de México (CONACyT), Fronteras de la Ciencia 1544 to E.S. Enrique Soto. CHZ was supported by CONACyT fellowship 669573.

Conflicts of Interest: The authors declare no competing financial interest. The data that support the findings of this study are available from the corresponding author upon reasonable request.

References

1. Boscardin, E.; Alijevic, O.; Hummler, E.; Frateschi, S.; Kellenberger, S. The function and regulation of acid-sensing ion channels (ASICs) and the epithelial Na(+) channel (ENaC): IUPHAR Review 19. *Br. J. Pharmacol.* **2016**, *173*, 2671–2701. [CrossRef] [PubMed]
2. Hanukoglu, I. ASIC and ENaC type sodium channels: Conformational states and the structures of the ion selectivity filters. *FEBS J.* **2017**, *284*, 525–545. [CrossRef] [PubMed]
3. Hanukoglu, I.; Hanukoglu, A. Epithelial sodium channel (ENaC) family: Phylogeny, structure-function, tissue distribution, and associated inherited diseases. *Gene* **2016**, *579*, 95–132. [CrossRef]
4. Kellenberger, S.; Schild, L. International Union of Basic and Clinical Pharmacology. XCI. Structure, Function, and Pharmacology of Acid-Sensing Ion Channels and the Epithelial Na+ Channel. *Pharmacol. Rev.* **2014**, *67*, 1–35. [CrossRef] [PubMed]
5. Ortega-Ramírez, A.; Vega, R.; Soto, E. Acid-Sensing Ion Channels as Potential Therapeutic Targets in Neurodegeneration and Neuroinflammation. *Mediat. Inflamm.* **2017**, *2017*, 3728096. [CrossRef] [PubMed]
6. Baron, A.; Lingueglia, E. Pharmacology of acid-sensing ion channels—Physiological and therapeutical perspectives. *Neuropharmacology* **2015**, *94*, 19–35. [CrossRef]
7. Cristofori-Armstrong, B.; Rash, L. Acid-sensing ion channel (ASIC) structure and function: Insights from spider, snake and sea anemone venoms. *Neuropharmacology* **2017**, *127*, 173–184. [CrossRef] [PubMed]
8. Cristofori-Armstrong, B.; Saez, N.; Chassagnon, I.; King, G.; Rash, L. The modulation of acid-sensing ion channel 1 by PcTx1 is pH-, subtype- and species-dependent: Importance of interactions at the channel subunit interface and potential for engineering selective analogues. *Biochem. Pharmacol.* **2019**, *163*, 381–390. [CrossRef] [PubMed]
9. Chassagnon, I.; McCarthy, C.; Chin, Y.; Pineda, S.; Keramidas, A.; Mobli, M.; Pham, V.; De Silva, T.M.; Lynch, J.W.; Widdop, R.E.; et al. Potent neuroprotection after stroke afforded by a double-knot spider-venom peptide that inhibits acid-sensing ion channel 1a. *Proc. Natl. Acad. Sci. USA* **2017**, *114*, 3750–3755. [CrossRef] [PubMed]
10. Burbach, J.P.; Grant, P.; Hellemons, A.J.; Degiorgis, J.A.; Li, K.W.; Pant, H.C. Differential expression of the FMRF gene in adult and hatchling stellate ganglia of the squid Loligo pealei. *Biol. Open* **2014**, *3*, 50–58. [CrossRef]
11. Golubovic, A.; Kuhn, A.; Williamson, M.; Kalbacher, H.; Holstein, T.W.; Grimmelikhuijzen, C.J.P.; Gründer, S. A peptide-gated ion channel from the freshwater polyp Hydra. *J. Biol. Chem.* **2007**, *282*, 35098–35103. [CrossRef] [PubMed]
12. Vick, J.S.; Askwith, C.C. ASICs and neuropeptides. *Neuropharmacology* **2015**, *94*, 36–41. [CrossRef] [PubMed]
13. Askwith, C.C.; Cheng, C.; Ikuma, M.; Benson, C.; Price, M.P.; Welsh, M.J. Neuropeptide FF and FMRFamide potentiate acid-evoked currents from sensory neurons and proton-gated DEG/ENaC channels. *Neuron* **2000**, *26*, 133–141. [CrossRef]
14. Catarsi, S.; Babinski, K.; Séguéla, P. Selective modulation of heteromeric ASIC proton-gated channels by neuropeptide FF. *Neuropharmacology* **2001**, *41*, 592–600. [CrossRef]

15. Deval, E.; Baron, A.; Lingueglia, E.; Mazarguil, H.; Zajac, J.; Lazdunski, M. Effects of neuropeptide SF and related peptides on acid sensing ion channel 3 and sensory neuron excitability. *Neuropharmacology* **2003**, *44*, 662–671. [CrossRef]
16. Xie, J.; Price, M.P.; Wemmie, J.A.; Askwith, C.C.; Welsh, M.J. ASIC3 and ASIC1 Mediate FMRFamide-Related Peptide Enhancement of H+-Gated Currents in Cultured Dorsal Root Ganglion Neurons. *J. Neurophysiol.* **2003**, *89*, 2459–2465. [CrossRef]
17. Sherwood, T.; Askwith, C.C. Endogenous Arginine-Phenylalanine-Amide-related Peptides Alter Steady-state Desensitization of ASIC1a. *J. Biol. Chem.* **2008**, *283*, 1818–1830. [CrossRef]
18. Reimers, C.; Lee, C.H.; Kalbacher, H.; Tian, Y.; Hung, C.H.; Schmidt, A.; Prokop, L.; Kauferstein, S.; Mebs, D.; Chen, C.C.; et al. Identification of a cono-RFamide from the venom of *Conus textile* that targets ASIC3 and enhances muscle pain. *Proc. Natl. Acad. Sci. USA* **2017**, *114*, E3507–E3515. [CrossRef]
19. Ostrovskaya, O.; Moroz, L.; Krishtal, O. Modulatory action of RFamide-related peptides on acid-sensing ionic channels is pH dependent: The role of arginine. *J. Neurochem.* **2004**, *91*, 252–255. [CrossRef]
20. Lingueglia, E.; Deval, E.; Lazdunski, M. FMRFamide-gated sodium channel and ASIC channels: A new class of ionotropic receptors for FMRFamide and related peptides. *Peptides* **2006**, *27*, 1138–1152. [CrossRef]
21. Chen, X.; Paukert, M.; Kadurin, I.; Pusch, M.; Gründer, S. Strong modulation by RFamide neuropeptides of the ASIC1b/3 heteromer in competition with extracellular calcium. *Neuropharmacology* **2006**, *50*, 964–974. [CrossRef]
22. Frey, E.N.; Pavlovicz, R.E.; Wegman, C.J.; Li, C.; Askwith, C.C. Conformational changes in the lower palm domain of ASIC1a contribute to desensitization and RFamide modulation. *PLoS ONE* **2013**, *8*, e71733. [CrossRef] [PubMed]
23. Bargeton, B.; Iwaszkiewicz, J.; Bonifacio, G.; Roy, S.; Zoete, V.; Kellenberger, S. Mutations in the palm domain disrupt modulation of acid-sensing ion channel 1a currents by neuropeptides. *Sci. Rep.* **2019**, *9*. [CrossRef] [PubMed]
24. Peeff, N.M.; Orchard, I.; Lange, A.B. Isolation, sequence, and bioactivity of PDVDHVFLRFamide and ADVGHVFLRFamide peptides from the locust central nervous system. *Peptides* **1994**, *15*, 387–392. [CrossRef]
25. Konno, K.; Kazuma, K.; Nihei, K. Peptide Toxins in Solitary Wasp Venoms. *Toxins* **2016**, *8*, 114. [CrossRef] [PubMed]
26. Petruska, J.C.; Napaporn, J.; Johnson, R.D.; Gu, J.G.; Cooper, B.Y. Subclassified acutely dissociated cells of rat DRG: Histochemistry and patterns of capsaicin-, proton-, and ATP-activated currents. *J. Neurophysiol.* **2000**, *84*, 2365–2379. [CrossRef] [PubMed]
27. Garza, A.; López, O.; Vega, R.; Soto, E. The Aminoglycosides Modulate the Acid-Sensing Ionic Channel Currents in Dorsal Root Ganglion Neurons from the Rat. *J. Pharm. Exp. Ther.* **2010**, *332*, 489–499. [CrossRef] [PubMed]
28. Donier, E.; Rugiero, F.; Jacob, C.; Wood, J.N. Regulation of ASIC activity by ASIC4-new insights into ASIC channel function revealed by a yeast two-hybrid assay. *Eur. J. Neurosci.* **2008**, *28*, 74–86. [CrossRef] [PubMed]
29. Benson, C.J.; Xie, B.; Wemmie, J.A.; Price, M.P.; Henss, J.M.; Welsh, M.J.; Snyder, P.M. Heteromultimers of DEG/ENaC subunits form H^+-gated channels in mouse sensory neurons. *Proc. Natl. Acad. Sci. USA* **2002**, *99*, 2338–2343. [CrossRef]
30. Xie, J.; Price, M.P.; Berger, A.L.; Welsh, M.J. DRASIC Contributes to pH-Gated Currents in Large Dorsal Root Ganglion Sensory Neurons by Forming Heteromultimeric Channels. *J. Neurophysiol.* **2002**, *87*, 2835–2843. [CrossRef]
31. Lingueglia, E.; de Weille, J.R.; Bassilana, F.; Heurteaux, C.; Sakai, H.; Waldmann, R.; Lazdunski, M. A Modulatory subunit of acid sensing ion channels in brain and dorsal root ganglion cells. *J. Biol. Chem.* **1997**, *272*, 29778–29783. [CrossRef] [PubMed]
32. Qiu, F.; Liu, T.T.; Qu, Z.W.; Qiu, C.Y.; Yang, Z.; Hu, W.P. Gastrodin inhibits the activity of acid-sensing ion channels in rat primary sensory neurons. *Eur. J. Pharmacol.* **2014**, *731*, 50–57. [CrossRef]
33. Sun, X.; Cao, Y.B.; Hu, L.F.; Yang, Y.P.; Li, J.; Wang, F.; Liu, C.F. ASICs mediate the modulatory effect by paeoniflorin on α-synuclein autophagic degradation. *Brain Res.* **2011**, *1396*, 77–87. [CrossRef] [PubMed]
34. Diochot, S.; Baron, A.; Rash, L.; Deval, E.; Escoubas, P.; Scarzello, S.; Salinas, M.; Lazdunsky, M. A new sea anemone peptide, APETx2, inhibits ASIC3, a major acid-sensitive channel in sensory neurons. *EMBO J.* **2004**, *23*, 1516–1525. [CrossRef] [PubMed]

35. Schroeder, C.I.; Rash, L.D.; Vila-Farrés, X.; Rosengren, K.J.; Mobli, M.; King, G.F.; Alewood, P.F.; Craik, D.J.; Durek, T. Chemical synthesis, 3D structure, and ASIC binding site of the toxin mambalgin-2. *Angew. Chem. Int. Ed. Engl.* **2014**, *53*, 1017–1020. [CrossRef]
36. Salinas, M.; Besson, T.; Delettre, Q.; Diochot, S.; Boulakirba, S.; Boulakirba, S.; Douguet, D.; Lingueglia, E. Binding site and inhibitory mechanism of the mambalgin-2 pain-relieving peptide on acid- sensing ion channel 1a. *J. Biol. Chem.* **2014**, *289*, 13363–13373. [CrossRef]
37. Rodríguez, A.A.; Salceda, E.; Garateix, A.G.; Zaharenko, A.J.; Peigneur, S.; López, O.; Pons, T.; Richardson, M.; Díaz, M.; Hernández, Y.; et al. A novel sea anemone peptide that inhibits acid-sensing ion channels. *Peptides* **2014**, *53*, 3–12. [CrossRef]
38. Chen, X.; Kalbacher, H.; Gründer, S. Interaction of acid-sensing ion channel (ASIC) 1 with the tarantula toxin psalmotoxin 1 is state dependent. *J. Gen. Physiol.* **2006**, *127*, 267–276. [CrossRef]
39. Baron, A.; Diochot, S.; Salinas, M.; Deval, E.; Noël, J.; Lingueglia, E. Venom toxins in the exploration of molecular, physiological and pathophysiological functions of acid-sensing ion channels. *Toxicon* **2013**, *75*, 187–204. [CrossRef]
40. Baconguis, I.; Gouaux, E. Structural plasticity and dynamic selectivity of acid-sensing ion channel-spider toxin complexes. *Nature* **2012**, *489*, 400–405. [CrossRef]
41. Salceda, E.; Garateix, A.; Soto, E. The sea anemone toxins BgII and BgIII prolong the inactivation time course of the tetrodotoxin-sensitive sodium current in rat dorsal root ganglion neurons. *J. Pharmacol. Exp. Ther.* **2002**, *303*, 1067–1074. [CrossRef] [PubMed]
42. Bevan, S.; Hothi, S.; Hughes, G.; James, I.F.; Rang, H.P.; Shah, K.; Walpole, C.S.; Yeats, J.C. Capsazepine: A competitive antagonist of the sensory neurone excitant capsaicin. *Br. J. Pharmacol.* **1992**, *107*, 544–552. [CrossRef] [PubMed]

toxins

MDPI

Article

Design and Production of a Recombinant Hybrid Toxin to Raise Protective Antibodies against *Loxosceles* Spider Venom

Paula A. L. Calabria, Lhiri Hanna A. L. Shimokawa-Falcão, Monica Colombini, Ana M. Moura-da-Silva, Katia C. Barbaro, Eliana L. Faquim-Mauro and Geraldo S. Magalhaes *

Laboratory of Immunopathology, Butantan Institute, São Paulo 05503-900, Brazil; paula.calabria@butantan.gov.br (P.A.L.C.); lhiri.hanna@gmail.com (L.H.A.L.S.-F.); monica.colombini@butantan.gov.br (M.C.); ana.moura@butantan.gov.br (A.M.M.-d.-S.); katia.barbaro@butantan.gov.br (K.C.B.); eliana.faquim@butantan.gov.br (E.L.F.-M.)

* Correspondence: geraldo.magalhaes@butantan.gov.br; Tel.: +55-11-2627-9777 or +55-11-98748-9390

Received: 16 January 2019; Accepted: 10 February 2019; Published: 12 February 2019

Abstract: Human accidents with spiders of the genus *Loxosceles* are an important health problem affecting thousands of people worldwide. Patients evolve to severe local injuries and, in many cases, to systemic disturbances as acute renal failure, in which cases antivenoms are considered to be the most effective treatment. However, for antivenom production, the extraction of the venom used in the immunization process is laborious and the yield is very low. Thus, many groups have been exploring the use of recombinant *Loxosceles* toxins, particularly phospholipases D (PLDs), to produce the antivenom. Nonetheless, some important venom activities are not neutralized by anti-PLD antibodies. Astacin-like metalloproteases (ALMPs) are the second most expressed toxin acting on the extracellular matrix, indicating the importance of its inclusion in the antigen's formulation to provide a better antivenom. Here we show the construction of a hybrid recombinant immunogen, called LgRec1ALP1, composed of hydrophilic regions of the PLD and the ALMP toxins from *Loxosceles gaucho*. Although the LgRec1ALP1 was expressed as inclusion bodies, it resulted in good yields and it was effective to produce neutralizing antibodies in mice. The antiserum neutralized fibrinogenolytic, platelet aggregation and dermonecrotic activities elicited by *L. gaucho*, *L. laeta*, and *L. intermedia* venoms, indicating that the hybrid recombinant antigen may be a valuable source for the production of protective antibodies against *Loxosceles* ssp. venoms. In addition, the hybrid recombinant toxin approach may enrich and expand the alternative antigens for antisera production for other venoms.

Keywords: phospholipases D; metalloproteases; *Loxosceles* spp.; recombinant toxins; hybrid immunogen; neutralizing antibodies; antivenoms

Key Contribution: The use of hybrid recombinant spider toxins to raise protective antibodies against *Loxosceles* spp. venoms may be helpful to decrease the number of antigens received by the animals during immunization. In addition, it may solve the problem of the limited amount of venom time-consuming extractions and animal handling.

1. Introduction

In view of the wide geographical distribution, the large number of individuals affected and the evolution of the clinical picture, the accidents with spiders of the genus *Loxosceles*, denominated loxoscelism, have received great attention from public health [1–3]. In Brazil, most of the human accidents are related to three main *Loxosceles* species: *Loxosceles gaucho*, *Loxosceles intermedia*, and *Loxosceles laeta* [3,4]. The loxoscelism is associated with a number of clinical symptoms including edema, an intense inflammatory reaction at the site of the bite, which can progress to a typical necrotic lesion on the skin with gravitational scattering, known as cutaneous loxoscelism [3,5–7]. In rare cases, cutaneous loxoscelism may progress to systemic manifestations (cutaneous-visceral loxoscelism) and the symptoms of this clinical condition usually begin 24 h after the spider bites, which is characterized by anemia, jaundice, intravascular hemolysis, platelet aggregation, and, in more severe cases, renal failure [8].

The venom of *Loxosceles* spp. is composed of numerous protein molecules with toxic and/or enzymatic activity [2,3,8–11], such as phospholipases D, metalloproteases, serine proteases, hyaluronidases, allergens, serine protease inhibitors, and peptides classified as cystine knot inhibitors [9,12–16]. Studies have shown that phospholipases D (PLDs) are the most abundant toxins able to elicit a cascade of adverse pharmacological events such as inflammation [13,17] dermonecrosis [11,13,18–21], platelet aggregation [21–23], hemolysis [13,23,24], and nephrotoxicity [25,26], among others.

Currently, the treatment used for human envenoming includes the use of anti-arachnid serum that in Brazil is obtained by immunizing horses with a mixture of venoms from *Loxosceles gaucho*, *Phoneutria nigriventer* spiders and the scorpion *Tityus serrulatus* (SAAr) or the use of anti-loxoscelic serum that is obtained with the mixture of *L. intermedia*, *L. laeta*, and *L. gaucho* venoms (SALox), usually associated with corticosteroids [1,27–32]. However, the extraction of the amount of venom needed for horse immunizations is expensive, laborious, and the yield obtained is very low. This fact has led some researchers to use recombinant toxins such as the PLDs [33–36] or even peptides from these toxins [30,37,38] to obtain the antiserum. Nonetheless, the antiserum obtained in this way is specific to PLD and did not neutralize all venom activities due to the synergistic action of other toxins that contribute to the deleterious effects of the venom [6,8].

In this sense, studies have shown that the astacin-like metalloproteases (ALMPs) are the second most abundant class of toxins in the venom glands of *L. laeta* [39] and *L. intermedia* [15] and appear to contribute to the envenomation picture since they hydrolyze some components of the extracellular matrix such as collagen [40], fibronectin [9,41,42], and fibrinogen [9,41,43–45]. Therefore, considering that the PLDs and ALMPs are the main toxins present in the venom of *Loxosceles* spp., in this work, we envisaged the construction of a hybrid recombinant toxin composed of the hydrophilic regions of a PLD and ALMP from *L. gaucho* to raise neutralizing antibodies in mice against of the venom of the three predominant *Loxosceles* spp. spiders that cause envenomation in Brazil. Therefore, this hybrid molecule might be an interesting tool to enhance and/or expand the possibilities to raise protective antiserum against *Loxosceles* spp. venom and this approach may also be applied to other venoms.

2. Results

2.1. Construction of the Hybrid Molecule LgRec1ALP1

In order to know the main toxin transcripts present in the venom gland of *Loxosceles gaucho*, a transcriptomic approach was performed and the analysis showed that 22.36% of all sequences gave match to toxins already described in the database. Among them, it was observed that phospholipase D (PLD) and astacin-like metalloprotease (ALMPs) were the most abundant, corresponding to 70.43 and 17.58%, respectively (Figure 1). Taking into consideration this result and the important activities of these toxins in the venom, they were chosen to make part of a hybrid immunogen construction.

Analyzing all the PLDs transcripts with identity greater than 97%, it was observed that the largest group contained 37% of all PLDs sequences, and a PLD called LgRec1 [20], present in this group was chosen to be part of the hybrid immunogen. Among the metalloprotease's transcripts with identity greater than 95%, the largest group contained 45% of all metalloproteinase transcripts, and a sequence called LgALP1 was selected from this group to be part of the hybrid immunogen.

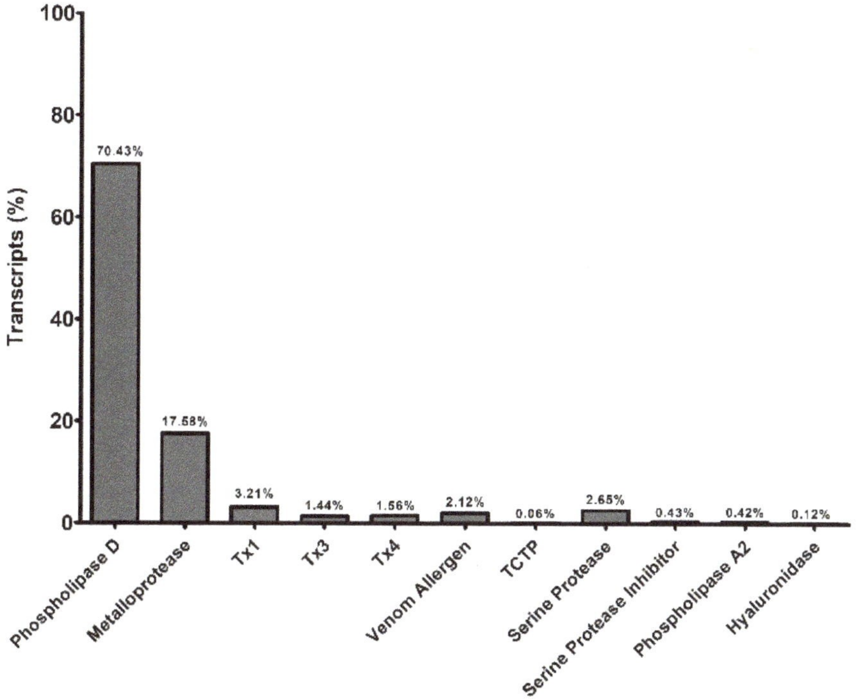

Figure 1. Graph showing the percentage of toxin transcripts in relation to the total toxins' transcripts found in *L. gaucho* venom gland. TX (similar to insecticide toxin); TCTP (similar to tumor-controlled translation protein).

The sequences of the two toxins were submitted to the ProtScale Tool program using the Hopp-Woods scale [46] to identify the hydrophilic regions of the molecules. This scale performs the prediction of potentially antigenic regions of polypeptides, where values greater than 0 are hydrophilic. After analysis, six and three hydrophilic peaks were found in the PLD LgRec1 (Figure 2A) and the metalloprotease LgALP1 sequences (Figure 2C), respectively.

The hydrophilic peptides found in the PLD LgRec1 (Figure 2B) and the ALMP LgALP1 (Figure 2D) are numbered and underlined. These peptides were then joined to form the hybrid immunogen that was called LgRec1ALP1 (Figure 2E). The exposures of these peptides on the surface of each toxin were also analyzed on the predicted tridimensional structure of the PLD LgRec1 (Figure S1) and the ALMP LgALP1 (Figure S2). To predict these structures, the crystal of a phospholipase D (3LRH) from *L. intermedia* [47] and the metalloprotease (3LQ0) from *Astacus astacus* [48] were used as templates by Phyre2 program. Since most of the hydrophilic peptides ended or stated in random coils, which are flexible loops from the original proteins, no linkers were used in the construction. In addition, to analyze the identity of the hydrophilic peptides with other spiders PLDs and metalloproteases, they were aligned against the PLDs LiRecDT1 (ABA62021) and Smase I (AAM21154) from *L. intermedia* and *L. laeta*, respectively, as well as with the metalloproteases LALP2 (ACV52010) and LLAE0237C (EY188609), also from *L. intermedia* and *L. laeta*, respectively. As can be seen, the peptides show higher identity with the PLDs (Table 1) and the metalloproteases (Table 2) from *L. intermedia*.

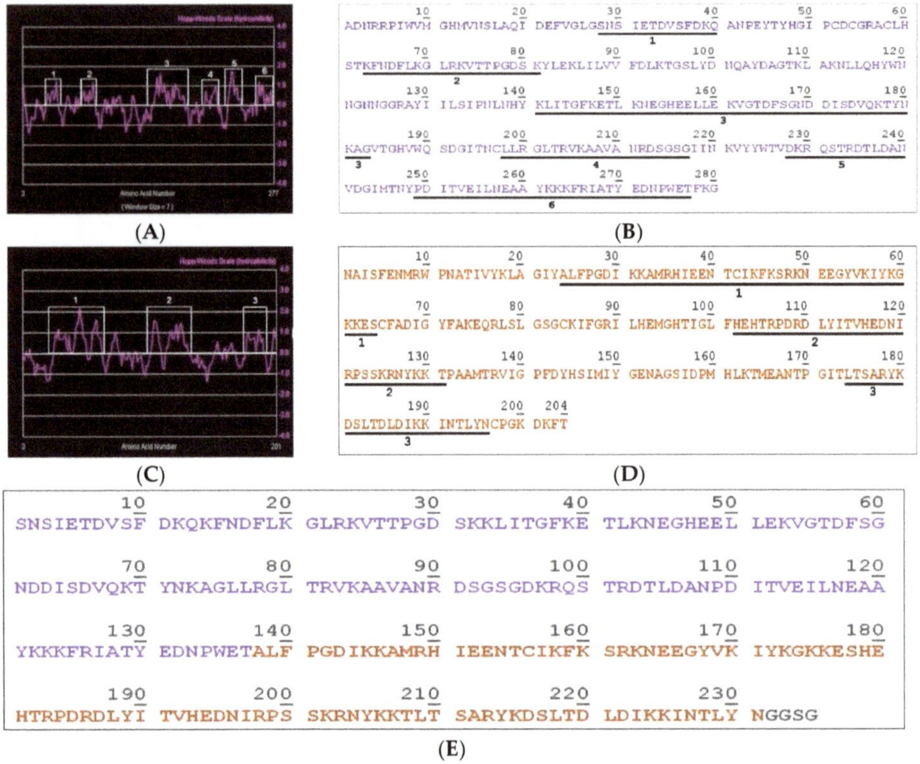

Figure 2. Sequence analysis of phospholipase D LgRec1 and metalloprotease LgALP1 to construct the hybrid immunogen LgRec1ALP1. Hydrophilicity plots of LgRec1 (**A**) and LgALP1 (**C**), deduced by the ProtScale program with Hopp–Woods scale, where the hydrophilic regions of each molecule are indicated with boxes. Sequence of LgRec1 (**B**) and LgALP1 (**D**) showing the predicted hydrophilic amino acids numbered and underlined. (**E**) Amino acid sequence of the hybrid immunogen LgRec1ALP1 containing only the hydrophilic regions of phospholipase D (PLD) LgRec1 (blue) and astacin-like metalloprotease (ALMP) LgALP1 (orange). Sequence numbers correspond to amino acid positions in the sequence.

Table 1. Amino acids identity analysis of the hydrophilic peptides of LgRec1 from *L. gaucho*.

L. gaucho	*L. intermedia*	*L. laeta*
PLD LgRec1 hydrophilic peptides	**PLD LiRecDT1**	**PLD Smase I**
SNSIETDVSFDKQ	78.6% *	50.0%
KFNDFLKGLRKVTTPGDSK	78.9%	63.1%
KLITGFKETLKNEGHEELLEKVGTDFSGNDDISDVQKTYNKAG	62.7%	55.8%
LLRGLTRVKAAVANRDSGSG	75.0%	40.0%
DKRQSTRDTLDAN	69.2%	38.4%
PDITVEILNEAAYKKKFRIATYEDNPWET	68.9%	51.7%

* Amino acids identity analysis (%) of the hydrophilic peptides of LgRec1 from *L. gaucho* with the PLDs LiRecDT1 (ABA62021) and Smase I (AAM21154) from *L. intermedia* and *L. laeta*, respectively. The identity alignment was obtained using the Clustal W Multiple Sequence Alignment tool.

Table 2. Amino acids identity analysis of the hydrophilic peptides of LgALP1 from *L. gaucho*.

L. gaucho	*L. intermedia*	*L. laeta*
Metalloprotease LgALP1 hydrophilic peptides	Metalloprotease LALP2	Metalloprotease LLAE0237C
ALFPGDIKKAMRHIEENTCIKFKSRKNEEGYVKIYKGKKES	90.4% *	48.7%
HEHTRPDRDLYITVHEDNIRPSSKRNYKKT	90.3%	46.6%
LTSARYKDSLTDLDIKKINTLYN	86.9%	47.8%

* Amino acids identity analysis (%) of the hydrophilic peptides of LgALP1 from *L. gaucho* with the metalloproteases LALP2 (ACV52010) and LLAE0237C (EY188609) from *L. intermedia* and *L. laeta*, respectively. The identity alignment was obtained using the Clustal W Multiple Sequence Alignment tool.

2.2. Expression and Purification of the Hybrid Immunogen LgRec1ALP1

The sequence of the hybrid immunogen LgRec1Alp1 was cloned into pET28a+ vector, transformed into chemically competent *E. coli* strain BL21 Star™ (DE3) and expressed at 30 °C for 4 h under induction of 1 mM of isopropyl-β-D-thiogalactoside (IPTG). The sodium dodecyl sulfate–polyacrylamide gel electrophoresis (SDS-PAGE) analysis (Figure 3A) indicates that the LgRec1Alp1 was successfully expressed as shown by the presence of an expected band with a molecular mass around 30 kDa after IPTG induction (lane 2). However, LgRec1Alp1 was expressed in the insoluble form, since after cell sonication the protein could only be seen in the pellet of cell lysed (lane 3). Therefore, the pellet was solubilized in 6 M urea and purified by immobilized metal affinity chromatography (IMAC) taking advantage of the 6xHis tag present at the C-terminus of LgRec1ALP1. After dialysis to remove urea, white clumps were observed in the dialysis bag, indicating that the recombinant LgRec1ALP1 was insoluble (lane 4). The purified LgRec1ALP1 was then subjected to identification by Western blot using an anti-His tag monoclonal antibodies (Figure 3B). The average yield of LgRec1ALP1 was 3.5 mg per liter of cell culture.

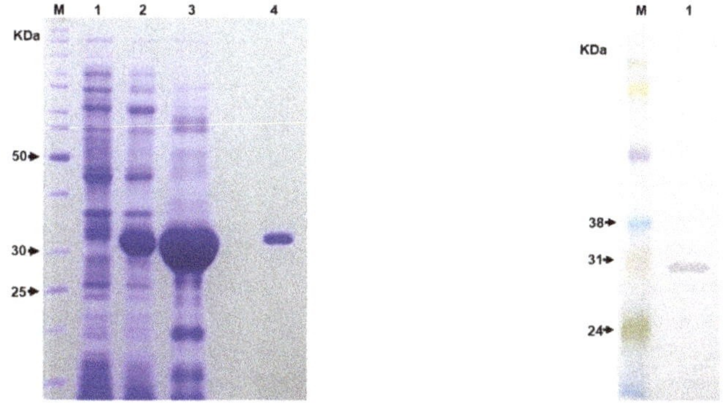

(**A**) (**B**)

Figure 3. Analysis of the recombinant hybrid immunogen LgRec1ALP1. Numbers on the left correspond to the position of molecular mass markers in kDa (M). (**A**) 12.5% sodium dodecyl sulfate–polyacrylamide gel electrophoresis (SDS-PAGE) gel showing expression and purification of the hybrid immunogen LgRec1ALP1 overexpressed in *E. coli* BL21 Star™ (DE3) at 30 °C. Protein was visualized on a 12.5% SDS/polyacrylamide gel under reducing conditions and stained with Coomassie blue. 1 and 2: Extract from BL21 Star™ (DE3) before and after isopropyl-β-D-thiogalactoside (IPTG) (1 mM) induction, respectively; 3: Bacterial pellet lysed by sonication; 4: LgRec1ALP1 solubilized in urea 6M and purified by IMAC. (**B**) Western blot analysis. 1: Purified LgRec1ALP1 was separated by 12.5% SDS-PAGE, transferred onto nitrocellulose membrane, incubated with monoclonal anti-polyhistidine antibody and revealed with 4-chloro-1-naphthol.

2.3. *Immunogenicity and Cross-Reactivity of Anti-LgRec1ALP1*

After dialysis, the recombinant LgRec1ALP1 in its colloidal state was mixed with Montanide and used via subcutaneous injection to produce polyclonal antibodies in mice. The immunoglobulins contained in the antiserum were then purified by Hi-Trap protein G affinity column. The titer of purified IgGs anti-LgRec1ALP1 was determined by ELISA using the recombinant LgRec1ALP1, *L. gaucho*, *L. laeta*, and *L. intermedia* venoms as coating antigens. The result shows, as expected, a higher titer for the recombinant LgRec1ALP1, followed by *L. gaucho*, *L. laeta*, and *L. intermedia* venoms (Figure 4A).

	Antigens			
	Hybrid immunogen	Venoms		
Antibody	LgALP1Rec1	*L. gaucho*	*L. intermedia*	*L. laeta*
Anti-LgALP1Rec1	1,024,000#	128,000	64,000	64,000

ELISA titer. Titers represent the reciprocal of the highest dilution that causes an absorbance greater than 0.050 at 492 nm, since non-specific reactions were observed below this value.

(A)

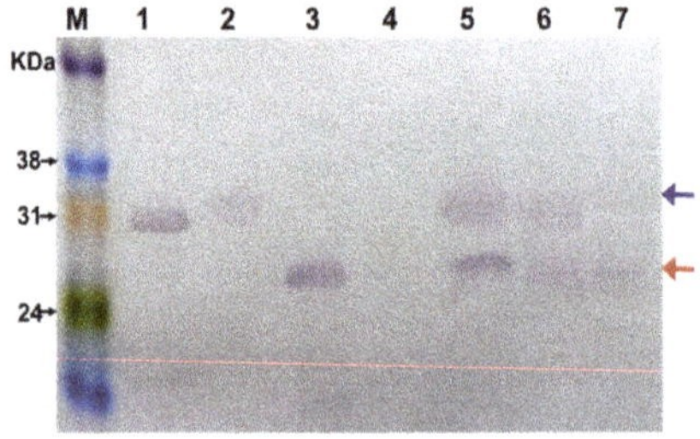

(B)

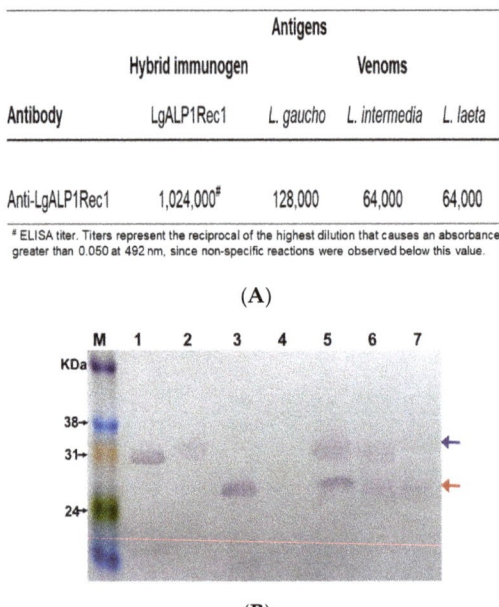

Figure 4. Evaluation of anti-LgRec1ALP1 by ELISA and Western blot. (**A**) Titration of LgRec1ALP1 antibodies by ELISA. The plates were coated with 5 μg/mL of the hybrid immunogen LgRec1ALP1, *L. gaucho*, *L. intermedia*, or *L. laeta* venoms. The absorbances of the samples were determined at 492 nm. (**B**) Recognition of anti-LgRec1ALP1 by Western blot. Proteins were separated by SDS-PAGE, transferred onto nitrocellulose membrane and incubated with anti-LgRec1ALP1. Numbers on the left correspond to the position of molecular mass markers (M). Recombinant hybrid immunogen LgRec1ALP1 (1); Recombinant PLD LgRec1 (2); Recombinant ALMP LgALP1 (3); Nonrelated recombinant protein EGFP (4); *L. gaucho* venom (5); *L. intermedia* venom (6); *L. laeta* venom (7). Blue and red arrows indicate the position for PLDs and ALMPs, respectively.

The specificity of the antibodies was also evaluated by Western blot using the recombinant PLD LgRec1 and the recombinant metalloprotease LgALP1 and the venoms of *L. gaucho*, *L. intermedia*, and *L. laeta*. The recombinant enhanced green fluorescent protein (EGFP) was used as non-related protein control. The result shows that the anti-LgRec1ALP1 recognized all recombinant toxins as well as the bands with approximate molecular mass expected for phospholipases D (blue arrow) and metalloproteases (red arrow) in all venoms. However, the bands corresponding to phospholipase D showed lower intensity in the *L. laeta* venom (Figure 4B).

2.4. Neutralization Assays

2.4.1. Neutralization of Fibrinogen Degradation Caused by *Loxosceles* spp. Venoms

To evaluate the ability of anti-LgRec1ALP1 to neutralize the proteolytic action of metalloproteases, the venoms of *L. gaucho*, *L. laeta*, and *L. intermedia* were pre-incubated with anti-LgRec1ALP1 and this mixture was then incubated with bovine fibrinogen. The samples were applied to SDS-PAGE (Figure 5A,B) and the percentage of neutralization of fibrinogen alpha chain degradation was evaluated with the ImageJ program (Figure 5C). The data show that 1.5 and 3.0 μg/μL of anti-LgRec1ALP1 was able to completely neutralize the degradation of the α subunit of fibrinogen (Figure 5A,B red arrows) caused by the *L. gaucho* venom (Figure 5B), 85–95% for *L. laeta* venom and 78–83% for *L. intermedia* venom (Figure 5C).

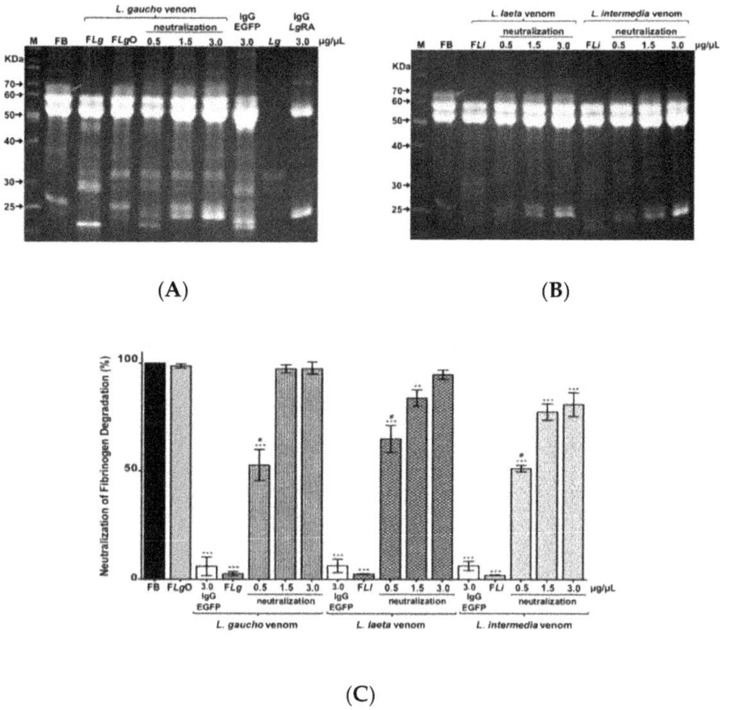

Figure 5. Evaluation of neutralization fibrinogen degradation (α subunit) by anti-LgRec1ALP1. Fibrinogen (FB) was incubated with 0.15 μg/μL of *L. gaucho* (FLg), *L. laeta* (FLl), or *L. intermedia* (FLi) venoms previously incubated or not with 0.5, 1.5, or 3.0 μg/μL of anti-LgRec1ALP1 (neutralization). Nonrelated IgG anti-EGFP (IgG-EGFP) pre-incubated with *L. gaucho*, *L. laeta*, or *L. intermedia* venoms were used as negative controls. FB: fibrinogen in Tris-HCl buffer; FLgO: fibrinogen incubated with *L. gaucho* venom and 1,10-phenanthroline (10 mM); IgG-LgRA: IgG anti-LgRec1ALP1. (**A**,**B**) SDS-PAGE gels showing the neutralization of fibrinogen α subunit (red arrow) degradation by anti-LgRec1ALP1. Samples were visualized on a 12% SDS/polyacrylamide gel under reducing conditions and stained with Coomassie blue. Numbers on the left correspond to the position of molecular mass markers (M) in kDa. (**C**) Graph showing the quantification of degradation of fibrinogen α subunit from SDS-PAGE analyzed by ImageJ densitometry software. Values given are the average ± SEM (n = 3). Significance was evaluated with an ANOVA one-way with the post-hoc Tukey test; (**) indicates $p < 0.01$, (***) indicates $p < 0.001$. # indicates statistical significance with $p < 0.001$ between samples of the venom's groups.

The role of metalloproteinases in the fibrinogen alpha subunit degradation was confirmed by incubating *L. gaucho* venom with the Zn^{2+} chelating metalloprotease inhibitor 1,10-phenanthroline (F*Lg*O), which completely abolished the degradation (Figure 5A,C). As a negative control, *L. gaucho*, *L. laeta*, and *L. intermedia* venoms were pre-incubated with a nonrelated IgG (anti-EGFP), which showed no neutralization activity (Figure 5C), represented by lane IgG EGFP in Figure 5A, where we can also visualize the bands related to *L. gaucho* venom (*Lg*) and IgG anti-LgRec1ALP1 (*Lg*RA).

2.4.2. Neutralization of Platelets Aggregation Caused by *Loxosceles* spp. Venoms

The activity of platelet aggregation is one of the main characteristics in *Loxosceles* envenomation. In order to neutralize this activity in vitro, platelet-rich plasma (PRP) was incubated with *L. gaucho*, *L. laeta*, and *L. intermedia* venoms previously pre-incubated or not with 0.1, 0.3, or 0.6 μg/μL of purified anti-LgRec1ALP1. The results show that 0.6 μg/μL of anti-LgRec1ALP1 was effective to neutralize ~100, 94, and 66% of the aggregating activity of *L. gaucho*, *L. intermedia*, and *L. laeta* venoms, respectively (Figure 6). In addition, 0.1 and 0.3 μg/μL of anti-LgRec1ALP1 were also effective to neutralize 91 and 93% of *L. gaucho* venom; 85 and 88% of *L. intermedia* venom and 41 and 56% for *L. laeta* venom, respectively. Platelet aggregation responsiveness was evaluated with 10 mM of adenosine diphosphate (ADP) agonist, and pre-incubation of *L. gaucho*, *L. laeta*, or *L. intermedia* venoms with 0.6 μg/μL of anti-EGFP antibody were used as negative controls (Figure 6, IgG EGFP).

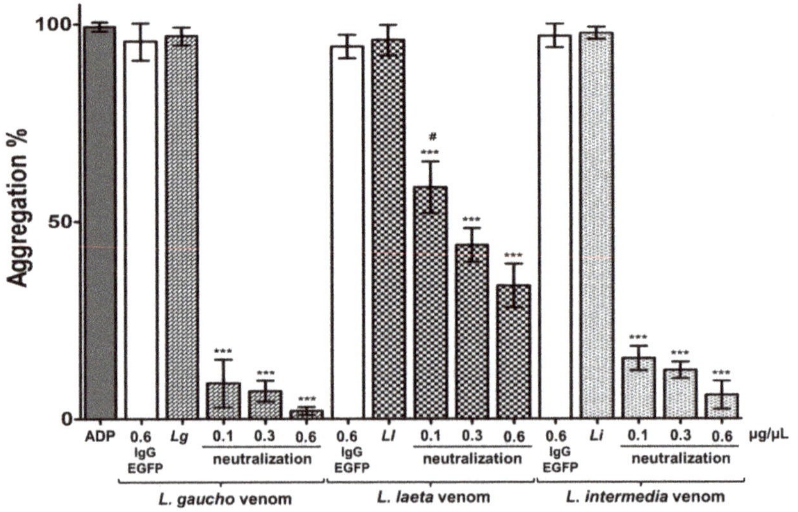

Figure 6. Analysis of platelet aggregation neutralization by anti-LgRec1ALP1. Platelet-rich plasma (PRP) was treated with 7.5 μg of the venoms *L. gaucho* (*Lg*), *L. laeta* (*Ll*), or *L. intermedia* (*Li*) previously incubated or not with 0.1, 0.3, or 0.6 μg/μL of anti-LgRec1ALP1 in a final volume of 100 μL (neutralization). Incubation of *L. gaucho*, *L. laeta*, or *L. intermedia* venoms with 0.6 μg/μL anti-EGFP (IgG-EGFP) were used as negative controls. Platelet aggregation was induced by adding 10 μM of adenosine diphosphate (ADP) in phosphate buffered saline (PBS) as a positive control. Aggregation was monitored by measuring the light transmittance for five minutes by an aggregometer ($n = 3$). Values given are the average ± SEM. Significance was evaluated with an ANOVA one-way with the post-hoc Tukey test; (**) indicates $p < 0.01$, (***) indicates $p < 0.001$. # indicates statistical significance with $p < 0.05$ between samples of the venom's groups.

2.4.3. Neutralization of Dermonecrosis and Edema Caused by *Loxosceles* spp. Venoms

Since local reactions such as edema and dermonecrosis are afflictions related to *Loxosceles* spp. envenomation, the neutralizing of this activity by the anti-LgRec1ALP1 were evaluated in rabbits′

skin. For this, 6 μg of the venoms *L. gaucho*, *L. laeta*, or *L. intermedia* were incubated with 0.4 μg/μL of anti-LgRec1ALP1 in a final volume of 150 μL and the area of lesions were measured 24 and 48 h after injection (Figure 7B). As seen in Figure 7A, the anti-LgRec1ALP1 was very effective to abolish all dermonecrosis caused by *L. gaucho* venom, 79% for *L. intermedia*, and 68% *L. laeta* venoms. The edema was also neutralized by the anti-LgRec1ALP1, although in less extent, showing neutralization of 73 and 76% for *L. gaucho*, 37 and 40% for *L. laeta* and 49 and 54% for *L. intermedia* venom in 24 and 48 h, respectively (Figure 7C).

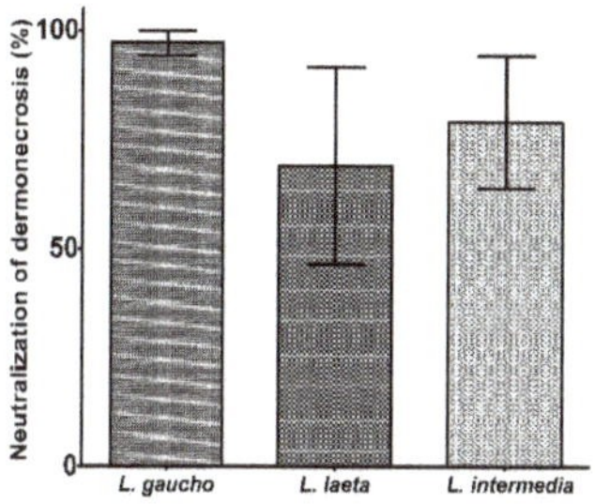

(A)

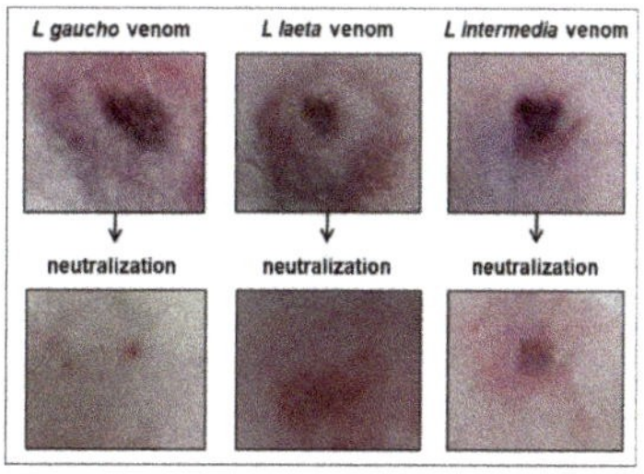

(B)

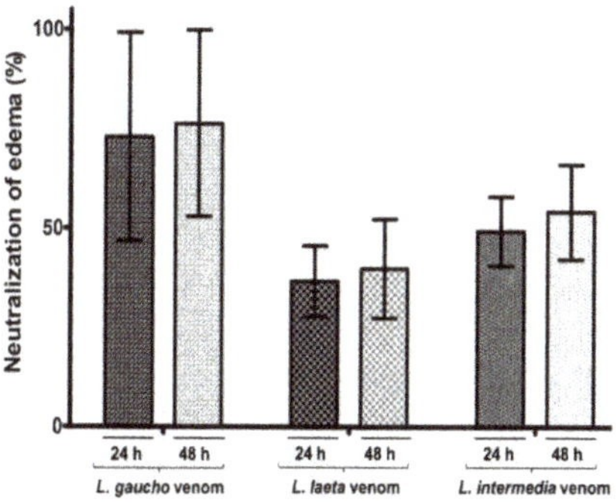

(C)

Figure 7. Neutralization of dermonecrosis (**A**) and edema (**C**) induced by *Loxosceles* spp. venoms after incubation with anti-LgRec1ALP1. (**B**) Rabbit's treated with *Loxosceles* venom or venoms incubated with anti-LgRec1ALP1. To the tests, 6 μg of the venoms *L. gaucho*, *L. laeta*, or *L. intermedia* were pre-incubated with 0.4 μg/μL of anti-LgRec1ALP1 in a final volume of 150 μL for 30 min at 37 °C, centrifuged and the supernatant injected i.d. into the rabbit dorsum. The animals were observed for 24 and 48 h. Size of the lesions was measured by ImageJ software and the results are expressed as the percentage reduction of the size of the lesions. Values given are the average ± SEM ($n = 2$).

3. Discussion

The search for new therapies and strategies for the treatment of people that suffer accidents with venomous animals is increasing every year and therefore it is considered a public health problem. In this sense, spiders of the genus *Loxosceles* spp. are of great medical importance, with several cases reported worldwide [49–53]. In Brazil, these spiders are responsible for thousands of accidents every year (Sistema de Informação de Agravo de Notificação, Ministério da Saúde) and the recommended treatment is the serum therapy [1,27–29]. However, due to the limited amount of venom extracted from the *Loxosceles* spp. that is used to produce the antiserum, many studies have been searching for alternatives such as the use of recombinant toxins. In this context, the recombinant phospholipases D (PLDs) or their peptides have been exploited [34–36,38,54,55] as these toxins are the main responsible for the symptoms related to the envenoming [11,13,21–23]. Nonetheless, antibodies against PLDs alone were not effective to neutralize some venom activities, presumably due to the presence of other toxins that can act synergistically with the PLDs.

Analyzing the transcriptomic profile of *L. gaucho* venom gland, we showed that the PLDs (70.43%) and the astacin-like metalloproteases (ALMPs) (17.58%) accounted for most of the toxin transcripts. Other toxins with lower expression were also found such as insecticidal peptides (TX) (6.21%) with action on Na^+ channels [56], venom allergens (2.12%) that elicit allergic response similar to other sources such as plant pollens, molds, and foods [57], translationally-controlled tumor protein (TCTP) (0.06%) that has been related to cause edema and vascular permeability [58] serine proteases (2.65%) described to have gelatinolytic activity [59]; serine proteases inhibitors (0.43%), which may be related to coagulation processes and fibrinolysis [39]; phospholipase A2 (0.42%) related to low myotoxic activity at high doses [12] and hyaluronic acid (0.12%), which have shown activity on hyaluronic acid and chondroitin sulfate [11,60]. In agreement with our results, the transcriptome of *L. laeta* [39] and *L. intermedia* venom gland [15] also showed a high level of expression of PLDs and ALMPs.

Because of their proteolytic activities on molecules such as fibronectin [41,42] and fibrinogen [9,44,45], these toxins may work synergistically with other toxins present in the venom, which may explain the local hemorrhage at the bite site, imperfect platelet adhesion and difficulties in wound healing. Therefore, in an effort to develop a new immunogen for raising broadly neutralizing antibodies against these two main toxins from *Loxosceles* venom, in this work we show the construction of a hybrid immunogen, called LgRec1ALP1, that was designed with the hydrophilic regions of the PLD LgRec1 [20] and the metalloprotease LgALP1 highly expressed in the *L. gaucho* venom gland. The rationale was that the hydrophilic regions are more exposed on the toxins surface and some of them might be essential to interact with receptors, therefore, antibodies raised against these regions could confer better neutralization activities.

The hybrid immunogen LgRec1ALP1 was successfully expressed as inclusion bodies and although some refolding protocols such as dialysis, dilution, and adsorption chromatography were performed [61], none of them seemed to work (data not shown). A plausible explanation might be the presence of peptides from astacin-like metalloprotease since most of the recombinant PLDs are soluble, previous work on metalloprotease expression from *L. intermedia* showed to be insoluble [45,62]. However, several other factors may contribute to the inclusion bodies formation [63] and it is very common during overexpression of heterologous genes in *E. coli*, particularly from animal origin. Although the biological activity of the protein in this state is impaired, some studies show that insoluble proteins can successfully be used to produce polyclonal antibodies [64–66]. In addition, the inclusion bodies may represent some advantages since they are less vulnerable to degradation and may remain longer in tissues, avoiding their fast clearance, which could, in theory, require fewer boosters or even the necessity of using adjuvants. In fact, some studies have been explored the use of inclusion bodies as a vaccine [67–69]. Therefore, after purification and dialysis, the LgRec1ALP1 was used to produce antiserum even in its insoluble state.

Antibodies raised against whole *Loxosceles* venoms have been described to have cross-reactivity among venoms [11,70], which indicates the presence of common epitopes in their toxins. In this regard, the alignment of the hydrophilic peptides of LgRec1ALP1 showed high identity with PLDs and metalloproteases from *L. intermedia* and average identity with these toxins' counterparts found in *L. laeta* venom (Table 1). Therefore, a cross-reactivity was expected for the anti-LgRec1ALP1. In fact, the ELISA showed that the higher titer of antibodies was against *L. gaucho* venom components, however, it was verified a significant cross-reactivity of this antiserum with *L. laeta* and *L. intermedia* venoms (Figure 4). In addition, Western blot analysis revealed that anti-LgRec1ALP1 was able to recognize PLDs and metalloproteases from all tested venoms, but only a very faint band was revealed for PLD from *L. laeta*, which might be due to the lower identity between *L. gaucho* and *L. laeta* PLDs (Table 1).

As discussed previously, the proteolytic action of ALMPs on some components of the extracellular matrix and fibrinogen [41,45,62] have brought attention to raise protective antibodies against these toxins. Lima and colleagues [71], for example, used the sequences of an ALMPs from *L. intermedia* to compose a chimera protein to raise neutralizing antibodies. However, in this study, the produced antiserum was tested only on *L. intermedia* venom, which used 100 μg of purified IgGs to achieve complete fibrinogenolytic neutralization. Taking into consideration the same amount of venom used in that study, here we showed that the anti-LgRec1ALP1 was more efficient, since 1.5 μg/μL of it was able to completely neutralize the fibrinogen degradation by *L. gaucho* venom and 3.0 μg/μL neutralized 95 and 83% of *L. laeta* and *L. intermedia* venoms, respectively. This result indicates that the identity shared among the LgRec1ALP1 hydrophilic peptides and the ALMPs from all tested venoms was able to raise antibodies with cross-reactivity neutralizing properties.

Platelet aggregation is another effect associated with *Loxosceles* spp. venoms and many studies indicate that this property is related to the PLDs [20,21,23,72,73]. Since there is no report showing the neutralization of this important activity, in this work the effectiveness of anti-LgRec1ALP1 was tested on three *Loxosceles* venom. The results were quite encouraging since the anti-LgRec1ALP1 was able to inhibit 100, 94 and 66% of platelet aggregation caused by *L. gaucho*, *L. intermedia*, and *L. laeta* venoms, respectively.

A very common clinical picture caused by the venom of *Loxosceles* spiders is the development of a notorious necrotic skin ulcer [74–76]. Therefore, the efficacy of anti-LgRec1ALP1 was evaluated to inhibit these activities on the rabbit´s skin. The results showed that the anti-LgRec1ALP1 was efficient in totally neutralizing the venom of *L. gaucho*, while this neutralization was around 79 and 68% for *L. intermedia* and *L. laeta* venoms, respectively. These differences in neutralization may be related to differences in the PLDs from the venoms. In fact, all works with antisera against recombinant PLDs demonstrate effectiveness in neutralizing the dermonecrotic action related to the species used to obtain the antiserum [34].

Another characteristic of *Loxosceles* envenomation is the evolution of edema that is difficult to neutralize when only antisera against PLDs are used [35,77], probably due to the contribution of other toxins present in the venoms as well as the evolution of the inflammatory picture [78]. Regardless of other factors that may be involved, the anti-LgRec1ALP1 was able to neutralize 76, 40 and 54% of this activity elicited by *L. gaucho*, *L. laeta*, and *L. intermedia* venoms, respectively. Although the edema was not fully abolished, the anti-LgRec1ALP1 showed to be promising since other studies using antiserum against recombinant PLDs or their peptides showed to be less effective. In this regard, Duarte and colleagues [36] reported that antibodies raised against the PLD LiD1 from *L. laeta* were able to neutralize only 17% of edema caused by this venom. In addition, using antiserum against PLDs peptides from *L. intermedia* and *L. laeta* venoms, Souza and colleagues [38] showed 40% edema neutralization of *L. intermedia* venom. Thus, the results obtained in the in vitro and in vivo tests with the three predominant *Loxosceles* spp. spiders in South America demonstrate the potential application for the constructed hybrid immunogen.

4. Conclusions

Taken together, the results shown in this work indicate that the hybrid immunogen LgRec1ALP1 might represent an interesting alternative antigen to produce neutralizing antibodies against the two main toxins present in the *Loxosceles* venom. The LgRec1ALP1 might also be useful to enrich the whole venom so less amount of it would be necessary which in turn would decrease the number of antigens received by the animals during immunization. In addition, this approach may be further extended to other toxins present in the venom to achieve complete neutralization. This approach may also be useful to solve the problem of the limited amount of venom, time-consuming extractions, and animal handling.

5. Materials and Methods

5.1. Ethics Committees

The procedures involving animals were conducted according to national laws and policies controlled by Butantan Institute Animal Investigation Ethical Committee. Experimental protocol in mice record n° CEUA 8172250816. Experimental protocol in rabbits records n° CEUAIB 886/12. The IBAMA (Brazilian Institute for the Environment and Renewable Natural Resources) provided animal collection permission n° 15383-2, while CGEN (Board of Genetic Heritage Management) provided the license for genetic patrimony access (02001.005110/2008). All manipulation of microorganisms has been developed in biosafety level P2 area, as authorized by CIBio and CTNBio (National Technical Commission on Biosecurity) (Record n° CQB-030/98 de 30/05/2011). All procedures involving human blood were approved by the Ethical Committee in Research from Municipal Secretary of Health of São Paulo, CAAE: 02990818.3.0000.0086.

5.2. Animals and Venoms

BALB/c male mice aged 7 to 8 weeks (18–22 g) and New Zealand adult rabbits (3 to 4 kg) were provided by the Butantan Institute Animal Husbandry. All animals received water ad libitum and food under controlled environmental conditions. The venoms were supplied by the Butantan Institute Venoms Center, resuspended in PBS (phosphate buffered saline). For the library of transcripts, 300 wild-type *Loxosceles gaucho* venom glands were collected as previously described [9] and macerated with 2 mL Trizol reagent (Invitrogen™, Thermo Fisher Scientific, Waltham, MA, USA) as recommended by the manufacturer. Subsequently, mRNA purification was performed using Dynabeads® mRNA Purification Kit (Dynal Biotech-Invitrogen™, Thermo Fisher Scientific, Waltham, MA, USA) and the cDNAs synthesized using the cDNA Synthesis System (Roche®, Sigma Life Science, Merck Corporation, Darmstadt, Germany) kit, both following manufacturer's guidelines.

5.3. Sequences and Analysis of Sequenced Transcripts

The preparation of cDNA libraries from the mRNA was performed by initial fragmentation of the sample with a $ZnCl_2$ solution's followed by purification of the desired fragments size and synthesis cDNA by cDNA Synthesis System (Roche®, Sigma Life Science, Merck Corporation, Darmstadt, Germany) kit, using Roche random primer. For the assembly of the sequences, it was used the 454 GS Junior Roche Life Science software (Branford CT, USA) of the Butantan Institute in the Special Laboratory of Applied Toxinology (LETA). The program used standards parameters except for the values of minimum identity (95%) and minimum length (50 pb). In this assembly an rRNA filter using the rRNA sequences for arachnids available in GenBank. Only the reads that met the criteria of quality and minimum size were used in the assembly to generate the isotigs. The identification of these transcript isotigs was performed using the Blast2GO platform [79], using the blastx algorithm [80] against GenBank nr (non-redundant) database (https://www.blast2go.com/). The hydrophilicity of the toxins was determined by the ProtScale Tool (http://web.expasy.org/protscale/) using the Hopp–Woods scale [46]. The molecular mass of the hybrid immunogen was calculated by the ProtParam Tool program (https://web.expasy.org/protparam/) and the alignments were performed with Clustal W tool (https://npsa-prabi.ibcp.fr/cgi-bin/npsa_automat.pl?page=npsa_clustalw.html). The tridimensional prediction of PLD LgRec1 and LgALP1 was performed by Phyre2 program in an intensive mode setting using the crystal of a phospholipase D (3LRH) from *L. intermedia* and the metalloprotease (3LQ0) from *Astacus astacus* as templates (http://www.sbg.bio.ic.ac.uk/phyre2/html/page.cgi?id=index). The models were visualized by Chimera software (http://www.cgl.ucsf.edu/chimera/download.html).

5.4. *Construction of the Hybrid Immunogen*

To construct the hybrid immunogen, six hydrophilic regions from the recombinant phospholipase D LgRec1: 1–SNSIETDVSFDKQ; 2–KFNDFLKGLRKVTTPGDSK; 3–KLITGFKETLKNEGHE ELLEKV GTDFSGNDDISDVQKTYNKAG; 4–LRGLTRVKAAVANRDSGSG; 5–DKRQSTRDTL DAN; 6– PDI TVEILNEAAYKKKFRIATYEDNPWET and three hydrophilic regions from the metalloprotease LgALP1: 1–ALFPGDIKKAMRHIEENTCIKFKSRKNEEGYVKIYKGKKES; 2–HEHTRPDRDLYITVH EDNIRPSSKRNYKKT; 3–LTSARYKDSLTDLDIKKINTLYN), were predicted by ProtScale Tool. The nucleotide sequence of each selected region was linked together and optimized for expression in bacteria by Invitrogen™ Gene Synthesis (GeneArt™), Thermo Fisher Scientific, Waltham, MA, USA. This sequence was then cloned into N-terminus of a 6xHis histidine tag between *Bam*HI and *Hind*III sites of pET-28a(+) (Novagen® Merck Corporation, Darmstadt, Germany) and called LgRec1ALP1.

5.5. *Recombinant LgRec1ALP1 Expression*

For expression of the hybrid immunogen LgRec1ALP1, chemically competent *E. coli* BL21 Star™ (DE3) cells (Invitrogen™, Thermo Fisher Scientific, Waltham, MA, USA) were transformed with the pET28a-LgRec1ALP1 construction and a colony grown on plate LB-agar containing 50 μg/mL of kanamycin for 16 h was transferred into liquid LB medium supplemented with 50 μg/mL of kanamycin and grown for 16 h at 30 °C under shaking at 250 rpm. An aliquot of this culture at the 1:50 dilution was added into LB medium supplemented with 50 μg/mL of kanamycin and incubated at 30 °C under agitation of 250 rpm until reaching the logarithmic exponential growth phase (DO 600, ~0.6). At this time, 1 mM of final isopropyl-β-D-thiogalactoside (IPTG) was added in culture and incubated for 4 h at 30 °C. After this period the cells were collected by centrifugation (10,000× *g*) for 15 min at 4 °C and either immediately used or stored frozen at −20 °C.

5.6. *LgRec1ALP1 Purification*

Cells were resuspended in binding buffer with urea 6 M (20 mM de sodium phosphate pH 7.0, 500 mM NaCl and 20 mM of imidazole) and lysed by an ultrasonication intermittently (amplitude of 20% with 3 s pulse and 4 s interval between each pulse) on ice for 90 s with 4 min intervals between each sonication for cooling purposes. This process was repeated five times. The lysate was centrifuged at 10,000 *g* for 10 min at 4 °C and the supernatant containing the solubilized protein was purified by immobilized metal affinity chromatography (IMAC) using 1 mL of Ni Sepharose® 6 Fast Flow GE® resin (Healthcare, Little Chalfont, UK) following the manufacturer's protocol. LgRec1ALP1 was eluted in elution buffer (20 mM sodium phosphate, 500 mM NaCl and 1 M Imidazole and 6M urea), dialyzed against TBS buffer (20 mM Tris, 150 mM NaCl, pH 7.5) with 3 mM DTT (Dithiothreitol) and analyzed on a 12.5% SDS-PAGE [81] under reducing conditions.

5.7. *SDS-Polyacrylamide Gel Electrophoresis*

Samples were analyzed with constant current of 25 mA on a 12.5% SDS-PAGE containing the same number of bacteria (determined by spectrometry) before and after IPTG induction or 20 μL of purified LgRec1ALP1 in sample buffer (62.5 mM Tris pH 6.8, 10% glycerol, 2% SDS, and 2.5% dithiothreitol) boiled for 5 min. The gels were stained with Coomassie R-250 blue. The molecular mass was estimated by PageRuler™ Prestained Protein Ladder (Thermo Fisher Scientific, Waltham, MA, USA) molecular weight standard.

5.8. *Quantification of Recombinant Proteins and Venoms*

The concentrations of the *L. gaucho*, *L. laeta* and *L. intermedia* venoms and the recombinant PLD LgRec1 and EGFP were determined in duplicate by the bicinchoninic acid method [82] using the Pierce™ BCA Protein Assay Kit (Thermo Fisher Scientific, Waltham, MA, USA) and BSA (Sigma Chemicals, St. Louis, MO, USA) as the standard curve following the manufacturer's protocol. The hybrid immunogen LgRec1ALP1 and the recombinant ALMP LgALP1, due to their insolubility, had their bands on the SDS-PAGE quantified by the freeware ImageJ, using different concentrations of bovine serum albumin (BSA) as a reference. ImageJ is a Java-based program developed by Wayne Rasband of the National Institute of Health (USA) and is available for download at http://rsb.info.nih.gov/ij/. The version used in this work was downloaded in 15/12/2018 (ImageJ bundled with 64-bit Java 1.8.0_112) using the Windows version [83].

5.9. Production of Anti-LgRec1ALP1 in Mice

To obtain polyclonal antibodies anti-LgRec1ALP1, a group of five BALB/c mice were immunized subcutaneously (s.c.) in the base of the tail (0.2 mL/animal) with 10 μg of LgRec1ALP1 in TBS buffer and emulsified in 0.2 mL of Montanide ISA50V. The animals were boosted i.d. 15, 30 and 45 days later with the same dose of antigen with an adjuvant. For the collection of the antiserum, the mice were euthanized in a CO_2 chamber, whole blood was collected by cardiac puncture and the serum obtained by centrifugation (4 °C, 10 min, 800 *g*). IgGs were purified by affinity chromatography using Protein G Sepharose™ 4 Fast Flow (GE Healthcare, Little Chalfont, UK), following the manufacturer's protocol. The concentration was determined in duplicate by the bicinchoninic acid method [82] using the Pierce™ BCA Protein Assay Kit (Thermo Fisher Scientific, Waltham, MA, USA) using the BSA (Sigma Chemicals, St. Louis, MO, USA) as the standard curve following the manufacturer's protocol. Purified mice IgGs against the recombinant enhanced green fluorescent protein (EGFP) were used as a control.

5.10. Immunoenzymatic Assay (ELISA)

Polyclonal anti-LgRec1ALP1 antibodies titer was determined by ELISA as described by Theakston and colleagues [84]. Thus, polystyrene plates (Polysorp, NUNC, Roskilde, Denmark) were coated with 5 μg/mL of LgRec1ALP1 diluted in urea 3 M or *L. gaucho*, *L. laeta* or *L. intermedia* venoms diluted in carbonate/bicarbonate buffer (0.05 M, pH 9.6). As a negative control, normal mouse serum was used. The intensity of the reaction was determined by reading the absorbance in ELISA plate reader (Multiskan Spectrophotometer EFLAB, Helsinki, Finland), where titers were determined as the reciprocal of the highest dilution which promotes a reading greater than 0.05 in the length of 492 nm since non-specific reactions should be below this value.

5.11. Western Blot Analysis

Samples of the recombinant LgRec1ALP1, LgRec1, LgALP1, EGFP and whole venoms of *L. gaucho*, *L. intermedia*, *L. laeta* were analyzed on a 12.5% SDS-PAGE under reducing conditions. Subsequently, the samples were transferred to nitrocellulose membranes using the Trans-Blot® SD Semi-Dry Transfer Cell (Bio-Rad® Laboratories, Hercules, CA, USA) following the manufacturer's recommendations. After transfer, the nitrocellulose membranes were stained with Ponceau S® (Merck Millipore Corporation, Darmstadt, Germany) 1:20 to verify the transfer of the proteins. To remove the dye, the membranes were washed with TBS-Tween (20 mM Tris, 150 mM NaCl, 0.05% Tween 20, pH 7.5) until complete removal. Subsequently, the membranes were blocked with incubation buffer (Tris/NaCl, pH 7.5 with 5% milk) for 2 h at room temperature and then washed 3 times with TBS-Tween. Afterward, the membranes were incubated for 2 h with mouse monoclonal anti-polyhistidine antibody (Sigma Life Science, Merck Corporation, Darmstadt, Germany) or anti-LgRec1ALP1 at a 1:1000 dilution in incubation buffer. After, the membranes were washed with TBS-Tween and incubated for 2 h with the peroxidase-labeled anti-mouse IgG (Sigma Life Science, Merck Corporation, Darmstadt, Germany) at a 1:5000 dilution in incubation buffer. Then a new wash cycle was performed and the antigenic components were revealed with 0.05% (*w/v*) 4-chloro-1α-naphthol in 15% (*v/v*) methanol in presence of 0.03% H_2O_2 (*v/v*).

5.12. Neutralization of Fibrinogen Degradation

For the neutralization tests of the proteolytic activity of the metalloprotease present in the *Loxosceles* sp. venoms, bovine fibrinogen (BF) was dissolved in Tris-HCl buffer (0.05 M HCl, 0.2 M Tris, 0.05 M $CaCl_2$, pH 7.4) at the final concentration of 3 μg/μL. In each test, 0.15 μg/μL of the *L. gaucho*, *L. laeta* or *L. intermedia* venoms were pre-incubated with 0.5, 1.5 or 3.0 μg/L of anti-LgRec1ALP1 in a final volume of 20 μL. These reactions were then incubated for 60 min at 37 °C and centrifuged for 5 min at 10,000× *g*. The supernatant of each sample was then mixed with 12 μL of the fibrinogen stock solution and the volume completed to 32 μL. All samples were then incubated for 16 h at 37 °C and analyzed on a 12.5% SDS-PAGE under reducing conditions. BF without venom was used as a control of the reaction and 1,10-ortho-phenanthroline (10 mM) was used to inhibit metalloprotease activity. As a negative control, BF was incubated with 0.15 μg/μL of *L. gaucho*, *L. laeta* or *L. intermedia* venoms previously incubated with 3.0 μg/μL of anti-EGFP. All samples were incubated for 60 min at 37 °C. After this period, all samples were analyzed on a 12.5% SDS-PAGE under reducing conditions and stained with Coomassie blue R-250. The densities of fibrinogen α subunit bands were quantified by the ImageJ freeware and the values were normalized. The experiments were performed in triplicate ($n = 3$) and reported as the mean ± SEM.

5.13. Neutralization of Platelet Aggregation

Human blood from healthy volunteers without using medications interfering with platelet activity for at least 10 days prior to testing was collected in 3.8% sodium citrate (1:9). Platelet aggregation using plasma rich in platelets (PRP) was performed as previously described [85]. For the aggregation assay, 7.5 μg of *L. gaucho*, *L. laeta* and *L. intermedia* venoms were pre-incubated or not with 0.1, 0.3 or 0.6 μg/μL of anti-LgRec1ALP1 IgGs in a final volume of 100 μL. The reaction was incubated for 60 min at 37 °C and then centrifuged for 5 min at 10,000 *g* before use. Platelet-poor plasma (PPP) was used as blank and 0.6 μg/μL of IgG anti-EGFP pre-incubated with 7.5 μg of *L. gaucho*, *L. laeta* or *L. intermedia* venoms in a final volume of 100 μL were used as a negative control. The agonist ADP (final concentration of 10 μM) was used as positive control for platelet aggregation. The experiments were performed in triplicate ($n = 3$) on a Chrono-Log Model 490 aggregator (Chrono-Log Corporation, Havertown, PA, USA) and reported as the mean ± SEM.

5.14. Neutralization of Dermonecrotic and Edema Activities by the Anti-LgRec1ALP1

To analyze the neutralization of edema and dermonecrotic activities induced by *Loxosceles* spp. venoms, samples of 6 μg of *L. gaucho*, *L. laeta* or *L. intermedia* venoms were incubated with 0.4 μg/μL of anti-LgRec1ALP1 in a final volume of 150 μL for 60 min at 37 °C. Thereafter, the mixtures were centrifuged, and the supernatant was injected i.d. into the rabbit dorsum. The same doses of venoms without antibody were used as a positive control and 0.4 μg/μL of anti-LgRec1ALP1 as a negative control. The animals were observed for 24 and 48 h to analyze the dermonecrosis and edema neutralization. Size of the lesions was measured by ImageJ software and the reduction of the size of the lesions was expressed in percentage. Values are the average ± SEM ($n = 2$).

5.15. Statistical Analyses

Statistical analyses were performed using analysis of variance (ANOVA) with the post-hoc Tukey test in the GraphPad Prism 5 software v5.01, 2007. (GraphPad Software, Inc. La Jolla, CA, USA). Significance was considered when $p < 0.05$.

Supplementary Materials: The following are available online at http://www.mdpi.com/2072-6651/11/2/108/s1, Figure S1: Multiple alignment analysis of deduced amino acid sequences of LgRec1 (AFY98967) from L. gaucho and with the sequence of a phospholipase (PDB: 3RLH) from L. intermedia used as a template to predict the 3D structure of LgRec1; Figure S2: Multiple alignment analysis of deduced amino acid sequences of LgALP1 from *L. gaucho* and the astacin metalloprotease (PDB: 3LQ0) from *Astacus astacus* used as a template to predict the 3D structure of LgALP1.

Author Contributions: Conceptualization, G.S.M. and P.A.L.C.; methodology, P.A.L.C.; L.H.A.L.S.-F.; E.L.F.-M. and M.C.; software analysis G.S.M. and P.A.L.C.; investigation, G.S.M. and P.A.L.C.; resources, G.S.M.; A.M.M.-d.-S. and E.L.F.-M.; data curation, G.S.M.; K.C.B.; A.M.M.-d.-S. and E.L.F.-M.; writing—original draft preparation, G.S.M. and P.A.L.C.; writing—review and editing, K.C.B.; A.M.M.-S. and E.L.F.-M.; project administration, G.S.M.; funding acquisition, G.S.M.

Funding: This study was financed by Fundação de Amparo à Pesquisa do Estado de São Paulo (FAPESP) 2014/23457-9 and 2017/1699-8 – G.S.M.; Coordenação de Aperfeiçoamento de Pessoal de Nível Superior - Brasil (CAPES) - Finance Code 001, P.A.L.C. scholarship and 88887.124146/2014-00 -PROCAD2013 research funds; and Conselho Nacional de Desenvolvimento Científico e Tecnológico (CNPq) (309392/2015-2 - E.L.F.-M. and 304025/2014-3 – A.M.M.-S. Fellowships).

Acknowledgments: We thank Inácio L. M. J. de Azevedo for his assistance in the use of the 454 GS Junior Roche Life Science software (Branford, CT, USA) from Butantan Institute in the Special Laboratory of Applied Toxinology (LETA) and Maria C. Caporrino for technical support.

Conflicts of Interest: The authors declare no conflicts of interest.

References

1. Hogan, C.J.; Barbaro, K.C.; Winkel, K. Loxoscelism: Old obstacles, new directions. *Ann. Emerg. Med.* **2004**, *44*, 608–624. [CrossRef] [PubMed]
2. Swanson, D.L.; Vetter, R.S. Loxoscelism. *Clin. Dermatol.* **2006**, *24*, 213–221. [CrossRef] [PubMed]
3. Gremski, L.H.; Trevisan-Silva, D.; Ferrer, V.P.; Matsubara, F.H.; Meissner, G.O.; Wille, A.C.M.; Vuitika, L.; Dias-Lopes, C.; Ullah, A.; de Moraes, F.R.; et al. Recent advances in the understanding of brown spider venoms: From the biology of spiders to the molecular mechanisms of toxins. *Toxicon* **2014**, *83*, 91–120. [CrossRef] [PubMed]
4. Málaque, C.M.; Castro-Valencia, J.E.; Cardoso, J.L.; Francca, F.O.; Barbaro, K.C.; Fan, H.W. Clinical and epidemiological features of definitive and presumed loxoscelism in São Paulo, Brazil. *Rev. Inst. Med. Trop. Sao Paulo* **2002**, *44*, 139–143. [CrossRef] [PubMed]
5. Pauli, I.; Puka, J.; Gubert, I.C.; Minozzo, J.C. The efficacy of antivenom in loxoscelism treatment. *Toxicon* **2006**, *48*, 123–137. [CrossRef] [PubMed]
6. Chaim, O.M.; Trevisan-Silva, D.; Chaves-Moreira, D.; Wille, A.C.M.; Ferrer, V.P.; Matsubara, F.H.; Mangili, O.C.; da Silveira, R.B.; Gremski, L.H.; Gremski, W.; et al. Brown Spider (*Loxosceles genus*) Venom Toxins: Tools for Biological Purposes. *Toxins* **2011**, *3*, 309–344. [CrossRef] [PubMed]
7. Malaque, C.M.S.; Santoro, M.L.; Cardoso, J.L.C.; Conde, M.R.; Novaes, C.T.G.; Risk, J.Y.; Franca, F.O.S.; de Medeiros, C.R.; Fan, H.W. Clinical picture and laboratorial evaluation in human loxoscelism. *Toxicon* **2011**, *58*, 664–671. [CrossRef]
8. Da Silva, P.H.; da Silveira, R.B.; Appel, M.H.; Mangili, O.C.; Gremski, W.; Veiga, S.S. Brown spiders and loxoscelism. *Toxicon* **2004**, *44*, 693–709. [CrossRef]
9. Da Silveira, R.B.; Dos Santos Filho, J.F.; Mangili, O.C.; Veiga, S.S.; Gremski, W.; Nader, H.B.; Von Dietrich, C.P. Identification of proteases in the extract of venom glands from brown spiders. *Toxicon* **2002**, *40*, 815–822. [CrossRef]
10. Appel, M.H.; da Silveira, R.B.; Gremski, W.; Veiga, S.S. Insights into brown spider and loxoscelism. *Invertebr. Surviv. J.* **2005**, *2*, 152–158.
11. Barbaro, K.C.; Knysak, I.; Martins, R.; Hogan, C.; Winkel, K. Enzymatic characterization, antigenic cross-reactivity and neutralization of dermonecrotic activity of five *Loxosceles* spider venoms of medical importance in the Americas. *Toxicon* **2005**, *45*, 489–499. [CrossRef]
12. Barbaro, K.C.; Sousa, M.V.; Morhy, L.; Eickstedt, V.R.D.; Mota, I. Compared chemical properties of dermonecrotic and lethal toxins from spiders of the genus *Loxosceles* (araneae). *J. Protein Chem.* **1996**, *15*, 337–343. [CrossRef]
13. Tambourgi, D.V.; Magnoli, F.C.; van den Berg, C.W.; Morgan, B.P.; de Araujo, P.S.; Alves, E.W.; Da Silva, W.D. Sphingomyelinases in the venom of the spider *Loxosceles intermedia* are responsible for both dermonecrosis and complement-dependent hemolysis. *Biochem. Biophys. Res. Commun.* **1998**, *251*, 366–373. [CrossRef]
14. Chaim, O.M.; Sade, Y.B.; da Silveira, R.B.; Toma, L.; Kalapothakis, E.; Chavez-Olortegui, C.; Mangili, O.C.; Gremski, W.; von Dietrich, C.P.; Nader, H.B.; et al. Brown spider dermonecrotic toxin directly induces nephrotoxicity. *Toxicol. Appl. Pharmacol.* **2006**, *211*, 64–77. [CrossRef] [PubMed]

15. Gremski, L.H.; da Silveira, R.B.; Chaim, O.M.; Probst, C.M.; Ferrer, V.P.; Nowatzki, J.; Weinschutz, H.C.; Madeira, H.M.; Gremski, W.; Nader, H.B.; et al. A novel expression profile of the *Loxosceles intermedia* spider venomous gland revealed by transcriptome analysis. *Mol. Biosyst.* **2010**, *6*, 2403–2416. [CrossRef]
16. Matsubara, F.H.; Gremski, L.H.; Meissner, G.O.; Constantino Lopes, E.S.; Gremski, W.; Senff-Ribeiro, A.; Chaim, O.M.; Veiga, S.S. A novel ICK peptide from the *Loxosceles intermedia* (brown spider) venom gland: Cloning, heterologous expression and immunological cross- reactivity approaches. *Toxicon* **2013**, *71*, 147–158. [CrossRef] [PubMed]
17. Manzoni-de-Almeida, D.; Squaiella-BaptistãO, C.C.; Lopes, P.H.; van Den Berg, C.W.; Tambourgi, D.V. *Loxosceles* venom Sphingomyelinase D activates human blood leukocytes: Role of the complement system. *Mol. Immunol.* **2018**, *94*, 45–53. [CrossRef]
18. Barbaro, K.C.; Cardoso, J.L.C.; Eickstedt, V.R.D.; Mota, I. Dermonecrotic and lethal components of loxosceles-gaucho spider venom. *Toxicon* **1992**, *30*, 331–338. [CrossRef]
19. Futrell, J.M. Loxoscelism. *Am. J. Med. Sci.* **1992**, *304*, 261–267. [CrossRef] [PubMed]
20. Magalhaes, G.S.; Caporrino, M.C.; Della-Casa, M.S.; Kimura, L.F.; Prezotto-Neto, J.P.; Fukuda, D.A.; Portes, J.A.; Neves-Ferreira, A.G.C.; Santoro, M.L.; Barbaro, K.C. Cloning, expression and characterization of a phospholipase D from *Loxosceles gaucho* venom gland. *Biochimie* **2013**, *95*, 1773–1783. [CrossRef]
21. Shimokawa-Falcao, L.; Caporrino, M.C.; Barbaro, K.C.; Della-Casa, M.S.; Magalhaes, G.S. Toxin Fused with SUMO Tag: A New Expression Vector Strategy to Obtain Recombinant Venom Toxins with Easy Tag Removal inside the Bacteria. *Toxins* **2017**, *9*, 82. [CrossRef]
22. Kurpiewski, G.; Forrester, L.J.; Barrett, J.T.; Campbell, B.J. platelet-aggregation and sphingomyelinase d activity of a purified toxin from the venom of loxosceles-reclusa. *Biochim. Biophys. Acta* **1981**, *678*, 467–476. [CrossRef]
23. Fukuda, D.A.; Caporrino, M.C.; Barbaro, K.C.; Della-Casa, M.S.; Faquim-Mauro, E.L.; Magalhaes, G.S. Recombinant phospholipase D from *Loxosceles gaucho* binds to platelets and promotes phosphatidylserine exposure. *Toxins* **2017**, *9*, 191. [CrossRef]
24. Forrester, L.J.; Barrett, J.T.; Campbell, B.J. Red blood cell lysis induced by the venom of the brown recluse spider: The role of sphingomyelinase D. *Arch. Biochem. Biophys.* **1978**, *187*, 355–365. [CrossRef]
25. Luciano, M.N.; Da Silva, P.H.; Chaim, O.M.; Dos Santos, V.L.P.; Franco, C.R.C.; Soares, M.F.S.; Zanata, S.M.; Mangili, O.C.; Gremski, W.; Veiga, S.S. Experimental Evidence for a Direct Cytotoxicity of *Loxosceles intermedia* (Brown Spider) Venom in Renal Tissue. *J. Histochem. Cytochem.* **2004**, *52*, 455–467. [CrossRef]
26. Kusma, J.; Chaim, O.M.; Wille, A.C.M.; Ferrer, V.P.; Sade, Y.B.; Donatti, L.; Gremski, W.; Mangili, O.C.; Veiga, S.S. Nephrotoxicity caused by brown spider venom phospholipase-D (dermonecrotic toxin) depends on catalytic activity. *Biochimie* **2008**, *90*, 1722–1736. [CrossRef]
27. Saude, M.D. Manual de Diagnóstico e Tratamento de Acidentes por Animais Peçonhentos. Available online: http://bvsms.saude.gov.br/bvs/publicacoes/funasa/manu_peconhentos.pdf (accessed on 26 November 2018).
28. Guilherme, P.C.; Fernandes, I.; Barbaro, K.C. Neutralization of dermonecrotic and lethal activities and differences among 32–35 kDa toxins of medically important *Loxosceles* spider venoms in Brazil revealed by monoclonal antibodies. *Toxicon* **2001**, *39*, 1333–1342. [CrossRef]
29. Pauli, I.; Minozzo, J.C.; Henrique Da Silva, P.; Chaim, O.M.; Veiga, S.S. Analysis of therapeutic benefits of antivenin at different time intervals after experimental envenomation in rabbits by venom of the brown spider (*Loxosceles intermedia*). *Toxicon* **2009**, *53*, 660–671. [CrossRef]
30. Dias-Lopes, C.; Guimarães, G.; Felicori, L.; Fernandes, P.; Emery, L.; Kalapothakis, E.; Nguyen, C.; Molina, F.; Granier, C.; Chávez-Olórtegui, C. A protective immune response against lethal, dermonecrotic and hemorrhagic effects of *Loxosceles intermedia* venom elicited by a 27-residue peptide. *Toxicon* **2010**, *55*, 481–487. [CrossRef]
31. Figueiredo, L.F.M.; Dias-Lopes, C.; Alvarenga, L.M.; Mendes, T.M.; Machado-de-Ávila, R.A.; McCormack, J.; Minozzo, J.C.; Kalapothakis, E.; Chávez-Olórtegui, C. Innovative immunization protocols using chimeric recombinant protein for the production of polyspecific loxoscelic antivenom in horses. *Toxicon* **2014**, *86*, 59–67. [CrossRef]
32. Karim-Silva, S.; Moura, J.D.; Noiray, M.; Minozzo, J.C.; Aubrey, N.; Alvarenga, L.M.; Billiald, P. Generation of recombinant antibody fragments with toxin-neutralizing potential in loxoscelism. *Immunol. Lett.* **2016**, *176*, 90–96. [CrossRef]

33. Tambourgi, D.V.; Pedrosa, M.D.F.; van den Berg, C.W.; Goncalves-de-Andrade, R.M.; Ferracini, M.; Paixao-Cavalcante, D.; Morgan, B.P.; Rushmere, N.K. Molecular cloning, expression, function and immunoreactivities of members of a gene family of sphingomyelinases from *Loxosceles* venom glands. *Mol. Immunol.* **2004**, *41*, 831–840. [CrossRef]
34. de Almeida, D.M.; Fernandes-Pedrosa, M.D.; de Andrade, R.M.G.; Marcelino, J.R.; Gondo-Higashi, H.; de Azevedo, I.; Ho, P.L.; van den Berg, C.; Tambourgi, D.V. A new anti-loxoscelic serum produced against recombinant sphingomyelinase D: Results of preclinical trials. *Am. J. Trop. Med. Hyg.* **2008**, *79*, 463–470. [CrossRef]
35. Guimarães, G.; Dias-Lopes, C.; Duarte, C.G.; Felicori, L.; Machado de Avila, R.A.; Figueiredo, L.F.M.; de Moura, J.; Faleiro, B.T.; Barro, J.; Flores, K.; et al. Biochemical and immunological characteristics of Peruvian *Loxosceles laeta* spider venom: Neutralization of its toxic effects by anti-loxoscelic antivenoms. *Toxicon* **2013**, *70*, 90–97. [CrossRef]
36. Duarte, C.G.; Bonilla, C.; Guimarães, G.; Machado de Avila, R.A.; Mendes, T.M.; Silva, W.; Tintaya, B.; Yarleque, A.; Chávez-Olórtegui, C. Anti-loxoscelic horse serum produced against a recombinant dermonecrotic protein of Brazilian *Loxosceles intermedia* spider neutralize lethal effects of Loxosceles laeta venom from Peru. *Toxicon* **2015**, *93*, 37–40. [CrossRef]
37. Felicori, L.; Fernandes, P.B.; Giusta, M.S.; Duarte, C.G.; Kalapothakis, E.; Nguyen, C.; Molina, F.; Granier, C.; Chávez-Olórtegui, C. An in vivo protective response against toxic effects of the dermonecrotic protein from *Loxosceles intermedia* spider venom elicited by synthetic epitopes. *Vaccine* **2009**, *27*, 4201–4208. [CrossRef]
38. Souza, N.A.; Dias-Lopes, C.; Matoso, Í.H.G.; de Oliveira, C.F.B.; ChàVez-Olortegui, C.D.; Minozzo, J.C.; Felicori, L.F. Immunoprotection elicited in rabbit by a chimeric protein containing B-cell epitopes of Sphingomyelinases D from *Loxosceles* spp. spiders. *Vaccine* **2018**, *36*, 7324–7330. [CrossRef]
39. Fernandes-Pedrosa, M.d.F.; Junqueira-de-Azevedo, I.d.L.M.; Gonçalves-de-Andrade, R.M.; Kobashi, L.S.; Almeida, D.D.; Ho, P.L.; Tambourgi, D.V. Transcriptome analysis of *Loxosceles laeta* (Araneae, Sicariidae) spider venomous gland using expressed sequence tags. *BMC Genom.* **2008**, *9*, 279. [CrossRef]
40. Williamson, A.L.; Lustigman, S.; Oksov, Y.; Deumic, V.; Plieskatt, J.; Mendez, S.; Zhan, B.; Bottazzi, M.E.; Hotez, P.J.; Loukas, A. Ancylostoma caninum MTP-1, an Astacin- Like Metalloprotease Secreted by Infective Hookworm Larvae, Is Involved in Tissue Migration. *Infect. Immun.* **2006**, *74*, 961. [CrossRef]
41. Feitosa, L.; Gremski, W.; Veiga, S.S.; Elias, M.C.; Graner, E.; Mangili, O.C.; Brentani, R.R. Detection and characterization of metalloproteinases with gelatinolytic, fibronectinolytic and fibrinogenolytic activities in brown spider (*Loxosceles intermedia*) venom. *Toxicon* **1998**, *36*, 1039. [CrossRef]
42. Veiga, S.S.; Zanetti, V.; Braz, A.; Mangili, O.C.; Gremski, W. Extracellular matrix molecules as targets for brown spider venom toxins. *Braz. J. Med. Biol. Res.* **2001**, *34*, 843–850. [CrossRef]
43. Young, A.R.; Pincus, S.J. Comparison of enzymatic activity from three species of necrotising arachnids in Australia: *Loxosceles rufescens*, *Badumna insignis* and *Lampona cylindrata*. *Toxicon* **2001**, *39*, 391–400. [CrossRef]
44. Zanetti, V.C.; da Silveira, R.B.; Dreyfuss, J.L.; Haoach, J.; Mangili, O.C.; Veiga, S.S.; Gremski, W. Morphological and biochemical evidence of blood vessel damage and fibrinogenolysis triggered by brown spider venom. *Blood Coagul. Fibrinolysis* **2002**, *13*, 135–148. [CrossRef]
45. Da Silveira, R.B.; Wille, A.C.M.; Chaim, O.M.; Appel, M.H.; Silva, D.T.; Franco, C.R.C.; Toma, L.; Mangili, O.C.; Gremski, W.; Dietrich, C.P.; et al. Identification, cloning, expression and functional characterization of an astacin-like metalloprotease toxin from *Loxosceles intermedia* (brown spider) venom. *Biochem. J.* **2007**, *406*, 355–363. [CrossRef]
46. Hopp, T.P.; Woods, K.R. Prediction of protein antigenic determinants from amino acid sequences. *Proc. Natl. Acad. Sci. USA* **1981**, *78*, 3824. [CrossRef]
47. de Giuseppe, P.O.; Ullah, A.; Silva, D.T.; Gremski, L.H.; Wille, A.C.M.; Moreira, D.C.; Ribeiro, A.S.; Chaim, O.M.; Murakami, M.T.; Veiga, S.S.; et al. Structure of a novel class II phospholipase D: Catalytic cleft is modified by a disulphide bridge. *Biochem. Biophys. Res. Commun.* **2011**, *409*, 622–627. [CrossRef]
48. Guevara, T.; Yiallouros, I.; Kappelhoff, R.; Bissdorf, S.; Stöcker, W.; Gomis-Rüth, F.X. Proenzyme structure and activation of astacin metallopeptidase. *J. Biol. Chem.* **2010**, *285*, 13958. [CrossRef]
49. Nicholson, G.M.; Graudins, A. Antivenoms for the Treatment of Spider Envenomation. *J. Toxicol. Toxin Rev.* **2003**, *22*, 35–59. [CrossRef]
50. Isbister, G.K.; Fan, H.W. Spider bite. *Lancet* **2011**, *378*, 2039–2047. [CrossRef]

51. Hubiche, T.; Delaunay, P.; del Giudice, P. A case of loxoscelism in southern France. *Am. J. Trop. Med. Hyg.* **2013**, *88*, 807–808. [CrossRef]
52. Coutinho, I.; Rocha, S.; Ferreira, M.E.; Vieira, R.; Cordeiro, M.R.; Reis, J.P. Cutaneous loxoscelism in Portugal: A rare cause of dermonecrosis. *Acta Med. Port.* **2014**, *27*, 654. [CrossRef]
53. Morales-Moreno, H.J.; Carranza-Rodriguez, C.; Borrego, L. Cutaneous loxoscelism due to *Loxosceles rufescens*. *J. Eur. Acad. Dermatol. Venereol.* **2016**, *30*, 1431–1432. [CrossRef]
54. Olvera, A.; Ramos-Cerrillo, B.; Estévez, J.; Clement, H.; de Roodt, A.; Paniagua-Solís, J.; Vázquez, H.; Zavaleta, A.; Salas Arruz, M.; Stock, R.P.; et al. North and South American *Loxosceles* spiders: Development of a polyvalent antivenom with recombinant sphingomyelinases D as antigens. *Toxicon* **2006**, *48*, 64–74. [CrossRef]
55. Fernandes Pedrosa, M.d.F.; Junqueira de Azevedo, I.d.L.M.; Gonçalves-de-Andrade, R.M.; van Den Berg, C.W.; Ramos, C.R.R.; Lee Ho, P.; Tambourgi, D.V. Molecular cloning and expression of a functional dermonecrotic and haemolytic factor from *Loxosceles laeta* venom. *Biochem. Biophys. Res. Commun.* **2002**, *298*, 638–645. [CrossRef]
56. De Castro, C.S.; Silvestre, F.G.; Araujo, S.C.; Gabriel de, M.Y.; Mangili, O.C.; Cruz, I.; Chavez-Olortegui, C.; Kalapothakis, E. Identification and molecular cloning of insecticidal toxins from the venom of the brown spider *Loxosceles intermedia*. *Toxicon*. **2004**, *44*, 3–273. [CrossRef]
57. Arlian, L.G. Arthropod allergens and human health. *Ann. Rev. Entomol.* **2002**, *47*, 395–433. [CrossRef]
58. Sade, Y.B.; Boia-Ferreira, M.; Gremski, L.H.; da Silveira, R.B.; Gremski, W.; Senff-Ribeiro, A.; Chaim, O.M.; Veiga, S.S. Molecular cloning, heterologous expression and functional characterization of a novel translationally-controlled tumor protein (TCTP) family member from *Loxosceles intermedia* (brown spider) venom. *Int. J. Biochem. Cell Biol.* **2012**, *44*, 170–177. [CrossRef]
59. Veiga, S.S.; Feitosa, L.; dos Santos, V.L.; de Souza, G.A.; Ribeiro, A.S.; Mangili, O.C.; Porcionatto, M.A.; Nader, H.B.; Dietrich, C.P.; Brentani, R.R.; et al. Effect of brown spider venom on basement membrane structures. *Histochem. J.* **2000**, *32*, 7–397. [CrossRef]
60. Da Silveira, R.B.; Chaim, O.M.; Mangili, O.C.; Gremski, W.; Dietrich, C.P.; Nader, H.B.; Veiga, S.S. Hyaluronidases in *Loxosceles intermedia* (Brown spider) venom are endo-β-N-acetyl-D-hexosaminidases hydrolases. *Toxicon* **2007**, *49*, 758–768. [CrossRef]
61. Hiroshi, Y.; Masaya, M. Refolding Techniques for Recovering Biologically Active Recombinant Proteins from Inclusion Bodies. *Biomolecules* **2014**, *4*, 235–251. [CrossRef]
62. Trevisan-Silva, D.; Gremski, L.H.; Chaim, O.M.; Da Silveira, R.B.; Meissner, G.O.; Mangili, O.C.; Barbaro, K.C.; Gremski, W.; Veiga, S.S.; Senff-Ribeiro, A. Astacin- like metalloproteases are a gene family of toxins present in the venom of different species of the brown spider (genus Loxosceles). *Biochimie* **2010**, *92*, 21. [CrossRef]
63. Upadhyay, A.K.; Herman, C.; Murmu, A.; Singh, A.; Panda, A.K. Kinetics of Inclusion Body Formation and Its Correlation with the Characteristics of Protein Aggregates in *Escherichia coli*. *PLoS ONE* **2012**, *7*, e33951. [CrossRef]
64. Novo, J.; Oliveira, M.; Magalhães, G.; Morganti, L.; Raw, I.; Ho, P. Generation of Polyclonal Antibodies Against Recombinant Human Glucocerebrosidase Produced in *Escherichia coli*. *Mol. Biotechnol.* **2010**, *46*, 279–286. [CrossRef]
65. Yang, H.; Zhang, T.; Xu, K.; Lei, J.; Wang, L.; Li, Z.; Zhang, Z. A novel and convenient method to immunize animals: Inclusion bodies from recombinant bacteria as antigen to directly immunize animals. *Afr. J. Biotechnol.* **2011**, *10*, 8146–8150. [CrossRef]
66. Lorch, M.S.; Collado, M.S.; Argüelles, M.H.; Rota, R.P.; Spinsanti, L.I.; Lozano, M.E.; Goñi, S.E. Production of recombinant NS1 protein and its possible use in encephalitic flavivirus differential diagnosis. *Protein Expr. Purif.* **2019**, *153*, 18–25. [CrossRef]
67. Jiang, X.; Xia, S.; He, X.; Ma, H.; Feng, Y.; Liu, Z.; Wang, W.; Tian, M.; Chen, H.; Peng, F.; et al. Targeting peptide-enhanced antibody and CD11c(+)dendritic cells to inclusion bodies expressing protective antigen against ETEC in mice. *FASEB J.* **2019**, *33*, 2836–2847. [CrossRef]
68. Kesik, M.; Saczyńska, V.; Szewczyk, B.; Płucienniczak, A. Inclusion bodies from recombinant bacteria as a novel system for delivery of vaccine antigen by the oral route. *Immunol. Lett.* **2004**, *91*, 197–204. [CrossRef]

69. Wedrychowicz, H.; Kesik, M.; Kaliniak, M.; Kozak-Cieszczyk, M.; Jedlina-Panasiuk, L.; Jaros, S.; Plucienniczak, A. Vaccine potential of inclusion bodies containing cysteine proteinase of Fasciola hepatica in calves and lambs experimentally challenged with metacercariae of the fluke. *Vet. Parasitol.* **2007**, *147*, 77–88. [CrossRef]
70. Such, D.R.; Souza, F.N.; Meissner, G.O.; Morgon, A.M.; Gremski, L.H.; Ferrer, V.P.; Trevisan-Silva, D.; Matsubara, F.H.; Boia-Ferreira, M.; Sade, Y.B.; et al. Brown spider (*Loxosceles* genus) venom toxins: Evaluation of biological conservation by immune cross-reactivity. *Toxicon* **2015**, *108*, 154–166. [CrossRef]
71. Lima, S.d.A.; Guerra-Duarte, C.; Costal-Oliveira, F.; Mendes, T.M.; Figueiredo, L.F.M.; Oliveira, D.; Machado de Avila, R.A.; Ferrer, V.P.; Trevisan-Silva, D.; Veiga, S.S.; et al. Recombinant Protein Containing B-Cell Epitopes of Different Spider Toxins Generates Neutralizing Antibodies in Immunized Rabbits. *Front. Immunol.* **2018**, *9*, 653. [CrossRef]
72. Tavares, F.L.; Peichoto, M.E.; Rangel, D.D.; Barbaro, K.C.; Cirillo, M.C.; Santoro, M.L.; Sano-Martins, I.S. *Loxosceles gaucho* spider venom and its sphingomyelinase fraction trigger the main functions of human and rabbit platelets. *Hum. Exp. Toxicol.* **2011**, *30*, 1567–1574. [CrossRef]
73. Appel, M.H.; Da Silveira, R.B.; Chaim, O.M.; Paludo, K.S.; Silva, D.T.; Chaves, D.M.; Da Silva, P.H.; Mangili, O.C.; Senff-Ribeiro, A.; Gremski, W.; et al. Identification, cloning and functional characterization of a novel dermonecrotic toxin (phospholipase D) from brown spider (*Loxosceles intermedia*) venom. *Biochim. Biophys. Acta* **2008**, *1780*, 167–178. [CrossRef]
74. Pezzi, M.; Giglio, A.M.; Scozzafava, A.; Filippelli, O.; Serafino, G.; Verre, M. Spider Bite: A Rare Case of Acute Necrotic Arachnidism with Rapid and Fatal Evolution. *Case Rep. Emerg. Med.* **2016**, *2016*. [CrossRef]
75. Mariutti, R.B.; Chaves-Moreira, D.; Vuitika, L.; Caruso, Í.P.; Coronado, M.A.; Azevedo, V.A.; Murakami, M.T.; Veiga, S.S.; Arni, R.K. Bacterial and Arachnid Sphingomyelinases D: Comparison of Biophysical and Pathological Activities. *J. Cell. Biochem.* **2017**, *118*, 2053–2063. [CrossRef]
76. Chaves-Moreira, D.; De Moraes, F.R.; Caruso, Í.P.; Chaim, O.M.; Senff-Ribeiro, A.; Ullah, A.; Da Silva, L.S.; Chahine, J.; Arni, R.K.; Veiga, S.S. Potential Implications for Designing Drugs Against the Brown Spider Venom Phospholipase-D. *J. Cell. Biochem.* **2017**, *118*, 726–738. [CrossRef]
77. Mendes, T.M.; Oliveira, D.; Figueiredo, L.F.M.; Machado-de-Avila, R.A.; Duarte, C.G.; Dias-Lopes, C.; Guimaraes, G.; Felicori, L.; Minozzo, J.C.; Chavez-Olortegui, C. Generation and characterization of a recombinant chimeric protein (rCpLi) consisting of B-cell epitopes of a dermonecrotic protein from *Loxosceles intermedia* spider venom. *Vaccine* **2013**, *31*, 2749–2755. [CrossRef]
78. Ribeiro, M.F.; Oliveira, F.L.; Monteiro-Machado, M.; Cardoso, P.F.; Guilarducci-Ferraz, V.V.C.; Melo, P.A.; Souza, C.M.V.; Calil-Elias, S. Pattern of inflammatory response to *Loxosceles intermedia* venom in distinct mouse strains: A key element to understand skin lesions and dermonecrosis by poisoning. *Toxicon* **2015**, *96*, 10–23. [CrossRef]
79. Conesa, A.; Götz, S.; García-Gómez, J.M.; Terol, J.; Talón, M.; Robles, M. Blast2GO: A universal tool for annotation, visualization and analysis in functional genomics research. *Bioinformatics* **2005**, *21*, 3674–3676. [CrossRef]
80. Altschul, S.F.; Madden, T.L.; Schäffer, A.A.; Zhang, J.; Zhang, Z.; Miller, W.; Lipman, D.J. Gapped BLAST and PSI-BLAST: A new generation of protein database search programs. *Nucleic Acids Res.* **1997**, *25*, 3389. [CrossRef]
81. Laemmli, U.K. Cleavage of Structural Proteins during the Assembly of the Head of Bacteriophage T4. *Nature* **1970**, *227*, 680–685. [CrossRef]
82. Smith, P.K.; Krohn, R.I.; Hermanson, G.T.; Mallia, A.K.; Gartner, F.H.; Provenzano, M.D.; Fujimoto, E.K.; Goeke, N.M.; Olson, B.J.; Klenk, D.C. Measurement of protein using bicinchoninic acid. *Anal. Biochem.* **1985**, *150*, 76–85. [CrossRef]
83. ImageJ, U.S. Available online: imagej.nih.gov/ij/ (downloaded on 15 December 2018)(ImageJ bundled with 64-bit Java 1.8.0_112 windows version).

84. Theakston, R.D.G.; Reid, H.A. Enzyme-linked Immunosorbent Assay (ELISA) in assessing antivenom potency. *Toxicon* **1979**, *17*, 511–515. [CrossRef]
85. Santoro, M.L.; Sousa-e-Silva, M.C.C.; Goncalves, L.R.C.; Almeida-Santos, S.M.; Cardoso, D.F.; Laporta-Ferreira, I.L.; Saiki, M.; Peres, C.A.; Sano-Martins, I.S. Comparison of the biological activities in venoms from three subspecies of the South American rattlesnake (*Crotalus durissus terrificus, C. durissus cascavella and C. durissus collilineatus*). *Comp. Biochem. Physiol. C: Pharmacol. Toxicol. Endocrinol.* **1999**, *123*, 293. [CrossRef]

toxins

MDPI

Article

Isolation and Characterization of Insecticidal Toxins from the Venom of the North African Scorpion, *Buthacus leptochelys*

Yusuke Yoshimoto [1], Masahiro Miyashita [1,*], Mohammed Abdel-Wahab [2], Moustafa Sarhan [2], Yoshiaki Nakagawa [1] and Hisashi Miyagawa [1]

1 Division of Applied Life Sciences, Graduate School of Agriculture, Kyoto University, Kyoto 606-8502, Japan; yoshimoto.yusuke.22v@st.kyoto-u.ac.jp (Y.Y.); naka@kais.kyoto-u.ac.jp (Y.N.); miyagawa@kais.kyoto-u.ac.jp (H.M.)

2 Zoology Department, Al-Azhar University, Assuit 71524, Egypt; manatee74@yahoo.com (M.A.-W.); moustafar@yahoo.com (M.S.)

* Correspondence: miyamasa@kais.kyoto-u.ac.jp

Received: 29 March 2019; Accepted: 22 April 2019; Published: 25 April 2019

check for updates

Abstract: Various bioactive peptides have been identified in scorpion venom, but there are many scorpion species whose venom has not been investigated. In this study, we characterized venom components of the North African scorpion, *Buthacus leptochelys*, by mass spectrometric analysis and evaluated their insect toxicity. This is the first report of chemical and biological characterization of the *B. leptochelys* venom. LC/MS analysis detected at least 148 components in the venom. We isolated four peptides that show insect toxicity (Bl-1, Bl-2, Bl-3, and Bl-4) through bioassay-guided HPLC fractionation. These toxins were found to be similar to scorpion α- and β-toxins based on their N-terminal sequences. Among them, the complete primary structure of Bl-1 was determined by combination of Edman degradation and MS/MS analysis. Bl-1 is composed of 67 amino acid residues and crosslinked with four disulfide bonds. Since Bl-1 shares high sequence similarity with α-like toxins, it is likely that it acts on Na^+ channels of both insects and mammals.

Keywords: scorpion venom; insecticidal peptide; mass spectrometric analysis; de novo sequencing

Key Contribution: Components of the *Buthacus leptochelys* scorpion venom were analyzed by mass spectrometric techniques. The primary structure of one of four peptides showing insect toxicity was determined.

1. Introduction

Scorpions are the oldest arachnids and can be traced back to the Silurian period [1,2]. Currently, over 2400 scorpion species are widely distributed on all continents except Antarctica [3,4]. Scorpions have adapted to different environments such as deserts, forests, grasslands, and caves because they can use toxic components in their venom to effectively capture prey and protect themselves from predators. Scorpion venom contains inorganic salts, amino acids, nucleic acids, peptides, and proteins, and some peptides show anti-insect and/or anti-mammal activities [5].

Scorpion peptides are structurally classified into two groups: disulfide bridge-containing peptides (DBPs) and non-disulfide bridge-containing peptides (NDBPs) [6,7]. Many DBPs specifically interact with neuronal ion channels, which are further classified into four families based on their targeting ion channels (Na^+, K^+, Cl^-, and Ca^{2+} channels) [8,9]. Sodium channel-specific toxins are long-chain peptides composed of 60–76 amino acid residues cross-linked with four disulfide bridges [10–12]. These toxins are divided into α- and β-toxins. The α-toxins inactivate Na^+ current by binding to the receptor site 3, whereas the β-toxins modify the voltage-dependent activation of sodium channels by binding to the receptor site 4 [13,14]. Potassium channel-specific toxins are composed of 20–70 amino acid residues cross-linked with three or four disulfide bridges. Most of these are short-chain peptides with fewer than 40 amino acid residues [15,16]. These toxins are classified into seven families, α-, β-, γ-, κ-, δ-, λ-, and ε-KTx, according to their sequence similarity and disulfide-bonding pattern [17,18]. Chloride ion channel-specific toxins are composed of fewer than 40 amino acid residues and contain four disulfide bonds [19,20]. Some toxins specifically act on calcium ion channels, which have varied structures and action sites [8,21]. On the other hand, many NDBPs adopt an amphipathic α-helical structure that can disrupt the cellular membrane structure to show antimicrobial and/or hemolytic activity [22].

These scorpion peptides have been identified from various scorpion species, but venoms of minor species remain largely unstudied. About 930 scorpion species inhabit Africa, most of which belong to the Buthidae family [23]. In this family, *Leiurus quinquestriatus* has been intensively studied because it contains medically important toxins [24]. The venom of the species of the genus *Buthacus* in the Buthidae family has been poorly investigated, and only two insecticidal toxins were isolated from this genus: Bu1 from *B. macrocentrus* and BaIT2 from *B. arenicola* [25,26]. In this study, we evaluated the insect toxicity of the venom of *B. leptochelys* and isolated four insecticidal peptides from the venom using a bioassay-guided HPLC fractionation approach. Finally, one of the insecticidal components in the *B. leptochelys* venom was identified by the combination of Edman degradation and MS/MS analysis.

2. Results and Discussion

2.1. Characterization of the B. leptochelys Venom

The venom showed significant toxicity against crickets (*A. domesticus*) with an LD_{50} value of 30 ng/mg body weight. This is 3-fold more potent than that of *Isometrus maculatus*, which has moderately toxic venom [27], but 1.5-fold less potent than that of *Tityus serrulatus*, which has highly toxic venom, although a different cricket species was used in the latter case [28].

The *B. leptochelys* venom was then subjected to mass spectrometric analysis using both MALDI-TOF MS and LC/MS to examine the molecular mass distribution of all the venom components (Figure 1). A total of 148 components, which are likely to be peptides, were detected in a molecular mass ranging from 500 to 12,000 Da (Table S1). About 80% of the components were detected in the range below 5000 Da. Regarding the components with molecular masses over 5000 Da, the number of those with molecular masses ranging from 7001–8000 Da is relatively high. These peptides are likely to be long-chain scorpion peptides, which could mainly contribute to the insect toxicity of the *B. leptochelys* venom as reported for other Buthidae scorpions [29,30].

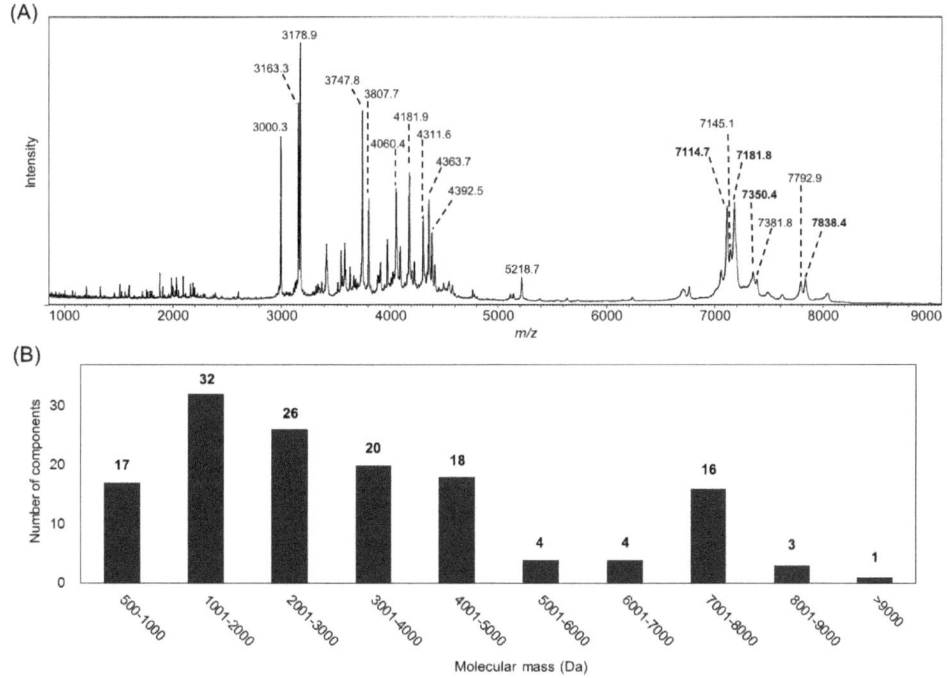

Figure 1. Components analysis of the *B. leptochelys* venom. (**A**) MALDI-TOF mass spectrum of the venom. Numbers shown in bold indicate the peptides isolated in this study. (**B**) Distribution of molecular masses of venom components detected by LC/MS analysis.

2.2. Purification of Insecticidal Peptides

The crude venom dissolved in distilled water was separated on a C_4 HPLC column (Figure 2A). Several fractions obtained based on the major chromatographic peaks were tested for insect toxicity using crickets. In this study, each fraction was injected at a dose equivalent to 160 ng venom/mg body weight, which is five times higher than the LD_{50} value, to specify peptides primarily responsible for the insect toxicity of the venom. Three fractions (I–III) were found to be highly toxic, and fraction I showed the strongest toxicity, which induced death or paralysis 48 h after injection in all insects tested. Fractions II and III showed relatively weak toxicity that induced transient paralysis in all insects tested. Differences in the insect toxicity between fractions could be attributed to the number and/or amount of active components in each fraction as well as to their intrinsic activity. These fractions were further separated on a C_{18} HPLC column to obtain single components. Four components (named Bl-1, 2, 3, and 4; Figure 2B–D) showed toxicity, and their monoisotopic molecular masses were determined as 7107.2, 7343.9, 7173.8, and 7828.1 Da, respectively (Figure S1). The N-terminal sequences of these peptides were determined by Edman method as shown in Table 1.

Table 1. Insecticidal peptides isolated from the *B. leptochelys* venom.

Name	N-Terminal Sequence (U = Unknown)	Similar Peptides	Toxin Classification
Bl-1	ARDGYISQPENCVYHCFPGS	Lqh3, Bom3	α-like insect and mammal toxin
Bl-2	URDGYLVDDUNCTFFCG	Lqh2, AaH2	α-mammal toxin
Bl-3	UVRDAYIADDKNCVYTCASN	OD1, Bu1	α-insect and mammal toxin
Bl-4	UKNGYAVDSSGKAPECILSNYCNNECTKV	AaHIT1, LqqIT1	β-insect toxin

A BLAST search revealed that Bl-1 is similar to α-like insect and mammal toxins such as Lqh3 from *Leiurus quinquestriatus hebraeus* [31] and Bom3 from *Buthus occitanus mardochei* [32]. Bl-2 is similar to α-mammalian toxins such as Lqq5 from *L. quinquestriatus quinquestriatus* [33] and AaH2 from *Androctonus australis* Hector [34]. Bl-3 is similar to α-insect and mammalian toxins such as OD1 from *Odontobuthus doriae* [35] and Bu-1 from *Buthacus macrocentrus* [25]. Bl-4 is similar to β-insect toxins such as AaHIT1 from *A. australis* Hector [36] and LqqIT1 from *L. quinquestriatus quinquestriatus* [37]. This suggests that the four insecticidal peptides isolated from the *B. leptochelys* venom may act on the insect Na^+ channel, although the selectivity of their action between mammals and insects may vary among peptides. The α- and β-toxins have been identified exclusively from the venom of the Buthidae scorpions, but the ratio between the number of α- and β-toxins in the venom is known to differ by species. For example, 9 α- and 12 β-toxins were identified from the venom gland transcriptome of *Lychas mucronatus* [38], whereas 1 α- and 12 β-toxin sequences were identified from the *I. maculatus* transcriptome [39]. In addition, only β-toxins were isolated as an insecticidal neurotoxin from the *I. maculatus* venom [40,41]. The fact that the insecticidal activity of *B. leptochelys* venom is relatively higher than that of *I. maculatus* may be attributed to the existence of multiple α-toxins.

2.3. Primary Structure of Bl-1

Bl-1 was further subjected to sequencing analysis to obtain its complete primary structure because it showed the most significant insect toxicity in this study. A 472 Da mass shift after carboxymethylation of Bl-1 is indicative of the presence of eight Cys residues (59 Da × 8) that form four disulfide bridges (Figure S2). Bl-1 was digested with endoproteinase Lys-C, and the resulting peptide fragments were purified by HPLC (Figure S3). The sequence of three fragments (L1, L2, and L3 with molecular masses of 3282.3, 3918.9, and 2686.3 Da, respectively) were determined by Edman and/or MS/MS sequencing analysis (Figure S4). Discrimination between Leu and Ile at several positions in the fragments during MS/MS analysis was achieved based on the side-chain fragmentation observed under HE-CID conditions in which the occurrence of key fragment ions (*d*-ions) allowed for its assignment (Figure S5). The sequences of L1 and L3 were determined as ARDGYISQPENCVYHCFPGSSG(CD/DC)TLCK and EGRGLACWCLELPDNVGIIVDIGK, respectively, by combination of Edman and MS/MS sequencing analysis (Figure 3). The N-terminal sequence of L2 was also determined as EKGGTGGHCGYKEGRGLA by Edman analysis, but other sequence information was not obtained by MS/MS analysis due to its large molecular mass. To assign the undefined sequence of cysteine and aspartic acid residues (CD or DC) in L1, Bl-1 was sequentially digested with Lys-C and chymotrypsin (Figure S3). The short fragment LC1 (molecular mass of 1628.6 Da) consisting of the C-terminal half of L1 was subjected to MS/MS analysis, and its sequence was determined as HCFPGSSGCDTLCK (Figure 3 and Figure S6). Moreover, carboxymethylated Bl-1 was digested with chymotrypsin, and the peptide fragment C1 (molecular mass of 2154.1 Da) was purified by HPLC (Figure S3). MS/MS analysis revealed the sequence of C1 as CLELPDNVGIIVDIGKCHT-NH_2 by considering the sequence of L3 (Figure 3 and Figure S6). Since C1 has the amidated C-terminus, it was assigned as the C-terminal end of Bl-1 (Figure 4). The fragment C2 (molecular mass of 5444.2) was also detected by LC/MS analysis, which confirms the connection between L1 and L2 based on its molecular mass and partially determined sequence (Figure S7). Finally, the complete primary structure of Bl-1 was successfully determined by integrating all the information obtained above (Figure 4).

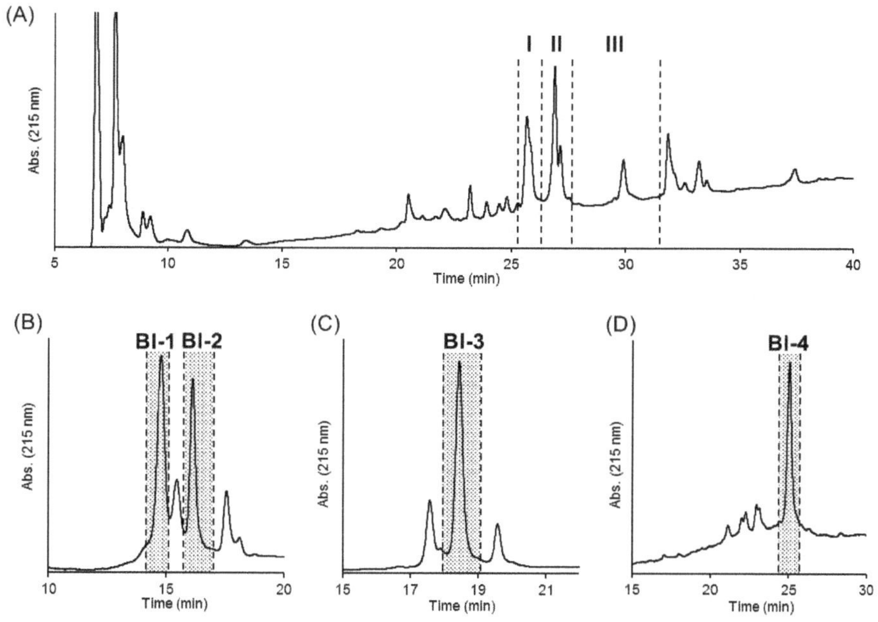

Figure 2. Isolation of the insecticidal peptides from the *B. leptochelys* venom. Separation of the crude venom on a C_4 HPLC column (**A**). Separation of fractions I (**B**), II (**C**), and III (**D**) on a C_{18} HPLC column.

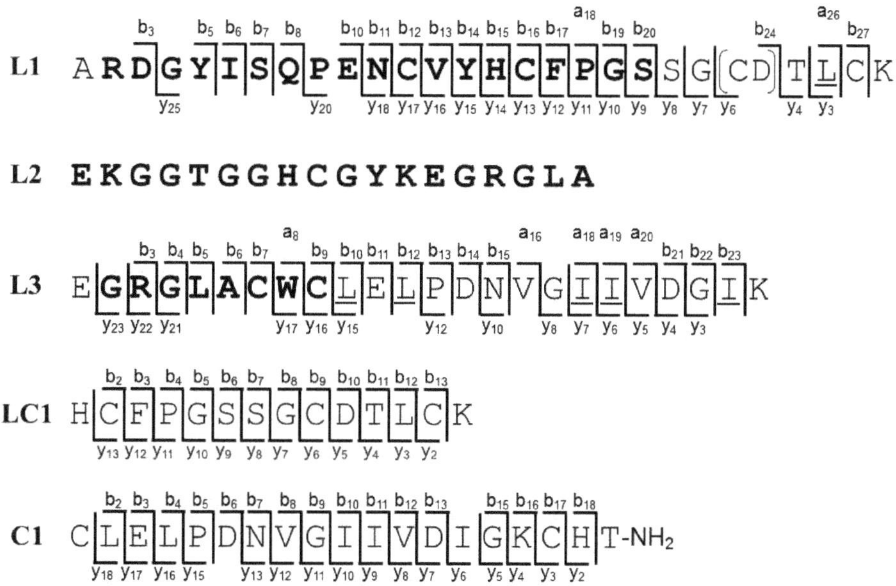

Figure 3. Amino acid seqences of digested fragments. Amino acid residues shown in bold were determined by Edman degradation. The MS/MS fragment ions that were used for sequence determination are shown. [CD] in the sequence of L1 indicates CD or DC. For L2, only the sequence determinated by Edman degradation is shown. Leu and Ile residues that are underlined were determined by MS/MS analysis inder the HE-CID conditon.

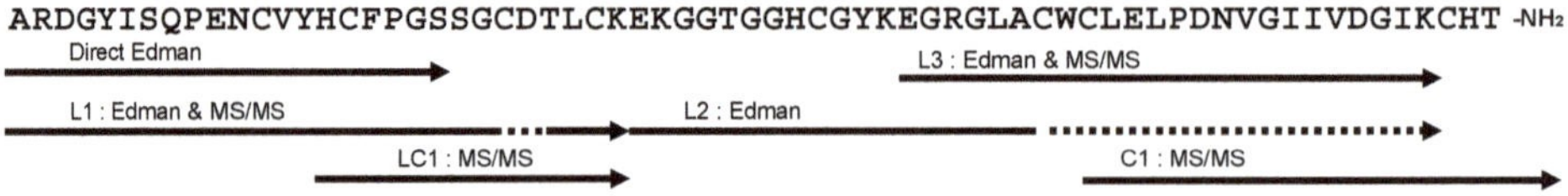

Figure 4. Primary structure of Bl-1. Solid lines indicate that the sequence was completely identified. Dashed lines show that the sequence was not or partically identified.

2.4. Sequence Comparison

A BLAST search for a full sequence of Bl-1 revealed that the peptide is similar to scorpion peptides classified as an α-like toxin, which can modulate both insect and mammalian Na^+ channels as described above (Figure 5A). This suggests that Bl-1 also shows toxicity against mammals, although mammal toxicity could not be evaluated due to the limited amount of the purified sample. Among the α-like toxins, the structure-activity relationship was comprehensively investigated for Lqh3 [42]. This study revealed that two distinct domains are particularly important for its binding to insect Na^+ channels. One (Core-domain) consists of three residues (His15, Phe17, and Pro18) preceding the α-helix and two residues (Phe39 and Leu45) in the β-strands. The other (NC-domain) is constituted by the C-terminal region, where Ile59, Lys64, and His66 contribute the activity (Figure 5B). These residues are also observed in Bl-1, except for Phe39. Since the aromatic ring of Phe39 is important for the activity, the substitution of Phe39 with Tyr in the case of Bl-1 may not affect the activity. To further confirm the structural similarity between Lqh3 and Bl-1, a three-dimensional structure of Bl-1 was constructed by homology modeling using Lqh3 as a template (Figure 5B). As expected, positions of all amino acid residues important for expression of full activity were almost identical between Lqh3 and Bl-1. This suggests that Bl-1 exerts its insect toxicity through the same mechanism as α-like toxins such as Lqh3.

(A)

		Identity
	`                 *  **                    *     *              *          `	
Bl-1	` ARDGYISQPENCVYHCFPGSSGCDTLCKEKGGTGGHCGYKEGRGLACWCLELPDNVGIIVDGIKCHT`	
Lqh3	`-VRDGYIAQPENCVYHCFPGSSGCDTLCKEKGGTSGHCGFKVGHGLACWCNALPDNVGIIVEGEKCHS`	56/67
Lqh7	`-VRDGYIAKPENCAHHCFPGSSGCDTLCKENGGTGGHCGFKVGHGTACWCNALPDKVGIIVDGVKCH-`	52/67
Bom3	`-GRDGYIAQPENCVYHCFPGSSGCDTLCKEKGATSGHCGFLPGSGVACWCDNLPNKVPIVVGGEKCH-`	49/67
Os3	`GVRDGYIAQPHNCVYHCFPGSGGCDTLCKENGATQGSSCFILGRGTACWCKDLPDRVGVIVDGEKCH-`	47/67

(B)

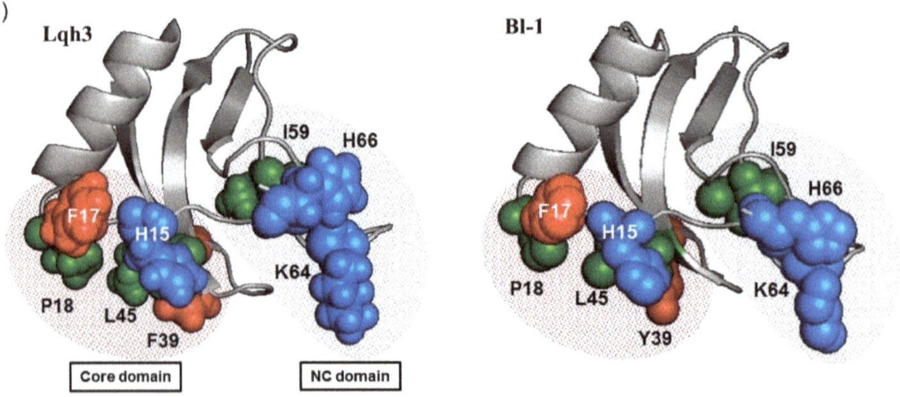

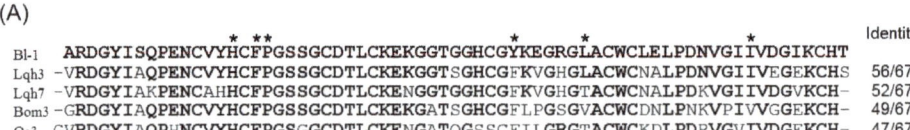

Figure 5. Comparison of the structure of Bl-1 with other toxins. (**A**) Multiple sequence alignment of Bl-1 with similar peptides found in the database. Asterisks indicate residues important for binding to insect sodium channels. (**B**) Three-dimensional structure of Lqh3 in PDB (ID: 1FH3) and Bl-1 constructed by homology modelings.

3. Conclusions

We characterized venom components of the North African scorpion, *B. leptochelys*, by mass spectrometric analysis and isolated the insecticidal peptides by the bioassay-guided fractionation approach. To our knowledge, this is the first report of the chemical and biological characterization of the *B. leptochelys* venom. Mass spectrometric analysis revealed that the venom components are mainly composed of two distinct groups based on the molecular mass ranges: one from 3000–5000 Da and the other from 7000–8000 Da, which is commonly observed for Buthidae scorpions. N-terminal sequences of four insecticidal peptides (Bl-1, Bl-2, Bl-3, and Bl-4) isolated from the *B. leptochelys* venom indicated that they are long-chain toxins that could specifically or non-specifically act on insect Na^+ channels. Among them, the primary structure of Bl-1 was completely determined to be an α-like toxin, which is likely to act on both insect and mammal Na^+ channels, by combination of Edman and MS/MS sequencing analysis. Insect toxicity is the common biological characteristic of scorpion venom, but the structure of insecticidal toxins and their combinations are diverse and complex among scorpion species. The results obtained in this study will provide a clue to understanding the synergistic role of α- and β-toxins in insecticidal activity in Buthidae scorpion venom.

4. Materials and Methods

4.1. Collection of Venom

Scorpions *B. leptochelys* were collected at the Western Mediterranean coastal desert of Marsa Matruh in Egypt. The venom was collected in a microtube by squeezing the venom glands using fine forceps and dissolving it in distilled water. The crude venom was centrifuged at 14,000 rpm for 10 min at 4 °C. The supernatants were pooled, lyophilized, and stored at −80 °C.

4.2. Bioassay

Insect toxicity was tested by injection of 1–2 μL sample solutions in distilled water into the abdominal cavity of crickets (*Acheta domesticus*, 50 ± 5 mg body weight). Distilled water was injected as a negative control. Several doses of the venom were injected, and ten animals were used for each dose. For evaluation of each HPLC fraction, six animals were used. The number of paralyzed or dead animals were counted 48 h after injection. The dose required to induce 50% mortality (LD_{50}) was calculated by statistical software GraphPad Prism 4 (GraphPad Software, San Diego, CA, USA). The research using experimental animals was approved by the Animal Experimentation Committee at Kyoto University (Permission number: 30-8; date of approval: 1 April 2018).

4.3. Mass Spectrometric Analysis

LC/MS and LC/MS^n measurements were carried out in the positive mode on an LCMS IT-TOF (Shimadzu, Kyoto, Japan) equipped with an electrospray ion source. HPLC separation was carried out on a reversed-phase C_{18} column (TSK-GEL, 1.0 mm ID × 150 mm, TOSOH, Tokyo, Japan). The column was eluted using a linear gradient from 5 to 60% solvent B (0.1% formic acid in acetonitrile) in solvent A (0.1% formic acid in water) for 110 min at a flow rate of 0.05 mL/min. The mass scale was externally calibrated using sodium trifluoroacetate cluster ions. Spectra were obtained over a mass range from *m/z* 400 to 2000, and the multiply charged molecular ions were manually deconvoluted to obtain molecular masses. The monoisotopic *m/z* values in each multiply charged ion were used for deconvolution.

MALDI-TOF/TOF MS measurements were carried out on an Autoflex III smart beam (Bruker Daltonics, Billerica, MA, USA) with a nitrogen pulsed laser (337 nm). Samples were dissolved in 0.1% TFA in 50% acetonitrile/water and mixed with a matrix solution containing 10 mg/mL of α-cyano-4-hydroxycinnamic acid (CHCA) in acetone. An aliquot (0.5 μL) of matrix/acetone solution was spotted onto the MALDI sample target to generate a thin layer of matrix crystal. Then, 1 μL of the matrix/0.1% TFA in 50% acetonitrile/water solution was spotted onto the thin layer and then dried at room temperature. External calibration of the mass scale was carried out using the molecular masses of the known peptides. Interpretation of the MS/MS spectra was conducted manually with the help of the open-source software mMass [43].

4.4. HPLC Purification

The crude venom (2.0 mg) was dissolved in distilled water and separated by HPLC on a reversed-phase C_4 column (Protein C_4, 10 mm ID × 250 mm, Grace Vydac, Deerfield, IL, USA). The column was eluted using a linear gradient from 15 to 60% solvent D (0.08% TFA in acetonitrile) in solvent C (0.1% TFA in water) for 50 min at a flow rate of 2 mL/min. Elution was monitored by UV absorbance at 215 and 280 nm. Seven fractions were obtained based on the major chromatographic peaks, and each fraction was subjected to the insect toxicity tests as described above. Fractions that showed insect toxicity were further separated by a reversed-phase C_{18} column (Everest C_{18}, 1.0 mm ID × 250 mm, Grace Vydac). The column was eluted with solvent C and D at a flow rate of 0.05 mL/min using a linear gradient from 20 to 50% solvent D for 45 min (fraction I), from 15 to 60% solvent D for 45 min(fraction II), and from 20 to 40% solvent D for 45 min (fraction III). Chromatographic peaks obtained from each fraction were subjected to insect toxicity tests to find the toxic component. The monoisotopic molecular mass of these components was obtained by LC/MS analysis as described above.

4.5. Determination of N-terminal Sequence

The peptide (200 pmol) was dissolved in the 0.2 M Tris (pH 8.0) buffer (30 μL) containing 6 M guanidine-HCl. To the solution was added 10 μL of 45 mM dithiothreitol (DTT) that was incubated for 1 h at 50 °C. Then, the reaction mixture was mixed with 10 μL of 100 mM iodoacetic acid to alkylate Cys side chains and incubated for 1 h at 28 °C in the dark. The peptide with carboxymethylated Cys residues was purified by HPLC and subjected to Edman sequencing analysis (PPSQ-21A, Shimadzu).

4.6. Enzymatic Digestion

For Lys-C digestion, the peptide solution after carboxymethylation reaction was diluted with a twofold volume of distilled water, which was mixed with Lys-C (Wako Pure Chemical Industries, Osaka, Japan) in an enzyme to a substrate ratio of 1:100 (*w*/*w*). After incubation for 18 h at 37 °C, digested peptide fragments were subjected to HPLC separation on a C_{18} column (TSK-GEL, 1.0 mm ID × 150 mm, TOSOH) eluted using a linear gradient from 15 to 60% solvent D in solvent C for 45 min at a flow rate of 0.05 mL/min. For chymotrypsin digestion, the peptide solution after carboxymethylation reaction was purified by HPLC on a C_{18} column (Everest C_{18}, 1.0 mm ID × 250 mm, Grace Vydac) eluted using a linear gradient from 5 to 90% solvent D in solvent C for 85 min at a flow rate of 0.05 mL/min. After lyophilization, the purified peptide was dissolved in 100 μL of distilled water and mixed with chymotrypsin (Roche Diagnostics K.K., Tokyo, Japan) in an enzyme to a substrate ratio of 1:100 (*w*/*w*). After incubation for 18 h at 37 °C, digested peptide fragments were subjected to HPLC separation on a C_{18} column (Everest C_{18}, 1.0 mm ID × 250 mm, Grace Vydac) eluted with solvent A and B at a flow rate of 0.05 mL/min using a linear gradient from 5 to 90% solvent B for 85 min. For sequential digestion with Lys-C and chymotrypsin, the peptide solution after Lys-C digestion for 18 h at 37 °C was mixed with chymotrypsin. After incubation for 18 h at 37 °C, digested peptide fragments were subjected to HPLC separation on a C_{18} column as described above.

4.7. Homology Modeling

To construct the three-dimensional model, homology modeling software Isolated-FAMS (In-Silico Sciences Inc., Tokyo, Japan) was used [44]. The primary sequence of Bl-1 was automatically aligned with that of Lqh3, and the structure of each toxin was optimized by simulated annealing method of FAMS-ligand using the coordinate of Lqh3 (PDB ID: 1FH3) as a template.

Supplementary Materials: The following are available online at http://www.mdpi.com/2072-6651/11/4/236/s1, Table S1. List of monoisotopic molecular masses of the venom components obtained by LC/MS analysis. Numbers shown in bold indicate the peptides isolated in this study. Figure S1. Mass spectra of Bl-1, 2, 3, and 4. Figure S2. Results of LC/MS analysis of native (**A**) and carboxymethylated Bl-1 (**B**). Figure S3. HPLC chromatograms of peptide fragments obtained by degestion with Lys-C (**A**), with chimotrypsin after Lys-C (**B**), and with chymotrypsin (**C**). Figure S4. Product ion spectra of L1 obtained by LC/MS/MS (**A**) and MALDI-TOF/TOF MS analysis (**B**). Product ion spectra of L3 obtained by LC/MS/MS (**C**) and MALDI-TOF/TOF MS analysis (**D**). Figure S5. Product ion spectra of L1 (**A**) and L3 (**B–F**) obtained by MALDI-TOF/TOF MS analysis under HE-CID condition. The mass region containing *d*- and *a*- ions necessary for Leu/Ile discrimination was shown. Vertical solid arrows show observed *d*-ions. Figure S6. Product ion spectra of LC1 (**A**) and C1 (**B**) obtained by MALDI-TOF/TOF MS analysis under HE-CID conditions. Figure S7. LC/MS/MS analysis of peptide fragments obtained by chymotrypsin digestion. (**A**) Total ion chromatogram of the fragments. (**B**) Product ion spectrum of C2. (**C**) Fragment ions of C2 observed by LC/MS/MS analysis.

Author Contributions: Conceptualization: M.M.; investigation: Y.Y.; resources: M.A.-W. and M.S.; supervision: H.M.; writing—original draft: Y.Y.; writing—review and editing: M.M. and Y.N.

Funding: This research received no external funding.

Acknowledgments: We are grateful to Fumihiko Sato and Kentaro Ifuku of Kyoto University for MALDI-TOF/TOF MS measurements, and Naoki Mori and Naoko Yoshinaga of Kyoto University for LCMS IT-TOF MS measurements.

Conflicts of Interest: The authors declare no conflict of interest.

References

1. Dunlop, J.A. Geological history and phylogeny of Chelicerata. *Arthropod. Struct. Dev.* **2010**, *39*, 124–142. [CrossRef]
2. Waddington, J.; Rudkin, D.M.; Dunlop, J.A. A new mid-Silurian aquatic scorpion-one step closer to land? *Biol. Lett.* **2015**, *11*, 20140815. [CrossRef] [PubMed]
3. Santibanez-Lopez, C.E.; Francke, O.F.; Ureta, C.; Possani, L.D. Scorpions from Mexico: From species diversity to venom complexity. *Toxins* **2015**, *8*, 2. [CrossRef] [PubMed]
4. The Scorpion Files. Available online: https://www.ntnu.no/ub/scorpion-files/intro.php (accessed on 20 March 2019).
5. Zlotkin, E. Scorpion venoms. In *Comprehensive Molecular Insect Science*; Gilbert, L.I., Iatrou, K., Gill, S.S., Eds.; Elsevier B.V.: Oxford, UK, 2005; Volume 5, pp. 173–220.
6. Santibanez-Lopez, C.E.; Possani, L.D. Overview of the Knottin scorpion toxin-like peptides in scorpion venoms: Insights on their classification and evolution. *Toxicon* **2015**, *107*, 317–326. [CrossRef] [PubMed]
7. Almaaytah, A.; Albalas, Q. Scorpion venom peptides with no disulfide bridges: A review. *Peptides* **2014**, *51*, 35–45. [CrossRef] [PubMed]
8. Zhijian, C.; Feng, L.; Yingliang, W.; Xin, M.; Wenxin, L. Genetic mechanisms of scorpion venom peptide diversification. *Toxicon* **2006**, *47*, 348–355. [CrossRef] [PubMed]
9. Housley, D.M.; Housley, G.D.; Liddell, M.J.; Jennings, E.A. Scorpion toxin peptide action at the ion channel subunit level. *Neuropharmacology* **2017**, *127*, 46–78. [CrossRef]
10. Possani, L.D.; Becerril, B.; Delepierre, M.; Tytgat, J. Scorpion toxins specific for Na^+-channels. *Eur. J. Biochem.* **1999**, *264*, 287–300. [CrossRef]
11. Rodriguez de la Vega, R.C.; Possani, L.D. Overview of scorpion toxins specific for Na^+ channels and related peptides: Biodiversity, structure-function relationships and evolution. *Toxicon* **2005**, *46*, 831–844. [CrossRef]
12. Yu, F.H.; Catterall, W.A. Overview of the voltage-gated sodium channel family. *Genome Biol.* **2003**, *4*, 207. [CrossRef]
13. Cestele, S.; Catterall, W.A. Molecular mechanisms of neurotoxin action on voltage-gated sodium channels. *Biochimie* **2000**, *82*, 883–892. [CrossRef]
14. Cestele, S.; Stankiewicz, M.; Mansuelle, P.; De Waard, M.; Dargent, B.; Gilles, N.; Pelhate, M.; Rochat, H.; Martin-Eauclaire, M.F.; Gordon, D. Scorpion alpha-like toxins, toxic to both mammals and insects, differentially interact with receptor site 3 on voltage-gated sodium channels in mammals and insects. *Eur. J. Neurosci.* **1999**, *11*, 975–985. [CrossRef]
15. Bergeron, Z.L.; Bingham, J.P. Scorpion toxins specific for potassium (K^+) channels: A historical overview of peptide bioengineering. *Toxins* **2012**, *4*, 1082–1119. [CrossRef]

16. Rodriguez de la Vega, R.C.; Possani, L.D. Current views on scorpion toxins specific for K^+-channels. *Toxicon* **2004**, *43*, 865–875. [CrossRef]
17. Chagot, B.; Pimentel, C.; Dai, L.; Pil, J.; Tytgat, J.; Nakajima, T.; Corzo, G.; Darbon, H.; Ferrat, G. An unusual fold for potassium channel blockers: NMR structure of three toxins from the scorpion *Opisthacanthus madagascariensis*. *Biochem. J.* **2005**, *388*, 263–271. [CrossRef]
18. Chen, Z.; Luo, F.; Feng, J.; Yang, W.; Zeng, D.; Zhao, R.; Cao, Z.; Liu, M.; Li, W.; Jiang, L.; et al. Genomic and structural characterization of Kunitz-type peptide LmKTT-1a highlights diversity and evolution of scorpion potassium channel toxins. *PLoS ONE* **2013**, *8*, e60201. [CrossRef]
19. DeBin, J.A.; Maggio, J.E.; Strichartz, G.R. Purification and characterization of chlorotoxin, a chloride channel ligand from the venom of the scorpion. *Am. J. Physiol.* **1993**, *264*, C361–C369. [CrossRef]
20. Froy, O.; Sagiv, T.; Poreh, M.; Urbach, D.; Zilberberg, N.; Gurevitz, M. Dynamic diversification from a putative common ancestor of scorpion toxins affecting sodium, potassium, and chloride channels. *J. Mol. Evol.* **1999**, *48*, 187–196. [CrossRef]
21. Quintero-Hernandez, V.; Jimenez-Vargas, J.M.; Gurrola, G.B.; Valdivia, H.H.; Possani, L.D. Scorpion venom components that affect ion-channels function. *Toxicon* **2013**, *76*, 328–342. [CrossRef]
22. Harrison, P.L.; Abdel-Rahman, M.A.; Miller, K.; Strong, P.N. Antimicrobial peptides from scorpion venoms. *Toxicon* **2014**, *88*, 115–137. [CrossRef]
23. Scorpiones.pl. Available online: http://scorpiones.pl/maps/#africa (accessed on 20 March 2019).
24. Loret, E.P.; Hammock, B.D. Structure and neurotoxicity of venoms. In *Scorpion Biology and Research*; Brownell, P.H., Polis, G.A., Eds.; Oxford University Press, Inc.: New York, NY, USA, 2001; pp. 204–233.
25. Caliskan, F.; Quintero-Hernandez, V.; Restano-Cassulini, R.; Batista, C.V.F.; Zarnudio, F.Z.; Coronas, F.I.; Possani, L.D. Turkish scorpion *Buthacus macrocentrus*: General characterization of the venom and description of Bu1, a potent mammalian Na^+-channel alpha-toxin. *Toxicon* **2012**, *59*, 408–415. [CrossRef]
26. Cestele, S.; Kopeyan, C.; Oughideni, R.; Mansuelle, P.; Granier, C.; Rochat, H. Biochemical and pharmacological characterization of a depressant insect toxin from the venom of the scorpion *Buthacus arenicola*. *Eur. J. Biochem.* **1997**, *243*, 93–99. [CrossRef]
27. Miyashita, M.; Sakai, A.; Matsushita, N.; Hanai, Y.; Nakagawa, Y.; Miyagawa, H. A novel amphipathic linear peptide with both insect toxicity and antimicrobial activity from the venom of the scorpion *Isometrus maculatus*. *Biosci. Biotechnol. Biochem.* **2010**, *74*, 364–369. [CrossRef]
28. Manzoil-Palma, M.F.; Gobbi, N.; Palma, M.S. Insects as biological models to assay spider and scorpion venom toxicity. *Venom. Anim. Toxins incl. Trop. Dis.* **2003**, *9*, 174–185. [CrossRef]
29. De Lima, M.E.; Figueiredo, S.G.; Pimenta, A.M.; Santos, D.M.; Borges, M.H.; Cordeiro, M.N.; Richardson, M.; Oliveira, L.C.; Stankiewicz, M.; Pelhate, M. Peptides of arachnid venoms with insecticidal activity targeting sodium channels. *Comp. Biochem. Physiol. C Toxicol. Pharmacol.* **2007**, *146*, 264–279. [CrossRef]
30. Gurevitz, M.; Karbat, I.; Cohen, L.; Ilan, N.; Kahn, R.; Turkov, M.; Stankiewicz, M.; Stuhmer, W.; Dong, K.; Gordon, D. The insecticidal potential of scorpion beta-toxins. *Toxicon* **2007**, *49*, 473–489. [CrossRef]
31. Sautiere, P.; Cestele, S.; Kopeyan, C.; Martinage, A.; Drobecq, H.; Doljansky, Y.; Gordon, D. New toxins acting on sodium channels from the scorpion *Leiurus quinquestriatus hebraeus* suggest a clue to mammalian vs insect selectivity. *Toxicon* **1998**, *36*, 1141–1154. [CrossRef]
32. Vargas, O.; Martin, M.F.; Rochat, H. Characterization of six toxins from the venom of the Moroccan scorpion *Buthus occitanus mardochei*. *Eur. J. Biochem.* **1987**, *162*, 589–599. [CrossRef]
33. Kopeyan, C.; Martinez, G.; Rochat, H. Amino acid sequence of neurotoxin V from scorpion *Leiurus quinquestriatus quinquestriatus*. *FEBS Lett.* **1978**, *89*, 54–58. [CrossRef]
34. Rochat, H.; Rochat, C.; Lissitzky, S.; Sampieri, F.; Miranda, F. Amino acid sequence of neurotoxin II of *Androctonus australis* Hector. *Eur. J. Biochem.* **1972**, *28*, 381–388. [CrossRef]
35. Jalali, A.; Bosmans, F.; Amininasab, M.; Clynen, E.; Cuypers, E.; Zaremirakabadi, A.; Sarbolouki, M.N.; Schoofs, L.; Vatanpour, H.; Tytgat, J. OD1, the first toxin isolated from the venom of the scorpion *Odonthobuthus doriae* active on voltage-gated $Na(^+)$ channels. *FEBS Lett.* **2005**, *579*, 4181–4186. [CrossRef]
36. Loret, E.P.; Mansuelle, P.; Rochat, H.; Granier, C. Neurotoxins active on insects—Amino acid sequences, chemical modifications, and secondary structure estimation by circular dichroism of toxins from the scorpion *Androctonus australis* Hector. *Biochemistry* **1990**, *29*, 1492–1501. [CrossRef]

37. Kopeyan, C.; Mansuelle, P.; Sampieri, F.; Brando, T.; Bahraoui, E.M.; Rochat, H.; Granier, C. Primary structure of scorpion antiinsect toxins isolated from the venom of *Leiurus quinquestriatus quinquestriatus*. *FEBS Lett.* **1990**, *261*, 423–426. [CrossRef]
38. Zhao, R.M.; Ma, Y.B.; He, Y.W.; Di, Z.Y.; Wu, Y.L.; Cao, Z.J.; Li, W.X. Comparative venom gland transcriptome analysis of the scorpion *Lychas mucronatus* reveals intraspecific toxic gene diversity and new venomous components. *BMC Genom.* **2010**, *11*. [CrossRef]
39. Ma, Y.B.; He, Y.W.; Zhao, R.M.; Wu, Y.L.; Li, W.X.; Cao, Z.J. Extreme diversity of scorpion venom peptides and proteins revealed by transcriptomic analysis: Implication for proteome evolution of scorpion venom arsenal. *J. Proteom.* **2012**, *75*, 1563–1576. [CrossRef]
40. Ichiki, Y.; Kawachi, T.; Miyashita, M.; Nakagawa, Y.; Miyagawa, H. Isolation and characterization of a novel non-selective beta-toxin from the venom of the scorpion *Isometrus maculatus*. *Biosci. Biotechnol. Biochem.* **2012**, *76*, 2089–2092. [CrossRef]
41. Kawachi, T.; Miyashita, M.; Nakagawa, Y.; Miyagawa, H. Isolation and characterization of an anti-insect beta-toxin from the venom of the scorpion *Isometrus maculatus*. *Biosci. Biotechnol. Biochem.* **2013**, *77*, 205–207. [CrossRef]
42. Karbat, I.; Kahn, R.; Cohen, L.; Ilan, N.; Gilles, N.; Corzo, G.; Froy, O.; Gur, M.; Albrecht, G.; Heinemann, S.H.; et al. The unique pharmacology of the scorpion alpha-like toxin Lqh3 is associated with its flexible C-tail. *FEBS J.* **2007**, *274*, 1918–1931. [CrossRef]
43. Strohalm, M.; Kavan, D.; Novak, P.; Volny, M.; Havlicek, V. mMass 3: A cross-platform software environment for precise analysis of mass spectrometric data. *Anal. Chem.* **2010**, *82*, 4648–4651. [CrossRef]
44. Ogata, K.; Umeyama, H. An automatic homology modeling method consisting of database searches and simulated annealing. *J. Mol. Graph. Model.* **2000**, *18*, 258–272. [CrossRef]

MDPI
St. Alban-Anlage 66
4052 Basel
Switzerland
Tel. +41 61 683 77 34
Fax +41 61 302 89 18
www.mdpi.com

Toxins Editorial Office
E-mail: toxins@mdpi.com
www.mdpi.com/journal/toxins

www.ingramcontent.com/pod-product-compliance
Lightning Source LLC
LaVergne TN
LVHW071936080526
838202LV00064B/6616